The Complete Recovery Room Book

The Complete Recovery Room Book

SIXTH EDITION

Anne Craig

Anaesthetist
Auckland City Hospital and Greenlane Surgical Unit
Auckland

New Zealand

Anthea Hatfield

Anaesthetist
New Zealand

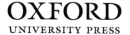
OXFORD
UNIVERSITY PRESS

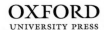
OXFORD
UNIVERSITY PRESS

Great Clarendon Street, Oxford, OX2 6DP,
United Kingdom

Oxford University Press is a department of the University of Oxford.
It furthers the University's objective of excellence in research, scholarship,
and education by publishing worldwide. Oxford is a registered trade mark of
Oxford University Press in the UK and in certain other countries

© Oxford University Press 2021

The moral rights of the authors have been asserted

First edition published in 1992
Second edition published in 1996
Third edition published in 2001
Fourth edition published in 2009
Fifth edition published in 2014
Sixth edition published in 2021

Published in the United States of America by Oxford University Press
198 Madison Avenue, New York, NY 10016, United States of America

British Library Cataloguing in Publication Data
Data available

Library of Congress Control Number: 2020934895

ISBN 978–0–19–884684–0

Printed and bound by
CPI Group (UK) Ltd, Croydon, CR0 4YY

Oxford University Press makes no representation, express or implied, that the
drug dosages in this book are correct. Readers must therefore always check
the product information and clinical procedures with the most up-to-date
published product information and data sheets provided by the manufacturers
and the most recent codes of conduct and safety regulations. The authors and
the publishers do not accept responsibility or legal liability for any errors in the
text or for the misuse or misapplication of material in this work. Except where
otherwise stated, drug dosages and recommendations are for the non-pregnant
adult who is not breast-feeding

Links to third party websites are provided by Oxford in good faith and
for information only. Oxford disclaims any responsibility for the materials
contained in any third party website referenced in this work.

Dedication

This edition is dedicated to Dr Sereima Bale. Sereima has been 'Head of Training' in Fiji since 1988. She has sent many young doctors and nurses out to the scattered Pacific Islands where they do an amazing job looking after patients during and after anaesthesia. All of them attribute their skill and achievements to Dr Bale.

Fifth Edition Dedicated To
Michael Tronson, the co-author of all the previous editions. One of the most imaginative and insightful doctors who ever practised anaesthesia.

Fourth Edition Dedicated To
The anaesthetists, surgeons and nurses of Box Hill Hospital Melbourne.

Third Edition Dedicated To
The staff of St Vincent's Hospital, Melbourne.

Second Edition Dedicated To
Staff working in isolated environments especially in the hospitals of the South West Pacific.

First Edition Dedicated To
Pamela Deighton, Palega Vaeau and Grant Scarf—the first recovery room team to visit Samoa.

Contents

Foreword

A patient's journey through a surgical intervention involves multiple steps, not just confined to the operating theatre, each of which requires attention to detail to optimize the final outcome. Failure to do so can undo previous good work to the patient's detriment.

Dedicated recovery room nursing was developed in the 1960s and has progressively become more specialized since. Patients are received in a vulnerable state and, as they transition, a multitude of potential complications occur. These can be related to the operative procedure, the anaesthetic or co-morbidity. Good management in the recovery room begins and ends with a well-communicated synoptic handover. Close monitoring and proactive care during this phase positively contribute to the final outcome.

It is 60 years now since the first Recovery Rooms were established. The understanding of the importance good recovery plays in the outcome of surgery for the patient has always been a passionate interest of Dr Anthea Hatfield and she is joined in this 6th edition by Dr Anne Craig who shares her enthusiasm for the overall well-being and successful outcome of surgery for all patients.

Stephen Kyle
Taranaki Base Hospital
New Zealand

Preface

Constant vigilance is the price of safety.

Patients believe they are asleep during their operation: they are not asleep, they are in a reversible drug-induced coma[1]. Emergence from general anaesthesia is a passive process and depends on the length of time, the amount and potency of the drugs given and the patient's physiology. The return to spontaneous respiration is one of the first signs of recovery. This corresponds to brain stem function returning. Eye opening is a late sign of recovery requiring cortical function. Most patients recover consciousness slowly and are unable to care for themselves. This is a period of extreme physiological insults: pain, hypothermia, hypoxia, acid–base disturbance and shifts in blood volume. Not only do the recovery room staff have to adeptly manage comatose and physiologically unstable patients, but also deal with the early postoperative care of surgical patients and attend to drips, drains and dressings. For this reason, two nurses should always attend patients arriving in the recovery room.

The recovery room is a *critical care unit* where necessary skills and equipment are gathered in the one place. Here the care of patients passes safely from the intensive monitoring in the operating theatre to the wards. Before recovery rooms became available, more than half the deaths in the immediate postoperative period occurred from preventable conditions such as airway obstruction, aspiration of stomach contents, and haemorrhagic shock.

It is most important that the nurse who scrubbed and assisted at the operation and the anaesthetist accompany the patient to the recovery room and each give a full handover to the recovery room nurses. Maintaining the chain of trust and care for the patient at this most vulnerable stage of their treatment cannot be overemphasized. From the first visit to the surgeon through all the preoperative 'work-up' and clinics many people have been part of this chain of care and the patient has been able to contribute or correct the commentary. The handover from operating theatre to the recovery room takes place without the patient participating and therefore must be performed most diligently. Do not accept that a scrub nurse is too busy preparing for the next case to handover. Insist on it for every patient.

This book is to help you to manage day-to-day problems that occur in recovery rooms. In teaching and specialist hospitals there are people around to ask for help or advice. But, at times in most hospitals, you will need to make difficult decisions on your own. Most recovery rooms will have computer access and can refer to FOAM[1] (Free Open Access Medical Education). Be aware there is no real-time peer review and medical knowledge is not always simple. This book should help you make these decisions. Begin to read the book anywhere. Each chapter is written to stand alone. Reading the chapters covering basic science which precede the practical sections will be worthwhile. Once you understand basic physiology and pharmacology it is easier to make sense of clinical disorders, anticipate problems and develop plans to avoid them.

The recovery room is one part of *perioperative practice*. In some sections the preoperative and operative procedure are described in detail, because what has happened before the patient reaches you is relevant to their management.

The opinions expressed in this book are our own. We intend them to convey common sense and humanity. There are no randomized blinded trials to prove that cuddling crying children comforts them. This is a guidebook, not a rulebook. Most of the facts incorporated in these chapters are commonly known. At the end of several chapters further reading is suggested. There is so much information available it is not possible to condense it all between these covers. We hope that reading this book will both enable you to look after your patients in an intelligent and thoughtful manner, stimulate you to further enquiry and give you much personal satisfaction.

Seek help from colleagues to understand fully what is happening to your patient.

Reference

1. **Carroll C**, *et al.* (2016). Social media and free open access medical education. *American Journal of Critical Care* **25**(1):93–96.

Acknowledgements

Thank you to everyone who has helped us wittingly or unwittingly. Searching the internet makes gathering opinions almost too easy. Sifting through this information with colleagues and experienced recovery room nurses, then deciding what can stay from previous editions means that many unacknowledged people have contributed a great deal to the final book 'between the covers'. We are grateful to all of you.

Special acknowledgements to the sixth edition

Edna Beech for her contribution to cardiopulmonary resuscitation. Kousaku Haruguchi for his innovative contribution to the chapter on design. Laura Foley and Lesley Caelli from ANZCA for computer and library research. Jane MacDonnell for help with computing. Stephen Kyle for the forward, his contribution to the chapter on surgical problems and for being a helpful and concerned colleague. Parma Nand for his review of the chapter on cardiovascular disease. Kaeni Agiomea for contributing to the information on oxygen concentrators. John Langrick for his contribution to the chapter on monitoring and equipment. Jin Wang for her contribution to the chapter on infection control.

20 Golden Rules

There is nothing more lethal than ignorance—or more frightful than a wilfully closed mind.

Johann von Goethe (1749–1832)

If you are in any doubt... ask somebody!

1. The confused, restless and agitated patient is hypoxic until proven otherwise.
2. Your patient may be hypoxic even though the oximeter reads 98%.
3. Never turn your back on a patient.
4. The blood pressure does not necessarily fall in haemorrhagic shock.
5. Never ignore a tachycardia or a bradycardia; find the cause.
6. Postoperative hypertension is dangerous.
7. Never use a painful stimulus to rouse your patient.
8. Nurse comatose children on their side in the recovery position.
9. If your patient is slow to wake up, or continues to bleed, consider hypothermia.
10. Noisy breathing is obstructed breathing, but not all obstructed breathing is noisy.
11. Let patients remove their airways when they are ready to.
12. Cuddle crying children; hold the hand of crying adults.
13. The opioids do not cause hypotension in stable patients.
14. When giving drugs to the elderly, start by giving half as much, twice as slowly.
15. If you do not know the actions of a drug, then do not give it.
16. Treat the patient, not the monitor.
17. Cold hands are a sign of a haemodynamically unstable patient.
18. Pain prevention is better than pain relief.
19. Do not discharge patients from the recovery room until they can maintain a 5-second head lift.
20. If confused read rule number 1!

Chapter 1

Recovery room routines

Introduction

In this chapter we will follow patients from the operating theatre to the recovery room, outline their care, describe routine procedures, and finally their discharge and transport to the ward.

The recovery room is the most important room in the hospital, for it is here that a patient is at most risk from inadvertent harm. Patients are in an unstable physiological state where critical events can develop rapidly. Most of these events are preventable, but detecting and treating them relies on skilled and vigilant nursing staff who can give constant and total care.

Immediate care

Things to check before the first patient arrives

Sign the recovery room's log book to confirm that:

- resuscitation trolleys are properly stocked;
- drug cupboards are restocked;
- disposable items are replaced;
- sharps and rubbish containers are empty and ready;
- suction equipment is ready, clean and working;
- oxygen supply is connected and working properly;
- Mapleson's C breathing circuit is connected;
- adequate supply of airways;
- monitoring equipment is all available and working;
- blood pressure machines and appropriate cuffs are available;
- intravenous drip hangers are ready;
- clean blankets and other linen are available;
- sufficient blankets in warming cupboard;
- working area is clean and uncluttered;
- alarm bells are working.

To see 'Recovery room step down', see Box 1.1.

Box 1.1 **Recovery room step down**

Stage 1 recovery

Patients who need Stage 1 recovery are those who are physiologically unstable, or who potentially may become so.

Patients in *Stage 1 recovery* must be attended by specialist staff proficient at advanced cardiac life support. (Advanced cardiac life support includes all the other skills, procedures and equipment needed to deal instantly with a deteriorating cardiorespiratory status, or arrest and include defibrillation.) Resuscitation equipment must be instantly available.

If you have any doubt about a patient's status then they should remain in Stage 1 recovery. Patients in Stage 1 recovery include those who are comatose; or require airway support, or continued frequent monitoring of their respiratory, cardiovascular, neurological or muscular function; or evaluation of their mental status; or assessment or management of core temperature, pain, nausea and vomiting, surgical drainage, blood loss or urine output. Patients transferred to the intensive care unit (ICU) remain in Extended Stage 1 recovery.

Whether a patient is likely to become physiologically unstable cannot be quantified, but experienced staff readily recognize those patients at risk.

While there is risk of harm
the patient remains in Stage 1 recovery.

Stage 2 recovery

At this stage the patients are conscious and fully able to care for their own airways. They are within the physiological limits defined by their preoperative evaluation. These patients must be attended by staff who are proficient at basic life support (this includes the basic ABC of resuscitation: maintenance of a clear airway, support of breathing and external cardiac massage). At this stage patients are fit to return to the ward, which by definition is Extended Stage 2 recovery and remains so for the whole period the patient is in the hospital. For *day case procedures* it refers to those who are waiting in a supervised area for discharge.

Stage 3 recovery

Following day procedures patients can be discharged into the care of a competent and informed adult who can intervene should untoward events occur. The carer may have no skills in life support, but must be capable of recognizing problems and know what to do about them. Stage 3 recovery also applies to patients who are discharged home from the ward, even after days or weeks in the hospital. Patients remain in Stage 3 recovery until they have completely recovered from their operation, and no longer need hospital care in any form (even as an outpatient).

How to transport the patient to the recovery room

You need at least three people to gently move the patient from the operating table on to a specially designed recovery room trolley. Staff need to adapt their techniques if the hospital has a no-lift policy. It is the anaesthetist's responsibility to look after the patient's head, neck and airway.

The trolleys must be capable of being tilted head up or down by at least 15°, carry facilities to give oxygen and apply suction and a pole to hang drains and intravenous fluids. As you move the patient take care not to dislodge catheters, drains and lines.

Position children on their sides with their operation site uppermost. Put the trolley sides up. Adults can be sitting up. Wheel patients feet first to the recovery room. The anaesthetist walks forward (never backward) maintaining the patient's airway. Put the trolley's sucker under the patient's pillow ready to use immediately if needed.

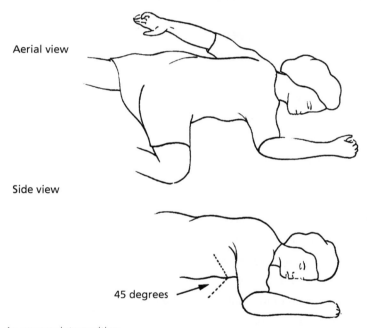

Aerial view

Side view

45 degrees

Figure 1.1 An appropriate position.

How to admit the patient to the recovery room

First check the patient is stable

The instant a patient is admitted to the recovery room, check that they are lying in an appropriate position (Figure 1.1). Check they are breathing quietly, put on an appropriate oxygen mask, check their pulse and blood pressure: only receive the handover when you are satisfied the patient's condition is stable. There are two handovers: the nurse's and the anaesthetist's.

The nurse's handover

The nurse's handover includes:

- surgeon's and anaesthetist's name;
- checking the patient's name against their medical records, and identity bracelet;
- care and placement of surgical drains;
- problems with skin pressure areas;
- relevant surgical detail, e.g. check flaps for blood supply and take care not to give too much fluid to patients with bowel anastomoses;
- organizing the patient's records;
- ensuring the correct charts and X-rays accompany the patient;
- care of the patient's personal belongings such as dentures and hearing aids.

The anaesthetist's handover

The anaesthetist's handover includes the:

- patient's name and age;
- indications for surgery;
- the type of operation;
- type of anaesthetic;
- relevant medical problems;
- conscious state;
- blood pressure during surgery;

Additionally the anaesthetist reports:

- untoward events occurring before and during surgery;
- analgesia given and anticipated needs;
- vascular monitoring lines;
- blood loss, and details of what intravenous fluids to give next;
- urine output during the procedure;
- drain tubes;
- patient's psychological state;
- additional monitoring if required in recovery room;
- how much oxygen, and how to give it;
- orders for any further investigations;
- and provides a recovery room discharge plan.

Before the anaesthetist leaves the recovery room the patient must be breathing, have good oxygen saturation, a stable blood pressure and pulse rate. Anaesthetists should tell the nursing staff where to find them if necessary, and they must remain close by while the patient is in the recovery room.

Maintain the patient's airway
during the handover.

Initial assessment

Immediate steps

Once the patient is transported to the recovery room, immediately apply an appropriate oxygen mask. First note the patient's conscious state. Then have an assistant attach the monitoring devices while you gain control by doing things in the following order of priority: A, B, C, D and E.

A Airway

B Breathing

C Circulation

D Drips, drains and drugs

E Extras

A = Airway

♦ Make sure patients have a clear airway, are breathing and air is moving freely and quietly in and out of their chest (Figure 1.2). Briefly, put one hand over their mouth to feel the airflow and the other hand on their chest to feel it rise and fall in synchrony.

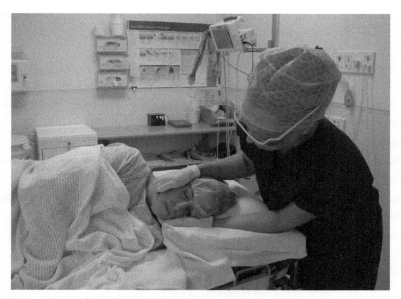

Figure 1.2 Attention to the patient's airway.

- Begin administering oxygen with a face mask at a flow rate of 6 L/min.
- Attach a *pulse oximeter* to obtain a baseline reading.
- If necessary gently suck out the patient's mouth and pharynx. Be gentle otherwise you may provoke *laryngospasm*.
- If the patient is still unconscious make sure an airway is properly located between the teeth and tongue, and the lips are not in danger of being bitten.
- If the patient has clamped his teeth shut and you are unable to insert an airway into the mouth, then gently slide a lubricated nasopharyngeal airway along the floor of the nose.

Hint

Tidal air exchange is best felt in the palm of your hand as you support the chin; now you can feel every breath taken. Do not remove the oxygen mask for more than a few breaths.

B = Breathing

- Check the chest is moving, and you can feel air flowing in and out of the mouth.
- Count the respirations for one full minute.
- Just because patients fog up their face masks, does not mean that they are moving adequate amounts of tidal air.
- Listen for abnormal noises as the patient breathes: wheezes, rattles, gurgles or snoring or crowing noises called *stridor*.
- Look at the strap muscles in the patient's neck; they should not tense with breathing. If they are contracting it suggests the patient is working hard to breathe. Check that the airway is not obstructed, and the patient is not wheezing. Airway obstruction is dangerous: notify the anaesthetist immediately.
- Look for signs of *cyanosis*. Cyanosis is a bluish tinge of the lips or tongue. It is a sign of severe *hypoxaemia*. If you are uncertain whether the patient is cyanosed then squeeze the tip of the patient's finger to engorge it with blood, and compare it with the colour of your own finger tip.
- Note in the patient's record the reading on the *pulse oximeter*. If the reading is less than 95%, change the oxygen mask to a rebreathing mask this will give a higher percentage of oxygen delivered than a Hudson mask.
- If the oxygen saturation does not improve rapidly then search for a reason. Seek help immediately if it is less than 90%.
- Chest movement does not always mean that breathing is adequate.

C = Circulation

- Once you are sure your patient is breathing properly and well oxygenated, measure the blood pressure, pulse rate and rhythm and record them in the chart.

- Record the patient's *perfusion status* in the notes.
- Check the patient is not bleeding into drains or dressings, or elsewhere. Look under the sheets.

D = Drugs, drips, drains and dressings

- Note the drugs given in theatre, particularly opioids that may depress the patient's breathing.
- Check whether the patient has any drug allergies or sensitivities.
- Note the intravenous fluids in progress, how much fluid, and what types have been given during the operation. Make sure the drip is running freely and is not sited across a joint (where it may be obstructed) or in the back of the hand (where it can be dislodged). Replace any pieces of sticky tape encircling the arm because they will cause distal ischaemia if the arm swells for any reason such as the drip fluid running into the tissues. If the cannula is sited across a joint, splint it until it is re-sited in a safer place away from the joint.
- Check the patency of drains and tubing; how much, how fast and what is draining out of them. Make sure the urinary catheter is not blocked, urine is dripping freely, and note the volume of the collecting bag's contents.
- Check vacuum suction devices are functioning properly.
- Check wound dressings and make sure blood or ooze is not seeping through them.

E = Extras

- Measure the patient's *temperature*. This is essential for babies and patients who have had major surgery.
- Measure the blood glucose of diabetic patients with a finger prick.
- If the patient has a limb in plaster, check the perfusion of the fingers or toes. Gently squeeze blood out of the tip of a finger or toe. It will turn white. If it does not turn pink again within 3 seconds of releasing the pressure then the limb is ischaemic; notify the surgeons. If the fingers or toes are congested and blue, this indicates venous obstruction; notify the surgeons immediately.
- Check peripheral pulses following vascular surgery.
- Check the circulation to graft sites.

Perfusion status

As the heart pumps blood to the tissues it must do so at sufficient pressure to ensure perfusion. There are two parameters involved: cardiac output and blood pressure. We do not routinely measure cardiac output in non-cardiac surgery, but we can estimate whether it is adequate from monitoring other variables such as blood pressure, peripheral perfusion, urine output, pulse oximetry and where necessary, acid base status and central venous pressures.

Measuring perfusion status

Poor peripheral perfusion is sometimes called *peripheral shutdown*, because circulation to the hands and feet is almost absent, the patients' hands are blue or even white and cold, and their radial pulse may be feeble or absent. Perfusion status is graded according to Table 1.1.

Table 1.1 Perfusion status

Observation	Adequate	Poor	No perfusion
Conscious state	Alert, oriented in time and place	Obtunded, confused, anxious or agitated	Unconscious
Skin	Warm, pink, dry	Cool, pale, clammy, sweating	Cool/cold, pale ± sweating
Pulse	60–100/minute	Either < 60/minute or > 100/minute	Absent or feeble pulse
Blood pressure	> 100 mmHg	< 100 mmHg	Unrecordable

Other signs of poor perfusion include:

- poor capillary return in fingernail beds;
- peripheral or central cyanosis;
- ischaemic changes on the electrocardiogram (ECG).

A useful way of testing perfusion is to press firmly for a moment on a patient's fingernail. When you let go the blood should blush back within a second or so. If the *capillary return time* (CRT) takes more than 3 seconds, your patient has poor peripheral perfusion.

During longer operations patients often cool down. This causes their skin perfusion to slow, so that when they first come to the recovery room their perfusion status is not a reliable indicator of how well their cardiopulmonary unit is functioning. In this case look at the perfusion inside their lips, rather than their fingertips. Even cold patients should not have central cyanosis, or a tachycardia.

Observations

There are no agreed criteria on how often to take patients' *vital signs* in the recovery room because it depends on the patient's clinical state. As a guide, if patients are stable, record their vital signs every 5 minutes for the first 15 minutes after their admission, and then every 10–15 minutes during their stay. If patients' vital signs are unstable then measure them at least every 5 minutes.

Recovery room records

The recovery room records are a direct continuation of the anaesthetic record. Keep them on the same chart.

*Good records are eloquent evidence
of your competence.*

Medical and legal responsibilities

Scrupulous and detailed records are your only medical and legal defence if problems should occur. If you do not write it down then it did not happen—it is a case of no record, then no defence. Remember that you may be called to a courtroom to account for an *adverse event* many years hence. Record only what you see and hear, and do not pass opinion unless it is directly applicable to the situation. 'The patient appears to me to be irrational' is an acceptable comment, but 'the patient is irrational' is passing a judgement you may not be able to substantiate years later.

Keep it legible, keep it relevant, and keep it factual. Only use abbreviations approved by your hospital and sign off on each entry.

The minimum information to document

Document your evaluation of the patient on their admission to the recovery room.

+ Record the time the patient comes to the recovery room.
+ Vital signs and levels of consciousness at specified times and intervals.
+ All drugs given, including the dose and route.
+ Amounts and types of intravenous fluids given.
+ An ECG rhythm strip if one was taken.
+ All unusual or untoward events.
+ Certify the vital signs are stable.
+ The patient can sustain the 5-second head lift test.
+ Details about planned follow-up of the patient.
+ Sign and date your entry.

Records and quality control

If you enter the recovery room scoring system on a standard spreadsheet computer program you can collect data and analyse it later. Use this data to identify potential problems, provide objective evidence about workloads, and help deploy staff effectively. Good data collection is an essential part of risk assessment and quality control.

Emergence from anaesthesia

Anaesthesia consists of three elements: coma, muscle relaxation, and abolition of unwanted *reflexes*.

Coma

The principal component of a general anaesthetic is a drug-induced and maintained coma. A useful definition of *coma* is a state of consciousness where the eyes are closed, and the patient does not respond to verbal or tactile stimuli. Practically, this means if the patient does not open their eyes when you gently shake them by the shoulder, and call their name, then they are by definition *comatose*.

But coma is more complex than this. To be conscious requires an intact *brainstem reticular activating system* (RAS), and intact cerebral hemispheres (or at least part of a hemisphere). As the RAS is sequentially suppressed, the coma deepens. A person can suffer extensive brain damage, but unless the reticular activating system is affected they will not lose consciousness. This is the reason why many patients with quite large strokes merely lose the movement of part of their body without becoming unconscious.

> *The reticular activating system continually prods the cortex to keep it awake.*

In the 1930s Dr Francis Guedel described four distinct stages of an ether anaesthetic, tracing the sequence of events as the reticular activating system was suppressed. The stages are not as easily identified with modern volatile anaesthetics as they were with ether because they happen so quickly, but the stages are more obvious (in the reverse order) as patients emerge from anaesthesia.

Assessing the level of coma

Figure 1.3 demonstrates a simple way to assess the levels of a drug-induced coma. For example, a patient with periodic breathing, divergent gaze and reactive pupils who responds in a semi-purposeful way to a firm squeeze on their triceps muscle is in a level 1 coma, and about to emerge from their anaesthetic.

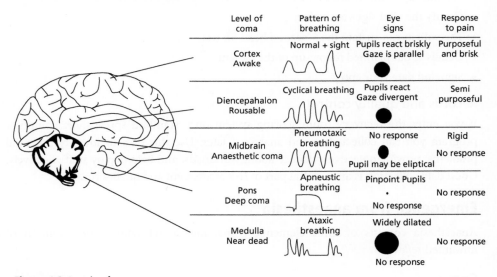

Figure 1.3 Levels of coma.

Stages of emergence

Stage 1—coma

Coma is one of the elements of a general anaesthetic. Patients do not respond to any stimuli. You cannot awaken patients from a coma. Be patient. Never use painful stimuli to try to rouse your patient.

Stage 2—responsive

As patients emerge from coma, they start to respond to stimuli. Although not awake their pupils constrict in reaction to light, but the direction of their gaze diverges. Then, a few moments before waking, their pupils suddenly dilate, and patients move their limbs, and perhaps begin to shiver or shake. Their pulse rate and blood pressure rise.

Stage 3—awake

Although now awake and responding appropriately to commands, their conscious state remains clouded. Later they will remember little, or nothing, about this stage. At this time, some patients become confused, restless, disoriented and possibly fearful, and you will not be able to reason with them. This *delirium* usually passes within a few minutes. If the delirium persists then exclude hypoxia and hypoglycaemia or a full urinary bladder as a possible cause.

Stage 4—alert

The patient is fully conscious but may well have difficulty in concentrating or making complex decisions. This fuzzy thinking normally resolves within 48 hours, but occasionally subtle changes in the patient's mental processes persist for months. This *postoperative cognitive disorder* is more likely in older people having major surgery.

How the patient views emergence

Hearing is the first sense to return. Voices are very loud, distorted and sometimes alarming. Louder noises, such as a telephone, can be frightening. Because their pupils are dilated, the lights seem unduly bright and vision is blurred. Their arms and legs feel heavy. Pain may be excruciating. Finally, their sense of locality and memory will return. The patient may feel disoriented, giddy and often asks: 'Where am I?'

What the patient worries about

In a study patients voted for the following outcomes that they preferred to avoid. Ranked in order from worst to best they are:

◆ vomiting;
◆ gagging on an airway;
◆ pain;
◆ nausea;
◆ recall without pain;
◆ residual weakness;
◆ shivering;
◆ sore throat;
◆ being drowsy and unable to think coherently.

Ongoing care

Why give oxygen?

Some drugs depress breathing

Opioids such as fentanyl and morphine given during the anaesthetic depress the brainstem's sensors for carbon dioxide and may cause shallow or slow breathing.

Volatile anaesthetic agents, such as isoflurane, sevoflurane, and especially desflurane, depress oxygen-sensitive chemoreceptors so that they do not respond to falling oxygen levels in the blood. As a consequence, the chemoreceptors will be unable to stimulate breathing.

Other reasons to give oxygen

Diffusion hypoxia occurs after general anaesthesia as nitrous oxide washes out of the blood into the lungs to displace air oxygen-containing air.

Shallow breathing, resulting in *hypoventilation*, causes carbon dioxide to build up in the lungs to displace oxygen containing air.

In patients who shiver or shake, oxygen consumption may increase seven- to tenfold. To supply oxygen to the shivering muscles the heart must increase its cardiac output substantially. If patients with heart disease are unable to meet the extra demand they will become hypoxic.

Patients who have had either spinal or epidural *neuraxial blocks* have vasodilated extremities. Normally the heart maintains the blood pressure by pushing blood against the *resistance* to flow offered by arterioles. If the arterioles dilate, then the heart has to pump harder to keep the blood pressure up. A hard-working heart needs more oxygen.

How to give oxygen

Low-dose oxygen

Low-dose oxygen is given by facemask. Different types of mask deliver different concentrations of oxygen. At flow rates less than 4.5 litres a minute some *rebreathing* occurs. Rebreathing occurs when the patient inspires a portion of their expired air, as you would do if you breathed into and out of a paper bag.

If the patient does not like wearing the oxygen mask cut off the top third, including the metal bar, with scissors. Do not use nasal prongs in the recovery room. Patients recovering from anaesthesia tend to breathe through their mouths.

High-dose oxygen

In an unintubated spontaneously breathing patient the only way to give high-dose oxygen is with a mask and reservoir bag (Figure 1.4). This will achieve an inspired oxygen concentration of about 85 per cent (FiO_2 = 0.85).

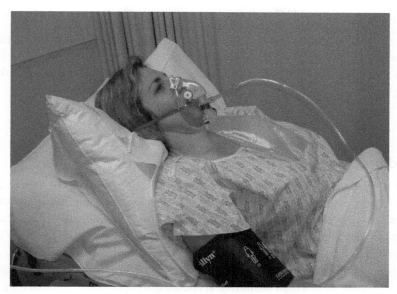

Figure 1.4 Oxygen mask with reservoir bag.

But, beware:

A recent systematic review and meta-analysis of more than 16,000 acutely unwell patients published in *The Lancet* gives high-quality evidence that liberal supplemental oxygen is harmful.[3]

Signs of hypoxia

Hypoxaemia is defined as an arterial partial pressure of oxygen (PaO_2) less than 60 mmHg (7.89 kPa).[1] An otherwise well person with an oximeter reading of 90 per cent or less is hypoxaemic (see Table 1.2). In contrast, *hypoxia* occurs when the tissues are so deprived of oxygen that they produce *lactic acid* from anaerobic metabolism. This can be measured, either as *pH* or lactic acid levels, or indirectly by checking the *anion gap*.

Table 1.2 Severe or critical hypoxia

Organ	Severe	Critical
Central nervous system	Agitation, restlessness, confusion	Seizures, coma
Cardiovascular	Hypertension, tachycardia, extrasystole	Hypotension, bradycardia
Skin	Cyanosis	Pallor, sweating
Urine output	10–30 ml/hr	< 10 ml/hr
Oxygen saturation	86–90%	< 85%

Early hypoxia

Early hypoxaemia can be difficult to detect clinically, but usually patients have a rising pulse rate, a decreasing perfusion status, and are unable to concentrate.

Monitors save lives

In the recovery room, about half of the life-threatening situations that occur are picked up by monitors. Monitors allow you to follow trends in blood pressure, pulse, heart function and in most units expired carbon dioxide, but they can fail to alert you when things go wrong or give false alarms. The best monitors are attentive staff.

Treat the patient,
not the monitor.

Blood pressure

When the patient is first admitted to recovery room, take the blood pressure and take it at 5-minute intervals for the first 15 minutes then every 10 minutes after that. If you have given a drug intravenously measure the blood pressure immediately and then every 5 minutes for the next 10 minutes. Non-invasive blood pressure monitors (NBP) give inaccurate readings if the pulse is irregular, for example with *atrial fibrillation* (AF). Do not rely on a non-invasive blood pressure reading if the systolic blood pressure is greater than 160 mmHg, or less than 80 mmHg. If you are not happy with the initial NBP reading check the blood pressure with a manual blood pressure machine. Keep at least one manual blood pressure machine in the recovery room.

To see some suggested stir-up exercises, see Box 1.2.

Pulse rate and rhythm

A normal pulse rate should be between 50 and 80 beats/min. Although a *tachycardia* is defined as a pulse rate greater than 100 beats/min, recovery room staff should be concerned if an adult's pulse rate rises above 80 beats/min.

Babies and infants have higher pulse rates than children and adults. In babies, infants and very old people it is easier to feel their hearts' apex beat than their peripheral pulses.

Record the pulse rate, rhythm and volume. If the pulse is irregular, suspect an arrhythmia. Attach an ECG. In young people, the most common cause of an irregular pulse is sinus arrhythmia where the pulse speeds up as they breathe in, and slows down when they breathe out: this is normal.

In older people the usual causes of an irregular pulse are atrial fibrillation or ventricular extrasystoles. If a patient develops ventricular extrasystoles it is a valuable early warning of cardiac ischaemia. The most common reasons for cardiac ischaemia are hypertension or tachycardia, or both.

Respiratory rate

The normal adult *respiratory rate* is between 12 and 14 breaths/min. Measure it by feeling the chest rise and fall under your hand, and not merely by watching the patient breathe. A rising respiratory rate is an excellent early warning sign of heart failure, developing *pulmonary oedema*, aspiration, sputum retention or rising temperature. After trauma or neurosurgery, a change in the rate or rhythm of breathing may be the first sign of a dangerous rise in intracranial pressure. The commonest cause of a slowing

Box 1.2 **Stir-up exercises**

Once patients are awake encourage them to do simple stir-up exercises. These exercises reduce the incidence of postoperative chest infections and deep vein thrombosis.

Deep breathing exercises

The aims of deep breathing exercises are to inflate segments of lung that inevitably collapse during general anaesthesia. Encourage the patient to take 2–3 very deep breaths every 5 minutes.

Coughing exercises

Coughing explosively clears the airways of mucus and dried secretions. Sit patients up if possible. If they have an abdominal wound then show them how to support their wound when they cough. Holding a small pillow to the site is helpful. Coughing exercises must not be done after open eye, middle ear, intracranial, facial or plastic surgery, as the cough may disrupt the surgery.

Leg exercises

Leg exercises help prevent deep vein thrombi forming. Get patients to move their feet up and down (to pump their calves), and to bend their legs at the knees (flex their quadriceps) and rotate their feet at least 20 times as soon as they are awake. Patients who are at risk from thromboembolism need good-quality compression stockings fitted before their surgery if calf compressing devices are not available (Figure 1.5).

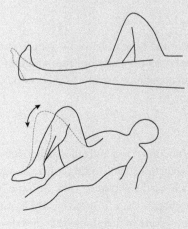

Figure 1.5 Most deep vein thrombosis begin in the recovery room.

respiratory rate is that the patient has received an opioid. See 'Patterns of breathing', Box 1.3.

*A change in the respiratory rate or pattern
means the physiological state of the patient has changed.*

Box 1.3 **Patterns of breathing**

You can gain a lot of information by simply monitoring the patient's breathing. Expose their chest. Put your hand on the sternum and feel it rise and fall. If there is mucus in the airways you will feel vibrations in the affected area. Listen to the tidal air exchange at the mouth for wheezes suggesting bronchial oedema, and the crackles of alveolar oedema. Sometimes *dyspnoea* is confused with a particular breathing pattern.

Kussmaul's breathing

Sometimes called *air hunger*, Kussmaul's breathing indicates metabolic acidosis. The patient breathes deeply, and feels breathless.

Cheyne–Stokes breathing

It is easy to recognize Cheyne–Stokes breathing (*periodic breathing*). The patient takes a series of breaths, and then slows or stops only to start again. In head injured patients, or after neurosurgery, periodic breathing is often a sign of rising intracranial pressure. Warn the anaesthetist immediately. Periodic breathing may occur in older patients who have received an opioid.

Pleuritic pain

Pleuritic pain occurs where the lung's pleura have been breached at surgery, or the patient has a pneumothorax. As they attempt to breathe in an intense stabbing pain stops them. To avoid the pain, patients breathe in shallow pants, and stop abruptly with a grunt as they feel the pain.

See-saw breathing

Normally the chest and the abdomen rise and fall together. *See-saw* breathing occurs after a life-threatening airway obstruction. While trying to breathe against the totally obstructed airway the patient's chest falls, as the abdomen rises. See-saw breathing is also known as *paradoxical breathing*. Young fit patients who try to breathe against a closed glottis may generate such violent swings of pressure in their lungs that they develop *pulmonary oedema*.

Obstructive and restrictive defects

Obstructive lung disease imposes a pattern of slow deep breathing; in contrast, restrictive lung disease imposes a pattern of rapid shallow breathing.

Temperature

The normal *core temperature* range is 36.5–37.2°C. Patients are often cold, so have warm blankets nearby. If their temperature is below 36°C then warm them with a forced air convection heater such as a BairHugger™, or a WarmTouch™. Advise the anaesthetist if the patient's temperature exceeds 37.5°C, or falls below 36°C.

Pulse oximetry

Put a *pulse oximeter* on every patient. Normal readings are between 96 and 100 per cent. If the reading falls to less than 92 per cent then seek a cause. At a reading of 90 per cent patients are hypoxaemic. Pulse oximeters do not work if the patient has poor circulation to their hands, or is wearing nail polish. To see when to alert the anaesthetist, see Box 1.4.

Box 1.4 **When to alert the anaesthetist**

Most reasons to call for assistance are obvious, but here are some subtle signs that give early warning of developing problems.

Notify the anaesthetist if:

◆ A previously stable blood pressure starts to decrease by more than 5 mmHg or more over each of three successive readings.

◆ A previously stable pulse rate rises to more than 100 beats/min.

◆ Pulse becomes irregular.

◆ Respiratory rate increases or decreases by more than 4 breaths/min.

◆ Pattern of breathing changes.

◆ Urine output falls to less than 30 ml/hr.

◆ Patient starts to sweat.

◆ Capillary return in their nailbeds slows.

◆ Conscious state deteriorates.

ECG

At the end of the surgery the anaesthetists may give you some rhythm strips from their monitors. This is especially likely if the patient's rhythm has altered during surgery. Paste the strips into the patient's record.

When the patient arrives in the recovery room attach an ECG monitor, especially to those at risk of cardiac arrhythmias or ischaemic heart disease. Write the initial cardiac rhythm in the recovery room chart. If the rhythm is abnormal, or is different from the cardiac rhythm recorded during the anaesthetic, then paste a sample of the rhythm strip taken from your monitor on the chart too. Remember to label, and put the date and time on each strip.

Recovery room scoring systems

Most recovery rooms use scoring systems for assessing and monitoring their patients to make sure they are safe to discharge and are comfortable. Many scoring systems have been published, some are more useful than others. Choose your scoring system carefully. Many are complex, some are confusing, and others misleading.

Table 1.3 Safety criteria

	Task	Score
Respiration	Needs assistance with ventilation	0
	Laboured or > 20 or < 10 breaths/min	1
	Normal rate: 12–15 breaths/min	2
O₂ sats	< 90% even with oxygen	0
	> 90% but requires oxygen to keep it there	1
	> 95% on room air	2
Power	Unable to lift head or move limbs on command	0
	Moves limbs but unable to sustain a 5-second head lift	1
	Sustains head lift for full 5 seconds	2
Circulation	BP ± 50% preoperative levels; or pulse > 120 or < 40 beats/min	0
	BP and pulse ± 20% preoperative levels	1
	Stable blood pressure and pulse with no changes in previous two sets of readings taken at 15-minute intervals	2
Sedation	Does not respond to shaking by shoulder	0
	Rouses when shaken by shoulder	1
	Awake, or awakes easily when spoken to, communicates coherently and coughs on command	2
Temp	Core temp < 35.5°C	0
	Core temp 35.5–36.5°C	1
	Core temp > 36.5°C and < 37.8°C	2
	Score out of 12	

The score sheet in Table 1.3 is simple. Each component can be used as a stand-alone module. For instance, the sedation score can be used to grade sedation during investigative procedures. The scoring system assesses two separate issues: first, is the patient safe to discharge from the recovery room and second, are they comfortable? Notify the anaesthetist of any patient who does not score at least 10 out of 12 points after 30 minutes.

Discharge from recovery room

How long should patients stay in recovery room?[2]

Stage 1 recovery

Patients stay in the recovery room while they are in Stage 1 recovery, unless they are transferred to the ICU.

Adults

As a rough guide adult patients stay in the recovery room for about an hour after general and regional anaesthesia and half an hour after local anaesthesia. Unstable patients stay longer, but once patients' vital signs are stable and their recovery room scores are satisfactory they can be discharged to Stage 2 recovery.

Children

Observe healthy children for at least 30 minutes if they have received inhalational anaesthesia by mask or laryngeal mask. If they have been intubated observe them for at least an hour. It may take this long for laryngeal oedema with its accompanying noisy breathing to become apparent.

Following tonsillectomy, adenoidectomy, cleft palate repair, pharyngeal or other major intra-oral procedures observe the patient for 90 minutes. Infants less than 12 months of age and those who have received naloxone are best observed for a minimum of two hours.

The anaesthetist, or a member of the medical staff, needs to review and certify in writing that their patient is fit to be discharged, and that some other member of the medical staff is properly briefed, and ready to take over responsibility for the patient's medical care.

Stage 2 recovery

1. Minimum criteria for discharge to Stage 2 recovery are:
   - the patient has a stable pulse rate, rhythm and blood pressure;
   - the patient is conscious and able to lift their head clear of the pillow for 5 seconds on demand;
   - patients are able to take a deep breath and cough;
   - oxygen saturation greater than 95%;
   - patients are able to touch the tip of their nose with their forefinger;
   - pain has been relieved;
   - there is no excessive loss from drains or bleeding from wound sites;
   - observation charts are completed;
   - the patient is clean, dry, warm and comfortable.
2. Remove all unnecessary intravenous lines and cannulas.
3. Remove ECG dots, and check the diathermy pad is not still attached.

4. Check that the medical and nursing staff have completed all the charts and notes and send them back to the ward with the patient.

5. Ensure the patient's recovery room record is complete. The ward staff need an accurate record to quickly identify any later deterioration.

6. Allow 20 minutes to elapse between the last dose of opioid analgesia and the patient's discharge from the recovery room.

7. Mandatory minimum stays in the recovery room are no longer necessary providing discharge criteria are met.

Local or regional anaesthesia

Patients recovering from local or regional anaesthesia need the same standard of care as those who have undergone general anaesthesia. Those patients still affected by spinal or epidural anaesthetic can be discharged to Stage 2 recovery provided all their other signs are stable. Patients with peripheral nerve block can be discharged home (Stage 3 recovery) even if full sensation has not returned, provided that they can walk steadily and meet the other discharge criteria.

How to handover to ward staff

The recovery room staff must be certain that the ward nurse understands the patient's medical problems, and current physical status, and is willing and competent to accept responsibility for the patient's care. Record the details of the handover on the patient's chart. Make sure that the ward staff have clear written instructions about infusion pump settings including drug doses.

How to transport patients to the ward

A nurse must accompany the patient when they return to the ward. Every trolley needs to carry portable oxygen and suction. Keep an emergency box containing a self-inflating resuscitation bag, airways and a range of masks on the trolley.

To prevent motion sickness, do not give your patients a fairground ride by swinging their head in a wide arc when turning corners on their way back to their ward. Sit them up at 45°. Wheel them forward with their feet first. When going around corners swing their feet and keep their heads as still as possible. This common-sense manoeuvre reduces subsequent vomiting in the ward by about 50 per cent.

Stage 3 recovery

Patients discharged home either from day case procedures; or after days or weeks in the ward remain in Stage 3 recovery. All patients remain in Stage 3 recovery until they no longer need the care of the hospital (including follow-up outpatient visits) and their welfare can be fully taken over by their family doctor or clinic. Even after going home patients can have complications as a result of the surgery or anaesthetic. These include deep vein thrombosis, pulmonary emboli, myocardial infarction, wound infection, and psychological problems.

Criteria for discharge to Stage 3 recovery

The patient must have had stable vital signs for at least 1 hour prior to discharge,[3] and be able to identify the time, place and relevant people.

As well as:

+ adequately controlled pain;
+ have no untoward nausea;
+ be adequately hydrated and able to drink without adverse consequences;
+ have minimal bleeding or wound drainage.

Note in the patient's record that discharge criteria have been met.

Day case procedures

Discharge from day case procedures

The patient must fulfil the criteria for discharge to Stage 3 recovery. In addition the following points are relevant:

+ The patient must be discharged into the care of a competent and responsible adult, who will accompany them home, and be able to report any untoward events.
+ The patient should not be alone that night.
+ The patient must have written instructions about diet, medication, acceptable physical activities, and a phone number to call in case of difficulties or emergencies. Bear in mind that about 15 per cent of the adult population cannot read even the simplest instructions. Staff should verify that the unit has the correct telephone number and address for a follow-up phone call. Usually this phone call is made on the evening of the procedure, and again the following day.
+ In most cases it is not necessary for patients to have passed urine before discharge, or demonstrated the ability to drink and retain clear fluids.

How to discharge a patient to the intensive care unit (ICU)

If the patient is going to the intensive care unit send for the bed, and check it has the following equipment with it:

+ a full cylinder of oxygen with flow meter;
+ a portable battery-powered ECG monitor and defibrillator;
+ a pulse oximeter;
+ suction;
+ emergency drugs, syringes, and needles in a closed sealed carrying box;
+ an anaesthetist, or member of the medical staff, to accompany patients returning to the intensive care unit.

Who needs to go to intensive care postoperatively?

In many cases patients who need emergency surgery are gravely ill. Because of the urgency of their surgical condition there may not have been time to fully assess medical illnesses, and optimize their vital signs before their anaesthetic. This is one reason emergency cases have higher morbidities and are more likely to die than elective patients.

Other patients who may need intensive care include those:

• who are already in ICU but are having an operative procedure, such as a tracheostomy;

• patients who were not fully assessed before their emergency surgery and have significant comorbidities;

• patients having uncomplicated surgery, but with severe intercurrent medical conditions, such as unstable diabetes, myasthenia gravis or unstable angina;

• patients having a major operation, such as oesophago-gastrectomy, liver or pancreatic surgery or prolonged plastic reconstructive surgery;

• patients where it may be anticipated complications will arise, such as head injured multiple trauma patients who are unable to protect their airway.

Elective postoperative ICU admissions

Patients who will have postoperative difficulties whatever their surgery, for example, the morbidly obese.

Families visiting the recovery room

Use your discretion here. Once you have stabilized your patient, especially a child, you may think it appropriate to have a relative come to the bedside. These concerned people are especially helpful if the patient is deaf, or disabled in some way. If possible meet these people before surgery and thoroughly brief the visitor. You will need guidelines on how to ensure the patient's confidentiality and privacy (and that of other patients in the recovery room).

Death in the recovery room

Sooner or later a patient will die in your recovery room. Have protocols to deal with this event. Guidelines should be in place about how to inform relatives, who is to be present at the interview, and where to hold the interview. It is most important that the most senior medical and nursing staff initially tell the relatives. It is most unfair and quite improper, to delegate this sad task to junior medical or nursing staff.

Telephone the patient's relatives to ask them to come to the hospital. It is unwise to tell them about the death over the phone; simply say there has been a problem. Suggest that they bring someone with them. It is better that a friend drives them to the hospital.

Litigation usually arises when relatives believe they are being deceived. Many legal problems can be avoided if this difficult duty is done in a humane, honest, sincere and sensible manner by the senior staff responsible for the patient's care.

Expected death

Occasionally, a patient who is expected to die following their surgery is brought into the recovery room. Care for the person in an area away from other patients. Out of respect and kindness, never let a patient die alone behind a closed curtain. Once the person has died make provision so that relatives can see the patient, and be consoled afterwards.

Unexpected death

Sometimes patients die unexpectedly despite the best care.[4,5] After the death the recovery staff may be upset, especially if the patient was young, or the circumstances distressing. Staff will need counselling, especially if they feel that more could have been done to save the patient's life.

There are also legal responsibilities. If a patient dies, nothing should be touched. A death in the recovery room must be reported to the coroner and evidence must be preserved for the coroner's inquest. Each country or state has its own requirements and these must be included in your hospital's protocol for death in the recovery room. Drips must remain attached, and endotracheal tubes left where they are. All drug ampoules must be kept, and the area quarantined until an investigation is complete. Carefully document the events leading up to the death because these notes may be required in the coroner's court. They must be detailed enough to record events in a way that does not rely on memory even years later.

Enhanced recovery pathways

Enhanced recovery after surgery (ERAS) programmes are multidisciplinary, evidence-based interventions in pre, intra and postoperative care that work synergistically to mitigate the undesirable effects of the surgical stress response. Implementation of ERAS pathways have been shown to reduce postoperative complications and accelerate recovery. They also allow standardization of perioperative care that minimizes variability and improves outcomes and should become standard of care for a variety of surgical procedures.

Overtreating and medication-related harm

Medication-related harms are unfortunately surprisingly common. They occur both in the hospital and in the community and cause a substantial burden on patients and the health care system.

Review your patients' medications before discharging them from the recovery room and if you are in any doubt as to why a patient is on a medication then ask. Too many patients just stay on medications because someone prescribed them and no one thought to stop them. This can result in unfortunate and unnecessary side effects or polypharmacy with drug interactions causing morbidity and mortality.[6]

If in doubt, ask.

References

1. **Ward DS, Karen SB,** *et al.* (2011) Hypoxia: a review. *Anaesthesia* **66** (Suppl 2):19–26.

2. **Clifford T** (2010) Reevaluation of the PACU patient before discharge. *Journal of PeriAnesthetic Nursing* **25**(6):416–417.

3. **Chu DK, Kim L,** *et al.* (2018) Mortality and morbidity in acutely ill adults treated with liberal versus conservative oxygen therapy (IOTA): a systematic review and meta-analysis. *The Lancet* **391**(10131):1693–1705.

4. **Sokol DK, McFadzean WA,** *et al.* (2011) Ethical dilemmas in the acute setting. *British Medical Journal* **343**:d5528.

5. **Frost PJ, Leadbeatter S,** *et al.* (2010) Managing sudden death in hospital. *British Medical Journal* **340**:c962.

6. **Robb G, Loe E,** *et al.* (2017) Medication-related patient harm in New Zealand hospitals. *New Zealand Medical Journal* **130**:1460.

Chapter 2

Recovery room procedures

Airway protection

- Airway control is an essential recovery room skill. Everyone caring for unconscious patients must be confident they can maintain the patient's airway, and recognize airway emergencies.
- Your most important tool is a high-capacity sucker, switched on and tucked under the patient's pillow where you can find it instantly.
- Have special trolleys (carts) ready and waiting for respiratory and other emergencies.
- Wherever possible nurse patients on their sides. Even conscious patients are safer in this position. As they wake up many patients will prefer to have their heads up. This is important in obese patients.

Those that look to heaven
go to heaven.

Airways

Oropharyngeal airways

Oropharyngeal airways (*Guedel airways*) are inserted to stop patients clenching their teeth and obstructing their airflow. They also open the mouth making it easier to clear the airway if required.

- If an airway is in place, then leave it there, and allow the patient to either spit it out or remove it themselves.
- In older people, especially if they have no teeth, try using a smaller rather than a larger size to maintain the airway.

Nasopharyngeal airways

Have a range of nasopharyngeal airways available (Figure 2.1). They are useful in those adults whose airways are difficult to maintain. Size 5, 6 and 7 will cover most needs. Commercially available nasopharyngeal airways are made of soft plastic with a flange to prevent them slipping in too far. They can, however, be made by cutting a 15 cm length of a blue polyvinyl chloride endotracheal tube. Push a safety pin through the outer end so that the tube cannot disappear into the nose. Lubricate well and insert by pushing them gently straight back, parallel with the floor of the nose. Do not push them upwards.

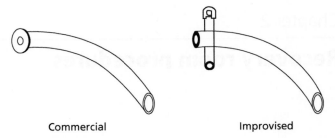

Commercial   Improvised

Figure 2.1 Nasopharyngeal airways.

Laryngeal mask airways

It is far easier to maintain an airway with a *laryngeal mask airway* (LMA) than with a normal face mask. Inserted through the mouth, laryngeal mask airways fit like a hood over the larynx. Inflating the cuff creates a loose seal in the pharynx to prevent air escaping (Figure 2.2).

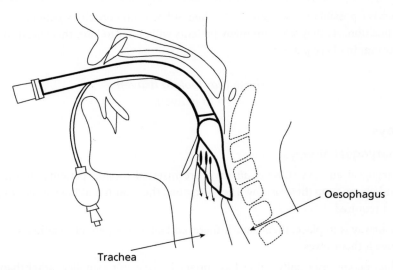

Oesophagus

Trachea

Figure 2.2 Laryngeal mask.

Advantages of laryngeal masks are that they:

- maintain a good airway, even in those who are difficult to intubate;
- are easy to use;
- do not traumatize or irritate the upper airway;
- are less likely to cause sore throats, coughing or bucking than an endotracheal tube;
- can be used to measure respiratory rate, minute ventilation and end-tidal CO_2 levels;
- do not require muscle relaxants to insert;

◆ can be useful if subsequent intubation is required by becoming a pathway for a bougie, endotracheal tube or fibreoptic bronchoscope.

Disadvantages of laryngeal masks are that they:

◆ require constant skilled supervision;

◆ do not protect the airway when stomach contents are vomited or regurgitated;

◆ if you attempt to ventilate a patient through them they may fill the stomach with gas under tension;

◆ are unsuitable for fat patients, who frequently have hiatus hernias, and may regurgitate gastric contents;

◆ are unsuitable for patients with high airway resistance such as asthmatics or those with bronchospasm;

◆ are sometimes impossible to insert, do not sit properly in place, or they fail to preserve the airway;

◆ do not prevent regurgitation and must only be used in fasted patients.

For instructions on how to clean and sterilize laryngeal masks see Box 2.1.

Box 2.1 **How to clean and sterilize laryngeal masks**

Most modern hospitals now have disposable laryngeal masks but not every hospital has the funds for this. If you are recycling the masks follow these instructions.

Put the dirty laryngeal mask straight into a bowl or jug of water. Dried secretions are difficult to wash off. Soak the mask thoroughly in soapy water. Use a bottle brush to gently clean the lumen and rinse it thoroughly in clean water.

Do not use glutaraldehyde (Cidex®), formaldehyde or ethylene oxide.

Autoclave the masks at low pressures and temperatures. Do not use the high-pressure high-temperature autoclave. To prevent the cuff from bursting as it is heated, deflate the mask almost completely before autoclaving.

Hints

◆ Patients coming from the operating theatre with a laryngeal mask in place can receive oxygen with a light T-Bag® attached to the oxygen tubing. This tubing can be moved from the transport oxygen cylinder to the wall oxygen once the trolley is settled in the appropriate bay.

◆ Leave the cuff inflated unless the anaesthetist suggests otherwise.

◆ Wait for patients to take out their own laryngeal masks.

◆ Undo the tie securing the laryngeal mask airway as soon as you receive the patient. You must be able to remove the airway instantly if the patient vomits or regurgitates.

- If the patient coughs or gags on the laryngeal mask airway remove it. Do not deflate the cuff. As you pull out the laryngeal mask the inflated cuff will drag most of the mucus and secretions with it.
- Be careful not to rip the laryngeal mask on the patient's teeth.
- Laryngeal masks do not sit well in babies, they have short, fat necks, and not much room in their pharynx. If the LMA keeps riding up, take it out and replace it with a Guedel airway.

Gas delivery circuits

T-Bag®

T-Bags® are light disposable devices that are easily attached to endotracheal tubes or laryngeal mask airways. T-Bags® reliably give an oxygen supply of 70 per cent at 6 L/min flow rate, and 50 per cent at 3 L/min with no rebreathing of expired air (Figure 2.3).

They are superior to T-piece circuits and outperform Hudson and other forms of high airflow entrainment masks.

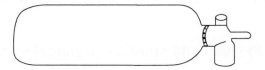

Figure 2.3 T-Bag®.

Mapleson circuit

The Mapleson C circuit is frequently used in the recovery room to ventilate patients and to administer high concentrations of oxygen. Use fresh gas flows. In spontaneously breathing patients the Mapleson C circuit causes unacceptable rebreathing with CO_2 retention. If you do use it on a spontaneously breathing patient remove the bag, leave the corrugated tubing attached to the valve and turn up the fresh oxygen supply to 8 L/min. This converts the circuit into a useful T-piece type extension (Figure 2.4).

Do not use a Mapleson C circuit on a
spontaneously breathing patient.

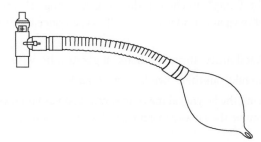

Figure 2.4 Mapleson C circuit.

Self-inflating resuscitation bags

Self-inflating resuscitation bags are portable and robust. The most commonly used are the Ambu® and the Laerdal Bag® (Figure 2.5). These bags are not easy to use; you may need to practise under supervision until you feel competent. They have a volume of about 1600 ml, but even with the biggest squeeze the maximum tidal volume you can deliver is about 1000 ml. Because they are self-inflating they automatically resume their shape after they have been squeezed, and do not depend on an oxygen or compressed gas supply.

If necessary you can deliver higher concentrations of oxygen by connecting them to an oxygen line. Attach a reservoir bag to increase the oxygen concentration of the inspired gas. Turn the oxygen on to a full flow of 10–15 L/min, using a flow less than this is no better than using room air.

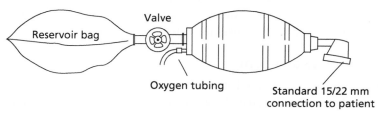

Figure 2.5 Laerdal resuscitation bag.

Intubation

Intubation in the recovery room is always an emergency. As soon as you hear the possibility mentioned bring your intubation trolley to the bedside. See emergency airway care Box 2.2.

Box 2.2 **Practical summary of emergency airway care**

1. Get help!
2. Keep a high-capacity sucker under the pillow.
3. Suck out the pharynx.
4. For laryngospasm consider 1.5 mg/kg lidocaine IV.
5. Always try bag and mask ventilation first.
6. A nasal airway if often useful.
7. If you can't 'bag and mask' ventilate then insert a laryngeal mask.
8. If you still can't ventilate then prepare to intubate.
9. If you can't intubate and you can't ventilate then prepare to insert a cricothyroid airway.

On the trolley

Keep the intubation trolley stocked and ready to wheel to a patient's side. Use the top shelf as a working area. On the bottom shelf keep everything you need for emergency airway management: laryngeal masks, cricothyroid puncture set, emergency tracheostomy kit, guide wires, bougies, and at least two spare working laryngoscopes. Your operating theatre suite should have a 'difficult intubation trolley' nearby with extra equipment such as a GlideScope® and fibreoptic laryngoscope. See Appendix 1.

Endotracheal tubes

You will need a range of sizes for different ages. Sizes are measured on their internal diameter. Children under the age of 10 do not require cuffed tubes, however above this age cuffs are needed for a good gas seal, and to prevent fluid entering the lower airways. Most modern airways will have a line indicating the position the tube should sit inside the lips. In the larger tubes a *Murphy eye*, which is a second hole near the distal end of the tube, prevents occlusion if the tip becomes obstructed.

How to intubate a patient

You will learn more about the intubation by seeing it done by an anaesthetist than you will from reading books. Practise your airway skills so that you are confident you will be able to ventilate the patient with the bag and mask until the anaesthetist arrives to help you. A Guedel airway, a nasal airway or a laryngeal mask are all useful in this situation and preferable to a failed intubation by an unexperienced operator.

How to prepare the equipment

Connect an Air-Viva™ or black Mapleson's C circuit to the oxygen supply. Have a selection of oropharyngeal tubes, nasopharyngeal airways and masks nearby. Assemble at least two endotracheal tubes (ETT), one the expected size, and the other a size smaller. Men take 8.5–9 mm endotracheal tubes, and women size 7–8 mm.

Take an endotracheal tube and inflate the cuff with a 10 ml syringe to make sure it has no leaks. Keep your fingers away from its sterile end. Squeeze a glob of water-soluble lubricant such as K-Y® Jelly onto a sterile gauze swab. Smear the endotracheal tube's cuff with jelly and put it in a sterile intubation tray where you can reach it later.

Check that all the equipment you need is close at hand:

- The patient is on a trolley that can be tipped quickly head down.
- A low pillow under the patient's head.
- A Yankauer sucker under the pillow, hissing and ready to use.
- A laryngoscope with a bright white light to inspect the larynx and vocal cords. A second laryngoscope of a larger size should also be available.
- A 10 ml syringe to blow up the cuff on the endotracheal tube.
- White cotton tracheostomy tape to secure the endotracheal tube.

- Magill forceps to remove chunks of matter in the airway or manipulate the endotracheal tube. Their handles curve out of the way so you can see what is happening at the tips.
- A lubricated gum-elastic *bougie* to railroad the tube along should there be any difficulty in getting the tip through the vocal cords.
- End-tidal CO_2 monitor to connect to confirm the tube is in the trachea.
- An intravenous infusion with warmed 0.9% saline.

Draw up the drugs and label the contents. Keep the ampoules to show the anaesthetist. The usual drugs are an induction agent such as propofol, an ultra-brief muscle relaxant (suxamethonium or mivacurium), and a longer-acting muscle relaxant such as rocuronium. Other drugs the anaesthetist might need include atropine, midazolam, lidocaine, and ephedrine. The anaesthetist then preoxygenates, sedates and paralyses the patient.

Offer the anaesthetist the laryngoscope. The anaesthetist will open the blade, place it in the patient's mouth and sweep the tongue away to the left giving a clear view of the larynx. Have the hissing Yankauer sucker ready for the anaesthetist to grab from your hand to suck out the pharynx if there are secretions. Have the lubricated endotracheal tube with the 10 ml syringe full of air already attached ready to hand to the anaesthetist.

The anaesthetist will pull the handle of the laryngoscope, moving the bottom jaw straight out to reveal the vocal cords as a little white V with the trachea disappearing like a tunnel beyond. The lubricated endotracheal tube is then slipped between the cords. To improve the view the anaesthetist may ask you to 'hold the corner of the mouth down'. To do this, put your gloved finger inside the right side of the patient's mouth. Pull the cheek outwards and downward towards you. You may also be asked to move the larynx, usually to the patient's right or left side.

To finish up

Once the tube is in place, hand the anaesthetist the catheter mount ('liquorice-stick') to connect the patient to the Air-Viva or Magill circuit. Not all anaesthetists will use this but have it available. Inflate the cuff and adjust the amount of air in the cuff until the leak just disappears. This usually takes 4–8 ml of air. Connect the endotracheal tube and the CO_2 monitor.

Hand the white tape to the anaesthetist who will use a clove hitch knot to secure the tape to the tube, being careful not to capture the pilot tube going to the cuff. Pass one end of the tape under the patient's neck.

Next the anaesthetist checks air entry into both sides of the lungs with a stethoscope. Note in the patient's record the size of the endotracheal tube, and its length at the incisors (it should be between 19 and 21 cm and up to 24 cm for very tall people).

Never tape or tie a nasogastric tube to the endotracheal tube, because if something snags on the drainage bag it will dislodge the tube.

How to manage an intubated patient

About 5 per cent of patients are still intubated when they come to the recovery room. Usually this is because they have *failed to breathe* adequately at the end of their anaesthetic and cannot be extubated safely at that time. Delayed extubation is more likely with prolonged operations, where the patient is hypothermic, in those with respiratory disease, in elderly patients and in sicker patients, or where the muscle relaxants have not yet reversed adequately. In this case, patients need to be ventilated until the muscle relaxant has worn off. Some patients may need to go to intensive care for further respiratory support, but in most cases the anaesthetist will continue to supervise the patient and extubate when appropriate. See 'Ten steps in extubation', Box 2.3.

Is it safe to extubate the patient?

It is always the anaesthetist's responsibility to extubate their patient. Before it is safe to extubate a patient they must fulfil three criteria:

1. They must be able to breathe adequately.
2. They must not be depressed by opioid or sedative drugs.
3. They must be able to able to protect their own airway against aspiration of material in their pharynx.

Box 2.3 **Ten steps in extubation**

1. Put the patient on high oxygen concentrations for 3 minutes before proceeding. Attach a *pulse oximeter*.
2. Check the larynx with a laryngoscope to make sure no foreign material is present, for example a throat pack, blood, or mucus.
3. Gently suck out the pharynx. Check the nasopharynx up behind the soft palate is clear too.
4. Lay the patients preferably on their left side.
5. Remove the ties and tape securing the endotracheal tube and deflate the cuff slowly with a 10 ml syringe.
6. Close the valve on the ventilation circuit and give the patient a good inspiration of oxygen. At the end of inspiration with one smooth movement, withdraw the tube.
7. Give the patient oxygen at a flow of 6 L/min through a face mask.
8. Encourage a few deep breaths and cough.
9. Check the oxygen saturation.
10. Watch for signs of postoperative hypoxia or hypercarbia.

Can the patient breathe adequately?

It is unsafe to extubate patients who have sputum in their airways or whose oxygen saturation is below 93 per cent. They must be able to take deep breaths on command through their endotracheal tube. Before extubation the tidal volume needs to be 4–7 ml/kg (about 500 ml) and the respiratory rate greater than 10 breaths/min.

Coughing

Coughing sharply raises the blood pressure, intracranial pressure and intra-ocular pressure, causing venous congestion in the head and neck. Vigorous coughing can fracture ribs in the elderly, or disrupt surgical stitches.

Coughing is the commonest cause of a raised intracranial pressure. Following neurosurgery, it is critically important that patients' intracranial pressure does not rise. It may cause catastrophic intracranial bleeding. Those with a spiking pattern on their intracranial pressure trace are especially at risk.

After open eye surgery coughing raises the intra-ocular pressure, and can detach retinas and/or dislocate lenses. Any of these events may cause irreversible blindness. Prevent coughing by giving 3–5 ml of 1 per cent lidocaine intravenously. Before doing this check with the anaesthetist that it is appropriate.

Injections

In the recovery room, drugs are usually injected intravenously, and sometimes intramuscularly.

Placing intravenous cannulas

This subject is controversial in many hospitals. We recommend that all nurses working in the recovery room learn to place intravenous cannulas and give intravenous injections.

Choose a suitable vein

Do not be tempted by those fragile little veins on the anterior aspect of the wrist, because the cannula will cut out in the next few hours. Beneath those veins are the flexor tendons to the hand as they enter the carpal tunnels. Extravasation here can cause permanent damage.

Take care putting drips in the cubital fossa. Lying very close to that large cubital vein are the brachial and radial arteries, and the median and radial nerves. Damage to these could mean impaired function of the patient's hand.

It is tempting to put drips and infuse drugs into the large veins in the back of the hand; but this is a bad place for a long-term infusion. Inflammation here may cause patients months of pain. If this happens, particularly to older people, they suffer every time they try to flex their fingers. If drugs extravasate in the back of the hand the consequences can be disastrous. The tendons that serve the fingers run close by; and a corrosive sloughing ulcer here may permanently damage tendons (or their sheaths) and cripple their hand.

Intramuscular injections

Give deep intramuscular injections only into the upper (outer) lateral quadrant of the thigh. Adults of normal weight and muscle mass can tolerate a maximum of 5 ml of fluid injected. Patients less than 45 kg can tolerate no more than 2 ml injected into muscle. In obese people, make sure your needle is long enough to reach the muscle. Unlike muscle, which is well perfused, fat is poorly perfused and drug absorption will be delayed. Apply skin prep to the site, and wait until it dries. Grasp the injection site firmly and insert your needle at 90° to the skin (Figure 2.6). Dart the needle in, aspirate slightly to make sure you are not in a blood vessel, and press the plunger slowly to avoid painful distension of the muscle. Do not massage the injection site, but encourage the patient to move their leg around.

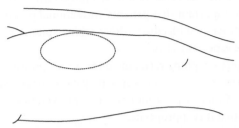

Figure 2.6 Safe area for intramuscular injections, on the upper outer lateral quadrant of the thigh.

Never give intramuscular injections into the buttocks of children because you might accidentally inject a drug into the sciatic nerve and permanently damage it causing the leg to become paralysed. Avoid injections into the deltoid muscle in children and young adults because you may damage the circumflex nerve.

Venothromboembolism

Deep vein thrombosis (DVT)

It is very important to check that effective thromboprophylaxis is in place for all postoperative patients.[1,2] Good management reduces the incidence of pulmonary embolism (PE) as well as post-thrombotic syndrome and pulmonary hypertension. Deep vein thrombosis is one part of a syndrome called *venothromboembolic disease* (VTE). Other components to the syndrome include pulmonary embolism and post-thrombotic venous disease.

If blood clots (thrombi) form in the great veins of the legs and pelvis, they can break off and lodge in the lung, plugging blood vessels like a cork. The effect is catastrophic. This is the number-one killer on the ward and in the weeks following discharge from hospital. Within a few seconds the patient collapses, becomes desperately short of breath, frightened and panics. They can have a cardiac arrest and die. A chest X-ray or ECG may reveal little or nothing at this early stage. Listening over the affected area with a stethoscope, you will hear a transient wheeze. Treatment involves giving oxygen, treating bronchospasm and anticoagulation with heparin.

DVT is particularly common after orthopaedic surgery, pelvic surgery and in patients with heart failure, cancer, or those who have had previous clots. Patients having prolonged surgery and those who are given a blood transfusion have a higher incidence. DVT becomes more common as people age, but it may occur spontaneously at any age. Changes in the vessel wall can occur in diabetics who become hyperglycaemic while in the recovery room. Blood glucose levels greater than 12 mmol/L cause vascular endothelial cells to shrivel up and pull away from their neighbours, exposing the basement membrane where clots readily form. Obese patients are also vulnerable. Women who are pregnant, or taking oral contraceptives, or hormone replacement therapy are also at risk of venothromboembolism. Take care with patients who have been on drugs that affect clotting such as antiplatelet agents or NSAIDs.

The incidence of DVT ranges from 36 to 84 per cent in patients who do not receive anti-coagulants after major hip surgery, in these patients, the risk of fatal pulmonary embolism is as high as 13 per cent. Even with DVT prophylaxis the rate of VTE is still 18–20 per cent although few of these progress to pulmonary emboli.

Why DVT occurs

Over one hundred years ago Professor Gustav Virchow described a triad of risk factors for deep vein thrombosis. They were changes in blood flow, changes in the vessel wall, and altered blood coagulability. All surgery changes the volume of blood supplying the legs. Postoperatively bandages or plasters impede flow. Physiological stress such as pain, or hypovolaemia, or even fear increases blood's tendency to clot.

Who needs prophylaxis?

Any patient over the age of 40 years who is having major surgery lasting longer than 30 minutes needs prophylaxis.

How to prevent DVT

Measures include:

* adequate hydration, leg exercises, and good analgesia to prevent hypercoagulopathy;
* maintain the blood glucose in diabetics to be in the range 7–10 mmol/L;
* check bandages and prevent any restriction to blood flow;
* check that suitable DVT prophylaxis and anticoagulation has been prescribed before the patient is discharged from the recovery room.

Aspirin and warfarin are also part of the DVT prevention in some patients. The risk of bleeding after surgery complicates the use of VTE prophylaxis. If you are unsure in the recovery room when you check the drug chart ask your surgeon or anaesthetist for guidance. The prescription is their responsibility but enquiring is a useful jolt to awareness too (see 'Antithrombotic drugs including anticoagulants', Box 2.4).

Graduated stockings

Properly fitted graduated stockings are clearly effective in reducing the incidence of deep vein thrombosis. Graduated pressure stockings apply graded degrees of pressure to the lower limb. The greatest pressure is at the ankle, and the pressure exerted by the stocking progressively decreases further up the leg. Graduated stockings prevent venous stasis increasing the rate of blood flow, protect from vessel injury and improving venous valve function. It is not known whether full thigh-length stockings are more effective than the

Box 2.4 **Antithrombotic drugs including anticoagulants**

Unfractionated heparin

Unfractionated heparin (UH) is a fast-acting anti-coagulant with a short half-life of about 90 minutes. The dose is 5000 units subcutaneously (s/c) twice daily. Its effect can be monitored with an activated partial thromboplastin time (aPTT). It can be reversed with protamine.

Low molecular-weight heparins

Low molecular-weight heparins (LMWH) are selective anti-coagulants causing less systemic effects than UH. There are number of LMWH, but the two most commonly used are enoxaparin and dalteparin, while fondaparinux is reserved for high-risk cases.

Enoxaparin is given once a day. The standard adult dose is enoxaparin 40 mg s/c. In patients weighing less than 50 kg, or those with renal failure use half of this dose.

Dalteparin is given twice a day. The standard adult dose is 5000 units s/c 1–2 hours preoperatively and repeated 12 hourly in high-risk patients. In patients weighing less than 50 kg, or those with renal failure use half of this dose.

Fondaparinux is a synthetic pentasaccharide derived from unfractionated heparin. It has a long half-life of 21 hours. It is more efficacious than warfarin, but not as safe. It is best reserved for patients with an extreme risk of DVT. The dose is 2.5 mg s/c injection for 5–9 days. Give the first dose 6 hours after surgery. It is unsafe to use in patients who have an epidural catheter in place.

shorter knee-length stockings. They are, however, not without risk, and must not be used on patients who have vascular disease affecting blood flow to the lower limb because they may cause limb ischaemia.

While in the recovery room get the patient to flap their feet up and down, and flex their knees at least 20 times every 15 minutes. For those with epidural anaesthesia, these exercises will have to be assisted by a nurse or physiotherapist in the ward until spontaneous movement returns.

Mechanical devices

Intermittent pneumatic compression (IPC) increase venous outflow and reduce venous stasis (see Figure 2.7). They are more effective used in combination with pharmacological prophylaxis and they can be continued in the ward.

If heparins are contraindicated use IPC, and graduated compression stockings. Do not use IPC in patients with severe peripheral vascular disease, severe peripheral neuropathy, lower limb oedema, or if the leg has a breach in the skin such as ulcers or eczema.

Intermittent calf compression

Devices that apply intermittent calf compression are useful where a LMWH is contra-indicated, for instance after intracranial, inner ear, or some forms of plastic procedures.

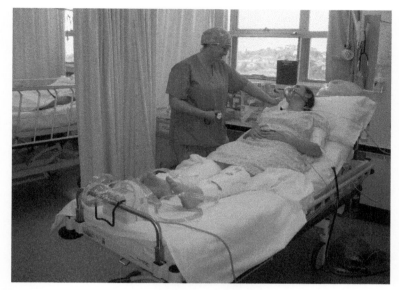

Figure 2.7 Intermittent pneumatic compression devices.

*Recovery room staff have
a major role in preventing VTE.*

A uniform enforced hospital policy on measures to prevent DVT gives the best results. However, even with the best regimes the relative risk reduction is probably only 60 to 80 per cent. Prophylaxis is no guarantee that thrombosis will not occur. Although PE is uncommon in the recovery room, deep vein thrombosis often starts here.

References

1. **Hill J, Treasure T**, *et al.* (2010) Reducing the risk of venous thromboembolism in patients admitted to hospital. *British Medical Journal* **340**:c95.
2. **Samama CM, Godier A** (2011) Perioperative deep vein thrombosis prevention. *Current Opinion in Anesthesiology* **24**:166–170.

Chapter 3

Design of the recovery room

Location of the recovery room

Shortly after the first anaesthetic was given in 1846, Florence Nightingale recognized the need for a special area, and special nursing care of patients recovering from ether anaesthesia. She wrote in her book *Notes on Hospitals* that the patient should be placed in a small room near to the ward, with clean fresh sand on the floor, clean bedclothes, and windows to admit the sunlight and fresh air.[1]

The recovery room is part of the operating theatre suite, located close to the operating theatre, but it should be readily accessible to medical staff who are in their street clothes. The staff tea room should be nearby so that the doctors having a break at the end of a case can quickly come to the patient if needed. It is also useful if there is a communicating window or door between the recovery room and the holding bay where patients arrive for theatre with their escorting nurses. Patients who are ready to leave can then be sent back with these nurses. It is best to have the intensive care unit on the same level and close to the recovery room.

Ideally there should be restricted as well as public access, and a separate entrance for goods to be delivered so that supplies do not take the same route as patients. There should be adequate space for administration. A computer-assisted drug narcotic dispensing unit saves a lot of time. Consider incorporating an isolation room for managing patients with infections, contaminated wounds, and those who are immunosuppressed. This room needs to have both negative- and positive-pressure air conditioning.

In hospitals with fewer than 200 beds it is useful to have the ICU adjacent to the operating theatre. The recovery room can then be a functional part of the ICU but remain a separate area away from the unit. Such an arrangement means that staff, facilities and equipment can be shared between the two areas. A further advantage is that after hours when there are fewer staff on the wards patients can be recovered in the ICU. The disadvantage is the risk of transferring infection from ICU patients to the surgical patient. This transmission of nosocomial infection is preventable but requires scrupulous care and iron-tight discipline. Wearing gowns and hand washing are crucial to this.

Plan for the recovery room

The minimum size of a recovery room should not be less than 164 m² for a department of eight theatres. Square recovery rooms are more efficient than long rectangular ones, because they keep traffic paths as short as possible and allow nurses to talk easily with each other. Plan an open and uncluttered room with no support structures obstructing your view (Figure 3.1). Avoid swing doors if possible.

The total overall area of the recovery room should be 18 m^2 for every trolley bay. Depending on the workload and expected turnover most hospitals will find that 1.5–2 trolley bays for each operating theatre is sufficient. However, those with high turnover and short cases (such as tonsillectomies) will require up to three beds per operating theatre.

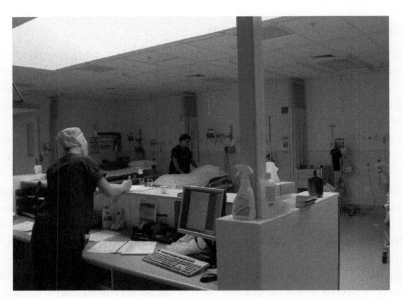

Figure 3.1 Plan of a typical recovery room.

Common mistakes when planning recovery rooms are to have too little storage space, insufficient power points (general power outlets), insufficient suction outlets and not enough room on either side of the patient for all the services that may need to be brought to the trolley side (Box 3.1). It is wise to consider provision for future technological advances.

Another consideration is privacy for the patients. Curtains are traditional but they are not ideal as they gather dust and always seem to be in the way when emergencies occur. There must be provision for rapid evacuation of the recovery room in an emergency. The provisions need to include strategies for evacuating comatose or unstable patients.

Where to from here?

Informational privacy could be improved for patients in the recovery room by the use of patient health information transmission systems and architectural solutions.[2]

The room illustrated in the photograph is typical of most recovery rooms but have a look at these imaginative designs from industrial designer Kousaku Haruguchi[3] (Figures 3.2 and 3.3).

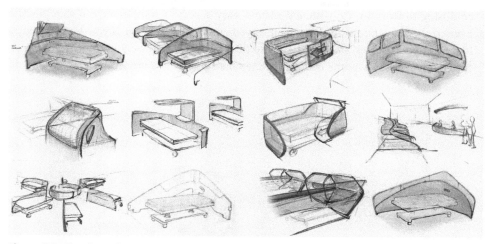

Figure 3.2 Sketches of recovery room areas emphasizing patient privacy. Reproduced with permission from Kousaku Haruguchi.

Box 3.1 **Standards**

There are many things to consider when planning and building a recovery room. Fortunately architects and engineers have access to help in the form of standards.

Standards are sets of specifications that cover almost everything to do with construction, design, safety, purchase and applications of buildings and equipment used in hospitals. Many countries, including Australia, the United Kingdom, the European community, and the USA have their own standards that specify such things as the design of buildings, the supply of piped gases, the quality of lighting, uniformity of fittings for anaesthetic apparatus, the formulation of drug names, electrical safety, hospital signage, medical records and so on. Eventually apparatus designed and used in one country will be used equally safely in another country; and all the various fittings, pipes, and colour codes will be uniform. Make sure that anything you design or build or buy complies with the accepted standards in your area.

The minimum number of trolley or bed spaces is 1.5 for each operating room. Operating suites with rapid turnover will require more spaces. There are statistical methods, such as the theory of queues, for helping decide the appropriate number of recovery room bays for each operating room.

Each recovery room trolley bay should be identical, with the same items of equipment in the same places. Do not design bays that are mirror images of each other, they are confusing to work in. Consistency ensures easy access to equipment and safe practice. Every trolley bay should be visible from anywhere within the room. If you design a central island for your nurses' station make sure the bench top is low enough for staff who are sitting down to see over the bench top. Keep flat surfaces to a minimum.

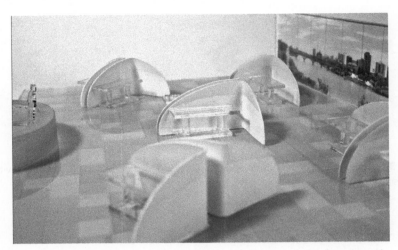

Figure 3.3 Model of an ideal recovery room. Reproduced with permission from Kousaku Haruguchi.

Make sure that patient trolleys can move easily around the room with the minimum number of corners to negotiate. Have two wide doors for access; one from the operating theatre and one to the wards, ideally these should be on opposite sides of the room.

As a rule trolley bays need to be at least 3.5 metres long with at least 2 metres on each side to allow equipment such as portable X-ray equipment, ventilators, and warming blanket to be brought to the patient. Nine square metres is the absolute minimum. Each trolley bay needs at least 1 cubic metre of storage space within the room, and at least 3 square metres of shelving and storage space outside the room, but nearby. Each recovery room trolley bay needs its own service utilities mounted on the wall at the head end of the patient trolley.

Trolley bay fixtures

Equipment needed for each trolley bay should include:

- two high-pressure oxygen outlets equipped with flow meters and nipples;
- two high-vacuum, high-flow suction outlets including receiver, tubing, rigid handpiece, and a range of suction catheters. These must conform with relevant national standards;
- two high-pressure medical air outlets;
- eight mains electric (*general*) *power outlets*;
- an emergency red panic button alarm on the wall above the patient's head;

- overhead runners similar to curtain rails with hooks are a useful way to hang drips— these must be high enough to allow the drip to run rapidly;
- have one freewheeling drip stand between each trolley bay. This should be on a wide base so that it will remain stable with a blood warmer or infusion pump attached to it. It must be easily raised to a suitable height when a rapid infusion is required in an emergency;
- one mobile examination light that can be swung to provide light at any point on the patient.

Appropriate electronic monitoring facilities mounted on the wall at eye level such as:

- ECG;
- carbon dioxide monitors;
- pulse oximeters;
- large underfloor conduits to carry communication cables to the central nurses' station;
- a blood pressure monitor attached to the wall at eye height to prevent errors caused by parallax;
- privacy screens; these are often curtains, but there are other options. Consider facing the patients towards the wall rather than into the centre of the room.
- two shelves with slightly raised edges to prevent things falling on the floor;
- handwashing facilities for scrubbing up, one between two is ideal;
- somewhere to keep the patient's chart;
- storage space or bins for a day patient's belongings.

Within the trolley bay keep:

- a good-quality stethoscope;
- oropharyngeal and nasopharyngeal airways;
- sterile disposable gloves (powder free);
- unsterile disposable protective gloves in all sizes;
- a pressure infusion bag for giving IV fluids rapidly;
- oxygen tubing with connectors;
- T-piece or T-bags® for delivering oxygen to spontaneously breathing patients who have a laryngeal mask or endotracheal tube in place;
- self-inflating bags (Laerdal® or Ambu®); and a Mapleson C circuit;
- bowels and kidney dishes;
- paper tissues;
- a good-quality reliable torch with spare batteries;
- scissors;
- tape; gauze and mouth swabs;
- sealable plastic bags for transporting potentially infectious material;

- containers for haematology and pathology specimens;
- blood gas syringes;
- a range of needles, syringes, and skin cleaning preparations.

Within the recovery room keep:

- a 12-lead ECG machine;
- a neuromuscular function monitor;
- a warming cupboard for blankets;
- a procedure light;
- basic surgical tray;
- bronchoscopy equipment;
- a ventilator;
- provision for inserting chest drains;
- blood gas and electrolyte measuring equipment;
- a refrigerator for storing heat-labile drugs.

Design your recovery room
so that you can see all the patients, all the time.

Emergency station

Establish an *emergency station*, where the defibrillator and trolleys (*crash carts*) for managing cardiac arrests and other emergencies are kept. Keep this in an easily accessible place. The emergency station needs a mains power supply to keep the portable equipment's batteries charged.

Emergency trolleys (crash carts)

Keep trays and trolleys set up for anaphylaxis, malignant hyperthermia, emergency airway care, emergency bronchoscopy, insertion of thoracic drains, minor surgical procedures, and vascular access. Attach the relevant protocols to the trolley. It helps to have a large, clear colour photograph of each set-up so that the trays can be checked quickly and are always put together in the same way. Photographs will tell you immediately what is missing. Consider sharing infrequently used trolleys such as those for malignant hyperthermia and bronchoscopy with the anaesthetic department.

Isolation rooms

Plan to incorporate isolation rooms into your recovery room; sterile ones to manage immunosuppressed patients, and non-sterile ones to manage patients with highly contagious airborne diseases such as tuberculosis (TB). Sterile isolation rooms, with airlocks, are kept at *positive pressure* with highly filtered air, so that organisms are not able to enter, whereas those where patients with infectious diseases are treated are kept at negative pressure so that organisms cannot escape.

Other facilities

Air conditioning

Air conditioning should maintain the temperature of the recovery room between 21° and 24°C with the capability of increasing it to 26°C. The relative humidity should be between 40 and 60 per cent under all conditions with at least 12 air changes per hour, which is the same as the operating theatres. Anaesthetic gas pollution can be high in the recovery room, because patients continue to exhale gases, especially the volatile vapours, for some time after leaving the operating theatre.

Clocks

A clock with a sweep second hand should be visible from all over the recovery room. Include battery replacement as part of your routine maintenance programme.

Use the 24-hour clock when noting time on charts and in the records.

For example:

Midnight	=	0.00 hr
10.20 a.m.	=	10.20 hr
Noon	=	12.00 hr
8 p.m.	=	20.00 hr

Cylinders

The gas in a cylinder is at extremely high pressure of 120,000 kPa or 2000 pounds per square inch. Handle cylinders with care. Do not drop them. They have been known to explode like a bomb. Use chains to make sure large cylinders stay upright and cannot fall over. Store them in a cool place well away from direct sunlight. Do not accept delivery if they show signs of rust.

Make sure you have the right key to turn them on and off. Cylinders have to be cracked before use. To *crack a cylinder*, gently turn it on for an instant to blow out any dust or grit that may be lodged in the cylinder's neck; otherwise the particles may damage apparatus.

Oxygen cylinders

Oxygen is neither explosive nor flammable, but it vigorously supports combustion. There are four sizes of oxygen cylinders normally available (see Table 3.1).

Table 3.1 Gas cylinders

Cylinder size	Litres	Cubic feet
J cylinder	6800	240
G cylinder	3400	120
F cylinder	1360	48
D cylinder	340	12

Defibrillator

Defibrillators are an essential piece of equipment. They are used to treat cardiac arrest and some forms of arrhythmias. Ideally have one with a pacing mode. In a small hospital it may be necessary to share one defibrillator with the whole theatre block. Keep it with the resuscitation trolley in the recovery room. There are many types, but the most useful are portable, lightweight, run on mains power or rechargeable batteries, and have an internal ECG monitor. Include its routine check in your maintenance plan.

Defibrillators put out large amounts of current; as much as 7000 volts at 4 joules. They are dangerous if they are not handled properly. Staff have been electrocuted while demonstrating its use. Practise using the defibrillator, but not while it is charged up. Defibrillators need special conductive jelly or conductive pads. Store these on the same trolley as the defibrillator. In hot climates slightly moisten the pads with saline if they are dry. Do not allow the saline to leave the area of the pad, or a short-circuit may occur. Do not use a non-conductive jelly (such as K-Y® Jelly) or water because it will cause a deep burn during cardioversion.

Decor

Paint walls and ceiling light neutral colours. Avoid colours such as blues, greens, pinks and yellows because they reflect misleadingly on patients' skins.

Drugs

Recovery rooms need a wide range of drugs. Sometimes they will be needed in a hurry. A set of recessed shelves with a door that can be rolled down is ideal. Organize your drug cupboard in alphabetical order according to generic name. Post an alphabetical list of both the trade names and generic names on the door. Consider having a third list of drugs arranged under their pharmacological actions, for instance a list of antibiotics, cardiac drugs etc.

Emergency power

A reliable power supply is crucial. An emergency power generator is essential in case the mains supply fails. This should automatically switch on if there is mains power failure. As an additional back-up in case both systems fail and the recovery room is plunged into total darkness, fit one or more emergency battery-powered torches that automatically switch on when mains power fails.

If there is a fire in any part of the hospital the fire brigade may cut off the electricity supply so they can use water to put the fire out.

Most cases of macroshock occur when someone touches a live electrical wire (see 'Electrical protection devices', Box 3.2), and the full mains current flows through their body to earth. Their heart goes into ventricular fibrillation (VF), which causes them to die from electrocution.

Box 3.2 **Electrical protection devices**

Ordinary wiring used in domestic houses has its electrical protection (Class A) limited to fuses, an earth wire in the cord or two levels of insulation (double insulation).

Recovery rooms are a *Body Protected Area* (Class B) giving protection against macroshock in the event of an accident. Macroshock protection is provided, preferably with an isolation transformer, or less preferably with core balance earth leakage devices.

Isolation transformers are fitted to the mains power supply and prevent a person being electrocuted if they touch an electric live (*active*) wire in the power supply while they are in contact with the earth. Such an event can easily happen for instance if someone accidentally spills fluid into an electrical device. Isolation transformers are expensive and require regular checking and maintenance.

Core balance earth leakage devices are a cheaper alternative. They detect a current flowing to earth and shuts down all the power on that circuit before enough current has passed to electrocute the person. For most recovery rooms this is sufficient, but it has the disadvantage of interrupting the power supply, which needs to be switched on again manually. To ensure that core balance works properly all earth points in the circuit need to have a common heavy copper grounding cable.

Modern recovery rooms are now designed to conform to cardiac-protected areas (Class Z). Class Z areas are similar to Class B areas but include special wiring to ensure that no exposed surfaces of plumbing, electrical equipment, or anything that can conduct electricity in the vicinity of the patient can create an electrical gradient sufficient to cause microelectrocution.

In contrast microshock occurs when tiny currents of a few millivolt pass through an electrolyte infusion or pacemaker wire to cause VF. Isolation devices protect against macroshock. Proper flooring, adequate humidity and properly earthed electronic devices guard, but do not completely protect, against microshock.

Emergency button

Site a large red panic button on the wall above each trolley bay to call for help. The best buzzer is one with an urgent repeating sequence that can be heard throughout the theatre complex, including the changing rooms. To prevent them being accidentally activated design them to pull on rather than push. Identify them with clear signs, and test them daily.

Flooring

Lay non-slip flooring with a non-absorbent surface of uniform colour that can easily be cleaned. Patterned or speckled flooring hides dirt, and makes it difficult to find small objects that fall on the floor.

Fire equipment

Fit fire-control equipment and smoke detection alarms in the recovery room.

Ensure fire extinguishers, fire hoses, and fire blankets, are installed in prominent places. Get advice from your local fire department. Remember to budget for regular maintenance of the equipment.

The best type of fire extinguisher for the recovery room is one that uses compressed carbon dioxide. This copes with fires involving wood, paper, burning plastic, live electrical equipment, flammable liquids, and oil.

Fire safety

Put up notices in conspicuous places giving clear instructions about what to do in case of fire (see Table 3.2).

Table 3.2 Fire safety

R	Rescue	Remove patient to a designated safe place.
A	Alarm	Sound alarm.
C	Contain	Close windows and doors to isolate the fire.
E	Extinguish	Only attempt to put the fire out if you know what you are doing.

Appoint specific staff as fire monitors, and take their photographs. Display their names, photographs, and duties at the entrance to the recovery room. These people will be in charge if a fire breaks out. All staff need regular training in case a fire does break out. Every member of staff should have written instructions on the back of their identification labels about what to do in the case of fire, or other emergencies requiring evacuation. Hold evacuation practices twice a year.

> *Hospitals do burn.*
> *And people do die.*

Put Anglia® or similar evacuation sheets under each trolley mattress. These tough sheets have handles, straps, and buckles to wrap the patients in a protective shell. It is easy to drag this shell along the floor, even down stairs if necessary.

Glucose meters

Glucose meters are small electronic devices that measure blood glucose concentrations from a drop of blood from a finger or heel prick. Keep their instructions with the meter. They use special reagent strips. Store them in a cool dry place. Do not take blood from the toes or feet of diabetics, or patients with vascular disease, because the puncture site is likely to get infected. Serious infections can cause the patient to lose a limb.

Handwashing basins

Ideally there should be one hand basin with hot and cold water running through an adjustable mixer system, liquid soap, paper towels, and a waste bin between adjacent trolley bays. Avoid hot air dryers because they are noisy, and spray germs and squames all over the room.

Haemoglobinometers

These compact cheap and accurate electronic devices read the concentration of haemoglobin on a reagent strip. Most are easy to use, but the microcuvettes used in some makes are damaged by humidity giving inaccurate results.

Humidifiers

Humidity is a measure of the mass of water vapour in a gas. Humidifiers increase the amount of water vapour in inhaled gases, helping prevent the tracheobronchial mucosa from drying out, and preserving the action of surfactant in the lungs. Humidification of inspired gas is especially important in those with acute or chronic respiratory disorders.

There are three principal types of humidifiers:

1. Condenser humidifiers. These are also known as heat and moisture exchangers (HMEs). They are effective, cheap and disposable. As the patient breathes out, the expired water vapour collects on baffles of the humidifier. When the patient breathes in, the dry air rushes over the baffles and becomes partially saturated with water vapour. Use HMEs only on patients who are on a ventilator. They are not designed for patients spontaneously breathing through an endotracheal tube or laryngeal mask because they are easily blocked by sputum and may then suffocate the patient. Special HMEs are available for tracheostomies. If their baffles become blocked with sputum the ends blow off so that the airway cannot obstruct.

2. Heated humidifiers are useful to help warm ventilated hypothermic patients. They deliver gas at 37–40°C at a relative humidity of 100%. They are expensive, need close attention and require regular maintenance. Only fill them with sterile water rather than tap water, because of the risk of transmitting pathogens such as *Legionella*. These humidifiers have a probe near the patient's airway to warn of overheating, because temperatures above 42°C cause tracheal burns.

3. Bubble-through humidifiers, where the gas passed through cold water are ineffective. Use only sterile water especially in warmer climates because tap water carries the risk of aerosol-acquired infections.

Infusion sets

Blood transfusions require special infusion sets with 120-micron filters. A useful type has an in-line squeeze pump for rapid transfusion. A Y-giving set is particularly useful for high-volume transfusions. These sets have an internal diameter of 3.2 mm. Special trauma sets for rapid transfusion have a 5.72 mm bore.

Infusion pumps and syringe drivers

Syringe drivers (such as the Atom®, Graseby®, Ohmeda® and Terumo®) use a turning screw to accurately deliver small volumes of fluids from a syringe. They are used to give small, but precise amounts, of concentrated fluids. Because of the compliance in the tubing, at flow rates of less than 10 ml/hr most have a slow start up time, and it may take 10 minutes or more before they are a delivering a steady flow. Inadvertently giving excess drug can occur if the fluid siphons into the patient, or if an obstructed line is suddenly released. To avoid errors only use the syringe recommended by the makers. Fatalities have occurred when syringe drivers are incorrectly set at the wrong flow rate. The most frequent error is wrongly setting the decimal point. Good syringe drivers have clearly marked figures with different-coloured marking on each side of the decimal point. Always get two trained staff to independently check drugs, dilutions and pump settings.

Infusion pumps

Infusion pumps (such as the IMed®) are drip-set regulators and deliver a set number of millilitres per hour through an infusion set. Always use them with a dedicated line. If you attach anything else to the line you must insert a one-way valve to prevent back flow. Multi-lumen central venous catheters are useful for running up to three separate infusions through a single catheter. However these catheters are more likely to be colonized by pathogenic microorganisms. If infusion pumps are not set up correctly they can deliver unintended amounts of fluid.

Imprest system

An imprest system for drugs and disposable items makes restocking easy. Under this system commonly used items are held in the recovery room. It is the duty of the pharmacist and supply officer to check and restock them to the agreed quantity every day.

Laryngoscopes

Laryngoscopes are essential equipment. Buy the same make and model, so that the blades, handles, batteries and globes can be interchanged. The parts of different brands are not interchangeable and if you get the bits mixed up, it becomes a jigsaw puzzle to reassemble them. Choose a brand with a detachable blade so that it can be easily washed, and cleaned. Do not autoclave blades with fibreoptic components because they will be destroyed. The handle may rust, so do not autoclave it; merely remove the batteries, wash the outside and dry it carefully. Sometimes the electrical contact between the blade and the contact on the handle corrodes. Clean it with a piece of steel wool or sandpaper until the brass contacts shine.

Part of your morning check should be to see that all the laryngoscopes' lights shine white and bright. If the light is dim or yellow check the batteries are fresh, and the brass electrical contacts are clean. A dim light is not due to a faulty light bulb: they either work, or they don't. Keep a supply of spare bulbs nearby because they blow easily especially if knocked or dropped.

The most useful blades are:

• MacIntosh curved blade. This comes in three sizes: child, standard and large. The standard is the most useful, but have at least one each of the others available.

• Kessel blades. These are essential for fat patients with short necks.

• Paediatric blades are straight. Choose a brand with the light as close as possible to the tip of the blade.

• A right-handed blade is useful if patients who need to be intubated are lying on their side.

Library and internet access

Have an unlocked bookcase built to house a small library of reference books, and your guidelines and protocols. Consider purchasing a practical reference book on drugs, a text-book of medicine such as *The Merck Manual*, and an ECG reference guide.

Internet access and a computer at the nurses' station will enable you to go online to check authoritative sources for certain problems.

Lighting

Consider the advantages of windows and natural light for both the patients and the staff. If natural daylight is not available, light the room with special colour-corrected fluorescent tubes. Do not use blue-light fluorescent tubes or incandescent light bulbs because these make it difficult to judge the patient's colour, and delay the diagnosis of cyanosis. The lights should provide 100 *candela* for every 10 square metres of floor space. Effectively this is enough light to read the printing on a drug ampoule at arm's length with one eye covered. For most purposes two 25-watt fluorescent tubes are enough to cover 10 square metres.

Linen and laundry

Make provision to collect soiled linen, and other contaminated waste. Plan for the orderly disposable of paper and clean plastic. Clear plastic bags for clean are preferable so that staff can easily see the contents.

Music

The recovery room should be kept as quiet as possible. Do not play music in the recovery room. Not only is music distracting, but it substantially delays the time it takes for staff to respond to alarms or other abnormal sounds such as a patient developing a wheeze. The human ear is excellent at detecting small changes in sound in the environment (like things that go bump in the night). Music, because it is constantly fluctuating, abolishes that ability. Patients say that waking from anaesthesia in a noisy environment is distressing.

Nerve stimulators

Nerve stimulators are used to assess the degree and type of neuromuscular block in patients who remain paralysed at the end of an anaesthetic. Do not use them in awake patients as they are painful. Test for muscle strength by asking the patient to squeeze your fingers.

Notice boards

It is useful to have a large white board and erasable pens for teaching, immediate notices and planning patient management at the nurses' station.

Oxygen concentrators

In regions where bottled oxygen is expensive or difficult to obtain oxygen concentrators can provide an economical supply of nearly pure oxygen from air. If you are working in an isolated hospital, oxygen concentrators are a most worthwhile proposition. The purchase price of a concentrator is about half the cost of a year's supply of the same amount of oxygen from cylinders. The compressors in these units run on mains electric current but in emergencies they will run on the output from a small generator. The power consumption of a concentrator is only 350 watt, even a petrol generator or a truck battery fitted with an oscillator will give 600 watt.

Room air is basically a mixture of two gases: 21 per cent oxygen and 79 per cent nitrogen. This air is drawn into the machine through a series of filters and compressed to a pressure of 4 atmospheres. It is then passed into a canister of manufactured zeolite (a form of aluminium silicate) which acts as a molecular sieve. Nitrogen binds to the zeolite and oxygen passes on to a storage tank. After about 20 seconds the zeolite sieve becomes saturated with nitrogen, and the supply of compressed air is automatically diverted to a second canister where the process is repeated. This gives a constant output of oxygen. While the pressure in the second canister is at 138 kPa the pressure in the first is reduced to zero. Most of the nitrogen then comes off the zeolite, and is released to the atmosphere. A small back flow of oxygen from the alternative cylinder assists the process.

The life of the zeolite crystals is about 20,000 hours, or about 10 years. The gas emerging from the two canisters and into the reservoir chamber is about 95 per cent oxygen. This oxygen can be drawn off at about 4 L/min without any loss in concentration. Higher flows result in lower percentages of oxygen. The concentrators are not suitable to drive ventilators or compressed gas anaesthesia machines such as a Boyles machine. Remember, if the power fails oxygen stored in the machine will only last for 2–3 minutes.

Servicing is required about every 5000 hours, it is not difficult and can be carried out by the user. Make sure you are given all the instructions for this when you purchase the machine. You should also be given at least 2 years' supply of spare parts.

If you are investing in oxygen concentrators you should buy two. Keep them clean and assign responsibility for them to one, named, person.

Patient trolleys

An absolute minimum of four patient transport trolleys are needed for each working theatre: one for attending to the patient in theatre, one for the patient in recovery room; and one for transporting the patient back to the ward and one in reserve. Only use trolleys built to the specification required by international standards.

Trolleys should:

- be quickly able to be tilted head or foot down by at least 25° from the horizontal;
- enable the patient to sit up with support;

and have:

- a frame to house portable monitoring equipment for transport;
- an adjustable footrest or bed-end to stop the patient sliding down;
- a firm base and mattress that will not sag should cardiac massage be needed;
- easily manoeuvred trolley sides or rails to stop the patient falling off;
- removable poles to carry drips;
- have large castor wheels with easily applied brakes;
- provision for portable suction and oxygen;
- a tray for carrying small articles such as the patient's history, dentures, and other belongings;
- provision for transporting ventilators, monitoring equipment, and drain bottles, and urine bags.

It is unnecessary to transfer patients from 'a sterile trolley' on to a 'non-sterile trolley' in the theatre block.

If your hospital has suitably designed beds, then patients having major surgery can be brought to the recovery room on their beds, although it is preferable for them to be on a narrower trolley.

Refrigerators

You will need two refrigerators: one for storing heat labile drugs, and other items, such as ice for testing the efficacy of local blocks, and another thermostatically controlled *blood fridge* for storing blood and vaccines. The blood fridge should have a clock-chart and an alarm to warn if the temperature has risen or fallen below set limits. If the alarm goes off check with the blood bank because you may need to discard all the biological items.

Security

The recovery room needs to be in a secure location so that passers-by cannot gain access. This is particularly important at night when there are not so many staff about. Usually the whole theatre block, including the recovery room, is secured by electronic sliding doors that are opened with a swipe card or numeric keypad.

Space blankets

Space blankets are thin shiny metallic sheets made of Mylar®. This material is an exceptionally strong (but easily torn) plastic sheet, which has a layer of silver a few molecules thick adsorbed on to it. Put the silver side next to the patient. They minimize radiant heat loss, however they conduct heat easily and need to be separated from the patient's skin by a sheet or blanket, which seals a layer of insulating air around the patient's body. They conduct electricity so keep them away from electrical apparatus. They are highly flammable and burn with intense heat to melt into a small red-hot plastic ball.

Spirit levels

Spirit levels are used for levelling transducers with the isophlebotic point on the body. You can easily make one from a 1.8-metre length of plastic tube whose ends are joined to make a loop. Half fill the tubing with coloured water (use ink), join the ends, seal it with tape, and label so it is not discarded.

Suction

A totally reliable high-capacity, high-volume suction system is lifesaving. In order to cope with blood and sticky mucus each sucker must be capable of sustaining a free flow of at least 80 L/min and achieve an occluded suction pressure of at least 60 kPa (460 mmHg) even if nearby suckers are working too.

To prevent the suction inlet from becoming blocked include a fluid trap (usually a 3-litre plastic container) between the sucker and the wall outlet. The tap collects the secretions, blood and other fluids and prevents the system becoming clogged with muck. The wall outlets are usually protected with a sintered brass filter. Unless these filters are cleaned daily they soon become clogged and the suction pressure falls.

Change the tubing between patients and replace the suction bottles as soon as they are contaminated.

Suction is your lifeline. Establish a maintenance routine where the hospital engineers clean, test and maintain the system daily.

Telephones

Noisy telephones disturb patients and demand to be answered. Use a quiet ring tone. The theatre receptionist or a secretary should filter trivial incoming calls.

Mobile phones are safe to use in the recovery room. It remains an urban myth that they generate sufficient electromagnetic fields to disrupt equipment.

If you are still concerned, then don't use them within 1 metre of electronic monitors.

X-ray screens

Many hospitals are switching over to electronic data transmission, but you will still need X-ray viewing screens for old sheet X-rays.

Isolated hospitals

Additional considerations

Nominate one member of your department to be in charge of the purchase, care and maintenance of equipment. This is an important and time-consuming job.

Work out why you need the equipment in the first place.

- Will it improve patient safety? For example, a pulse oximeter.
- Will it help staff work more efficiently by doing routine chore better? For example, a non-invasive blood pressure machine.
- Can it do something that was impossible before? For example, an oxygen concentrator.
- Does it need a special power source? A gas-powered ventilator is useless unless there is a reliable and cheap source of compressed gas to run it. Many isolated hospitals have to work with an erratic and unreliable power supply.

Equipment must be robust and reliable. Robustness is important, and reliability essential. Equipment is useless if it constantly needs maintenance, or has to be sent a long distance for repairs. Before purchasing any piece of equipment, find out how often it breaks down. In engineering terms this is known as the *mean time between failures* (MTBF). The best of the oxygen concentrators have an MTBF of 6000 hours of operating time.

What happens when your piece of equipment does break down? Does it break down in a safe way?

If in doubt about the reliability of the equipment, or its suitability for the task, telephone your nearest university teaching hospital and consult either the Biomedical Engineering Department or the Department of Anaesthesia. They should be able to give you helpful and unbiased advice.

When buying expensive equipment, such as electronic monitors or ventilators, involve the engineering staff in the planning phase. Consider their advice on technical matters about the choice of equipment, and what sort of training they need; and particularly, the manufacturer's ability to provide support such as manuals, maintenance contracts, spare parts, and training films or familiarity courses.

Servicing equipment in a remote hospital

Of all the areas in which the isolated hospital has problems, servicing equipment causes the most difficulty. Lying around departments of most isolated hospitals is broken down or unusable equipment. Thoughtful planning avoids such waste.

Sending equipment away for repairs or servicing can take many months and is expensive. Often a local technician can do the work if he has access to the workshop manuals. Do not buy equipment unless the company is willing to release circuit diagrams, and detailed workshop manuals of the equipment. Get at least two copies of the operator's manual and the maintenance manual; one for the hospital's biomedical engineers, and one to keep in the department. Check the manuals are complete, relevant, clearly written and illustrated (surprisingly often, this is not the case). Poor instruction manuals indicate that the company selling it is not reliable.

Where do spare parts come from? Importing spare parts from another country can take months. Make sure there is an after-sales service, with a reliable supply of spare parts. It is a good idea to order appropriate spare parts when the equipment is purchased. Even with normal wear and tear some pieces will begin to break down almost immediately; for example the rubber bulbs on blood pressure machines, or rubber straps on an electro-cardiograph, and blood pressure cuff bladders. This is especially true in tropical climates where rubber perishes quickly.

Most equipment requires simple servicing by the people who use it. Establish a regular programme of checking the equipment with clear orders on what is to be done, and enforce them or else it may not happen! Every time a service is carried out, enter it in a book kept with the equipment.

This includes:

◆ daily, or pre-use checks;

◆ routine calibration;

◆ daily or pre-use cleaning and the reporting of faults;

◆ ensuring accessories are serviceable and complete;

◆ consumables are available.

Regular checks should be done by the biomedical engineers. To make things proceed smoothly the following questions need to be considered:

◆ what is to be maintained?

◆ how is it to be maintained?

◆ when is it to be maintained?

◆ is the maintenance effective?

To answer the first question draw up an inventory or register of equipment that needs maintenance. Commission equipment before putting it into use. Commissioning involves setting up a maintenance programme and training staff to use and care for the equipment. The regular maintenance schedule must balance the manufacturer's recommendations with how often the equipment is used. The more often the equipment is used, the more frequently it should be checked.

Documentation is crucial, and card index systems are best in a smaller hospital. We hesitate to recommend computer-based systems in an isolated hospital because they require expert staff to run them. If the computer breaks down (and proper back-ups have not been made) all your data can be lost.

Some items of biomedical equipment such as blood gas machines require periodic calibration by an outside agency. Try as far as possible to calibrate the apparatus on the spot to avoid long periods without the equipment, and the risk of damage during transport. Bring the technician to the machine, try not to send the machine to the technician.

If servicing and maintenance is beyond the resources of your biomedical engineers it is possible for regions or even countries to co-operate to share a technician at regular intervals. This reduces cost, and increases efficiency.

If it cannot be repaired, then condemn broken biomedical equipment. Do not leave it lying around in your department. Ask the Supply department to organize its disposal, and attend to the proper inventory and accounting procedures. Consider modifying the equipment to extend its useful life, or using parts of it for other things.

Disposables

It is tempting to buy disposable items, because they release staff from the chores of cleaning and sterilization. Disposables save wages, and time, and reduce the chance of cross-infection. However, they are expensive, and need lots of storage space. If you are working in an isolated hospital think carefully before you discard, or stop using reusable items such as stainless steel dishes, metal suckers and linen drapes. Circumstances can make disposable unobtainable. Once the routines for cleaning and sterilizing reusable items are abandoned, it is hard to start again.

An inventory system is needed to automatically re-order disposables. Delegate this clerical function to either the pharmacy or the supply office.

Reusing disposable items is a controversial issue. Many disposable items which have not been exposed to blood, or body fluids, can be washed, and then sterilized and safely reused. In many countries, medicolegal problems make the reuse impracticable.

Budgets

Most hospitals require every service area, such as the recovery room to have their own budget with the freedom, within set limits, to purchase and maintain their equipment. Until you are familiar with the budgets it is worthwhile sitting down with a hospital administrator to check through the figures to see how the department is managing financially.

References

1. **Nightingale F** (1863) *Notes on Hospitals* (3rd edn). London: Longman, Green, Longman, Roberts, and Green.
2. **Koivula-Tynnila H**, et al (2018). Informational privacy in the recovery room-patients' perspective. *J Perianesth Nurs* **33**(4):479–489.
3. Kousaku Haruguchi's website. <http://kousaku-haruguchi.com>

Further Reading

Australian and New Zealand College of Anaesthetists (2018). *PS04 Statements on the Post-Anaesthesia Care Unit*. <http://www.anzca.edu.au/resources/professional-documents/documents/professional-standards/professional-standards-4.html/>

Chapter 4

Monitoring and equipment

Introduction

The best monitor in the recovery room
is an observant, informed and vigilant nurse.

Monitors warn of approaching problems, but they are not a substitute for carefully observing your patient. Do not automatically assume monitors give you accurate information. If you are concerned that the monitor is misleading you, then reassess the patient's condition: their colour, pulse rate, perfusion, and breathing. Measure their blood pressure manually and take their temperature.

Treat the patient, not the monitor.

Much modern equipment is so complex that it can confuse the most competent staff. Staff need to understand their monitoring equipment, know its limitations, and especially what can go wrong with it. Although well-designed monitors are intended to be used intuitively, it is easy to get lost in their hierarchical menus. It is worthwhile having a continuing education programme for newcomers, and to refresh the memory of more experienced staff. Keep the instruction manuals nearby.

Recovery room monitors should be compatible, and if necessary interchangeable, with the monitors used in the operating theatres. For most otherwise healthy patients undergoing minor elective surgery a pulse oximeter, blood pressure monitoring and a record of temperature, pulse and breathing are all you need.

Routine monitoring

Making routine observations and collecting data helps you establish trends to assess whether your patient is improving, is stable, or is deteriorating. The data gives you an objective assessment—things that you can measure—of your patient's response to treatment.

All patients need certain parameters measured and recorded regularly. These involve:

◆ conscious state;

◆ pulse rate;

◆ blood pressure;

◆ perfusion status;

- oxygen saturation;
- respiratory rate;
- temperature.

Record the data at 5-minute intervals for 15 minutes; then if your patient remains stable every 10 to 15 minutes thereafter until the patient returns to the ward. With sicker or unstable patients, the nurse, the surgeon and the anaesthetist should review their progress and make a comprehensive management plan for the following 24 hours before you discharge patients to the ward. This plan might include transferring the patient to the ICU or a high dependency unit.

Additional monitoring

Sicker or unstable patients, or those who have had long or physiologically stressful surgery need additional monitoring that may include:

- ECG;
- end-tidal carbon oxide monitoring;
- intra-arterial blood pressures;
- central venous pressures;
- urine output;
- volume and nature of wound drainage;
- haematology;
- chemical pathology;
- blood gas estimation.

If your patient's observations deviate from the defined limits set by the surgical team, then seek help immediately. If in doubt, play it safe: ask a senior colleague or the anaesthetist to review the patient and go over the data with you.

Pulse oximetry

Pulse oximeters are the most useful monitors in the recovery room. Correctly used on well-perfused skin they are reliable and accurate.

Pulse oximeters give an early warning of *hypoxaemia*. The device consists of a light-emitting diode and a photo detector applied to a fingertip or ear lobe. They measure the differential absorption by haemoglobin of two wavelengths of *pulsed* light, red and infrared, and then calculate the proportion of oxygen saturated haemoglobin (SaO_2) in the capillaries, and display the result as a percentage on a screen.

Normal arterial blood is more than 97 per cent saturated with oxygen (see Table 4.1). If the saturations fall to 90 per cent or less, then the patient is hypoxaemic. Use an oximeter on every patient until they are fully awake, and have a consistent SaO_2 over 96 per cent.

Table 4.1 Oxygen saturations

Status	Oxygen saturation
Normal	> 96%
Abnormal	< 96%
Hypoxaemia	< 90%

Do not discharge patients to the ward if their oxygen saturations are less than 93 per cent without discussing it with the anaesthetist. If your patients have a persistently low oxygen saturation they need oxygen by mask during transport to the ward, and mandatory oxygen in the ward.

You can use the pulse oximeter readings to estimate the arterial PaO_2, but to do this you must know the patient's *pH*. pH is a measure of hydrogen ion activity. Excessive hydrogen ion activity distorts the shape of haemoglobin, altering its ability to take up and release oxygen, and in so doing determines the pressure (PO_2) at which oxygen is pushed into the tissues. To see the haemoglobin oxygen dissociation curve, see Figure 4.1.

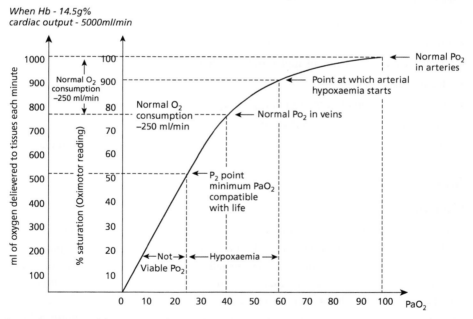

Figure 4.1 Haemoglobin oxygen dissociation curve.

You need to understand the graph in Figure 4.1 if you are to make sense of how oxygen gets into the tissues. The graph matches the haemoglobin's saturation with oxygen (on the vertical axis) to the pressure it exerts as it attempts to leave the haemoglobin (on the horizontal axis). For example if haemoglobin is 90 per cent full of oxygen, the push oxygen exerts as it leaves the haemoglobin is about 60 mmHg (7.9 kPa). For oxygen to get into, and be used by the cells, it has to be delivered both in sufficient quantity and with enough pressure. The partial pressure of oxygen in capillaries provides the force to drive oxygen from the red cells into the tissues, then on through the cell membrane, through the cell's cytoplasm and into its mitochondria.

The shape of the curve changes with the pH of the blood, and the patient's temperature. Patients in recovery room are often moderately acidotic and hypothermic. Acidosis causes the arterial PaO_2 to be higher than normal at a given haemoglobin oxygen saturation. This is a good thing, as the extra pressure increases tissue oxygenation. On the other hand hypothermia decreases tissue oxygenation, but also reduces the tissue's oxygen consumption.

Once the saturation falls to 90 per cent the signs and symptoms of hypoxia accelerate. A PaO_2 less than 60 mm Hg (7.9 kPa) is dangerous, and a PaO_2 less than 35 mmHg (4.6 kPa) is potentially lethal even in healthy people.

Purchasing a pulse oximeter

Points to check when purchasing a pulse oximeter

- size, weight and portability;
- power: mains power or rechargeable batteries;
- display: easy to see from all angles and in all lights;
- alarms: easy to set;
- probes: robust, easy to repair or cheap to replace;
- finger probes: come in various sizes;
- ear probes are useful for babies and patients who are cold or have poor circulation.

Blood pressure

Physiology

Blood pressure is the force per unit area that the blood exerts on the vessel wall at right angles to direction of the flow. Arterial blood pressures are measured in millimetres of mercury (mmHg). Venous pressures are usually measured against column of water in centimetres of water (cm H_2O). Since pressure varies with the depth of the fluid, blood pressures are measured against a reference point called the *isophlebotic point*, which is at the same level as the right atrium. In a supine patient the isophlebotic point is located where the fourth intercostal space crosses the midaxillary line.

Blood pressure is maintained by a balance between the volume of blood ejected by the heart with each beat (*stroke volume*) and the *impedance* (resistance) the arterioles impose to blood flowing through the vascular bed. By convention, we measure the peak or *systolic blood pressure* (when the heart contracts), and the trough or *diastolic blood pressure* (when the heart relaxes), however it is the *mean arterial blood pressure* (MAP) that determines tissue blood flow.

Clinical aspects of blood pressure

Blood pressure (BP) is an important measure of a patient's physiological well-being. Blood pressure can be measured *non-invasively* with:

- a mercury sphygmomanometer;
- an anaeroid clock face device;
- an automated oscillotonometer;

or *invasively* with an intra-arterial cannula attached to an electronic *transducer*.

Non-invasive blood pressure monitoring

Because blood pressure is such an important physiological parameter you must measure and record it accurately. An automated oscillotonometer is available in most recovery rooms but older devices can still be used and will give accurate results.

Manual blood pressure monitors

Mercury-filled sphygmomanometers: Using the mercury column measure the blood pressure with the monitor at eye level to prevent parallax errors (Figure 4.2).

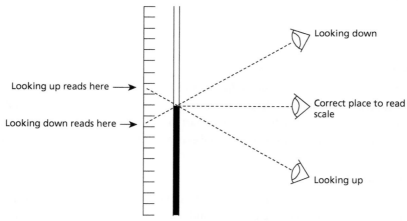

Figure 4.2 The position of a mercury blood pressure machine may cause errors in the readings.

It takes some skill to get consistent results with a sphygmomanometer, so let us go step by step through the technique. Select the appropriate cuff size. Warn your patients what you are about to do. Check that their radial pulse is regular. Then with your finger on the radial pulse, quickly inflate the cuff to above the expected systolic pressure. Let the cuff deflate gradually. Note the pressure at which the pulse returns. Now, having found the approximate systolic pressure, reinflate the cuff to above the previous reading. Listen with the diaphragm (but not the bell) of your stethoscope over the brachial artery in the cubital fossa. Deflate the cuff by no more than 5 mmHg per second. The systolic pressure is the point where you hear the first pulse. The diastolic pressure is the point where the sounds disappear completely (and not where they become muffled).

Conventionally systolic pressures are measured to the nearest 5 mmHg, and diastolic pressures to the nearest 2 mmHg. The most common error is to allow the pressure in the cuff to plummet rapidly so that you miss the actual blood pressure between hearing adjacent beats.

Check the blood pressure in both arms if the patient is elderly, has vascular disease or diabetes because *pseudo hypertension* may deceive you. Here the cuff cannot compress the rigid calcified arterial walls to occlude blood flow, so that you can still feel the pulse even though the cuff is above systolic pressure.

Different sized cuffs are available (see Table 4.2): larger ones for obese adults and smaller ones for children.

Table 4.2 What is the correct cuff size?

	Cuff width (cm)	Cuff length (cm)	Arm circumference (cm)
Child	8–10	20–24	Up to 25
Adult	12–13	24	Up to 33
Large adult	13–15	35	Up to 38
Obese adult	15–18	35	Up to 42

Anaeroid devices

Anaeroid clock face devices are fairly reliable, but lose their calibration if they are not maintained regularly. These manual devices need to be calibrated against a mercury sphygmomanometer at least once a month. Before you start to measure the blood pressure, ensure the needle is on zero. The mechanism in some makes of anaeroid device rusts in humid climates.

Automated devices

Automated non-invasive blood pressure (NBP) devices detect changes in the pressure-wave form as it oscillates between systolic and diastolic pressure. The result is fed into a microprocessor that calculates and displays the systolic, mean and diastolic blood pressures on a screen. The devices are popular because they measure blood pressure at regular intervals and give warnings if the blood pressure rises or falls beyond set limits, and free up staff to attend to other duties.

An NBP monitor is useful in most situations. Once the systolic blood pressure falls below 80–90 mmHg, these devices become unreliable. If they constantly recycle check the blood pressure manually. They are also likely to give misleading results if the pulse is irregular, patients are moving their arms about or the wrong-sized cuff is used. The mean pressure is most accurate. Wrinkled cuffs may bruise the skin. Repeated cycling can damage nerves or even cause ischaemic injury to the arm, especially in diabetics and those patients with vascular disease.

Invasive blood pressure monitoring

Arterial monitoring is used for haemodynamically unstable patients, or where infusions of vasoactive drugs are needed to control the blood pressure.

Invasive blood pressure (IBP) monitoring involves inserting a small cannula into an artery (usually the radial) and connecting it to a *transducer* with a plastic catheter. The signal is processed and the systolic and diastolic pressure, as well as the waveform, are displayed on a screen.

Check at least the first few readings
with a manual blood pressure device.

One might assume that intra-arterial monitors measure blood pressure accurately, but if the fluid dynamics of the set-up are not properly balanced they are prone to errors of up to 70 per cent or more. To avoid these errors, follow the manufacturer's recommendations and use properly matched catheters and cannulas, otherwise the pressure wave will not be faithfully transmitted to the transducer. Damping problems occur when pressure waves ricochet willy-nilly around inside the tubing (an *under-damped signal*) or are cushioned by pliant or excessively long tubing (an *over-damped signal*).

The transducer should be positioned at the level of the heart. Make sure it is zeroed.

Keep the cannula patent by flushing it with 1 ml of 0.9 per cent saline when your patient is first admitted to the recovery room. Usually a special valve trickles in saline at 3 ml per hour from a filled bag pressurized to 300 mmHg. Do not add heparin to the saline because it may cause *heparin-induced thrombocytopenia* (HITs).

Do not disturb the dressings around the arterial cannula. If a cannula accidentally falls out, then press firmly over the site with a gauze pad for at least 5 minutes. Arterial bleeding does not stop as readily as venous bleeding. Mark the arterial lines with red marker tags at both ends, and in the middle to ensure that drugs are not inadvertently injected into them.

Radial artery thrombosis after an arterial line occurs in 2 to 15 per cent of cases. To prevent this complication use arterial lines for as short a time as possible, especially if you are giving vasoconstricting drugs.

If your patient has an arrhythmia,
then check the blood pressure manually.

Central venous pressure

Central venous pressure (CVP) is the pressure of the blood in the vena cava at the entrance to the right atrium. Central venous lines (CVL) are often used in acutely ill patients coming to surgery.

They are used:

♦ for measuring central venous pressure;

♦ as a guide to intravenous fluid therapy;

♦ for giving drugs that would injure peripheral veins; for example, adrenaline and nor-adrenaline infusions, parenteral nutrition fluids, and 50% glucose;

♦ to assess how effectively the heart is pumping.

The catheters are radio-opaque and about 20 cm long. There are single lumen and multiple lumen catheters available. With multi-lumen catheters, each lumen opens at a different point along the catheter: distal (at the tip of the catheter), medial (in the middle) and proximal (just inside the vein). In most multi-lumen catheters the distal lumen (brown port) has a wider bore for giving high volumes, viscous fluids, colloids or for measuring the central venous pressure. The middle lumen (blue port) is used for giving intravenous drugs, or parenteral nutrition. The proximal lumen (white port) is used for giving drugs or withdrawing blood.

Some types of catheters also have an on–off switch or clamping device to prevent air accidentally entering the system.

Inserting the catheter

Before inserting the catheter the patient is tipped about 10° head down, and the site prepped and draped. Inserting a catheter is a strictly aseptic procedure requiring gloves, gown, and mask. The anaesthetist usually inserts the catheter in the right internal jugular vein, but occasionally will use a subclavian approach. Each lumen is then flushed with 2 ml of normal saline. Once the procedure is over, the catheter is securely stitched in place, covered with a clear dressing so that you can see if the catheter becomes kinked, and its position is then checked with a chest X-ray. If the drip abruptly stops, then check that the catheter is not kinked where it enters the skin.

Measuring the central venous pressure

Measurements are made against one of two reference points: either at the *sternal angle*, or at the *isophlebotic point*. Once you have decided which point to use, then mark it with a waterproof pen so that staff know it is the *zero point*.

Unlike arterial blood pressure, which is measured in millimetres of mercury, central venous pressures are measured in centimetres of water using either a graduated fluid manometer, or a pressure transducer attached to an electronic monitor which has been 'zeroed' to the reference point, and attached to your electronic monitor.

The old way of measuring the central venous pressure with a fluid-filled manometer is still used in isolated hospitals (Figure 4.3). First, establish a zero point on the manometer with either a spirit level, or a loop of plastic tubing partially filled with coloured water. The aim is to make sure the *reference point* on the patient is exactly at the same level as the zero mark on the manometer. Fill the manometer from a bag of intravenous fluid. Close the three-way tap to the IV bag and allow fluid from the manometer to run into the patient until it stops. At this point, the top of the column of fluid should swing up and down slightly as the patient breathes. Record the halfway point as the fluid swings. This is the *mean central venous pressure*.

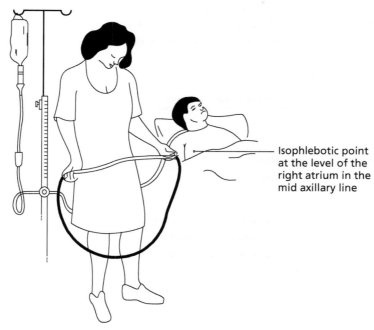

Isophlebotic point at the level of the right atrium in the mid axillary line

Figure 4.3 Measuring central venous pressure with reference to the isophlebotic point.

The normal central venous pressure lies between 0 to 5 cm H_2O at the angle of the sternum, or between 5 to 10 cm H_2O at the isophlebotic point in the midaxillary line.

Complications

Complications during insertion include:

- pneumothorax when the lung is punctured;
- haemothorax where a major vessel or the heart is perforated;
- *chylothorax* if the lymphatic duct is damaged. This duct carries milky-coloured lymph back to the circulation;
- cardiac dysrhythmia if the catheter irritates the myocardium;
- accidental arterial puncture causing haemorrhage into the soft tissue around the site;
- nerve damage to the brachial plexus.

Complications during use include:

- air emboli;
- pulmonary emboli from sleeve clots or clots forming on the catheter tip;
- infection.

How to interpret central venous pressures

In adults and children the normal blood volume is about 70 ml/kg. For a 70 kg person this amounts to about 5 litres of blood. Of these 5 litres (at any given moment) 1 litre of the blood is in the heart and lungs, 2 litres are in the arteries and capillaries, and 3 litres are in the veins. To see how to interpret the central venous pressures, see Table 4.3.

Table 4.3 How to interpret the central venous pressure

Problem	Central venous pressure	Arterial blood pressure
Blood loss	Low	Low
Cardiac failure	High	Low
Cardiac tamponade	High	Low
Overhydration	High	High

The *great veins*: the vena cava and the larger veins in the limbs are *capacitance vessels* (Figure 4.4). They act as collapsible reservoirs of blood. Unlike the arteries whose volume remains more or less constant, the volume of blood in the great veins increases or decreases as the total blood volume rises or falls. Once blood loss exceeds 500 ml the pulse rate starts to rise, however the central venous pressure does not alter until about 800 ml of blood is lost.

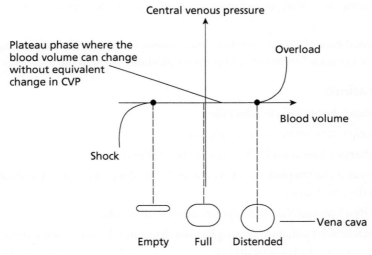

Figure 4.4 Cross-sectional shape of the great veins as they follow the blood volume.

If we transfuse blood into a normal person, the great veins expand to accommodate it. After receiving about 400 ml of blood they can expand no further, and at this point the central venous pressure begins to rise. We can use this phenomenon to work out whether the patient's hypotension is caused by hypovolaemia or something else.

A *CVP stress test* is done by quickly giving the patient 250 ml of colloid, such a 5 per cent albumin or blood. If the central venous pressure does not rise by 5 cm of water or more then wait 5 minutes and give another 250 ml of colloid. You can cautiously repeat this, until either the blood pressure rises, or the central venous pressure rises by 5 cm H_2O.

Care of lines

Catheters are prone to set up havens for bacteria in the little clots that form at the tips of the lumens. These bacteria can leak out into the blood causing systemic sepsis, so take care to maintain sterility when you are injecting anything into a central line, and when changing infusions. Usually central lines are kept patent with a pressurized bag of 0.9 per cent *saline* slowly dribbling through a valve at about 3 ml an hour. Do not use heparinized saline because you may cause a delayed immune reaction called *heparin-induced thrombocytopenia* (HITs).

> *Never inject anything into patients*
> *unless they are lying flat.*

Keep the lines free of bubbles and never allow air to enter them. Air emboli can be fatal. Given an opportunity, air is sucked into a central venous line astonishingly rapidly. If a patient with a central venous line collapses, always consider air embolism as a cause. Immediately tip the patient 20° head down, check that the lines have not become disconnected and call for help. Use Luer-locks on central venous lines so that they cannot accidentally come apart. Be sure that you understand exactly how a three-way tap works (Figure 4.5).

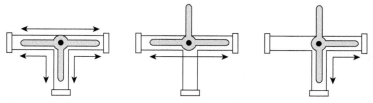

Figure 4.5 Direction of flow in a three-way tap.

Special precautions

Do not give anything through a central venous catheter until a chest X-ray has confirmed the catheter tip lies 2–4 cm above the right atrium. On the chest X-ray this point is level with the *carina* at the junction of the left and right main bronchi.

Each lumen should be fitted with a *positive fluid displacement valve* (PFD). Infuse each fluid through its own lumen. Label the ports.

Monitoring respiration

Clinically, the best way to monitor patients' breathing is to place your hand on their chest, count the rate and feel what is going on. The normal respiratory rate is 12 to 14 breaths/

min for adults, and slightly faster for children. Seek advice if the respiratory rate exceeds 20 breaths/min or falls below 8 breaths/min.

Feeling your patient's chest can give you a lot of information. You can gauge the rate and rhythm as the chest rises and falls: normal inspiration should be half the length of expiration. You can feel whether their intercostal muscles are contracting (they should not). Furthermore, you may be able to feel the fine vibrations of wheeze, or the coarser vibrations of loose sputum rattling in the airways.

Modern recovery room monitors sense the respiratory rate from the changes in voltage of the ECG. Sensory pads are available that detect apnoeic periods in babies under 12 months of age.

Routinely feel the patient's chest move with your hand.

Capnography

Capnography[1] is useful to monitor ventilation. With each breath, capnographs measure carbon dioxide concentrations in the expired air. During expiration, the last little bit of air expelled from the lung comes from the alveoli. This *end-tidal CO_2* gives a good estimate of the *partial pressure* of carbon dioxide ($PACO_2$) in the lungs, and reflects the partial pressure of carbon dioxide in arterial blood ($PaCO_2$). When the patient is intubated this monitoring is easy to carry out and the results are accurate. When the patient is in the recovery room with an oxygen mask or nasal prongs the results gained from monitoring end-tidal CO_2 are less reliable and cannot be substituted for careful observation.

Respirometers

Respirometers (also called *anemometers*) measure gas flows. You can attach them to a tight-fitting facemask, laryngeal mask, or endotracheal tube to measure tidal and minute volumes on patients in the recovery room. There are two main types of mechanical devices: The Wright's respirometer® and the Dragermeter®. The Wright's respirometer is the more sensitive of the two, but it is also delicate. Never blow into a Wright's respirometer because you will shred the gears and tear the vanes. The more robust Dragermeter® can be autoclaved if necessary. Electronic anemometers are also available.

Arterial blood gases

Arterial blood gases (ABG) measure the partial pressure of oxygen in arterial blood, the partial pressure of carbon dioxide, and the pH of the blood. From these measurements other parameters are calculated including the standard bicarbonate, and base excess.

Arterial blood gases are best taken from an arterial cannula, or failing that the radial or femoral artery. Do not use the posterior tibial or dorsalis pedis arteries except in *neonates*.

Brachial or femoral artery punctures in patients with diabetes of vascular disease may dislodge an atheromatous plaque, which if it lodges in a distal vessel, may infarct the limb causing gangrene. Avoid using the ulnar artery because it provides the collateral circulation to the hand, and never take blood from arteriovenous fistulae in patients on renal dialysis.

To collect arterial blood you need a blood gas syringe, an alcohol swab, 23 gauge needle, a pressure bad, protective eyewear and non-sterile gloves, a patient identification label, and a sharps disposal container within reach.

Commercial kits of needles and syringes are available to collect blood gases. If you do not have these, then lightly smear the inside of a 5 ml glass syringe with heparin. Attach a 23 gauge needle to collect the blood. Once you have collected the blood press firmly on the puncture site with a pad for 5 minutes by the clock. Remove the pad, and check that the bleeding has stopped. Reapply the pressure if necessary. It is better not to tape a cotton-wool swab over the site; simply leave it uncovered so that you can periodically check whether it is bleeding or swelling.

Things to check after performing an arterial puncture include: bleeding, bruising, swelling around the puncture site, nerve injury, impaired circulation to the hand or fingers, or pain. Store the blood immediately in melting ice, and send it quickly to the laboratory for analysis. Unless the blood is processed within 10 minutes of collection, the results will be unreliable. Make sure the laboratory knows the patient's temperature and the inspired oxygen concentration so they can adjust their calculations to compensate.

Nerve stimulators

Nerve stimulators use an electrical pulse to stimulate a nerve (usually the ulnar nerve) to cause the hypothenar muscles to contract. With each stimulus the thumb moves towards the little finger. Ignore any movements in the other fingers. Nerve stimulators are used to assess the degree and type of paralysis caused by neuromuscular blocking drugs in intubated patients. Do not use them on conscious patients—they hurt.

If a nerve stimulator was repeatedly used during the anaesthetic patients may sometimes complain of pins and needles—*paraesthesia*—around their little finger and down the inner aspect of their arm. The paraesthesia resolves in a few hours.

X-ray

Portable X-ray may be needed in recovery room in patients with:

◆ a suspected pneumothorax;

◆ respiratory distress;

◆ to check the position a CVP line or a pulmonary artery catheter;

◆ suspect aspiration;

◆ heart failure;

◆ renal surgery: where the pleural space has been breached.

Electrocardiography

Electrocardiography (ECG) is an essential monitor in the recovery room. It warns of arrhythmias and myocardial ischaemia, but not hypoxaemia, or hypercarbia or hypotension.

The ECG monitor gives a continuous picture of the heart's electrical activity. Apart from screen monitors, the recovery room needs at least one machine capable of taking a full 12-lead ECG and printing out a hard copy of the trace. Electrodes placed at strategic points on the skin track the passage of myocardial *action potentials* as they pass through the heart. Each electrode views the potential from a different vantage point. As the current passes towards an electrode it causes an upward (*positive*) wave on the trace, and when travelling away it causes a downward (*negative*) wave. By studying the amplitude and form of the waves at each electrode an experienced observer can build up a three-dimensional picture of the where, when and how the current is travelling.

Who to monitor?

Myocardial ischaemic and arrhythmias commonly occur in patients in the recovery room, particularly if they have pre-existing risk factors (see Table 4.4). So use ECG monitoring with all patients who have, or are at risk of having cardiac instability, or who have had major surgery, but especially in those at risk of ischaemic heart disease.

Table 4.4 Monitor patients with these risk factors

Age > 50 years	Smoked for > 10 years
Family history	Hypertension
Diabetes	Dyslipidaemia
Depression	Peripheral vascular disease
Cerebrovascular disease	Chronic kidney disease

About 40 per cent of patients with ischaemic heart disease have a normal preoperative resting ECG, but *postoperative adverse cardiac events* (PACE) only occur in 2 per cent of these patients. However, in those patients with an abnormal preoperative ECG, about a quarter will have adverse cardiac events (arrhythmias, ischaemia, or hypotension) either while they are in the recovery room, or later in the ward.

It is important to detect ECG abnormalities in the recovery room because arrhythmias or signs of ischaemia forewarn of cardiac problems in the coming days. These patients will need careful surveillance in the ward.

ST-depression or elevation are hallmarks of ischaemia, but the absence of ST changes on the ECG does not guarantee that there is no ischaemia present. Most modern cardiac physiological monitors can detect ST changes and warn you as they occur. Make a note in the patient's records of any arrhythmias or ST changes—even if they are only transient.

If arrhythmias or signs of ischaemia occur, notify the anaesthetist, and do a 12-lead ECG. Give a hard copy to the anaesthetist, and save another copy for the patient's notes. Compare the hard copy to the preoperative one.

How to apply the electrodes

Put a diagram on the wall so that everyone knows exactly where to put the sticky ECG electrodes. Some staff use the mnemonic 'Ride Your Bike' to put the colours in the correct place. Put the red electrode on the upper part of the manubrium, the yellow electrode on the left shoulder, and the black electrode over the heart's apex beat, which is usually near the anterior axillary line between the fourth and fifth rib. Now select lead II. This arrangement is called the CM5 lead, and it is the most useful single lead to pick up arrhythmias, and most ST depression. Sometimes you may not be able to use the normal electrode positions, in which case place the electrodes anywhere as long as they roughly form an equilateral triangle around the heart. If necessary, you can put the red electrode on the forehead, the yellow on the left arm and the black electrode over the lower back (Figure 4.6).

A single lead CMV5 trace detects about 75 per cent of ischaemic episodes. In contrast, if your monitor can display a three-lead trace with lead II, lead V4 and lead V5 then you can detect 98 per cent of ischaemic events.

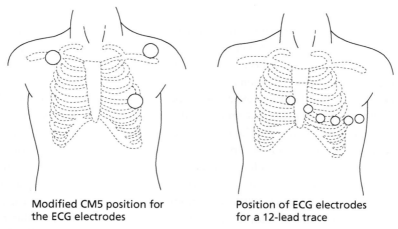

Modified CM5 position for
the ECG electrodes

Position of ECG electrodes
for a 12-lead trace

Figure 4.6 Where to put the electrodes.

How to get a good trace

To get a good trace the electrodes must have excellent contact with the skin. You may need to shave the area, but always clean the skin with an alcohol wipe. Poorly applied electrodes cause noisy ECG traces, especially when the patient moves.

The ECG leads may also pick up other noise such as electromagnetic interference ('AC hum'). If the leads are lying across power cables, or are in contact with metal AC hum may blur the trace. Move the leads away from nearby electrical devices. Plugging the ECG monitor and other nearby electrical apparatus into the same power socket (*general power outlet*) usually eliminates the problem. Still having trouble? Try loosely coiling the ECG cable to stop it acting as an aerial.

ECG monitors

To make servicing and maintenance easier, buy all your ECG monitors from the same company as your other equipment. The better ECG monitors have a clear display, easily read from 2–3 metres away, audible pulse monitoring and pulse rate display. There should be a cascade mechanism to view the last 30 seconds of trace and a screen freeze function to analyse a pattern. You will need a paper printout to record arrhythmias for later analysis. Printouts must be properly calibrated. On the vertical axis 1 cm = 1 millivolt; and on the horizontal axis 1 large square = 0.2 seconds.

Most modern monitors have the facility to measure multiple parameters including blood pressure and oximetry, as well as the ECG. Keep all the manufacturer's instructions and electronic technicians' phone numbers, in a convenient place.

ECG leads are easily damaged, so treat them gently. Store spare cables and sensors loosely coiled in a dry dark place. If you are in a tropical climate, seal the storage unit against moisture.

Glucose monitors

Measure the blood sugar of diabetic patients as soon as possible after they arrive in the recovery room. Every recovery room must have a glucose meter (*glucometer*) on hand. These small cheap electronic devices measure blood glucose concentration by using a drop of blood from a finger or heel prick. Keep the instructions on how to use the device in the box with the instrument. Store the reagent strip in a cool dry place.

Hypoglycaemia, like hypoxia, quickly causes brain damage and kills unless it is detected in time. Those at risk of hypoglycaemia include: neonates and babies, diabetics, patients who drink excessive alcohol, or who have liver disease. Make it part of your protocols to measure the blood glucose in these patients as soon as they come to the recovery room. Notify the anaesthetist if the blood glucose is less than 3.8 mmol/L (*hypoglycaemia*) or greater than 12 mmol/L (*hyperglycaemia*). It is not well known that in patients with diabetes even brief episodes (as little as 20 minutes) of hyperglycaemia in the recovery room increases, by several fold, the risk of postoperative myocardial infarction and stroke.

Remember not to take blood from the feet or toes of diabetics or patients with peripheral vascular disease because they may get an infected ulcer at the site.

Monitoring temperature

When patients come to the recovery room routinely check their *temperature*. This is essential for babies who get cold on the operating table.

Humans tightly maintain their *core temperature* around a *set point* of 37 ± 1°C. The core of the body, the heart, liver, kidneys, lungs and brain are warmer than the skin and limbs. Skin temperature depends principally on ambient air temperature; in contrast the metabolic rate determines the core temperature. Normally the skin temperature is about 33°C or 91°F, but this varies enormously from site to site. For this reason, axillary temperature is highly misleading. It does not reflect core temperature and should never be used in the recovery room.

How to measure temperature

Mercury thermometers are unsafe and should not be used in recovery rooms. Apart from being fragile, they do not register temperatures below 35.8°C. Clinical thermometers have been replaced by user-friendly *thermistor* electronic temperature probes.

The most popular electronic probes are hand-held devices (such as Thermofocus® and the Exergen Temporal Scanner®). When pointed towards the patient the device collects infrared emissions from the skin without actually touching it. The large temporal artery supplies the blood to the forehead, a convenient place to measure body temperature. Additionally the head, with its rich blood supply, is the first region of the skin to change temperature with fever.

Infrared tympanic thermometers reliably estimate core temperature. The tympanic membrane in the ear shares the same blood supply as the body's thermoregulatory centre in the *hypothalamus*. Be gentle when you insert a probe into the ear. They need to be placed precisely to get an accurate result.

Adult skin temperature sensors have small thermistors set in hypoallergenic sticky pads that can be placed anywhere on the body surface, but the only place to get a reliable estimate of the core temperature is over the temporal artery. If the patient becomes sweaty, the pads can fall off. Other forms of measuring skin temperature, such as thermoresponsive crystal sensors, are not as reliable.

Body temperature can also be measured with rectal, oesophageal or pharyngeal probes, or with a thermistor incorporated into pulmonary artery flotation catheters. Rectal temperature probes are not as reliable as once thought. They can be cooled by blood returning from the legs, or warmed by up to 1°C by heat generated by thermogenic bacteria in the faeces.

Hyperthermia

Hyperthermia is uncommon in the recovery room and is always serious. Causes include blood transfusion reactions, a pre-existing febrile state or a thyroid crisis. The most sinister cause is malignant hyperthermia. This condition is fatal if not treated quickly.

Hypothermia

Hypothermia is defined as a core temperature of 36°C of lower. About 60 per cent of patients arrive in the recovery room with a low body temperature. An even larger number who have had their chest or abdomen opened become hypothermic during surgery. Feel your patient's chest with the palm of your hand. If it feels cool to touch then recheck the patient's temperature.

Hypothermia is a gravely underappreciated problem. It is the principal cause of blood failing to clot after surgery; drug *metabolism* is delayed, and it is a major predictor of postoperative infection and wound breakdown.

Warming blankets

Convection warming blankets work by blowing warm air into a light plastic envelope enclosing the patient. They are highly effective in preventing further heat loss and help rewarm cold patients in recovery room. One of the most popular makes of warming blanket is the BairHugger™; it can increase the body temperature by 1.5°C per hour when set on high.

Air-warming devices are not without risk, they may contribute to cross-infection and it is possible to cause burns if the blankets are not properly attached to the hose. You are likely to burn your patient if you simply place the hose under the sheet or blanket.

Reference

1. **Odom-Forren J** (2011) Capnography and sedation: a global initiative. *Journal of PeriAnaesthesia Nursing* **26**(4):221–224.

Chapter 5

Pain

What is pain?

Pain is a subjective experience; its intensity depends on how one interprets what one is feeling. The intensity of pain is influenced by the neural stimuli received from damaged tissue, the memory of previous pain, the expected outcome, and psychological factors, predominantly anxiety.

Individuals perceive and respond to pain in different ways. It is not easily described in words and even less easily measured. For instance, your splitting headache is not necessarily the same as my pounding headache. How can I possibly explain to you what I am feeling and how much it hurts? This problem remains unsolved.

Pain has survival value. This unpleasant sensation and emotion helps prevent further injury. A widely accepted definition of pain is 'a sensory and emotional experience from actual or potential tissue damage, or described in terms of such damage' (to see various types of pain, see Table 5.1). In more practical sense, pain is what the patient says hurts, and when the patient says it hurts—this is a most important concept to grasp. Pain is a combination of what your patients feel, and their emotional response to it.

Table 5.1 Various types of pain

Type of pain	Description
Clinical	
Somatic pain	Well-localized, sharp, acute pain arising from skin, muscles, joints.
Visceral pain	Deep, diffuse, ill-localized arising from an organ.
Pathological description	
Neuropathic pain	Arises from injured nerves.
Nociceptive pain	Occurs where inflammation stimulates pain receptors.

Why pain is harmful

Uncontrolled pain is harmful because it:

- causes restlessness, which increases oxygen consumption; this in turn increases cardiac work, and can result in hypoxia;
- contributes to postoperative nausea and vomiting;

- increases the blood pressure, with the risk of precipitating cardiac ischaemia;

- decreases hepatic and renal blood flow, delaying the metabolism and excretion of drugs, and promoting fluid retention;

- prevents the patient from taking deep breaths and coughing, especially following thoracic or upper abdominal operations. This increases the risk of postoperative sputum retention and pneumonia;

- discourages patients from moving their legs slowing blood flow. The venous stasis contributes to the formation of deep vein thrombi, and pulmonary embolism;

- increases the postoperative stress response, with greatly increased cortisol secretion. This delays wound healing, and predisposes to infection;

- increases metabolic rate, protein breakdown, and the catabolic effects of injury;

- delays the return of normal bowel function;

- impairs the bonding of a mother with her newborn child if the mother is in pain after Caesarean section; and

- demoralizes the patient, disrupts sleep, and causes distressing anxiety and despair.

Uncontrolled pain can delay healing,
and increase the risk of infection.

The greatest physiological risk of untreated pain is to frail patients, those with heart or lung disease, the very young and the very old, and those undergoing major procedures such as aortic, abdominal, or major orthopaedic surgery.

How we perceive pain

How we perceive pain involves two inputs: the injury that hurts (*noxious stimulus*) and the anxiety or fear (*affective feelings*) that goes with this. These interact in a complex way to form the sensation of pain.

If you stubbed your toe against a door, you would probably not feel very anxious about it. You know the pain will soon go away, and there should be no consequences. Your logical analysis involves experience, knowledge, memory and foresight.

If you were to wake suddenly in the night with a terrible abdominal pain you would rightly be alarmed, and your physiological and psychological response quite different. The emotional responses to pain can be harmful. Emotions may range through acceptance, apprehension, fear or even terror. Fear of physical deformity is particularly evident in patients who have been burnt, or who are undergoing disfiguring operations such as mastectomy or amputation. The young tend to be more fearful than older people. Sincere empathy, reassurance and skilled nursing reduce destructive emotional responses substantially.

Emotional stress activates the sympathetic nervous system: blood pressure rises, the heart beats faster and more forcibly and the brain becomes hypervigilant about its surroundings and what is happening to the body. If this stress remains unmodulated then enough cortisol is secreted from the adrenal gland to jeopardize wound healing and predispose to infection.

Pain physiology

Those organisms that can recognize that they have been injured and then avoid further injury are far more likely to survive long enough to pass on this ability to their offspring. One billion years of evolution have refined this aptitude endlessly. We are the beneficiaries of eons of physiological adaptations by these survivors, our ancestors, and we have inherited their complex ways of recognizing and reacting to pain. The following description is the barest outline of this process, but should give you a feeling for its complexity, and how we can use this knowledge to modify the response.

Sensory nerves to the spinal cord and brain carry pain sensations. Here they are integrated and modified to produce a coordinated response and remembered for later analysis. 'What part of me is hurting?' 'Am I in danger?' 'How much does it hurt?' 'Have I felt it before?' and so on. Meanwhile the subcortical areas of the central nervous system recruit background responses such as an increase in blood pressure and heart rate, the amount of sweating and the size of the pupils.

Nociceptors

Inflammation causes pain

Pain receptors in the tissues are called *nociceptors*. Under a microscope nociceptors have no distinct structure, but appear as a woven network of free bare nerve endings distributed everywhere through the tissues; they are found in viscera, in periosteum, in connective tissue and around blood vessels.

Inflammation is ultimately the original cause of all pain. Where there is one, you will find the other; nevertheless, under some circumstances, when the inflammation resolves, the pain persists. This *neuropathic pain* can be unremitting and can eat away people's lives. The sad thing is that in most cases neuropathic pain is preventable if the original pain is treated early and vigorously.

Inflammation is caused by thermal damage, mechanical trauma, or chemical irritation. Surgery also damages tissue. The dead and damaged cells release pain-producing (*algogenic*) chemicals including eicosanoids, potassium ions, and bradykinins. The nerve endings also release *substance P*. All these biochemicals cause vasodilation, and oedema at the site of injury. Ischaemic injury does likewise, but adds hydrogen ions to the inflammatory soup. Soaked in inflammatory mediators, the capillary beds in the area leak protein-rich fluid (*exudate*) into the tissues. The exudate carries more bradykinins and other algogenic chemicals such as histamine, *serotonin* and noradrenaline into the area.

Macrophages and white cells flock to the site to mop up the damaged cells, to deal with invading micro-organisms and start the repair process. They send out distress messengers in the form of cytokines, histamine, serotonin, bradykinin, purines and many others. All these biochemicals further stimulate pain receptors.

Analgesics such as aspirin and the *non-steroidal anti-inflammatory drugs* (NSAIDs) impair the synthesis of some inflammatory mediators, and reduce pain and the inflammatory response.

Pain thresholds

What you feel depends on the type of sensory ending stimulated, and its connections to the spinal cord and the brain. The stimulus, such as a burn, a stab or a bite, must have enough strength (*to exceed threshold potential*) to trigger a response; in contrast a signal of insufficient strength is said to be *subthreshold*. A mosquito bite is subthreshold and passes unnoticed, in contrast a dog bite certainly exceeds the threshold potential.

Nociceptors fire more easily, at a lower threshold, if they are exposed to repeated high-intensity stimulation, or irritated by inflammatory biochemicals. This process is called *sensitization*. If anyone has slapped your sunburnt back you will recognize sensitization. *Allodynia* is the name for the pain where a stimulus that does not normally cause pain, begins to do so.

Substantia gelatinosa

Once a painful stimulus exceeds the threshold level, the impulse is carried to the substantia gelatinosa (SG) in the dorsal horn of the spinal cord. The substantia gelatinosa crudely analyses the intensity and quality of the pain. Like a gatekeeper it acts to control which impulses are important enough to pass and where to pass them. Are you wearing a watch? Normally you are unaware of it, but once your conscious self (in your *cerebral cortex*) interrogates your substantia gelatinosa it will direct attention to the appropriate wrist, and allow a previously subthreshold stimulus to pass back to your consciousness (Figure 5.1).

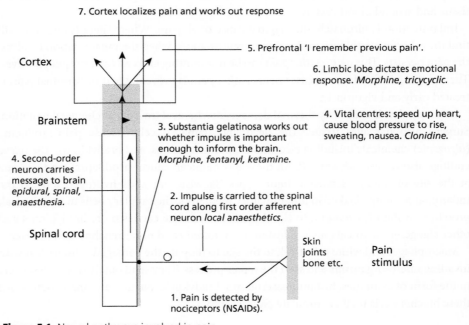

Figure 5.1 Neural pathways involved in pain.

If you touch a hot stove you will immediately pull your hand away—a *withdrawal reflex*—about 0.6–0.8 seconds before you consciously know anything has happened, and hopefully before too much damage is done. The *substantia gelatinosa* in the spinal card instantly recognized the supra-maximal stimulus, and directed an impulse down your motor nerves to get your hand out of the way of danger. This simple *reflex* response avoids wasting about 1.8 to 2 seconds needed to pass messages back and forth to obtain directions from your conscious self (to see an experiment in neuronal transmission see Box 5.1).

Box 5.1 **An experiment**

Without having to actually burn yourself, you can demonstrate the effects of the fast (A-delta fibres) and the slower (C fibres) neuronal transmission. Take your Achilles tendon at the back of your heel between your forefinger and thumb. Now, quickly squeeze it hard. You will feel two pains; the first is sharp, well-localized and brief, and the second dull, deep, diffuse, persistent, and uncomfortable.

Consider walking barefoot along a stony path. The substantia gelatinosa, receiving impulses arising in the prefrontal region in the brain, readjusts the threshold potential in the SG to tolerate jabs and pricks on the sole of your foot. Now, if you stand on a thorn, the adjusted threshold stimulus is exceeded and the withdrawal reflex pulls your foot out of the way.

To some degree you can consciously override a response to pain, such as when you make a grab to pull the plug out of a sink full of hot water. Although the pain threshold is exceeded, you expected the pain, and for that moment you can override the withdrawal reflex.

Peripheral nerves

First-order neurons carry sensation from skin, muscle, bone and the organs to the spinal cord. If you have ever burnt your hand on a hot stove you might, with dispassionate analysis, have noticed two sorts of pain. First a fast onset pain that only last for a short time and pricks, stabs or lances. Large myelinated A-delta nerve fibres carry this pain sensation. Second, a slower onset pain is duller, and lasts longer. Small unmyelinated C fibres carry this pain impulse. Both these first-order neurons carry impulses from the periphery to the spinal cord.

Endorphins

All these responses to pain are regulated by local neurotransmitters, which open and close neural gates in the substantia gelatinosa. Open gates allow pain impulse to pass, and closed ones do not. Inhibitory neurotransmitters close the gates and excitatory ones open them. One of these inhibitory substances is a member of a group of naturally occurring opioids called β-*endorphin*. This acts on opioid μ-receptors near pain *synapses*, hyperpolarizing the neuronal cell membrane so that it takes a bigger stimulus to make them fire. Opioids, given with epidural or spinal anaesthetics, mimic β-endorphins and impede the passage of pain impulses to the brain.

Ketamine[1] blocks the effects of an excitatory neuropeptide, *glutamate*, in the substantia gelatinosa. This slams the gate shut to stop pain impulses reaching the central nervous system. Ketamine also profoundly affects how the brain perceives pain.

Second-order neurons

Once through the gate, the pain impulses are relayed to second-order neurons that splay out in the spinal cord to carry information to the brain. Some impulses pass up to the *thalamus* in easily identifiable contralateral spinothalamic tracts. Others enter the diffuse spinoreticular tracts that connect with *vital centres* in the brainstem's reticular formation. These vital centres coordinate innate responses such as heart rate, blood pressure, sweating, pupil size, respiratory rate and depth.

Thalamus

Astride the top of the midbrain sits the *thalamus*. It acts as the body's administrative headquarters coordinating the body's automatic functions such as temperature control, respiration, and blood pressure maintenance. In the spinal cord the *spinothalamic tracts* lie laterally and the paleospinothalamic tracts lie medially. The neospinothalamic tract passes up the spinal cord to the posterior thalamus to carry and process information about the location, duration and intensity of pain. The paleothalamic tract sends its fibres to the medial thalamus and is associated with the autonomic and emotional aspects of pain.

Third-order neurons

In the medial thalamus the quality of the pain touches consciousness for the first time. Messages pass on through third-order neurons to the prefrontal lobes (foresight and previous experience) and the limbic lobe (emotion) where we analyse the memory and the emotional implications of the pain. In other words 'I have felt this before, it hurts—it's a burn'.

Meanwhile messages from the lateral thalamus pass on to the postcentral gyrus in the sensory cortex, where we integrate all the messages to discover 'my left hand is burning'. Now we know our hand is burnt we can organize other appropriate and complex behavioural responses such as finding water to cool it.

How pain is modified

We are genetically programmed to forget some types of acute pain. This is fortunate, otherwise a woman would never go through childbirth for the second time. Sometimes we need to cope with, or even ignore, pain. In the brainstem the periaqueductal grey matter (PAG) monitors emergencies. If roused it blocks pain impulses on their way to the brain. This is why people injured in war, or on the sports field, often do not feel pain until they are safe.

When the thalamus perceives the situation is an emergency it induces the hypothalamus and pituitary gland to secrete β-endorphin. These endogenous opioids impede inward-bound pain impulses through the PAG so that they are not passed on to consciousness.

Plasticity and wind-up

Plasticity

Once barraged by pain, stimuli sensory nerves recruit help from their neighbours by producing neuropeptides including substance P, neurokinin A, and calcitonin gene-related peptide (CGRP). These substances also pass up the axon to the cell body, which then remodels its connections in the substantia gelatinosa.

With repetitive painful stimuli nerves establish more peripheral pain receptors, send out new dendrites to their neighbours, and increase the number of receptors in the post-synaptic endplates in the substantia gelatinosa. At the distal end of the nerve the overall effect is to increase local sensitivity to inflammation, while at the proximal end in the substantia gelatinosa the nerve radically improves its communication with the central nervous system.

Now alerted to the problem, the neurons in the central nervous system establish new connections, allow others to lapse, and then increase their production of peptide neurotransmitters (*glutamate, aspartate*, and *substance P*). All this ability to change, to remodel, nerve connections and to adapt biochemical responses according to need is termed plasticity.

Plasticity does not only occur with pain. Just studying this book will actually remodel parts of your brain. Repetition reinforces the process; hence the observation that practice makes perfect.

> *Unrelieved severe pain can evolve*
> *into permanent chronic pain.*

How wind-up leads to chronic pain

Continuous severe pain changes the structure and function of sensory nerves. If the neural circuits in the substantia gelatinosa are barraged with pain impulses then calcium channels in the nerve membranes become jammed open. Calcium ions flood into the nerve cells and stimulate certain genes to act (express themselves). The genes programme the microsomal protein factories to produce many more neuropeptide transmitters, new receptors and cell membrane pumps. With all this new equipment for detecting pain, the cell now responds massively to stimuli that would previously have passed unnoticed.

With good pain relief we can prevent a catastrophe: unrelieved severe pain can cause so much calcium to enter the nerve cells of the dorsal horn that they die. Once this happens the neural gate mechanism in the substantia gelatinosa is permanently jammed open. Pain becomes entrenched so that even a minor stimulus now causes a massive response. Unhappily this response continues long after the precipitating injury has healed. An example of this phenomenon is the severe pain of post-hepatic neuralgia following an attack of shingles.

Ketamine prevents chronic pain

We can predict that some injuries, such as pelvic fractures or surgery like rib resection, will be so painful that *wind-up* is likely to occur. In such cases ketamine is useful for preventing the onset of chronic pain syndrome.

Ketamine blocks polysynaptic reflexes in the spinal cord and functionally dissociates the thalamus so that it cannot pass on impulses from the *limbic system* (which recognizes pain) to the cortex (where the pain impulses are consciously analysed). This means the pain never reaches a conscious level.

Reference

1. **Urban MK, Ya Deau JT** (2008) Ketamine as an adjunct to postoperative pain management. *HSS Journal* 4(1):62–65.

Chapter 6

Postoperative pain

Introduction

It is not only distressing to emerge from anaesthesia in agony, it is harmful.[1] Pain is physiologically damaging,[2] and mostly preventable (see 'Ten pain principles', Box 6.1). Managing postoperative pain optimally is one of the most important functions of the recovery room. In the recovery room pain can be rapidly controlled by titrating opioids intravenously. There are also many modern and sophisticated procedures available.

Box 6.1 **Ten pain principles**

1. Pain has many elements and you must treat them all.
2. Assessment is the key to treating pain.
3. Attack pain at more than one point on its path from the tissues to consciousness.
4. Be aware that uncontrolled *acute pain* can develop into disastrous chronic pain.
5. Cuddle crying children.
6. Opioids do not cause hypotension in stable patients.
7. Inappropriate pain needs investigation.
8. If you do not know all the actions of a drug, do not use it.
9. In elderly patients, use smaller doses.
10. Use multimodal analgesia.

How pain is modified

We are genetically programmed to forget some types of acute pain. This is fortunate, otherwise a woman would never go through childbirth for the second time. Sometimes we need to cope with, or even ignore, pain. In the brainstem the periaqueductal grey matter (PAG) monitors emergencies. If roused it blocks pain impulses on their way to the brain. This is why people injured in war, or on the sports field, often do not feel pain until they are safe.

When the thalamus perceives the situation as an emergency it induces the hypothalamus and pituitary gland to secrete β-endorphin. These endogenous opioids impede inward-bound pain impulses through the PAG so that they are not passed on to consciousness.

Plasticity and wind-up

Plasticity

Once barraged by pain, stimuli sensory nerves recruit help from their neighbours by producing neuropeptides including substance P, neurokinin A, and calcitonin gene-related peptide (CGRP). These substances also pass up the axon to the cell body, which then remodels its connections in the substantia gelatinosa.

With repetitive painful stimuli nerves establish more peripheral pain receptors, send out new dendrites to their neighbours, and increase the number of receptors in the post-synaptic endplates in the substantia gelatinosa. At the distal end of the nerve the overall effect is to increase local sensitivity to inflammation, while at the proximal end in the substantia gelatinosa the nerve radically improves its communication with the central nervous system.

Now alerted to the problem, the neurons in the central nervous system establish new connections, allow others to lapse, and then increase their production of peptide neurotransmitters (*glutamate, aspartate*, and *substance P*). All this ability to change, to remodel, nerve connections and to adapt biochemical responses according to need is termed plasticity.

Plasticity does not only occur with pain. Just studying this book will actually remodel parts of your brain. Repetition reinforces the process; hence the observation that practice makes perfect.

Unrelieved severe pain can evolve
into permanent chronic pain.

How wind-up leads to chronic pain

With good pain relief we can prevent a catastrophe: unrelieved severe pain can cause so much calcium to enter the nerve cells of the dorsal horn that they die. Once this happens the neural gate mechanism in the substantia gelatinosa is permanently jammed open. Pain becomes entrenched so that even a minor stimulus now causes a massive response. Unhappily this response continues long after the precipitating injury has healed. An example of this phenomenon is the severe pain of post-hepatic neuralgia following an attack of shingles.

Ketamine helps prevent chronic pain

We can predict that some injuries, such as pelvic fractures or surgery like rib resection, will be so painful that *wind-up* is likely to occur. In such cases ketamine is useful for preventing the onset of chronic pain syndrome.

Ketamine blocks polysynaptic reflexes in the spinal cord and functionally dissociates the thalamus so that it cannot pass on impulses from *limbic system* (which recognizes pain) to the cortex (where the pain impulses are consciously analysed). This means the pain never reaches a conscious level.

Misunderstandings about pain

Patients tend to assume:

- pain is inevitable after surgery; or
- that modern surgery is absolutely pain free;
- pain is simply something they have to put up with;
- pain is not hazardous merely uncomfortable;
- staff know when they are in pain;
- if they wait a while it will get better;
- if they complain, they will be thought to be making a fuss.

Preventing acute pain from becoming chronic pain

Acute pain must be treated aggressively to prevent it from developing into chronic pain. The transition from acute to chronic postoperative pain is a tragedy for the patient and everything possible must be done to prevent it.[3,4] Psychological factors also play a part including preoperative anxiety and depression. A sense of loss after mastectomy can trigger residual pain in the resulting scar.

Effective and early treatment of postoperative pain is the best way to reduce the risk of chronic pain developing. Gabapentin and pregabalin are useful drugs for patients at risk[5] as are clonidine and ketamine. (Gabapentin and pregabalin should be given preoperatively.)

Acute pain service

Most hospitals have an acute pain team to take over pain management once the patient has left the recovery room. These specialist teams provide consistent and superior pain management. Refer your patients who are difficult to recover because of their pain to this team.

How to manage pain

Although pain is a complex phenomenon, acute pain is relatively easy to assess and treat. First, ask patients about their pain, and then give enough analgesic to alleviate it. The recovery room is the logical place to assess, plan, organize, and start the treatment of coordinated postoperative pain management.

C—Cause of pain.

A—Assess the pain.

R—Reassure and comfort your patient.

E—Effective and appropriate analgesia.

R—Reassess pain and side effects.

C = Causes of pain

Tissue damage causes pain, but how the pain is interpreted depends on psychological and emotional factors and whether the patient has previous pain issues.

Tissue damage

Postoperative pain is initially caused by the inflammatory response associated with tissue damage, but not all pain is due to the surgery. Long incisions cutting through bone, muscle and nerves (for example, thoracic and abdominal incisions) are more painful than short incisions elsewhere. Small incisions are one of the reasons that laparoscopic surgery is less painful. Donor sites for split-skin grafts are surprisingly painful.

Sharp well-localized (somatic) pain comes from the skin and muscle incision, and deep poorly localized gnawing (visceral) pain comes from the deeper structures.

Psychological factors

Tissue damage is only part of the story. Pain is a subjective experience, and so depends on how patients interpret what they are feeling.[6] It is not only determined by the neural stimuli from the damaged tissue, but also the patients' expectations and other psychological factors, of which anxiety is easily the most predominant. Fear exacerbates pain. Fear can cause an alternative pathway in the brain for pain. Some people are more stoical than others and tend not to complain. Some cultures expect a stiff upper lip while in others it is fine to scream one's head off. Individuals respond differently to analgesics. Young healthy people usually require higher doses of opioids than older people.

Pain is less likely to be distressing if the patient:

+ expects pain;
+ knows how long it will last;
+ feels it is less severe than expected;
+ has been involved in deciding the options for pain management;
+ has been taught relaxation methods before surgery;
+ has good coping skills;
+ and most importantly is not anxious about the outcome of the surgery.

Pain control is likely to be good if the staff:

+ understand how patients perceive pain;
+ know the profound damage uncontrolled pain can cause;
+ do not consider reports about pain to be a psychological weakness in the patient;
+ know the properties of the drugs they are using;
+ use preventative analgesia;

- know how to treat nausea and vomiting;
- know how to treat respiratory depression and hypotension;
- are not worried that the patient may become a drug addict;
- formulate a sound plan for continuing analgesia after they leave the recovery room.

Non-surgical causes of pain

Not all postoperative pain is caused by surgery. Pain is an important sign that something is wrong. Ask the patient to point to where it hurts.

Consider non-surgical causes of postoperative pain.

- Sore throat from endotracheal tubes, laryngoscopy or metal suckers.
- Headache is particularly common after anaesthetic especially if they have been given ondansetron or tramadol.
- Pressure on peripheral nerves during the operation.
- Poor positioning on the operating table, stretching ligaments and causing joint pain.
- Tight bandages or plasters, nasogastric tubes and catheters.
- Intravenous placement.
- Muscle shearing caused by the use of suxamethonium.
- Poor position on the operating table causing severe back or joint pain.
- Pre-existing comorbidities.

Myocardial ischaemia

One very important cause of pain that may occur in the recovery room is myocardial ischaemia. This can present as poorly localized pain or more often aching discomfort, anywhere above the umbilicus. It does not have to be retrosternal, and may be in the jaw, neck, back or even the top of the head.

A = Assess the pain

Subjectively, if the patient says it hurts, then they are in pain. Believe what the patient tells you. Objectively, it is difficult to measure pain, because there are no biochemical tests to confirm its presence.

Gauge the severity of pain

Attempts to quantify pain have produced many ingenious pain scales, but none do the job perfectly. The best technique of all is to simply ask whether your patient is in pain, and if so whether it hurts a little, or a lot, or is terrible. If your patient has a history of chronic pain, consider an early referral to the pain team (if you have one).

Visual analogue pain scale

There is no point in trying to explain a visual analogue scale for the first time to a patient in recovery room because they will not be able to concentrate sufficiently to understand it.

Unless the scale has been explained to patients before they come to theatre, the scales are almost useless. The scale is simply a 10 cm long line drawn on a piece of paper. The right-hand end of the line is labelled 'worst pain ever', and the other end 'no pain'. It is called an analogue scale because it has no units marked on it, and therefore patients need not fret about the numerical magnitude of their pain.

Numeric scales

Many recovery rooms use numeric scales to assess pain once the patient is awake. With these scales staff ask the patients to rate their pain using a 0 to 10 scale. If you do elect to use a numeric scale then aim for a pain score of less than 4 out of 10. Numeric scales assume the patient is numerate, understands English, is not deaf, or has impaired vision and has no cognitive disorder. Patients in pain who are often sedated and distracted by other unfamiliar sensations find abstract intellectual tasks difficult.

What to document

Pain assessment includes location of the pain, its intensity using a pain score, verbal descriptions (sharp, burning, aching), physical signs (hypertension, sweating, tachycardia, pupillary dilation), clinical signs (limitation of breathing or moving, abdominal rigidity or guarding), affective emotional response (distressing, annoying, irritating), psycho-logical response (acceptance, anxiety, fear), and biochemical response (hyperglycaemia).

Pain charts

Some hospitals, especially those with pain teams, use pain indicator and assessment charts (PINDA) to record a standardized assessment of the patient's pain. PINDA charts are useful for pain audits and include details of the analgesic agent, the method of delivery, the effect of the analgesia using a pain score, whether nausea and vomiting are a problem, a sedation score, and how pain limits patients' normal activities. Sometimes PINDA charts are started in the recovery room.

How to assess pain in the elderly

It is difficult to assess pain in elderly patients who have cognitive impairment or who cannot communicate well. Elderly people cannot process the standard pain scores, but are easily able to tell you whether their pain is 'very bad', 'bad', 'moderate', 'just a little', or 'no pain'; and whether their pain is better after an analgesic. Even the terms 'severe' and 'minimal' are too complicated for some demented patients to understand after their anaesthetic.

Behavioural pain assessment

Patients who have had strokes, or have major intellectual impairment, or are too sedated or sick to respond will not be able to tell you that they are in pain. In this case you need to assess their body language. If you stroke the patient and they scream or wince then you know they have pain. If you like working to tables, you can try the CALMS scale in Table 6.1.

Table 6.1 The CALMS Scale

	0	1	2
C Comfort	Responds quietly when touched	Reassured when hand is held, or brow stroked	Difficult to comfort
A Activity	Deep breathes, cough and moves limbs freely	Reluctant to deep breathe, cough or move limbs	Moves only minimally when asked
L Looks	Relaxed or sleeping	Grimaces only when moved	Screwed up face and clenched jaw
M Moves	Relaxed	Tenses muscles when moved	Continuous clenched grasp, or rigid, may writhe around
S Speaks	Quiet	Moans only when moved	Continually grunts or whimpers
Score out of 10			

Source data from Healey, E.C. (2012) CALMS Assess for School-Age Children Who Stutter, University of Nebraska-Lincoln, USA.

How to assess pain in the intellectually impaired

These patients usually come with a caregiver or there will be extensive notes attached to the patient's chart, written by a qualified expert. The caregiver can be very helpful if they are with them in recovery room. Some intellectually impaired patients, especially those with Down's syndrome, may have a lower tolerance for drugs such as the benzodiazepines and opioid analgesics. Start with a half dose of analgesic based on their lean body mass.

How to assess pain in neonates

Even the most premature *neonates* respond to pain. Diagnosing pain in neonates is easy if they cry, but sick neonates may be too weak to cry. Look for a furrowed brow, flared nostrils, and an open mouth with a taut tongue. Their chins may quiver and their tongue may protrude.

There is overwhelming evidence that pain does great harm to the newborn, and because of the plasticity of the developing nervous system, there are likely to be adverse long-term consequences. They could be sensitized to pain for their entire lifetime. Neonates mount a qualitatively much greater neurohumoral response than adults. Cruel procedures, such as circumcision without anaesthesia, disturb bonding, disrupt feeding patterns and cause behavioural changes that persist for days or weeks and can even affect development of the central nervous system permanently. In some cases very painful procedures have been known to cause a neonate's blood pressure to rise high enough to cause an intracranial haemorrhage.

How to assess pain in children

It is also difficult to assess pain in children, and no single method works every time. Many children are comforted by their 'security blanket': a familiar and loved toy or object. You can use such toys to assist with explaining things and assessing how the child feels.

Toddlers

Children over the age of 2 years will tell you it hurts and where it hurts. Toddlers often express pain by rubbing the affected part; or by kicking, biting and hitting at staff (*combative behaviour*) in an attempt to escape the situation. They also cry and seek comfort from people they trust.

Children from 3 to 5 years

Even pre-school children will reliably tell you when something hurts and where it hurts, but unlike toddlers they can tell you how much it hurts—'a little bit', or 'a lot'. Believe what they say. If they say they are not in pain then you can believe that too.

Children from 6 to 9 years

School-age children are able to tell you more about the quality and intensity of their pain. It feels 'sharp like a knife' or 'dull' like after someone has punched you. They will also be able to tell whether the pain is worse or better than it was previously. They should be able to grade the pain into 'hurts a lot', 'hurts a bit', and 'doesn't hurt at all'. There are charts for you to use if you prefer them in many hospitals.

Older children

Older children can be assessed in the same way as competent adults.

R = Reassure the patient

Patients who have had disfiguring operations, or those with cancer, are far more likely to focus on the site of surgery and suffer more pain.[5] Anxious patients suffer more with pain than those who are calm. A recovery room nurse can give a patient in pain two great gifts. The first is empathy (the ability to respond with genuine compassion to your patient's reality), while the second is effective analgesia.

Almost all patients at or beyond middle age fear cancer. Many men and women affectionately remember the recovery room nurse who held their hand briefly, and told them everything went well. They say that with those few words their pain simply went away.

E = Effective analgesia

There are four main ways of controlling postoperative pain:

1. Parenteral drugs.
2. Regional or neuraxial local anaesthetic blockade.
3. Infiltrating the wound with local anaesthetic.
4. Oral analgesia.

It is best to use drugs intravenously. If drugs are given subcutaneously or intramuscularly they may be absorbed erratically, and act unpredictably. Giving drugs by mouth requires the patient to drink, swallow, not to vomit, and for the medication to be absorbed reliably.

Why various analgesics are used

Visceral pain

Visceral pain is diffuse, deep, aching pain arising from injury to, or distention of, an internal organ such as bowel. Patients localize it with the flat of their hand. Visceral pain responds best to opioids.

Somatic pain

Somatic pain is sharp, *acute pain* arising from skin, muscles, bone, joints, connective tissue and parietal pleura. Patients can accurately localize it with the tip of their fingers. Somatic pain responds best to non-steroidal anti-inflammatory drugs (NSAIDs).

Spasmodic pain

Spasmodic pain occurs when patients have operations on tendons or have diseases like muscular sclerosis. If opioids are not giving relief the anaesthetist may ask you to give diazepam. There are suppositories available that are useful in children.

Gabapentin and pregabalin are useful drugs for this type of pain but they take time to work.

Colic

Colic will respond to pethidine or diclofenac if morphine seems ineffective.

Tonsillectomy

Benzydamine is the active ingredient in a spray to ease the pain after tonsillectomy. It contains alcohol which is probably the most active of its ingredients so it should be used sparingly in small children. Follow the instructions on the container carefully.

Pre-emptive analgesia

Experienced recovery room nurses know that once pain is established far more opioid is needed to relieve it than if the opioid is given before the pain starts. If one drug, even morphine, seems ineffective it is better to try a different drug than persist in giving more and more.

The basis of pre-emptive analgesia is preloading the patient with pain-relieving drugs and techniques before they emerge from anaesthesia. Local anaesthetic techniques used during surgery substantially reduce the amount of opioids needed to control pain in the recovery room. Even under general anaesthesia surgical pain causes changes in the way neurons in the spinal cord behave, and the way these neurons relay pain impulses to the brain. Once the changes become established, it is difficult to suppress this hyperexcitable state with analgesics.

Patients who have been given remifentanil during their anaesthetic sometimes appear to suffer hyperalgesia in the recovery room. Magnesium sulfate[7] is sometimes given during the anaesthetic to help prevent this problem occurring. Morphine is the preferred drug to transfer a patient from remifentanil postoperatively. A single dose of pre-emptive analgesia given before the incision provides no more analgesia than the same dose given after surgery, but repeated doses of opioids used during surgery certainly have a good effect.

If the patient is difficult to settle in the recovery room adding clonidine in increments of 30 micrograms is helpful. Check the blood pressure between boluses as clonidine has antihypertensive properties. Low-dose ketamine is also useful in these patients. 10–20 mg/hour is often effective.

Multimodal analgesia

Advances in receptor pharmacology have identified exactly where in the pain pathway various drugs work. The rationale of *multimodal analgesia* is to block the pain at more than one point on its path from receptor to consciousness. For example, a patient who has had a radical nephrectomy might have a combination of a thoracic epidural, or intercostal blocks, to treat the *somatic pain* from muscle and skin; as well as morphine to control the *visceral pain* from the peritoneum and an NSAID to quieten the inflammatory response at the site of injury.

R = Reassess

Never send a patient back to the ward in pain. Adequate pain control means the patient can move with ease about the trolley or bed, take deep breaths, cough effectively, and feel comfortable. Just before discharging the patient to the ward record your assessment of their pain in their clinical record.

Patients with nerve blocks

Patients with nerve blocks are unlikely to report pain in recovery room. Check their postoperative drug chart.[8] These blocks do wear off and the patient needs to be warned of this. Some form of pre-emptive pain relief such as a long-acting NSAID and paracetamol will soften the blow of returning sensation. Patients who have had major orthopaedic surgery will often require opioids once their block wears off so make sure this is prescribed before the patient leaves you. A useful drug for pain relief after major orthopaedic surgery such as knee replacement is gabapentin, or even better if it is available pregabalin. These drugs started the day before surgery and continued for several weeks postoperatively help these patients to exercise and move their painful postoperative joints. They cause some patients to feel dizzy or drowsy. They will not experience this in the recovery room but you can warn them once they are fully awake.

Day surgery patients

Day surgery patients are discharged into the care of a responsible adult after their procedure. Because the day surgery patient is in hospital for a short time, their discharge needs to be planned at the time they are first assessed for their anaesthetic. The plan should include how to control pain, and what to do about potential postoperative problems. Patients should be offered a few analgesic tablets to take home with them. Paracetamol is often sufficient, to tide them over the next day or so. Sometimes nausea and vomiting prevent the patient leaving hospital. Ideally they will have been warned of this possibility in the preoperative visit.

Patients may ask if they will be fit to go back to work the next day. Reassure patients that most people do not go to work the following day and that they should only return to work if they feel fit to do so.

Slow release opioids and addiction potential

There has been a lot of publicity in the last year on the opioid crisis in America which has highlighted several important issues regarding the prescribing of slow-release opioids.

The take-home message is that slow-release opioids should not be used to treat acute pain. Patients should not go home on these postoperatively.

The acute risk of giving slow-release opioids is that it is similar to adding a background infusion to a patient-controlled analgesic (PCA) but worse as it cannot be switched off if the patient is over-sedated. This can lead to respiratory depression or more accurately, opioid induced hypoventilation syndrome. This can be fatal in opioid naïve patients, the elderly or other at-risk patients.[9]

The chronic risk of giving slow-release opioids is that they may lead to dependence and addiction. A significant proportion of patients who are started on an opioid for acute pain are still on it 1–2 years later and this association is stronger with slow-release opioids.

The other important point to note is that acute pain peaks immediately after surgery, i.e. in the recovery room, and then rapidly declines over the first two days postoperatively. If slow release opioids are taken this puts the patient at risk of overdose as time goes by and pain decreases.

Importantly for recovery, there is also a huge patient variability in opioid requirements and metabolism so the 'correct' dose for slow-release opioids is just not known. It is far safer to titrate small doses of immediate release opioids to manage acute pain.

If a slow-release opioid is prescribed, it must be on a case-by-case basis with regular review and reduction of the dose over the first 48 hours. It must have a cut off prescribed (usually 4–6 doses) and the prescriber must liaise with the GP to make sure it is not continued to reduce dependence and addiction potential.

For the chronic pain patient who comes for surgery already on a slow-release opioid, it must be continued with the addition of short-acting opioids for the postoperative period. A follow-up plan must be made for reducing it and stopping it with the GP and involvement of a chronic pain team if possible.

References

1. **Wu CL, Raja SN** (2011) Treatment of acute postoperative pain. *The Lancet* **377**(9784):2215–2225.
2. **Mei W, Seeling M**, *et al.* (2010) Independent risk factors for postoperative pain. *European Journal of Pain* **14**:149.e1–149.e7.

3. **Grosnu I, de Kock M** (2011) Strategies to prevent chronic postoperative pain. *Anesthesiology Clinics* **29**(2):311–327.

4. **Shipton EA** (2011) The transition from acute to chronic post-surgical pain. *Anaesthesia and Intensive Care* **39**:824–836.

5. **Gilron I** (2007) Gabapentin and pregabalin for chronic neuropathic and early postsurgical pain. *Current Opinion in Anaesthesiology* **20**(5):456–472.

6. **Ghandi K, Heitz JW**, *et al.* (2011) Challenges in acute pain management. *Anesthesiology Clinics* **29**(2):291–309.

7. **Song JW, Yoon KB**, *et al.* (2011) Magnesium sulphate preventing post-operative hyperalgesia. *Anesthesia and Analgesia* **113**(2):390–397.

8. **Phillips DP, Knizner TL**, *et al.* (2011) Acute pain management. *Anesthesiology Clinics* **29**(2):213–232.

9. **Chou R, Gordon D, de Leon-Casasola O**, *et al.* (2016) Guidelines on the management of post-operative pain: a clinical practice guideline from the American Pain Society, the American Society of Regional Anesthesia and Pain Medicine, and the American Society of Anesthesiologists' Committee on Regional Anesthesia, Executive Committee, and Administrative Council. *The Journal of Pain* **17**(2):131–157.

Further Reading

Gartner R, Kroman N (2010) Multimodal prevention of pain, nausea and vomiting. *Minerva Anestesiologica* **76**(10):805–813.

Chapter 7

Analgesics

Analgesics are drugs used to relieve pain

Three principal groups of drugs are used for parenteral pain relief:

1. Opioids.
2. Non-steroidal anti-inflammatory drugs (NSAIDs).
3. Adjuvants.

Opioids

Opioid analgesics include morphine, diamorphine, pethidine, fentanyl, alfentanil, remifentanil, codeine, oxycodone, methadone and tramadol. To use opioids effectively we need to know their properties thoroughly. Opioids are the best parenteral drugs we have to control moderate to severe pain.

Remifentanil is a very short-acting opioid and is usually given as an infusion. Before it is discontinued at the end of an anaesthetic a loading dose of morphine should be given to the patient about 1 hour before the patient is woken. If the patient wakes from an anaesthetic using remifentanil without this morphine load they will experience very severe pain. This can go on to become persistent post-surgical pain; this is hyperalgesia induced by the remifentanil.[1] If this problem should arise in your recovery room, treat it vigorously with fentanyl initially and then morphine. A small dose of ketamine or clonidine will also be useful to settle the patient.

Tramadol is not a typical opioid. Although it is an analgesic, many of its properties differ from other opioids.

Pharmacology of opioids

Opioids are analgesic drugs that work on the same receptors as our own intrinsic pain-killers called *β-endorphins*. Endorphins are a group of naturally occurring opioid *peptides* synthesized in the hypothalamus. When people are in pain, their hypothalamus releases β-endorphin into the cerebrospinal fluid, and the pituitary gland releases it into the circulation. β-endorphin latches on to opioid receptors in the spinal cord and brain. In the spinal cord, β-endorphin inhibits pain impulses passing through the *substantia gelatinosa* to reach the brain. In the brain opioid receptors are found in the periaqueductal grey matter (involved with the subconscious gauging of the level of pain), in the thalamus (where the decision is made whether or not to alert 'the conscious you' about the pain) and the limbic system (responsible for our emotional response to pain). Opioid receptors are also scattered throughout the gut (causing constipation) and *adrenal medulla*. They are widely spread in tissues, on lymphocytes and associated with pain receptors where they have anti-inflammatory activity.

Pharmacodynamics

Opioids work by binding to receptors on nerve cell membranes where they pull a series of biochemical levers to restrain nerves from reacting to incoming pain stimuli.

The opioids are classified by how they act on the various opioid receptors. There are three main groups of opioid receptors: mu (μ), delta (δ) and kappa (κ). The mu receptor is named after morphine, the kappa receptor after the only known pure *agonist*, ketocyclazocine; while the delta receptor is so named because it was first found in rat vas deferens.

The mu receptor is the most effective for pain relief, but unfortunately it is also the one responsible for respiratory depression. Importantly, the mu receptor gives opioids their wonderful ability to dissolve anxiety. As anxiety dissipates, patients report that although they still feel the pain, it doesn't hurt anymore.

Although delta and kappa receptors give *analgesia*, stimulating them has unfortunate effects. Stimulating delta receptors causes vomiting; while stimulating kappa receptors causes feelings of profound unease. These properties are not desirable in an analgesic. So it is hardly surprising that the effective pain-relieving morphine, diacetylmorphine (diamorphine), and pethidine are highly effective stimulators of mu receptors. Unfortunately their ability to temporarily wipe away the cares of this world makes them candidates to become drugs of addiction.

On the other hand, kappa receptor analgesic drugs (such as buprenorphine) or those with low mu receptor affinity are unlikely to cause addiction.

> *Patients in pain are unlikely to experience*
> *severe respiratory depression.*

Pharmacokinetics

Once an opioid is injected into a vein it is first rapidly carried to regions of the body that have a good blood supply: this process is called uptake. The opioid concentration in the blood then falls away in an exponential fashion as the drug is distributed through less well-perfused body tissue compartments. Meanwhile the liver and the kidneys start to eliminate the drug from the body. Only a tiny fraction of the dose of opioid gets through the blood–brain barrier to act on receptors in the central nervous system and spinal cord.

Clinical properties of the opioids

All the opioids have common properties, but there are also important differences. One opioid is not superior to another, but some opioids are better suited to some patients and procedures.

Effective dose

The effective dose of an opioid varies greatly from patient to patient. This variation is greatest in the elderly.

Opioids depress respiration

Respiratory depression causes either the patient's rate or depth of breathing, or both, to lessen. Opioids may slow the rate of breathing from 12–14 breaths per minute to 8 breaths or fewer per minute. Initially, as the respiratory rate slows, the patient takes bigger breaths, but eventually breathing becomes shallow. Given enough opioid, a patient will stop breathing altogether. Addicts who die from heroin overdose usually just stop breathing. Combining an opioid with a benzodiazepine, such as diazepam or midazolam, compounds respiratory depression.

Careful titration in recovery room should avoid respiratory depression. There is, however, a trap where a patient in severe pain has received a large dose of an opioid and subsequently is given a local anaesthetic block. Unopposed by pain, the opioid is likely to cause severe respiratory depression.

In patients who are not in pain even low doses of opioids suppress the innate desire to take a breath. People affected by opioids can voluntarily hold their breath long enough to become cyanosed. Equi-analgesic doses of all the opioids tend to cause about the same amount of respiratory depression.

On arriving in the recovery room many patients, although rousable, seem to forget to breathe, only taking a breath when reminded to do so. This phenomenon is called *Ondine's curse*. For a short time you can help a patient over this hurdle of respiratory depression, by simply waking them and reminding them to take each breath. This helps avoid the risks of giving naloxone.

Respiratory depression, if it is going to occur, takes place within the first 3–5 minutes after giving an intravenous opioid. Carefully observe the depth of breathing, count the respiratory rate and do not turn your back on your patient during this period. Sedation and respiratory depression occur in parallel. Once a patient becomes drowsy they have had enough opioid, but watch for developing respiratory depression with a decline in respiratory rate. Patients who become drowsy with lower doses of opioids in the recovery room need lower doses of opioid, and a longer interval between doses in the ward.

Equipment for monitoring expired carbon dioxide may be available in your recovery room. If so, this is an appropriate time to use it.

With respiratory depression the $PaCO_2$ rises, and this causes:

+ raised intracranial pressure;
+ raised intraocular pressure;
+ drowsiness (but not confusion);
+ peripheral vasodilation;
+ hyperglycaemia;
+ respiratory acidosis.

With respiratory depression accumulating carbon dioxide spills over into the lungs, displacing oxygen to cause hypoxaemia. If you are giving the patient an opioid ensure the oximeter reading is at, or above, 92 per cent. Send patients who are at risk of respiratory depression back to the ward on supplemental oxygen by mask.

If you are using an opioid continue
monitoring respiration and sedation levels.

Opioids and blood pressure

Opioids do not significantly alter a stable, well-perfused patient's blood pressure, although they may cause the heart rate to slow. You cannot blame opioids for hypotension without excluding other causes.

Hypotension occurs when an opioid lessens the sympathetic response to some other insidious problem such as hypovolaemia, *cardiac failure*, hypoxia, or septicaemia. Postoperatively, the most common reason for a falling blood pressure is hypovolaemia.

Hypotension? Exclude hypovolaemia

Even sick patients tolerate small doses of morphine given cautiously and slowly intravenously. Start with a low dose, say morphine 2 mg diluted in saline slowly intravenously, and wait 5 minutes to gauge the results.

Opioids, such as morphine and fentanyl, do not cause significant myocardial depression or hypotension and do not predispose to arrhythmias; but pethidine is an exception to this rule. Pethidine, being a vasodilator and myocardial depressant, often drops the blood pressure when given intravenously. If pethidine unmasks hypovolaemia or cardiac failure, the blood pressure will fall within a minute or two.

Neonates and infants may drop their blood pressure with morphine, and almost certainly will do so with pethidine.

The short-acting opioids fentanyl (and its daughter sufentanil, and son alfentanil) can cause bradycardia and profound respiratory depression. Titrate them carefully and remember their pain-relieving qualities are short-lived so make sure they go to the ward with a suitable ongoing prescription.

Opioids sedate patients

Opioids cause drowsiness. Patients tend to lie quietly and not move much unless prompted. When asked what they are thinking about they report a non-dreaming sleep-like state, but they are aware of their surroundings. Time appears to pass more quickly. This inability to structure thoughts, to anticipate or plan, and the disinclination to move is called *psychomotor retardation*. Do not tell patients important information while they are under the influence of opioids. They almost invariably forget it. This includes instructions about their care after surgery.

Opioids cause nausea and vomiting

Twenty to thirty per cent of patients who receive opioids during their anaesthetic become nauseated, or vomit in the recovery room. Equivalent doses of all opioids trigger nausea in certain patients, but those with kappa effects (such as tramadol) do so more readily. Opioids make patients susceptible to motion sickness by increasing their sensitivity to inputs from the vestibular apparatus in their middle ear: they get giddy easily. Pain itself can cause nausea and vomiting.

Opioids dissolve anxiety

Opioids promote an overwhelming feeling of well-being. They make it difficult to worry about anything and anxiety melts away. As the threatening feelings of alarm and fear dissolve, so does the activity of the sympathetic nervous system: tachycardia, hypotension and the other metabolic effects all fade away. Pain becomes less threatening, and although it is often still present it does not cause the patient much concern. As one patient said, 'Yes, I still have pain, but it doesn't hurt anymore'.

Opioid-induced pruritus

Opioids cause itchy noses, and patients sometimes rub them vigorously when emerging from anaesthesia. This unpleasant sensation is probably coming from a central stimulus. It is very unpleasant indeed for the patient who has been given morphine in a spinal anaesthetic if they develop widespread itching.

Pruritus becomes a real problem after eye or nose surgery, and facial plastic surgery. A small dose of intravenous promethazine 0.3 mg/kg takes their mind off the problem and they stop scratching. Another drug to try is ondansetron, but this may cause a headache. A small dose of naloxone or droperidol is also worth trying.

Opioids and urinary retention

Not only do opioids reduce the desire to pass urine, they cause the bladder's vesicle sphincter to tighten while relaxing detrusor muscle. In older men this can cause problems. Patience, encouragement and the sound of running water often help; or try a small dose of naloxone 0.04 mg. Failing that, they will need a catheter.

Opioids and pinpoint pupils

Opioids cause pinpoint pupils (miosis). This will be most evident in those patients who also have slowed their breathing and are heavily sedated. They are a sign that the patient is experiencing opioid overdose.

Opioids can cause allergy

Like many low molecular-weight drugs, some opioids displace histamine from mast cells. This is not an immune response, but it may cause the patient to develop itchy welts near the site of injection. This resolves within a few minutes. True allergic (IgE- or IgG-mediated responses) to opioids are rare, but not unknown. Usually morphine is the culprit. In theory morphine may precipitate bronchospasm in asthmatics, but in the recovery room this is not a problem provided the morphine is given slowly.

Tolerance and addiction

There are two groups of patients where opioids may cause problems in the recovery room: patients who are on long-term opioids, and narcotic-dependent people such as heroin addicts.

Patients with disseminated cancer presenting for surgery are frequently taking long-term opioids, usually fentanyl patches, oral morphine solutions or oxycodone. Because they develop tolerance they will need much more opioid than an 'opioid naïve' patient to control their postoperative pain. In the recovery room ketamine and clonidine are useful drugs to reduce the opioid required postoperatively.

Tolerance and opioids

With frequent administration opioids gradually lose their effect, and larger and larger doses are needed to achieve the same response. This tolerance to opioids takes a few days to develop. Tolerance is a problem in patients presenting for repeated painful procedures, such as debriding or grafting burns, or those with cancer pain.

It is cruel to withhold opioids because you fear a patient may become addicted to them. Patients in pain rarely become psychologically dependent (*addicted*) to opioids.

How to manage heroin addicts

Heroin addicts, and opioid-dependent patients, need proper analgesia, just like anybody else. In 'recovering addicts' there is no evidence that opioid analgesia will trigger a relapse, but many would prefer not to receive opioids for analgesia, because they fear the consequences.

Heroin addicts on a methadone programme are already taking an opioid and will have cross-tolerance with other opioids. Addicts on a methadone programme need their usual dose of methadone on the day of surgery. This will prevent them suffering the symptoms of withdrawal. Do not attempt to withdraw their drugs before surgery. The best option is to simply maintain their baseline methadone regime, and use other options to control their pain such as NSAIDs, or regional anaesthesia. If you do elect to use opioids, anticipate using a larger than normal dose.

Some patients may come to the recovery room wearing low-dose transcutaneous patches impregnated with buprenorphine. These are applied every four or seven to provide analgesia for low back pain or osteoarthritis of hips and knees. Sometimes patients forget to take them off. Because the buprenorphine trickles into the circulation so slowly, it has less than 15 per cent receptor occupancy. This means that 85 per cent of the opioid receptors are still unoccupied. Consequently, for these patients, you can use normal doses of morphine or other opioids for postoperative analgesia.

Opioid withdrawal syndrome

In the recovery room, you may occasionally see a patient who has been taking long-term opioids (including heroin addicts) experiencing a *withdrawal syndrome*. In its severe form this causes sweating, shaking, shivering, a runny nose, abdominal cramps, headache, nausea, and dilated pupils. Although unpleasant, it is rarely fatal, unlike alcohol. Mild withdrawal usually brings on nothing more than a headache, and an itchy nose. Some patients feel apprehensive, shaky and jittery. Signs of opioid withdrawal in the neonate include convulsions, excessive crying, and hyperactive *reflexes*.

How to use opioids

Intravenous administration is best

In the recovery room the only reliable and predictable way to give drugs is intravenously. After surgery the muscles are usually poorly perfused, consequently intramuscular drugs are unreliably absorbed and may take more than 30 minutes to work. This unacceptable delay aggravates the physiological and emotional stresses caused by pain.

Intravenous opioids are safe even with unstable or shocked patients. Small increments of well-diluted opioids given intravenously start to have an effect within 3–5 minutes, and measures can be taken instantly to compensate for changes in blood pressure. On the other hand it is risky giving large irretrievable doses of opioid into poorly perfused muscle where the absorption and uptake is erratic. In this case unwitnessed respiratory depression may occur back in the ward many hours after the patient has left the recovery area.

How to give an opioid

Start by putting your patient on 35 per cent inspired oxygen by mask. Make up 10 mg of morphine to 10 ml in saline. To build up effective blood levels, load the patient with a slow intravenous injection of 2 ml of this solution over a 5-minute period. Use the pain algorithm set out in this chapter to guide you. Wait 5 minutes for the drug to be distributed through well-perfused tissues and then continue to give the opioid until the pain is either relieved, or the patient becomes drowsy with droopy eyelids and pupils about 2–3 mm in diameter. Stop giving the opioid if the respiratory rate drops to 8 breaths/min or less. In adults, the age of the patient is a better predictor of opioid requirements than weight, but the response varies widely and some patients need larger doses.

What to do next

Once the loading dose of opioid is effective begin the patient-controlled analgesia (PCA) or instigate the ongoing plan for pain relief in the ward. For duration of effect of the opioid analgesics, see Table 7.1.

Do not wake patients
to ask if they are in pain.

Table 7.1 Duration of effect of the opioid analgesics

Opioid analgesic	Duration of action
Fentanyl	20 minutes
Morphine	3–4 hours
Pethidine	2–3 hours
Diamorphine	3–4 hours
Oxycodone	4–6 hours

If opioids do not relieve pain

Opioids are powerful analgesics. They are excellent at removing the anxiety component of pain, especially deep visceral or bone pain, but they are relatively ineffective against pain originating in skin, or with some forms of headache: in this case use either paracetamol or a NSAID.

Use ice

Figure 7.1 illustrates a sophisticated device for continuous cooling but a plastic bag filled with ice cubes can be very helpful to alleviate the pain after painful surgery.

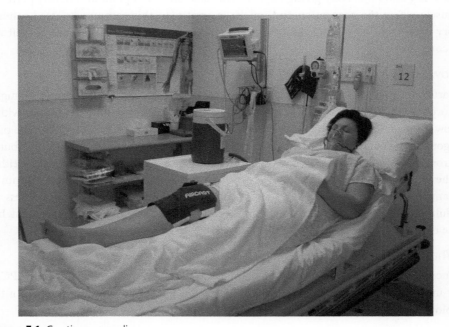

Figure 7.1 Continuous cooling.

Try clonidine

For restless patients, especially if they are hypertensive, a small dose of clonidine 150 micrograms in 10 ml of saline given in 2 ml increments, that is clonidine 30 micrograms, is often effective. Clonidine spares opioids as well as reducing their anxiety. Because clonidine causes the blood pressure to fall, measure the blood pressure after each increment.

Or ketamine

Ketamine is also useful as an anxiolytic when patients are not settling with opioids. Small increments of 10 mg are suitable. It is also advisable to give 1–2 mg of midazolam when you use ketamine in this way.

Consider a surgical cause

If pain persists despite normal amounts of an opioid, consider a surgical cause for the pain. Persistent pain after a *laparoscopy* or colonoscopy may be the first sign of a perforated bowel, or pain after an arthroscopy may be a sign of bleeding into a joint. Pain following manipulation of a fracture under anaesthetic (MUA) means the plaster might be too tight. Inform the surgeon about any persistent pain.

> *Persistent pain?*
> *Consider a surgical cause.*

Hypersensitivity

This is also a possible cause of restlessness. Consider using a different opioid. Changing to pethidine or fentanyl may solve the problem. Or at least give you breathing space to reassess your patient for causes of their ongoing pain.

Special precautions with opioids

Patients who eliminate opioids slowly

Some patients eliminate opioids slowly. This is likely if they have chronic kidney disease, liver disease, are elderly, or are less than 2 years old; or if they have been hypovolaemic at any stage before or during their surgery. Opioid requirements can vary by up to tenfold in elderly people. Some elderly patients tolerate morphine well and consequently may receive inadequate pain relief. The message is give it slowly, use incremental doses, and watch for the effects.

Enzymes in the liver convert codeine to morphine. About 12 per cent of Caucasians and most Chinese people lack the necessary enzymes and consequently may receive no analgesia at all from codeine or tramadol.

Opioids in shocked patients

It is safe to use small doses of morphine in shocked patients. Morphine does not usually depress myocardial contractility, but pethidine most certainly does.

It is hazardous to give large irretrievable doses of opioid into poorly perfused muscle where the absorption and uptake is erratic, and adverse reactions may occur hours after patients leave the vigilance of the recovery area.

Opioids in children

Neonates, and especially premature babies up to the gestational age of 22 months, or those with neurological or pulmonary abnormalities, have a high risk of respiratory depression and apnoea if given opioids. Apnoea and respiratory depression are dose-related. If opioids are used in children they must go from the recovery room to an area where they can be monitored with apnoea alarms for at least 24 hours.

Babies require lower doses and longer intervals between doses. As with the elderly, it is best to give small doses incrementally. Infants under the age of 3 months need about a quarter of the dose per kilogram recommended for older children.

Opioids in pregnancy

Opioids are safe to use in pregnant patients, but excessive doses in labour may cause respiratory depression in the newborn. Remifentanil infusions used for pain relief will not have residual effects as remifentanil has a very short half-life. Pethidine used in some hospitals might cause a problem.

Opioids and lactation

All the opioids, along with many anaesthetic drugs, enter breast milk and may be transferred to the baby. If the baby is tiny or vulnerable it is best for the mother to express her milk before surgery and store it in the refrigerator. She can also express and discard the first feed after surgery.

Opioids in hypothermic patients

Hypothermic patients metabolize and excrete opioids slowly, although opioid requirements do not seem to be affected by mild postoperative hypothermia. Patients with temperatures less than 35.5°C may stop breathing if given normal doses of opioids. Use small doses intravenously with great caution.

When to avoid opioids

Avoid opioids in patients with chronic obstructive pulmonary disease, unstable asthma, cor pulmonale, and severe liver disease; also refrain from using opioids in those with suspected raised intracranial pressure; and in patients who have had neurosurgery, inner or middle ear surgery, and open eye surgery.

Consider alternatives to opioids

Keep in mind that other techniques, and drugs apart from the opioids, can be used to *facilitate* pain relief: paracetamol, NSAIDs, a regional nerve block, clonidine or ketamine. Occasionally relaxation techniques are useful for acute postoperative pain, but the patient needs to be familiar with these before coming to the operating theatre.

*A kind caring sympathetic nurse
can reduce the pain score*

Opioid drugs

Morphine

Advantages

Morphine effectively controls moderate to severe pain. It attaches to mu receptors and works better with deep-seated ill-defined (visceral) pain, than sharper well-localized (somatic) pain. Patients who only experience pain when they move are unlikely to get pain relief from morphine.

Morphine is a safe drug even in patients with heart failure. It is unlikely to cause hypotension and tachycardia, however if they do occur then you must find the reason (first eliminate hypovolaemia). Morphine suppresses the cough reflex. It is the only safe opioid to use to relieve the symptoms of acute *pulmonary oedema*. It is unlikely to have serious adverse reactions with other drugs.

If you give morphine to people who are not in pain many report they feel nauseated or dizzy especially if they move their head around. They have difficulty in concentrating, feel vague and uneasy (dysphoria), and they perspire. Objectively they are pale, with pinpoint pupils, they look sweaty and their rate and depth of breathing decreases. Most would prefer not to receive the drug again.

Liver disease

Where possible avoid opioids in patients with *hepatic impairment*. These drugs may cause hypoventilation, hypoxia and acidosis and precipitate liver failure. Although morphine metabolism is not overly prolonged in most patients with stable cirrhosis, it is best to start with 50 per cent of the normal loading dose of morphine. For subsequent doses give only 50–75 per cent of the initial dose, and increase the interval between doses by 50 per cent. For instance, for the first dose give 5 mg of morphine (instead of 10 mg) and for subsequent doses give 2.5 mg (instead of 5 mg) and give it 6-hourly (instead of every 4 hours). You can always give more morphine if necessary.

Chronic kidney disease

Morphine is metabolized to morphine 6-glucuronide (M6G), which itself is much more potent than morphine. M6G is excreted by the kidneys and will accumulate in patients with chronic kidney disease. If the estimated glomerular filtration rate is less than 30 ml/min/1.73 m^2 then halve the loading dose and reduce subsequent doses by 75 per cent. You can always top-up the dose in small increments if necessary.

Pethidine is metabolized to 6-pethidinic acid (6PA) which has no analgesic activity. 6PA is toxic and if it accumulates it causes agitation, muscle twitching, seizures, coma, and even death. 6PA is excreted by the kidneys and accumulates in patients with chronic kidney disease. Some anaesthetists avoid morphine completely but it can be used with caution. Avoid pethidine in renal patients, and certainly if the estimated creatinine *clearance* is less than 30 ml/min/1.73 m^2.

Pethidine

Advantages

Although seldom used now, pethidine (called meperidine in the USA) has many properties similar to morphine, but it also has some very important differences. Being a potent mu agonist it is useful for rapid control of moderate to severe pain. Given intravenously it works within 2–3 minutes, which is faster than morphine, but it causes more hypotension, and tachycardia. When surgery causes smooth muscle spasm, for example, on the Fallopian tubes, pethidine is more effective than morphine.

Disadvantages

Pethidine has a low *therapeutic index*. This means the toxic dose (which is a dose that exceeds 150 mg in an adult) is close to the therapeutic dose (50–100 mg). Pethidine adversely interacts with many drugs and may precipitate the serotonin syndrome in patients taking:

- tramadol;
- SSRI inhibitors;
- tricyclic antidepressants;
- MAOI type A inhibitors (moclobemide);
- MAOI type B inhibitors (phenelzine or tranylcypromine).

> *Do not give pethidine or tramadol to people
> taking psychiatric medication.*

Dose

Titrate the dose of pethidine to the patient's needs. In some patients the effective dose can be high, especially if the patient has been on long-term opioids for the relief of cancer pain, or is a recovering heroin addict taking methadone.

In patients with chronic kidney or liver disease, pethidine is not as safe as morphine.

Top-ups

As with morphine, patients need a smaller dose to bring the levels back within the effective therapeutic range. An appropriate dose would be pethidine 75 mg slowly injected intravenously over 5 minutes while watching for drowsiness, and a decrease in the rate and depth of breathing.

Fentanyl

Fentanyl is a potent opioid working predominately on mu receptors.

Advantages

Fentanyl is an excellent analgesic, quick acting and unlikely to cause hypotension (even in hypovolaemic patients). Metabolized entirely by the liver, and not depending on the kidneys for its elimination, fentanyl is safe to use in renal disease.

Disadvantages

Fentanyl is not a good analgesic by itself in the recovery room, it is very short acting and the patient's pain scarcely settles down before another dose is required. Because it causes profound dose-related respiratory depression it can bring on *Ondine's curse* with a vengeance, where the patient is awake, but not breathing. Children are especially likely to stop breathing with fentanyl.

Fentanyl can cause unpredictable respiratory depression some hours after a patient returns to the ward. This is more likely in the elderly, especially after endoscopic procedures, where fentanyl sequestrated in muscle vascular beds is released back into the circulation when the patient begins to move about.

Occasionally higher doses of fentanyl cause glottal spasm making it impossible to ventilate a patient with a bag and mask. Until recently, chest wall rigidity was thought to cause this phenomenon. In large doses fentanyl causes bradycardia.

Diamorphine

Although diamorphine (heroin) is an illegal drug in most parts of the world, it is widely used in the United Kingdom. In many ways it is the ideal opioid. It has a quick onset, is highly effective, and is unlikely to cause hypotension. It reputedly causes less nausea and vomiting than morphine. The dose is 0.015 mg/kg intravenously. The liver quickly metabolizes diamorphine into an active metabolite, which may well be the principal analgesic.

Methadone

Methadone, a long-acting opioid, is equipotent with morphine. It works for about 30 hours. This means a 10 mg dose of morphine given every 4 hours is equivalent to 10 mg of methadone given daily. Because of its long action, methadone does not allow for flexibility in dosing regimes.

Codeine

Codeine is a useful analgesic, especially when combined with paracetamol for ambient patients. It is not a suitable drug to give in the recovery room. Patients who are staying in hospital should not be given codeine as it has a powerful effect on immobilizing their bowel function.

Tramadol

Tramadol is an unusual opioid analgesic. Not only does its metabolite bind weakly to opioid mu receptors in the brain and spinal cord, but tramadol also inhibits the uptake of noradrenaline and *serotonin* into nerves. This gives it some of the properties of tricyclic antidepressants (which are sometimes used to manage chronic pain).

Unlike morphine, which has high mu activity, tramadol's affinity for the mu receptor is 6000 times less than morphine's. As a result tramadol does not have the anxiety-relieving properties of morphine or pethidine and it certainly is not as effective as morphine against acute severe pain. It is worth trying as an alternative to morphine in patients who have had adverse reactions. If the patient is 'tramadol naïve', give the first dose very slowly as many patients respond with sweating, restlessness, and nausea.

Tramadol is contraindicated in epileptics or those at risk of seizures (alcoholics, heroin or cocaine addicts, head injuries, liver disease and possibly diabetics). Naloxone only partly reverses its effects, and may increase the risk of seizures.

Unlike morphine, tramadol adversely interacts with many drugs, especially almost all psychotropic medication (SSRIs, tricyclic antidepressants, and MAOIs) where there is an appreciable risk of the serotonin syndrome (see more on serotonin syndrome in Box 7.1). The analgesic effect of tramadol is decreased when ondansetron has been given due to the inhibition of the 5HT$_3$ receptors.

Although many patients dislike tramadol's effects, it remains popular with clinicians who feel that, in contrast to morphine, people are more unlikely to abuse tramadol; there is little respiratory depression, and less constipation than with other opioids.

*Do not use pethidine or tramadol in patients taking
psychotropic drugs.*

Dose

Give the initial dose of tramadol of 100 mg diluted in 100 ml of normal saline by slow intravenous injection over 20 minutes. Top-up doses are 50 to 100 mg every 4 to 6 hours, up to a total daily dose of 600 mg. It takes effect in 12 to 15 minutes. It is not known if tramadol is safe to use in children so it is best to avoid it.

Box 7.1 **Serotonin syndrome**

Serotonin is a monoamine neurotransmitter in the central nervous system. (Serotonin is another name for 5-hydroxytryptamine, or 5-HT.) Many drugs have serotoninergic activity. Clinical depression is sometimes treated with selective serotonin *re-uptake* inhibitors (SSRIs). These include sertraline, citalopram, fluoxetine, paroxetine and fluvoxamine. Other drugs, such as pethidine, tramadol, venlafaxine and some tricyclic antidepressants, or monoamine oxidase inhibitors also release serotonin and noradrenaline in the brain. If these drugs are used concurrently with SSRIs then within minutes to hours the excessive serotonin in the patient's brain causes them to develop the *serotonin syndrome*. They develop mental changes (becoming confused, agitated and mentally clouded); neuromuscular excitation (with jerky clonic muscle movements, abnormal muscle twitches and shakes); and autonomic stimulation (with hypertension, and tachycardia, and ventricular extrasystoles). Excessive muscle movement causes the body temperature to rise, with sweating and flushing.

Treat the serotonin syndrome by stopping the offending drug, treat each symptom as it arises. In severe cases it may be necessary to use serotonin antagonists such as cyproheptadine and methysergide.

Newer opioid drugs

The quest for the ideal analgesic continues in the hope of finding a strong analgesic that is not addictive, not a respiratory depressant and is cardiac stable. New opioid drugs are introduced every few years, prescribed with enthusiasm, and then fall by the wayside. The drugs have included buprenorphine, pentazocine, dipipanone, meptazinol, nalbuphine and others.

Although morphine has unpleasant and annoying side-effects, inconvenient pharmacokinetics, needs to be locked away in a cupboard, and is a bad drug from many points of view, all the others are worse. For a summary of the use of opioids see Box 7.2.

Box 7.2 **Opioids**

1. Diamorphine is the best analgesic of all.
2. Morphine is good for deep, diffuse, poorly localized pain.
3. Pethidine works faster, but can be toxic.
4. Use opioids intravenously in recovery room.
5. Use tramadol cautiously.
6. Avoid naloxone if possible.
7. If patients are over 55 years and receiving opioids, then give supplemental oxygen.

Opioid antagonists

Naloxone

Naloxone is a highly potent opioid mu receptor antagonist. Given intravenously it rapidly (within 1 to 2 minutes) reverses respiratory depression. If not titrated to effect it also reverses all the analgesic and *narcotic* effects of the opioid (and the patient's own endorphins too). Usually patients are catapulted into agonizing pain and their blood pressure may rise abruptly. The hypertension in turn may cause myocardial ischaemia, and the first sign might be the onset of *ventricular premature beats* on the ECG monitor. Naloxone works in an 'all or nothing' manner.

The sudden onset of agony can result in a strong adrenergic jolt, which is severe enough to cause the pulmonary vascular pressures to surge abruptly resulting in acute *pulmonary oedema*. Patients start to wheeze, and their oxygen saturations fall. Naloxone has caused sudden death in this manner.

Naloxone reverses the respiratory depression caused by opioids for about 35 minutes, and then its effect wears off. If, after this period, patients still have effective levels of the opioid in their brain they will relapse into respiratory depression. After a single dose of naloxone continue to observe your patients for about an hour to ensure that they do not relapse. If you have given naloxone and the patient does not respond, then there is probably another cause for their respiratory depression or altered mental state.

If the patient does not respond to naloxone then you may need to use the non-specific stimulant doxapram, or if this fails the patient may need to be ventilated. Assisted ventilation is the safest option, and gives time to reassess what might have gone wrong.

Naloxone does not reverse myocardial depression caused by pethidine or tramadol, nor the bradycardias caused by fentanyl, or the seizures caused by norpethidine or tramadol.

Patient-controlled analgesia (PCA)

Since only the patients know how much pain they have, it seems reasonable to allow them to control their own *analgesia*. *Patient-controlled analgesia* infusion devices use a minicomputer to give a bolus dose of an opioid when the patient presses a button. This is followed by a lock-out time where no further drug is given no matter how often the button is pressed. Patients will not press the button if they are drowsy, asleep, or not in pain.

PCA has proved an effective and safe way to administer opioids, while keeping opioid doses to a minimum. The technique has fewer complications than intermittent intramuscular injections of opioids.

PCA is a maintenance technique;
it is not useful for delivering a loading dose.

Some devices give a background maintenance infusion. Background infusions are hazardous unless the patient is going to a high dependency area. There is no evidence that they are helpful, and there are many reports of respiratory depression. A constant background infusion does not reduce the night-time demands for analgesia, nor ensure better sleep. For a list of the advantages vs. disadvantages of PCA, see Table 7.2.

Table 7.2 Advantages vs. disadvantages of PCA

Advantages of PCA	Disadvantages of PCA
Patient feels in control	Drowsiness, nausea and itching
Frees up nursing staff	Costly equipment
Respiratory depression less	Nurses need training in its use
Fewer sleep disturbances	Ties patient to bed with the IV line
Can be used in children > 6 years	No use in demented patients
Elderly patients, capable of using PCA suffer less postoperative confusion	May mask pain warning of postoperative complications such as angina, pulmonary embolism, too tight plasters, or full bladder

Start PCA in the recovery room. The staff can give the first few loading doses, as they have the training to recognize adverse effects and gauge the drug's efficacy.

Morphine is the best drug for PCA. Pethidine is not a safe drug to use for PCA, because it has a low *therapeutic index* and there is a risk of norpethidine toxicity.

Fentanyl can be used as PCA in patients who cannot tolerate morphine. The dose and lock out intervals need adjusting individually.

How to reduce mishaps

There have been many reports of accidents and mishaps with automated PCA devices: they are good, but not foolproof. Monitor your patients carefully. There are many different makes of PCA device on the market, so make sure you are familiar with the devices available in your hospital.

Age is the best predictor for opioid requirements. In the elderly double the lock-out time to start with. You can always increase the doses later if more is needed.

The best way to avoid problems is to use a standard protocol and a standard order form in every ward. Most slips occur when setting up the infusion, such as prescription errors, errors in administering the drug, and patient factors.

Prescription errors

Prescription errors include wrong dose, wrong lock-out time, and wrong infusion rate.

The prescription sheet should clearly set out:

- drug dose and dilution;
- dose increments (the dose given when the patient presses the button);
- allowable number of doses per hour;
- lock-out time;
- maximum amount of drug allowable in any 4-hour period;
- how often nurses need to make observations;
- acceptable limits of blood pressure, and respiratory rate.

The protocol should include details about:

- who is responsible for setting up the infusion;
- disposal of unused solutions;
- how to treat side-effects;
- where to find medical support staff (pager and telephone number).

Administration errors

Simple mistakes in setting up the apparatus are the source of most problems. These include preparing the wrong concentration of drug, not reading the prescription form accurately, setting up the equipment incorrectly, and accidentally injecting the drug while changing the infusion apparatus.

- Make sure your hospital uses only one type of PCA device so that every ward uses identical devices.

- Have a checklist (just like an airline pilot) and go through it step-by-step with another member of staff.

- Design your forms to be clear. A common source of error is where doses can be either written as milligrams or millilitres. Design your PCA form to eliminate this error. The orders need to be written exactly as they appear on the machine.

- Use a dedicated intravenous line. Opioids infusions need their own separate intravenous line; nothing else should run through this line. Piggy-backing it on another line risks the drug being pushed backward if the cannula becomes blocked. When the cannula is unblocked the large dose that has backed up in the line will run into the patient.

Do not start PCA in patients who are still having opioid infusion into their *epidural space*. In this case respiratory depression is almost inevitable.

Patient factors

Sick or confused patients are unable to use PCA. Occasionally problems occur because visitors and staff press the button for the patient. One variation on the theme of PCA is parent-controlled analgesia where an anxious parent, worried their child is in pain, unnecessarily presses the button. Some patients, especially those with a dependent or anxious personality, dislike PCA. Respect their wishes.

Sleep apnoea

Many obese patients have a sleep apnoea syndrome. If they receive opioids, they sometimes simply stop breathing, often in the early hours of the morning when the ward is 'nice and quiet'. Patients with sleep apnoea have less active respiratory drives, and opioids turn down the response even further. Sedated with morphine, propped up on pillows, and becoming even drowsier as their $PaCO_2$ rises, their head lolls forward to quietly obstruct their upper airway. A couple of attempted gasps, and it is all over. The nurse finds them an hour later—dead. *Ondine's curse* strikes again.

Anti-inflammatory drugs

Inflammation, with its biochemical mediators, causes nearly all pain. Inflammation is a result of tissue damaged by trauma (including surgery) or infection. The COX (cyclo-oxygenase) enzymes use *arachidonic acid* (which is in part derived from the *phospholipids* in damaged cell membranes) to produce a whole zoo of biochemical inflammatory mediators collectively called *eicosanoids*. These biochemicals stimulate pain nerve-endings to send pain signals to the brain and are also responsible for producing fever.

Non-steroidal anti-inflammatory drugs (NSAIDs) inactivate COX enzymes, and in doing so dampen the inflammatory response, reduce pain and decrease fever.

COX-2 inhibitors

COX-2 inhibitors have largely had their heyday. They are certainly effective, but have serious side-effects in a tiny minority of patients. There are two principal isoforms of COX enzymes in the tissues: COX-1 and COX-2. The isoform COX-1 does useful things: it produces certain *prostaglandins* to dilate bronchi, protect the stomach against its hydrochloric acid, and dilate arterioles in the kidney. In contrast, COX-2 produces another separate set of prostaglandins to turbo-charge the inflammatory response.

Conventional NSAIDs, such as aspirin, diclofenac, ibuprofen, naproxen, indometacin, and piroxicam, inactivate both the isoforms of COX enzymes. Apart from taking the pain out of the inflammatory response they also aggravate asthma, peptic ulcers, and renal impairment.

Highly selective COX-2 inhibiting drugs, celecoxib and meloxicam, do not cause as many peptic ulcers, or impair platelet aggregation, but they have adverse effects on renal blood flow and are not widely used.

Parecoxib, an injectable form of a COX-2 inhibitor, is occasionally used in the recovery room, but not in patients with ischaemic heart disease, or following coronary artery bypass surgery. This parenteral COX-2 inhibitor is given intramuscularly or intravenously as a once-only dose. It is moderately effective for acute pain having a ceiling effect equivalent to 4 mg of morphine. When combined with a low dose of opioid it is a useful analgesic. It has no effect on blood clotting. The intramuscular dose is 40 mg by deep slow injection. Do not use in patients who are sensitive to aspirin, or are likely to have renal impairment. There are reports of an increased incidence of postoperative myocardial infarction, stroke, and pulmonary embolism curtailing the use all COX-2 inhibitors. Make sure there is an interval of 12 hours before any prescription for regular non-steroidal medication on the patient's chart begins.

Non-steroidal anti-inflammatory drugs (NSAIDs)

Advantages of NSAIDs

NSAIDs (pronounced 'enn-sade') are popular for the management of mild to moderate postoperative pain because they do not cause respiratory depression, sedation or tolerance. They also reduce fevers, and make patients feel better. They are not effective as the sole agent after major surgery, but they do reduce opioid requirements and improve the quality of opioid analgesia. Optimization of pain with simple analgesia of paracetamol and a NSAID is the first step of managing all post-surgical pain.

Disadvantages of NSAIDs

Reduce kidney blood flow

All the NSAIDs can seriously jeopardize renal blood flow, especially in the elderly or in patients who are, or have recently been, hypovolaemic. Young people are not necessarily immune to this effect. Depending on the half-life of the NSAID the effect can persist for hours or days after the drug has been stopped. Do not use them in patients whose preoperative *estimated glomerular filtration rate* (eGFR) is less than 60 ml/min/1.73 m^2.

Impair blood coagulation

NSAIDs block prostaglandin production and *thromboxane* synthesis, and consequently the ability of platelets to aggregate to form a clot. It is unclear to what extent NSAIDs aggravate bleeding, but many surgeons prefer to stop them at least 4 days before surgery where bleeding may be a problem. For most NSAIDs platelet aggregation returns to normal after 3 to 4 half-lives have elapsed. Aspirin, however, permanently destroys platelets' ability to function for the whole of their 10-day life span; and it takes at least 4–6 days before the bone marrow can manufacture enough platelets to restore blood clotting to normal.

Aggravate asthma

Some patients, particularly those who have a hypersensitivity to aspirin, are likely to get severe bronchospasm if given an NSAID. Again this is due to their ability to block the production of bronchodilating *prostaglandins*. NSAIDs are better avoided in asthmatics. Asthma may be aggravated by any of the NSAIDs, but aspirin, naproxen, indometacin, and ibuprofen are particularly bad offenders. Check with the patient if they experienced previous problems before giving the medication.

Cause peptic ulcers

Parietal cells in the stomach mucosa produce quantities of strong hydrochloric acid. All NSAIDs inhibit the production of prostaglandins that protect the gastric mucosa from the damage caused by hydrochloric acid. Avoid them in patients with peptic ulcer disease. If the patient is already taking proton pump inhibitors (PPIs) such as esomeprazole and pantoprazole, then you can use an NSAID. PPIs partially alleviate the damage by preventing the stomach from making hydrochloric acid; in contrast the 5-HT3 inhibitors, such as ranitidine, are not so effective.

May cause hypersensitivity

NSAIDs cause hypersensitivity reactions in certain patients causing angio-oedema, rhinitis, and urticaria. These are not truly immune-mediated hypersensitivity reactions, but are caused by the overproduction of a group of inflammatory mediators produced by *lipoxygenase* enzymes.

Other precautions

NSAIDs should not be used in patients with pre-eclamptic toxaemia, hypovolaemia, suboptimally controlled *hypertension*, or abnormal clotting studies.

> *Only give NSAIDs to healthy patients having*
> *straightforward surgery.*

Adverse drug interactions

Do not use NSAIDs in patients taking thiazide diuretics (such as hydrochlorothiazide, or indapamide); loop diuretics (furosemide); beta blockers (such as metoprolol, atenolol); and *ACE inhibitors* (end in '-pril' e.g. enalapril) or angiotensin receptor blockers (end in '-sartan' e.g. candesartan).

Varieties of NSAIDs

A large number of NSAIDs are available. Despite strong drug company promotion, no drug is demonstrably superior to the others; all have their problems. There is evidence that NSAIDs impair bone healing.[2] Orthopaedic surgeons prefer not to use NSAIDs for postoperative pain relief in their patients.

Aspirin

Aspirin alone is used rarely in the recovery room. Aspirin in combination with paracetamol is effective against mild to moderate pain, and certainly more effective than paracetamol alone, or paracetamol and codeine for pain arising from joints or ligaments. The dose is 300–600 mg 4–6 hourly. It is contraindicated in children under the age of 17 years, and in breastfeeding mothers because of the remote risk of Reye's syndrome (encephalopathy and liver damage) in her infant.

Diclofenac

Diclofenac is most useful for the control of ureteric colic, pelvic gynaecological surgery and pain after the insertion of ureteric stents. It is sometimes used as eye-drops after eye surgery to suppress inflammation. It is rapidly absorbed from the gut and has a half-life of 1 to 2 hours.

Ibuprofen

Ibuprofen has the lowest incidence of side-effects of any of the non-specific NSAIDs. It is an effective analgesic, but its anti-inflammatory effect is weaker. It is useful for the pain following dental extractions and *laparoscopy*. Give it preoperatively to allow it time to act. It is rapidly cleared with a half-life of 1 to 2 hours. The dose of ibuprofen is 200–400 mg 6-hourly. For a summary of the duration of effect of all NSAIDs, see Table 7.3.

Table 7.3 Duration of effect of NSAIDs

NSAID	Duration of effect in hours
Aspirin	4
Ibuprofen	8
Indometacin	8
Ketorolac	6
Meloxicam	18
Parecoxib	12
Naproxen	24
Piroxicam	24
Atypical NSAID	
Paracetamol	4

Ketorolac

Ketorolac can be given intravenously or intramuscularly. It gives moderate pain relief, and remains popular in day-surgery cases because it does not cause the problems of opioids. Do not use repeated doses if there is any chance of surgical bleeding. Start with 0.2 mg/kg and then use 10–30 mg 6-hourly. The maximum daily dose is 90 mg in those under 50 years and 60 mg in those between 50 and 65 years.

Avoid using ketorolac in children or those over the age of 65 years; or those with coagulopathy hypovolaemia, renal impairment, diabetes, peptic ulcer disease, or those who are older smokers. Anaphylaxis can occur with ketorolac, and it must not be used in patients who are sensitive to aspirin or any of the NSAIDs. There are reports they can cause renal failure even in young people.

Paracetamol

As a first choice, paracetamol (called acetaminophen in the USA) is the best and safest drug for mild acute pain. Paracetamol, especially when combined with codeine or NSAID, is an effective analgesia. Unlike other NSAIDs it has no anti-inflammatory properties. It does not aggravate asthma, disturb renal function or prolong bleeding. Larger doses can be hepatotoxic so use it cautiously in alcoholics or patients with liver disease. The optimal dose is 1 g 4–6 hourly. Its ceiling effect means that increasing the dose does not increase its efficacy. To get better analgesia increase the frequency of dosing rather than the dose. It works better if taken regularly rather than when required (prn). The maximum safe dose for an adult is 4 g per day (8 × 500 mg tablets), but in this dose it may cause nausea. In overdose, it causes fulminating potentially fatal liver damage which requires expert treatment with acetylcysteine infusion.

In children, suppositories of paracetamol 20–30 mg/kg are effective, but in adults suppositories may not achieve effective *plasma* levels. Intravenous paracetamol is available in most countries and it is very effective in the recovery room where patients may be unable to take oral medication. It is more effective than oral paracetamol.

Tips about using NSAIDs

- Ibuprofen is the drug with the least troublesome side-effects.
- Used as a sole agent, NSAIDs do not effectively control pain after major surgery, but may do so after minor surgery. They are more effective if combined with paracetamol.
- NSAIDs are best used in combination as one of the modes in multimodal analgesia. Add an opioid. You can then reduce the dose of the opioid by one-third, with the added benefits of decreasing nausea and respiratory depression.
- Paracetamol and NSAIDs are valuable components in multimodal analgesia.
- NSAIDs need time to work. They are more effective if given 3 to 5 hours before the pain is expected.
- NSAIDs are a useful pre-med for patients having laparoscopic surgery.

- ◆ Do not use NSAIDs in pregnant or breastfeeding women.
- ◆ NSAIDs are effective with biliary pain and renal colic.
- ◆ Avoid NSAIDs (particularly ketorolac) in patients who are likely to have renovascular disease such as diabetics, the elderly, smokers, and those with heart failure (especially if they have, or had, peripheral oedema).
- ◆ Do not use aspirin in children under the age of 16 years.
- ◆ There is no advantage in using more than one type of NSAID.
- ◆ Intravenous NSAIDs are no more effective than the same drug given orally.
- ◆ Avoid NSAIDs in elderly patients who are taking drugs with a low *therapeutic index*, such as digoxin or aminoglycosides.
- ◆ If parecoxib is given during anaesthesia further NSAIDs should be withheld for 12 hours.

For a summary of the use of NSAIDs see Box 7.3.

Box 7.3 **NSAIDs**

1. Ibuprofen is best, but it takes 3 hours to act.
2. Paracetamol works if there is no inflammation, otherwise use ibuprofen.
3. Do not use NSAIDs in people over 70.
4. Do not use NSAIDs in patients with chronic kidney disease.

Adjuvants

Ketamine

Ketamine is a non-barbiturate, non-narcotic, dissociative anaesthetic agent that acts on the spinal cord and at many places in the brain. Its principal action is to prevent pain impulses being relayed to consciousness. Ketamine blocks the NMDA receptor which is central to development of hyperalgesia and tolerance. Ketamine should be used cautiously. Even with a low dose there is a risk of psychomimetic or psychological adverse effects.

In anaesthetic doses

In anaesthetic doses, ketamine produces a *dissociative anaesthesia* where patients appear to be in a trance with their eyes wide open, but not responding to any stimulus (*catalepsy*). Their eyes may flick from side to side. Their muscle tone is increased slightly. Patients remember nothing of the procedure (amnesia). The blood pressure usually rises except in severely shocked patients. Ketamine causes a tachycardia.

Patients usually salivate profusely, and may develop transient *laryngospasm* and apnoea immediately after receiving the drug. It is prone to cause postoperative nausea and vomiting.

In analgesic doses

Given judiciously by infusion ketamine is superb for controlling agonizing postoperative pain. It is useful to manage the pain after burns debridement, and amputations. It is also useful when phantom limb pain reappears during or after spinal anaesthesia, or with severe metabolic stress.

Used alone ketamine often causes unpleasant visual and tactile hallucinations. Patients see weird things, often in vivid colours, and occasionally feel strange things crawling over their skin. These hallucinations can be frightening. To prevent them many anaesthetists add a benzodiazepine (such as midazolam or diazepam). To achieve effective plasma concentrations, give a loading dose of 0.1 mg/kg of ketamine and follow this with an infusion of 12 mg/kg/hr. Good analgesia occurs within an hour, but if no loading dose is given, it takes about 48 hours for plasma concentrations to reach effective levels. Usually, at these doses, hallucinations and dysphoria are not a problem.

Ketamine reduces opioid requirements
in opioid-tolerant patients.

Gabapentin

Gabapentin, an antiepileptic drug, is one of a new class of analgesics. Given preoperatively it enhances the effects of morphine, does not depress breathing, however it may cause drowsiness. Gabapentin should be given preoperatively. It is not appropriate as a rescue drug in recovery. Gabapentin has been shown to lower pain scores but also to delay discharge from the recovery room.[3]

Clonidine

Clonidine is a centrally acting alpha-2 agonist used occasionally to treat severe hypertension. It is becoming popular because it usefully potentiates the effects of other analgesics. It appears to work on the spinal cord. It can be given orally, intravenously, or as a skin patch. Most of these uses are *off-label*. Clonidine causes sedation, lessens anxiety, reduces shaking, nausea and vomiting in doses of 3 micrograms/kg made up to 10 ml in saline and given intravenously in 2 ml increments. Being an anti-hypertensive drug it may cause hypotension.

Recent advances

Improved knowledge of how pain works at the molecular level have given us multimodal treatment and we have new drugs, and new ways of using older drugs to treat postoperative pain. These include:

Capsaicin

Capsaicin (8-methyl-N-vanillyl-6-nonenamide) is a non-narcotic alkaloid and it acts peripherally as a TRPV-1 agonist. The activation of the TRPV receptors releases substance P, which results in an initial sensation of burning. There is a subsequent decrease in C fibre activation. Other pain fibres are not affected.

It can be used as a cream and also as an injectable analgesic. The injectable form is not widely available as it is still undergoing tests in some countries. This cream could be useful for the elderly patient who is not able to take NSAIDs and at risk of respiratory depression with opioids.

Dexmedetomidine

Dexmedetomidine is a highly selective central alpha-2 agonist. Given in doses of 0.5–2 micrograms/kg it causes sedation without respiratory depression. It does not affect the blood pressure or heart rate and it reduces shivering. It is very useful as a morphine sparing drug which nausea is a problem.

Tapentadol

Tapentadol is a centrally acting analgesic with dual action. It is an agonist at the μ-opioid receptor and also a noradrenaline reuptake inhibitor. The opioid effect of the drug is more powerful than morphine but this is modified by the noradrenaline reuptake inhibition. The result is a drug with a potency similar to oxycodone. You will probably not administer it in the recovery room as it must be taken orally but you may see it prescribed.

Tapentadol can be given 4–6 hourly up to a maximum dose of 700 mg in 24 hours. It is well tolerated and does not cause as much nausea and vomiting or constipation, problems that commonly occur with morphine. There are no renal or hepatic side effects (none reported so far.) Tapentadol is contraindicated in patients with asthma and in patients taking monoamine oxidase inhibitors (MAOIs).

Extended-release epidural morphine (EREM)

It does seem a worthwhile goal to give a drug locally that will give long-acting relief after very painful joint surgery. EREM DepoDur™ can last for 48 hours. Patients need to be closely monitored during this time as they are at risk of respiratory depression. Opioid side-effects like pruritus and nausea can also be troublesome. These side-effects can be treated with opioid antagonists.

Fentanyl intradermal iontophoretic system (ITS)

Fentanyl intradermal iontophoretic system (ITS) gives similar analgesia to IV morphine PCA but through the skin. It can bring another set of problems with itchy painful skin and all the normal side-effects of opioids occur with nausea the most common one. Using this system patient can move about easily and do not have to continue with the intravenous line and the PCA pump. The drug is delivered by the application of a low-intensity electric field.

The patient-controlled fentanyl hydrochloride iontophoretic transdermal system (fentanyl ITS) was designed to address these concerns. Fentanyl ITS is an innovative, needle-free, self-contained, pre-programmed drug-delivery system that uses iontophoretic technology to deliver fentanyl through the skin by application of a low-intensity electrical field. It has not been approved by the U.S. Food and Drug Administration (FDA) for current clinical use; however, clinical studies have been conducted on human subjects to evaluate it for efficacy, safety, and tolerability.

Efficacy of fentanyl ITS

The efficacy of fentanyl ITS in treating acute postoperative pain was first established in three phase 3 double-blind placebo-controlled clinical trials. More importantly, fentanyl ITS now has been demonstrated to have efficacy and safety equivalent to morphine IV-PCA in four randomized controlled trials, a subgroup analysis, and a meta-analysis. It is thought that 40 per cent of the administered dose is absorbed in the first hour of treatment and the system reaches 100 per cent efficacy in 100 hours.

Panchal et al.[4] evaluated the incidence of analgesic gaps resulting from system-related events (SREs) for patients using the fentanyl ITS vs. morphine IV PCA for postoperative pain management. Fentanyl ITS was associated with a significantly lower incidence of analgesic gaps than morphine IV PCA.

Safety and tolerability of fentanyl ITS

The safety and tolerability of fentanyl ITS have been found to be acceptable by several studies and pooled data analysis. Adverse events associated with fentanyl ITS are similar to those reported with IV opioid administration, including nausea, vomiting, pruritus, headache, and mild-to-moderate dizziness. Nausea was the most common adverse event.

Disadvantages

As with all transdermal systems, skin hypersensitivity, skin redness, and hyperpigmentation are potential problems. The system has not been adequately studied in children. It should be used with extreme caution for in-patients with severe hepatic dysfunction, head injuries, sleep apnoea, and impending respiratory failure and in patients with increased intracranial pressure of any aetiology.

The system lacks programmability and a basal infusion rate that may be important in opioid-dependent and opioid-tolerant patients. The number and timing of attempts by the patient also cannot be determined. The system has to be disposed only after disassembly by the pharmacist. The most important disadvantage at the current time is the availability of fentanyl ITS, since it is not currently being produced due to technical problems. Perhaps technological modifications, including recording the number and timing of the attempts and the addition of a basal rate, may make it more advantageous in the future.

References

1. **Song JW, Lee YW**, *et al.* (2011) Magnesium sulfate prevents remifentanil-induced postoperative hyperalgesia. *Anaesthesia and Analgesia* 113(2):390–397.

2. **Cohen DB, Kawamura S,** *et al.* (2006) Indomethacin and celecoxib impair rotator cuff tendon-to-bone healing. *The American Journal of Sports Medicine* **34**:362–369.

3. **Siddiqui NT,** *et al.* (2018) The effect of gabapentin on delayed discharge from the postanaesthesia care unit: a retrospective analysis. *Pain Pract* **18**(1):18–22.

4. **Panchal SJ, Damaraju CV,** *et al.* (2007) System-related events and analgesic gaps during postoperative pain management. *Anesthesia and Analgesia* **105**(5):1437–1441.

Further Reading

Vadivelu N, Mitra S, *et al.* (2010). Recent advances in postoperative pain management. *Yale Journal of Biology and Medicine* **83**(1):11–25.

Chapter 8

Postoperative nausea and vomiting

Nausea and vomiting are feared

Postoperative nausea and vomiting (PONV) is common. Its severity ranges from mild queasiness through to a distressing, prolonged, life-threatening event requiring resuscitation with intravenous fluids. Postoperative nausea and vomiting delays discharge from the recovery room, and increases nurses' workload. About 1 per cent of day surgery patients have to stay in hospital overnight because of uncontrollable nausea and vomiting; this makes it an expensive complication.

In many cases patients
fear PONV more than pain.

Nausea

Nausea is an unpleasant feeling of the need to vomit. It may be accompanied by sweating, pallor, bradycardia, and salivation.

Vomiting

Vomiting (*emesis*) is an involuntary active protective *reflex* for evicting ingested toxins from the gut. The patient usually realizes a few seconds beforehand that they are about to vomit. Vomiting begins with a deep inspiration, the glottis closes, and diaphragm and abdominal muscles contract violently, ejecting the stomach contents.

Vomiting is hazardous because it:

♦ can cause pneumonitis if aspirated into the lungs;

♦ damages the cornea if it gets into the eyes;

♦ damages facial skin flaps;

♦ raises intra-ocular and intracranial pressure;

♦ may tear suture lines;

♦ causes bradycardia in patients with ischaemic heart disease;

♦ causes hypotension in patients with peripheral vascular disease;

♦ leads to hypokalaemia and saline depletion if prolonged;

♦ may rupture the oesophagus in a few susceptible individuals.

Regurgitation

Regurgitation is a passive process where fluid matter refluxes up the oesophagus from the stomach. It occurs without warning, and can cause aspiration pneumonitis in a comatose or mentally *obtunded* patient. Regurgitation is likely to occur in a patient with:

- full stomach;
- decreased level of consciousness e.g. due to intoxication with drugs or alcohol;
- hiatus hernia;
- obesity;
- distended abdomen;
- intestinal obstruction;
- ascites;
- pregnancy.

Aspiration

Mendelson's syndrome

Aspiration during pregnancy is called Mendelson's syndrome, although the term is now more widely used to cover all patients who have aspiration pneumonitis. All pregnant patients are at risk, and if it occurs in pregnancy the pneumonitis is peculiarly fulminant, and often fatal. Pregnant patients are most at risk during induction of general anaesthesia, but nausea at any time during their recovery, even after spinal or epidural anaesthetics, must be treated quickly to prevent this complication.

Aspiration pneumonitis

Aspiration pneumonitis is a severe inflammation of the lungs caused by inhaling gastric contents into the lower airways. Severe aspiration is said to occur in about 3 in 10 000 anaesthetics, but it is probably less than that. Even the longest fast does not abolish the risk of aspiration because the stomach is never completely empty. Water is cleared exponentially from the stomach; half is gone after 12 minutes, and about 60 minutes later it has all gone leaving only acidic gastric juice behind. A fasted stomach contains about 30 ml of fluid composed of hydrochloric acid and peptic *enzymes*, which are strong enough to blister skin. Subtle micro-aspiration in the recovery room soon after patients emerge from anaesthetic is probably responsible for many postoperative chest infections.

If serious aspiration occurs, patients may need their respiratory function closely observed in ICU. Initially give them oxygen by mask, and if their oxygen saturation deteriorates they may need intubation and ventilation. If the oxygen saturation is above 90 per cent intubation can be avoided. An endotracheal tube abolishes the patient's ability to cough and deep breathe. X-ray changes revealing inflammation may take several hours to develop and usually first appear in the right lower lobe. Bronchial lavage, steroids and antibiotics are not useful in the early stages. If solid food has been inhaled then a bronchoscopy may be needed to remove the larger lumps.

Physiology

Vomiting

Vomiting is a *reflex* that evolved to eject ingested toxins, and the unpleasant nausea is a reminder not to ingest that toxin again. There are three components to the vomiting reflex: emetic detectors, coordinating centres, and motor outputs. Retching involves the same processes, but no stomach contents are ejected.

Input

The *vomiting centre* (VC) lies protected inside the blood–brain barrier in the brainstem. In contrast, the *chemoreceptor trigger zone* (CTZ) lies outside.

Processors

The centres coordinating vomiting in the brainstem have neural inputs from the stomach, the vestibular apparatus in the ear, emotional centres, in the cortex and from direct stimuli by toxins carried in the blood (Figure 8.1).

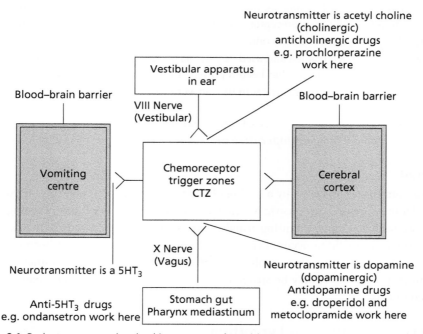

Figure 8.1 Brainstem centres involved in nausea and vomiting.

The vomiting centre coordinates the control of the complex vomiting reflex. Rich in cholinergic receptors, it receives incoming signals from the pharynx, gastrointestinal tract and mediastinum via the vagus nerve; and from the vestibular portion of the eighth cranial nerve and the chemoreceptor trigger zone. It is interconnected with centres controlling various activities of the autonomic nervous system such as salivation, sweating, bradycardia, and blood pressure control.

The receptors

There are three principal types of receptors involved in stimulating nausea and vomiting. Once stimulated they relay information to the vomiting centre, which then initiates and coordinates vomiting.

Dopamine D_2 receptors are mostly found on afferent input pathways from the vagus nerve serving the abdominal viscera, pharynx and genitals. Anti-dopaminergic drugs, such as metoclopramide, and droperidol, partially block these receptors.

Cholinergic receptors are mostly found in the pathways from the vestibular apparatus. Anti-cholinergic drugs such as hyoscine, some antihistamines and prochlorperazine block them. Opioids tend to sensitize the vestibular apparatus, and essentially cause motion sickness.

Toxins and impulses from nerves stimulating the chemoreceptor trigger zone are relayed across the blood–brain barrier to the vomiting centre which then coordinates all the processes needed for vomiting.

Serotonin (5-HT$_3$) receptors are mostly involved in the final common pathway relaying information from the chemoreceptor trigger zone to the vomiting centre. They are blocked with 5-HT$_3$ antagonists such as ondansetron or cyclizine. *Neurokinin-1* (NK1) receptor inhibitors[1] have been trialled and used in patients on chemotherapy with good results but an increase in infection rates has been reported. They have a long onset of action so they are not suitable for rescue treatment in the recovery room.

> *NSAIDs do not cause*
> *postoperative nausea and vomiting.*

Output

Most vomiting is preceded by a feeling of nausea, however patients with raised intracranial pressure or acute gastric distension may simply vomit without warning. Once the stomach is empty, vomiting usually ceases unless it is caused by toxins in the gut. Then dry retching occurs because the stimulus to vomit has not been removed. Dry retching and vomiting involve violent contractions of the abdominal wall and diaphragm. The effort may be strong enough to fracture ribs in elderly patients with osteoporosis.

Causes of nausea and vomiting

Postoperative nausea and vomiting occurs in all types of patients, and with all types of operations and anaesthetics. There are, however certain groups of people, and certain types of procedures where vomiting is more likely.

Surgical factors

The following procedures are associated with more nausea and vomiting:

- intra-abdominal operations where the peritoneum is stretched, or the gut's perfusion or oxygenation is compromised;
- biliary surgery;
- breast augmentation surgery;
- thyroid surgery;
- gynaecological laparoscopic surgery;
- ophthalmic operations, especially squint surgery;
- ENT surgery; especially tonsillectomy and middle ear surgery;
- urological surgery; especially if the spermatic cord is involved;
- emergency surgery, especially for fractures.

Patient factors

Children vomit more frequently than adults. Women are more likely to vomit than men and elderly patients over 70 years do not often vomit. There is no evidence that obese patients are more likely to vomit than thin patients. Patients who get motion sickness are at high risk. There is also a strong psychological factor: those people who think that they are likely to vomit, or who have a history of doing so, are three times more likely to vomit after subsequent operations. Smokers are less likely to vomit than non-smokers.

Supplemental oxygen helps prevent postoperative nausea and vomiting.

Anaesthetic factors

Opioids

Opioid drugs are a potent cause of nausea and vomiting. Opioids act directly on the brainstem centres, and are more likely to cause vomiting if the patient is moving around. They sensitize the vomiting centres to input from the vestibular apparatus. Opioids given as premedication, and during operations more than double the incidence of vomiting. Oxycodone causes less nausea and vomiting than morphine.

Anaesthetic agents

All the inhalational anaesthetic agents and many induction agents (thiopental, ketamine, and particularly etomidate) can cause nausea and vomiting.

Propofol decreases the risk of vomiting. Benzodiazepines and muscle relaxants have no effect on the incidence of nausea and vomiting. The best anaesthetic option to prevent the nausea and vomiting is total intravenous anaesthesia (TIVA) with propofol. Neostigmine given to reverse muscle relaxants at the end of surgery may cause vomiting on waking.

Type of anaesthetic

Patients who have a general anaesthetic with volatile agents are more likely to have PONV than those who have TIVA or regional anaesthesia. Patients who breathe spontaneously during the operation are less likely to vomit than those who are ventilated. This may be related to the greater use of opioids in the ventilated group.

Patients who are hypotensive during or after their anaesthetic are highly likely to feel nauseated and vomit. This is probably related to suboptimal oxygen supply to the gut. If the gut becomes hypoperfused or hypoxic, its neural network almost instantly releases serotonin ($5HT_3$) which initiates nausea. Even brief periods of hypotension quickly cause nausea and then vomiting. Anticipating and treating hypotension, e.g. for Caesarean section patients having regional anaesthesia is important. Giving higher concentrations of supplemental oxygen almost halves the incidence of PONV after major abdominal surgery. The length of surgery has little effect on the amount of postoperative vomiting.

Recovery room factors

In the recovery room nausea and vomiting may be induced by:

- severe pain, which tends to produce nausea rather than vomiting;
- hypotension;
- hypoxia;
- hypovolaemia;
- anxiety;
- early mobilization;
- swallowed blood;
- water intoxication syndrome.

Transport causes motion sickness

Moving patients around after giving them an opioid is a potent cause of nausea and vomiting postoperatively. When transporting patients on their trolleys sit your patients up, and face them forward. Turn the trolley from the foot end. Do not swing the head in a wide arc (as occurs in stomach-churning fairground rides) when turning corners. These simple measures reduce vomiting in the first hour after returning to the ward by about half.

Nausea after epidural, or spinal anaesthesia?
Eliminate hypotension.

How to manage nausea and vomiting

Identify those at risk

Not everyone is likely to vomit. Patients at risk of postoperative nausea and vomiting are frequently given anti-emetic drugs before they come to the recovery room and these drugs have side effects. A very common side effect of ondansetron is headache.

Prophylaxis against nausea and vomiting

With high-risk patients, strategies to prevent nausea and vomiting should begin long before the patient comes to the recovery room.

Prolonged preoperative fasting causes *dehydration*. If the patient is not well hydrated during or after anaesthesia they will become hypotensive, especially when you move them. Hypotension is a potent cause of nausea.

Although the optimal fasting period for solid food is 4–6 hours, most patients should be allowed to drink water until 2 hours before their surgery. Water is exponentially cleared from the stomach, half being absorbed within 12 minutes, and it is all gone within 1 hour, leaving behind normal stomach fluids. During the procedure the anaesthetists will give a base line infusion of 15–20 ml/kg of crystalloid fluid, for example Plasma-Lyte®. If the anaesthetist has not given fluid, and your patient is nauseated, then consider giving them an infusion of crystalloid before using anti-emetic drugs.

Once the patient comes to the recovery room, prevent nausea and vomiting by:

+ avoiding hypotension;
+ giving high concentrations of oxygen;
+ treating pain;
+ avoiding sudden movement.

> *Not all patients need PONV prophylaxis but*
> *for patients with risk factors for PONV, it is essential.*

Immediate management

In semi-conscious patients who are about to vomit, roll them on to their side, take their pillows away, and turn their head so that the vomitus can drain from their mouth.

Once they have finished vomiting gently suck out their mouth and pharynx with a wide-bore sucker. Be gentle, or you will stimulate further vomiting.

Patients who are expected to be susceptible to either regurgitation or vomiting after major surgery usually leave the theatre with a nasogastric tube draining freely. A nasogastric tube will not prevent regurgitation, nor reduce the risk of aspiration pneumonia. It may even predispose to regurgitation.

Children

Children are very susceptible to the dystonic side-effects from certain anti-emetic drugs. If it is necessary to use an anti-emetic in children droperidol 20 micrograms/kg is unlikely to cause problems. This drug often stops vomiting, and does not cause prolonged sedation. Ondansetron is also safe to use in children.

Anti-emetic drugs

Anti-emetics include several classes of drugs that relieve the symptoms of nausea and vomiting (for an overview see Table 8.1). There are many controlled studies of the efficacy of anti-emetic drugs, but they often contradict each other, the results are confusing, the trials are bedevilled by problems of *heterogenicity* and some studies are arguably fraudulent. This makes it difficult to arrive at valid conclusions.

The following facts, however, emerge:

- anti-dopaminergic anti-emetics seem to work best against inputs from the vagus nerve;
- anti-cholinergic drugs appear to work best against cholinergic input from the labyrinth (vestibular apparatus) in the ear;
- anti-serotonin (anti-5-HT$_3$) antagonists work well against both but are only effective prophylactically in large doses;
- it is best to give two or three antiemetics from different groups if a patient is high risk for PONV. This is best done prophylactically by the anaesthetist in the OR;
- antiemetic stickers on the drug chart with protocols for the treatment of PONV are useful in PACU.

Table 8.1 Anti-emetic drugs

Group	Drug	Best for
Phenothiazines	Promethazine	Opioid-induced PONV
Antihistamine	Prochlorperazine	Opioid-induced PONV
5-HT$_3$ antagonist	Cyclizine	All PONV
	Ondansetron	Gut and gynaecological surgery
	Granisetron	Major tissue damage
Steroids	Dexamethasone	All PONV
Benzamide	Metoclopramide	Gut and gynaecological surgery
Butyrophenones	Droperidol	All PONV
Anti-cholinergic	Hyoscine	Opioid-induced PONV

Dexamethasone

Dexamethasone is a steroid related to cortisol.[2] It reduces the incidence of postoperative nausea and vomiting while potentiating the effects of other anti-emetics. It has no obvious side-effects. It is given as a single dose at the start of the anaesthetic and should not be repeated.

It's been shown that intravenous dexamethasone provides effective anti-emetic prophylaxis during the first 24 hours postoperatively in patients receiving long-acting neuraxial opioids.[3]

It probably inhibits *prostaglandin* synthesis and gives patients a feeling of well-being. The recommended dose is 150 micrograms/kg for children and 4–8 mg for adults. Since it takes at least 2 hours to work, it is best given on induction of anaesthesia, rather than in the recovery room. Its effect persists for up to 24 hours.

*If the anti-emetic you have given to the patient is not effective,
try one from another group.*

Serotonin antagonists

Serotonin (5-hydroxytryptamine) antagonists include ondansetron, granisetron, dolasetron, and tropisetron. Serotonin is a neurotransmitter involved in activating vagal afferent pathways, principally from the gut and reproductive organs. These drugs are all equally effective and equally safe. They are more effective when used at the end of the anaesthetic, and are the most effective drugs to give if the patient is actually vomiting. Given prophylactically, as it often is, means that the drug is metabolized before the serotonin is released. Cyclizine is an older drug in this group but it can be used instead if you have it.

Repeated doses of the serotonin antagonists are not any more effective. If this first dose is not effective then do not persist; instead use an agent from another class of anti-emetics such as promethazine 12.5 mg.

Granisetron

Granisetron is probably the best of this group of drugs. It is equally if not more effective as ondansetron and has similar side-effects and disadvantages, but granisetron is much cheaper. Furthermore, because it is not metabolized by CYP 2D6 enzymes in the liver, granisetron is less likely to cause drug interactions than other 5-HT$_3$ antagonists. Granisetron 1 mg IV can be given at the end of the anaesthetic, or if not then, in the recovery room. Apart from an occasional annoying headache, granisetron has few side-effects, and it does not cause extrapyramidal syndrome.

Ondansetron

Ondansetron was the first of this group. Give ondansetron 4 mg IV over 90 seconds. Repeat after 5 minutes if necessary. Higher doses are (8mg of ondansetron) are sometimes needed. They are then more likely to cause headache, and disturbed liver function. Ondansetron is more than twice as effective as metoclopramide for treating postoperative nausea and vomiting in intestinal and gynaecological surgery.

Note: both tramadol and ondansetron are metabolized by the liver CYP 2D6 enzymes, if the patient has already taken one, it may aggravate the effects of the other.

Antihistamines

Antihistamines block H$_1$ receptors, in the brain and periphery. Their anti-emetic effect is probably due to their anti-cholinergic blocking activity. Cyclizine and promethazine are two antihistamines without significant anti-dopaminergic activity.

Cyclizine is a safe and most effective anti-emetic against opioid-induced nausea and vomiting, and the dizziness associated with motion sickness (incurred during the trip back to the ward). It is a potent histamine receptor blocker. Cyclizine also has anti-cholinergic properties. It makes patients drowsy, but less so than either prochlorperazine or promethazine. Cyclizine is equally as effective in treating nausea and vomiting as ondansetron but it causes a feeling of light headedness which older patients find unpleasant. Cyclizine is only available in some countries (not in Australia or the USA). The dose is 25–50 mg intravenously in adults and 1 mg/kg IV in children. Later, in the ward, it can be given as a tablet.

Promethazine, an antihistamine (one of the phenothiazine group), is sometimes used to treat nausea and vomiting, but it makes patients drowsy, delays emergence, and can drop their blood pressure by causing peripheral vasodilation. It works mainly through its anticholinergic action on the chemoreceptor trigger zone. The adult dose is 12.5–25 mg IM, 4–6 hourly. It is worth considering 'when all else fails'.

Phenothiazines

Phenothiazines are anti-emetics primarily because, as dopaminergic D_2 antagonists they act on the chemo-trigger receptor zone. They are only slowly cleared as they are long-acting with a half-life of more than 30 hours. In elderly or debilitated patients they are prone to cause hypotension, agitation, apprehension, and sleep disturbance. In addition, extrapyramidal syndrome can be an issue and this is outlined in Box 8.1.

Box 8.1 **Extrapyramidal syndrome**

Children, young adults, and debilitated elderly patients are susceptible to extrapyramidal syndrome (dystonia and nystagmus). This is frightening for the patient, who develops muscle rigidity, and marked oscillations of the eyes, (nystagmus) known as an *oculogyric crisis*. With phenothiazines the incidence is about 0.3 per cent, but a quarter of these reactions occur after a single parenteral dose. Treat this with benzatropine 1 mg IV, and repeat in 10 minutes if necessary.

Prochlorperazine is effective for postoperative nausea and vomiting, particularly if the stimulus is coming from the vestibular apparatus in the ear. An appropriate dose is 0.1–0.2 mg/kg IM, but it causes a dry mouth and its sedative effects make it unsuitable for day case surgery. It is long-acting, so do not repeat the dose in less than 6 hours. Box 8.2 outlines neuroleptic malignant syndrome (NMS).

Box 8.2 **Neuroleptic malignant syndrome**

NMS is a result of extreme dopamine blockade. It occurs when here is an excessive or abnormal response to metoclopramide, droperidol, and phenothiazines such as prochlorperazine, promethazine, and particularly perphenazine. It presents just like quick-onset Parkinson's disease. The patient starts to move slowly (bradykinesia) as their muscles stiffen up, they then become immobile and seem unresponsive. In reality they are locked-in because their vocal cords and voluntary muscles are too stiff to move. They also become febrile, their blood pressure rises and blood tests show muscle damage reflected in a raised plasma phosphokinase (CPK) levels. Neuroleptic malignant syndrome is treated with bromocriptine.

Anti-dopaminergics

Droperidol and metoclopramide are dopamine D_2 antagonists. Do not use them in patients who have Parkinson's disease because they will precipitate rigidity. Anti-dopaminergic drugs can cause an unpredictable *extrapyramidal syndrome*, particularly in children and young women. They also may cause *serotonin syndrome* in patients who are taking selective serotonin reuptake inhibitors (SSRIs). Do not use them in patients taking long-term psychotropic medication—such as lithium or any of the phenothiazines—because they have been reported to cause the *neuroleptic malignant syndrome* (NMS).

Droperidol

Droperidol has strong anti-dopaminergic activity, and blocks input to the chemoreceptor trigger zone. It is an alpha-blocker, and in larger doses causes *postural hypotension*.

Droperidol is among the most effective of the antiemetics, but in higher doses it can cause hypotension and can cause severe *dysphoria* and motor retardation. The dysphoria makes patients feel as though they are locked inside their body where they feel agitated and frightened, yet are unable to tell anyone about it. This horrible effect may persist for 6 or more hours.

> *If the patient has had one dose of droperidol,*
> *do not repeat it.*

The most appropriate antiemetic dose of droperidol is 10–20 micrograms/kg. It is best given at the beginning of the anaesthetic as it takes 1–2 hours to be effective and lasts for about 6 hours. To see droperidol's 'black box warning' see Box 8.3.

Box 8.3 **Droperidol's 'black box warning'**

In December 2001 the American Food and Drug Administration (FDA) issued their highest grade 'black box warning' about the use of droperidol after some reports of deaths from the cardiac arrhythmia torsades de pointes when it was used in high doses. Some authorities convincingly argued this warning was based on flimsy hearsay evidence. No report of an adverse cardiac event has ever been published in a peer-reviewed journal since its introduction for the management of PONV. It is estimated that adverse cardiac events following the use of droperidol is about 74 cases in 11 million. Consequently, the FDA modified its warning to allow droperidol to be used in anaesthesia as an anti-emetic.

Metoclopramide

Metoclopramide has a place in treating nausea and vomiting where the bowel, uterus or ovaries have been manipulated; or after laparoscopy or where blood has been swallowed. Its reputation for being ineffective is due to the inadequate dose of 10 mg often given. The effective dose is 15–20 mg slowly intravenously. In some patients it may cause bradycardia. Do not repeat metoclopramide, try a different anti-emetic drug. Being anti-dopaminergic metoclopramide will precipitate acute parkinsonism in patients taking anti-parkinsonian drugs such as levodopa, or bromocriptine.

Other drugs

Hyoscine

Hyoscine is an anti-cholinergic drug. It blocks the cholinergic muscarinic receptors in the brain and in the periphery. Because it is centrally acting it blocks input from the vestibular apparatus in the ear to the chemoreceptor trigger zone; this makes it effective against motion sickness. Hyoscine is not used very often but it can be given safely to children if they are vomiting after squint or tonsil surgery.

Ephedrine

Ephedrine is sometimes used in day case surgery. A dose of 0.5 mg/kg IM can be very effective. It probably acts by preventing *postural hypotension* but there may be a central mechanism. Keep your patients well hydrated, this will be effective in preventing a drop in blood pressure when you sit them up or move them on the trolley.

Complementary techniques

Acupressure

Acupressure techniques are well worth trying for postoperative nausea and vomiting (Figure 8.2). The pressure point (P6 or Neiguan point) is in the midline on the anterior aspect of the left forearm about a Chinese inch above the proximal skin crease of the wrist. (A Chinese inch is the length of the interphalangeal joint of the thumb.) Firmly probe about with the tip of your thumb between the tendons until you find a point of deep ache. It has to cause an ache to be effective. Press firmly here and the nausea may abate, let go and it will return. Instruct patients to find their own pressure points. Acupressure is ineffective once vomiting has started.

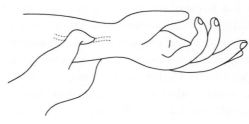

Figure 8.2 Acupressure.

References

1. **Diemunsch P, Joshi GP**, *et al.* (2009) Neurokinin-1 receptor antagonists in the prevention of postoperative nausea and vomiting. *British Journal of Anaesthesia* **103**(1):7–13.
2. **Elston MS, Conaglen HM**, *et al.* (2013) Duration of cortisol suppression following a single dose of dexamethasone in healthy volunteers. *Anaesthesia Intensive Care* **41**:596–601.
3. **Grape S**, *et al.* (2018) Intravenous dexamethasone for prophylaxis of postoperative nausea and vomiting after administration of long-acting neuraxial opioids: a systematic review and meta-analysis. *Anaesthesia* **73**(4):480–489.

Chapter 9

Regional analgesia

Introduction

Patients who have had regional anaesthesia, epidurals, spinals and various nerve blocks come to the recovery room. They may be awake and appear easy to care for, but problems do occur. This chapter will enable you to assist the anaesthetist to insert regional anaesthetics, monitor patients with regional analgesia, identify problems and deal with them.

*The recovery room must be equipped to handle
complications of regional anaesthesia.*

Epidural anaesthesia

Advantages of epidurals

- Epidurals give excellent pain relief from pain in skin and muscle.
- Postoperative nausea and vomiting is minimized.
- Epidural blockade reduces the bad effects of postoperative stress syndrome.
- Wounds heal faster, wound infections are less prevalent, and the metabolic insults caused by surgery are less.
- Deep vein thrombosis and pulmonary emboli are reduced because the blood flow through the lower body and legs is increased.
- Low-dose aspirin (100 mg) daily is unlikely to cause problems with bleeding into the epidural space.
- They improve blood flow to the legs following vascular surgery, and reduce the rate of graft occlusion.
- Dressings and other surgical manipulations can be done without causing pain or requiring additional analgesia.

Disadvantages of epidurals

- They may cause *postural hypotension*, in which case the patient will feel faint or nauseated when they try to sit up.
- They cannot be used in patients who have recently received *low molecular-weight heparins* (LMWH), dabigatran or who are anticoagulated with warfarin and have an INR > 1.2. They should not be placed in patients with a platelet count of less than 100.

- Low-dose aspirin (less than 100 mg) daily is unlikely to cause problems with bleeding into the *epidural space*.
- Patients must have a urinary catheter, because they will not know when their bladder is full.
- Pressure sores can become a problem if the patient lies in one position for too long. You will need to help adjust the patient's position to relieve pressure areas every 30 minutes.
- Continuous epidural infusions need specifically designed pumps.
- Patients must receive supplemental oxygen.
- The patient must have an intravenous drip running.
- Education of those caring for patients with epidurals. In some hospitals this means admission to a high dependency unit.

Looking after a patient with an epidural

If your patient feels nauseated, check his blood pressure. It often means they are becoming hypotensive. Increase the rate of the IV infusion. Give oxygen. Lift their legs on to pillows; but never tip the patient head down. Epidural opioids also cause nausea and vomiting. Check the blood pressure before giving antiemetics. Have ephedrine 30 mg diluted in 10 ml of normal saline close by when you are looking after these patients. If the blood pressure drops, give a 2 ml (6 mg) bolus.

Nausea warns of hypotension.

Dermatomes

Dermatomes are areas on the skin innervated by a spinal sensory nerve originating in a single posterior spinal segment. They are labelled sequentially: cervical C1–5, thoracic T1–10, lumbar L1–5, and sacral S1–4. As they enter the spinal cord, each sensory nerve trunk usually contains separate fibres that spread out to enter their own spinal segment. Dermatomes overlap considerably at their edges, as shown in Figure 9.1.

Useful landmarks

Useful dermatome landmarks are S1, which is the groin area; T10, which is the level of the umbilicus (think of it as the 0 in T10); and the tip of the xiphisternum is at the level of T6 (Figure 9.1). Once the local anaesthetic reaches T5 it starts to affect the sympathetic outflow to the heart, which may cause the blood pressure to fall. The intercostal muscles necessary for coughing are served by motor fibres from T1–10, the muscles and skin in the arms from C5–8, while C3, C4, and C5 'keep the diaphragm alive' (the phrenic nerve).

If a spinal or epidural is causing tingling or weakness in your patient's arms or hands it has reached the cervical level. Monitor them carefully, because they may complain they are finding it difficult to breathe. Sitting them up is helpful.

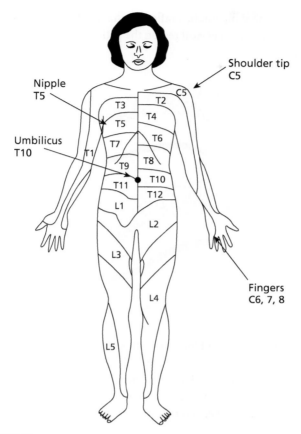

Figure 9.1 Dermatomes.

Problems with high blocks

Local anaesthetic is soaked up by nerves in much the same way as ink is soaked up by blotting paper. The initial spread of local anaesthetic in the *epidural space* is affected by the position of the patient. If the patient is sitting up, then most of the local anaesthetic solution will sink to the bottom of the *epidural space*, affecting the dermatomes in the lower part of the body.

> *If a patient with an epidural cannot cough effectively then notify the anaesthetist immediately.*

If you immediately lay the patient flat, the local anaesthetic moves along the epidural space towards the nerves serving the upper body (Figure 9.2). Fortunately the spine is S-shaped, and the local anaesthetic is unlikely to rise up the thoracic curve. However, should you tip patients head down, the local anaesthetic progressively anaesthetizes the intercostal muscles making it more and more difficult for the patient to breathe. Once it reaches T4, it blocks the sympathetic outflow to the heart so that the cardiac output falls, and should it reach the upper cervical region the patient will be completely paralysed and unable to breathe.

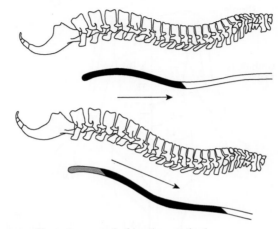

Figure 9.2 How posture affects the spread of local anaesthetic.

Anaesthetists adjust the dose of local anaesthetic they inject into the space to catch the nerves to the painful area. After a single shot of local anaesthetic, it takes about 10 minutes for the anaesthetic to fully soak into the nerves. Warning signs the block is too high are that the patient finds it hard to take a deep breath; or more alarmingly their arms become weak or their little fingers go numb.

> *Do not tip patients with an*
> *epidural head down.*

How to test the level of block

Use ice to test the level of a block because the sensations of cold travel in the same nerve pathways as pain. Put a piece of ice in a disposable glove and touch your patient's forehead with it so that they know what to expect. Then starting at T2, just under the clavicle, slowly move the ice down until the patient says the sensation has changed—this is the level of the block.

Never test for pain with pinpricks, because you will damage the skin and may introduce infection—and quite justifiably, when the epidural wears off the patient will complain about the pinpricks.

What to monitor

Pain score

Use the linear pain analogue to monitor a pain score. Check pain when the patient is at rest, when they are moving about the bed, and when they deep breathe and cough. The therapeutic aim is that the patient has no pain at rest.

Blood pressure and pulse

The anaesthetist will set the parameters for blood pressure and pulse on the epidural order sheet. Check that these limits are still appropriate before discharging the patient to the ward.

Level of the block

Unless the block is sufficiently high the patient will experience breakthrough pain. For most abdominal operations this level is about T6 and for surgery below the waist about T8.

Motor power

Record the patient's ability to bend each their legs at the knee, and waggle their feet up and down. Any deterioration of this ability may be an early warning sign of a developing epidural abscess or haematoma.

Sedation score

There are many sedation scores, but the most useful is the one used on the recovery room assessment score sheet.

How to rescue breakthrough pain

If the patient is in pain, the first priority is to rescue the patient. With breakthrough pain it may be possible for the anaesthetist to give a 5 ml bolus of 2 per cent lidocaine, and increase the infusion rate in increments of 4 ml up to a maximum of 20 ml/hr. If this fails the anaesthetist may elect to use an alternative block, or offer other analgesics.

Problems with epidurals

When to notify the anaesthetist

The local anaesthetic may extend beyond the intended area, or the opioid may cause respiratory depression. Both events can cause problem, notify the anaesthetist if the patient:

- block reaches T4 level—the nipple line;
- complains of weakness in their arms or numbness in their hands or little fingers;
- has difficulty in taking a deep breath or coughing;
- blood pressure falls by more than 20%;
- pain remains unrelieved, or skips certain areas;
- respiratory rate falls to 10 breaths/min or less.

Hypotension

The local anaesthetic blocks the sympathetic outflow serving the lower body. The consequent arteriolar vasodilation will cause the blood pressure to fall. Once the local anaesthetic reaches thoracic T4 level it will totally block the sympathetic outflow to the heart. When this occurs the heart cannot increase its output to prevent the blood pressure falling.

Avoid epidurals in patients with aortic or mitral stenosis, hypertrophic obstructive cardiomyopathies, cardiac *tamponade*, or restrictive pericarditis because they will become alarmingly hypotensive.

Do not overlook other causes for hypotension such as bleeding or volume depletion. If the patient has cold hands this is a highly suspicious sign of another cause for the hypotension. If the patient's blood pressure falls by more than 20 mmHg when you sit them up at 45° then suspect they are bleeding or hypovolaemic.

Nausea is an early warning sign that the blood pressure may be falling. Check the blood pressure. Lay your patient flat. Lift their legs onto a pillow. DO NOT TIP YOUR PATIENT HEAD DOWN. Increase the intravenous infusion rate and prepare to give a dose of ephedrine.

How to manage hypotension

Hypotension usually occurs within 10–15 minutes of a top-up. If the patient's blood pressure falls by more than 20 mmHg then lay the patient flat, and lift their legs on to pillows. Never tip the patient head down. Give oxygen and infuse 250–500 ml of IV fluid, e.g. Plasma-Lyte®.

If the blood pressure does not rise give ephedrine. Dilute ephedrine 30 mg in 10 ml of sterile saline and give 6 mg (2 ml) increments every 2 minutes until the blood pressure returns to a safe level. Monitor the blood pressure every 5 minutes to ensure the hypotension does not recur.

Respiratory depression

Respiratory depression can occur when the patient has received an opioid in their epidural. The incidence of respiratory depression is about 0.2–0.4 per cent. It can occur within 30 minutes, or be delayed for any time up to 24 hours. Typically, the patient's respiratory rate falls slowly to 6–8 breaths/min (or even less) over an hour or more. The patient becomes drowsy, sweaty, and may even become cyanosed. Respiratory depression usually outlasts the analgesia. Respiratory depression may develop up to 2 hours after a single dose of fentanyl. Keep patients under close supervision for at least 3 hours after epidural fentanyl.

Use smaller doses of opioid where there is an increased risk of respiratory depression, such as in the elderly, the very frail or in patients with significant chronic obstructive airway disease. If the patient is receiving opioids into the *epidural space* never use intravenous or intramuscular opioids, because the patient may stop breathing.

> *Epidural opioids exclude
> the use of systemic opioids.*

Delayed respiratory depression is more likely with morphine than more highly lipid-soluble opioids such as fentanyl. Instead of quickly binding to opioid receptors in the spinal cord, morphine remains in solution in the *cerebrospinal fluid* (CSF). As the CSF slowly circulates, the dissolved morphine moves up to the brainstem where it may depress the respiratory centres.

Once the patient's respiratory rate falls to 10 breaths/min, attach a pulse oximeter, and check for signs of hypoxia. Treat respiratory depression if the respiratory rate falls below 8 breaths/min or the oxygen saturations fall below 94 per cent. Naloxone 100–200 micrograms intravenously will usually cause an immediate improvement, but it only lasts for 30 minutes. For established opioid induced respiratory depression use a naloxone infusion: it will require about 10 micrograms/kg/hr intravenously. This dose reverses the analgesic effects of morphine, but not necessarily the analgesia of epidural fentanyl.

Postdural puncture headache

The dural membrane can be punctured if the epidural needle is advanced too far. Once punctured, the CSF continues to leak into the epidural space, putting tension on blood vessels around the brain and spinal cord causing a severe headache. Accidental dural puncture occurs in 1 to 2 per cent of epidural blocks. It is less common with an experienced anaesthetist.

Large-bore needles are more likely to cause headache than smaller ones. Typically the patient gets an excruciatingly severe frontal headache, which gets worse when the patient moves, or tries to sit up. Diagnostically, it is relieved when the patient lies flat. Other features include photophobia, nausea and even vomiting.

If the headache does not resolve with simple measures such as hydration and analgesia within 4 hours, then it may be necessary to stop the leak with a *blood patch* (see Box 9.1). Sumatriptan, a 5HT agonist, could be given as an early option. Also try caffeine but most patients will require a blood patch.

Box 9.1 **Blood patch to control headaches**

Although dural puncture during epidural anaesthesia is uncommon in experienced hands, there is an overall incidence of 1–4 per cent. To plug the hole in the dura 10–20 ml of blood is taken from the patient's arm and injected into the epidural space at the level of the skin hole. Lay the patient flat for 2 hours. The blood will clot over the hole to block the leak. In most cases the headache eases almost immediately.

The procedure needs two operators; one takes blood from the patient's arm, while the other locates the epidural space. Use the strictest of sterile precautions. Infection of the clot in the epidural space risks abscess formation and irreversible paraplegia could follow.

Do not use a blood patch if the patient has unexplained neurological symptoms; any sepsis or chance of sepsis (such as immediately after urological or bowel surgery or draining an abscess), or localized sepsis near the site of injection.

Patchy epidurals or one-sided blocks

Sometimes epidural analgesia skips segments, yet everything around the area may be numb. The block may extend beyond the intended dermatomes.

In some people the epidural space is broken up into compartments by thin membranes which causes erratic spread of the local anaesthetic. Furthermore patients who have had previous epidurals may have the scars from old blood clots in their epidural space that prevent the local anaesthetic spreading correctly.

If the local anaesthetic does not diffuse uniformly enough to soak into the nerve roots within 5 minutes, then sometimes simply rolling the patient so that the unblocked side is downwards fixes the problem.

Occasionally a *unilateral block* occurs where one side of the affected area is analgesic and the other side is not adequately blocked. Usually this is caused by septa or scarring inside the epidural space. Simply rolling the patient so that their unaffected side is downwards often solves the problem. Gravity encourages the local anaesthetic to flow down to reach the nerves.

Bloody tap

Sometimes the needle penetrates an epidural vein. Blood then comes back into the syringe. In this case the needle is withdrawn and the epidural re-attempted in an adjacent space.

Itch

Morphine commonly causes itch. With fentanyl, the itch is minimal.

Risks of epidurals

Nerve damage

Although some patients complain of patchy areas of skin numbness for up to 6 weeks after an epidural anaesthetic, major neurological sequelae are rare. The big risk of neurological damage occurs with epidural haematoma or infection, or in attempts to place an epidural in a patient who has already had a laminectomy where the *epidural space* no longer exists.

Backache

Backache is common after spinal and epidural anaesthetics (Figure 9.3). Recovery room staff can help prevent this by supporting the lumbar arch with a small pillow, or a rolled-up towel to prevent the arch sagging and unintentionally stretching the interspinous ligaments. The lumbar spine has a natural arch. Once the epidural takes effect the muscles sustaining the arch lose their protective tone, the arch sags and stretches these ligaments. Although you are unlikely to encounter it in the recovery room, always remember that back pain is also a sign of potentially disastrous epidural haematoma or infection.

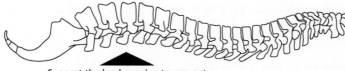

Support the lumbar spine to prevent
stretching of the ligaments

Figure 9.3 How to prevent post-epidural back pain.

Epidural haematoma

Bleeding into the epidural space is a grave but fortunately rare complication. Alarmingly, with the introduction of the newer anticoagulants the incidence of epidural haematomas is increasing.

Haematomas are more likely in elderly women undergoing hip or knee replacements, but particularly if they have been given low molecular-weight heparins such as enoxaparin or dalteparin as prophylaxis against deep vein thrombosis.

The epidural space is not empty; it is filled with an engorged network of venous plexuses and scattered fatty tissue. Continued bleeding into the confined space will compress the spinal cord and unless this is recognized and treated the patient will become paraplegic. To have a reasonable chance of complete or partial neurological recovery, surgical decompression must be performed as soon as possible and certainly within 8 hours.

Spinal cord compression
is an emergency.

The signs and symptoms of spinal cord compression are:

- the onset of new, severe or persistent back pain;
- tingling or persistent numbness in the legs;
- muscle weakness in the lower limbs;
- urinary or faecal incontinence.

A recently reported sign of a developing haematoma is that the patient's sensory block alters to become denser, which is soon followed by a progressive motor block leading to a point where the patient cannot move their legs.

It is critically important to notify the anaesthetist immediately if you notice any back pain, or any deterioration in the patient's motor or sensory function. Your hospital's epidural protocols must have provision to 'red flag' these events and automatically obtain an urgent MRI or computed tomography (CT) myelogram and immediate neurosurgical referral. Unfortunately these signs of a developing haematoma are absent in 20 per cent of cases.

Epidural infections

Infection is a rare but devastating complication. If bacteria, especially staphylococci or streptococci, get into the space they can produce an abscess. The signs are similar to epidural haematomas with the added sign of a possible fever and raised white cell count.

Epidural abscesses are more likely in diabetics, immune-compromised patients, those on steroid therapy, where the patient has already been in hospital for more than 48 hours before the catheter was placed, and where the catheter is to be left in for longer than 3 days. You may need to start appropriate antibiotic prophylaxis in the recovery room in patients with these risk factors.

Total spinal

If the tip of the epidural needle is advanced too far it will pierce the dural mater, and CSF will gush back into the syringe. If this dural tap is not recognized, and more than a few millilitres of local anaesthetic is accidentally injected into the CSF it causes total spinal anaesthesia. The patient abruptly collapses, loses consciousness, becomes unresponsive to pain, develops widely dilated pupils, profound hypotension, and stops breathing. With urgent intubation, ventilation and ionotropic support and dopamine to maintain the blood pressure, and with suitable care the patient usually recovers with no sequelae within 24 hours. Fortunately total spinal anaesthesia is rare, and at worst most dural taps cause a postdural puncture headache.

Local anaesthetic toxicity

There is a risk of toxicity if local anaesthetic is injected into an epidural vein. Should enough local anaesthetic reach the heart or brain it will rapidly cause coma and cardiac failure. The patient's blood pressure falls and they lose consciousness (signs and treatment of toxicity are outlined in Table 9.1). Bupivacaine especially can cause 'stone heart' where the heart simply stops and remains unresponsive. This may respond to intravenous infusion of lipid emulsions (Intralipid®), however if this fails cardiac bypass may be required for several hours.

Table 9.1 Signs and treatment of toxicity

Stage	Signs	Treatment
1	Numbness of face, visual disturbances, confusion	Give oxygen by mask; encourage deep breathing; summon help
2	1	Turn into coma position; clear airway, assist breathing; attach oximeter and ECG; check pulse and BP
3	Convulsions	Thiopental 1–3 mg IV
4	Hypotension	Give IV fluids, inotropes

The earliest feature of systemic toxicity is numbness or tingling of the tongue and around the mouth. The patient may become light-headed, anxious, or drowsy, with slurred speech or complain of tinnitus.

Epidural infusions

Patients find continuous epidural infusion highly effective to control acute pain after surgery to the chest, abdomen, pelvis or lower limbs. Once an infusion is established measure the vital signs: blood pressure, pulse and respiratory rate, and oxygen saturation every 10 minutes for the first hour. Watch carefully for any trends in patients' respiratory rates especially if they have been given epidural opioids. Once patients are pain-free encourage them to deep breathe and cough. Record the neurological signs of pupil size and reaction to light, and the level of consciousness.

With specifically trained nursing staff, clear protocols, and anaesthetic staff on duty in the hospital epidural analgesia can be continued quite safely in the ward.

Although epidural infusions are generally safe, there is always the possibility of adverse events including respiratory depression, hypotension, epidural haematoma or abscess. When you transfer a patient with an epidural to the ward ensure that:

- there are clearly written protocols. Your hospital should have a standard form, with precise limits for vital signs and infusion rates. The form needs clear instructions on what to do if the limits are exceeded;
- your handover to the ward staff follows the guidelines;
- if opioids are used then a stat dose of naloxone is ordered in the drug chart;
- the epidural system is completely closed and must not be breached;
- the epidural lines are clearly identified with the yellow marker tag;
- there are always suitably trained nursing staff on the ward to monitor the patient closely;
- the ward has facilities for resuscitation, and that there is a resuscitation team available at all times;
- suitably trained medical staff are on-call and nearby.

How to remove an epidural catheter

- Wait until at least 12 hours have elapsed since the last dose of enoxaparin or dalteparin.
- Ease the catheters out gently.
- If you meet resistance, then call for skilled assistance. These fine catheters can occasionally break off in the epidural space while being removed.
- Once you have removed the catheter make sure it is intact, and record this fact in the patient's notes.
- Apply a dressing over the hole.
- If a piece of catheter is left behind usually it causes no problems, but the patient must be warned in writing, because it can become a focus for infection at any time in the future.

Drugs used for epidural analgesia

Local anaesthetic drugs anaesthetise the somatic nerves as they leave the spinal cord, and the opioids interrupt the transmission of pain impulses within the spinal cord itself. This gives analgesia for the incision, the nearby skin, and muscle, and will almost completely relieve postoperative pain. Ill-defined deep visceral pain from the organs may persist, because visceral pain impulses are transmitted through the vagus nerve, and do not travel in the spinal cord.

The choice of drugs used for analgesia depends on the indication for the epidural. Bupivacaine and epidural opioids are the agents most frequently used drugs. Lidocaine is too short-acting to be useful for postoperative analgesia.

To avoid the inconvenience of continually having to top up the epidural use a volumetric pump to infuse epidural opioids when the patient returns to the ward.

Bupivacaine

Bupivacaine hydrochloride is an amide local anaesthetic. Compared to lidocaine it has a relatively slow onset, but a long action. In a single shot it lasts 3–4 hours for epidural block, and may last 12–24 or more hours with brachial plexus and some other nerve blocks. It is more cardiotoxic than lidocaine or ropivacaine. The maximum dose is 2 mg/kg.

Ropivacaine

Ropivacaine is an amide local anaesthetic chemically closely related to bupivacaine, but it is less lipid soluble, less toxic and less potent. It is cleared from the body 40 per cent faster than bupivacaine. The maximum safe dose is about 3 mg/kg. It does not act for as long as bupivacaine.

Fentanyl

Fentanyl is the most commonly used opioid in epidural anaesthesia. It comes in pre-prepared packs in concentrations of 2–4 micrograms/ml infused at 5–15 ml/hr with one or other of the local anaesthetic agents. Since it does not cause a motor block it allows the patient to move around after surgical procedures, and deep breathe and cough. Because fentanyl causes neither sympathetic blockade nor peripheral vasodilation, it should not cause hypotension. Profound respiratory depression, however, can occur as much as 2 hours after a single dose of epidural fentanyl. Patients should be under close observation for at least 3 hours after a dose of epidural fentanyl.

Diamorphine

Diamorphine 50–100 micrograms/ml infused at 5–15 ml/hr is used in the United Kingdom but not elsewhere.

Other blocks

Intercostal blocks

Intercostal blocks give pain relief after upper abdominal operations such as cholecystectomy and thoracotomy. The patient lies with the side to be blocked uppermost and 2–3 ml of local anaesthetic with adrenaline are infiltrated behind each rib into the neurovascular groove. The two main dangers are accidental puncture of the pleura causing a pneumothorax, and intravascular injection of local anaesthetic causing toxicity.

Thoracic paravertebral blocks

Thoracic paravertebral blocks are useful to relieve the pain of thoracotomy. A catheter is placed in the paravertebral space and may be left in for up to 5 days. The risk of infection is less than a catheter in the epidural space.

Transversus abdominis block (TAP block)

The transverse abdominis plane can be located using ultrasound and a diluted solution of local anaesthetic injected giving effective analgesia for many laparoscopic procedures.[1] If you have a patient with this block they may not experience any pain in the recovery room but they must be warned that the block will wear off and given adequate non-steroidal anti-inflammatories (NSAIDs) or similar oral medication to take in the ward or when they leave the hospital.

Brachial plexus blocks

Brachial plexus blocks are useful for upper limb surgery. There are two approaches, the axillary and the supraclavicular. Both are effective, but the supraclavicular approach carries a high risk of pneumothorax and nerve damage. Horner's syndrome is occasionally seen after a supraclavicular block. With fully successful blocks patients lose all muscle power in their arms. Since biceps flexion is sometimes spared, warn patients not to bend their arm or try to look at their hand, because it might fly out of control and hit them in the face. If the patient has a plaster on their arm, they can break their nose. Bupivacaine may cause the block to last for 18 hours or more. Use long-acting local anaesthetics only if such a long-lasting effect is required.

Intra-articular local anaesthetics

Arthroscopies can be painful and bupivacaine injected into the joint space provides effective analgesia. Patients should not be discharged until one hour after intra-articular injection of bupivacaine, because peak plasma levels are delayed by slow absorption from the joint, and any side-effects may take this long to become apparent.[2]

Spinal anaesthesia

Spinal anaesthetics are rarely inserted in the recovery room, but many patients will have them for their surgery, and come to the recovery room still affected by them.

Spinal (intrathecal) anaesthesia has many features in common with epidural anaesthesia, but there are some differences. Epidurals can be topped up whereas spinals cannot. Spinals are used for many operations below the waist and provide good conditions for painful procedures. It is the anaesthetic of choice for elective Caesarean sections, and transurethral prostate resection. Spinal anaesthesia is sometimes used for surgery on premature babies and reduces the incidence of life-threatening apnoea.

Spinal anaesthesia is safe, and complications are few. As with epidural anaesthesia backache may be a problem, and mild pain can last for a week or so after the injection. The principal reason for backache, as it is with epidural anaesthesia, is inadequate support of the lumbar arch during and after surgery.

Criteria for discharging a patient after a spinal

It is not always possible for recovery rooms to keep otherwise stable patients until their spinal block has worn off. Because the sensation of cold and pain are carried in similar neural pathways you can easily test the level of sensory block with a piece of ice. The patient can be discharged to the ward if the level of sensory blockade is below T10 (the umbilicus) and the patient's cardiovascular and surgical state is otherwise stable and adequate. The nurses on the ward must be experienced in looking after patients with a spinal anaesthetic, and must know how to respond to various complications that might arise (for a protocol for ward care of the patient after spinal anaesthetic see Box 9.2).

Box 9.2 A protocol for ward care of the patient after spinal anaesthetic

Standard post-anaesthetic observations

Sensation should return within 4 hours. If after 4 hours the patient remains numb, and there are no 'pin-and-needles' sensations, notify the anaesthetist immediately because delayed return of feeling is a warning sign of epidural haematoma.

Analgesia. Severe pain may return suddenly once the spinal block has worn off. Give analgesia at the first complaint of pain.

Fasting. Fasting is not necessary unless it is a surgical requirement, such as after abdominal operations.

Posture. The patient should be able to sit up as soon as the analgesia has worn off.

Ambulation. If not surgically contraindicated, the patient may get out of bed 2 hours after the return of normal sensation, but only with assistance. Before getting the patient out of bed, sit him up slowly and check his blood pressure. If the systolic blood pressure falls more than 20 mmHg, or if the patient feels faint, dizzy or nauseated, then lie the patient down again.

Potential complications

Postural hypotension. Lie the patient in bed, and notify the anaesthetic registrar on duty who will increase the fluid intake.

Urinary retention. Encourage the patient to void when sensation returns. If the patient has not voided within 4 hours, or his bladder can be palpated, he will require a catheter.

Obviously if the patient is going home the spinal block must have worn off and the patient must be able to walk and void. In most units this means in most day case surgery spinal anaesthetic is only used for morning cases.

References

1. **De Oliveira GS Jr, Fitzgerald PC**, *et al.* (2011) A dose-ranging study of the effect of transversus abdominis block. *Anesthesia and Analgesia* **113**(5):1218–1225.
2. **Noyes FR** (2012) Intraarticular pain pump causes chondrolysis. *American Journal of Bone and Joint Surgery* **94**:1448–1457.

Chapter 10

Special problems

Allergy

Allergy is an immunological response to foreign molecules. It is marked by urticarial rash (hives), oedema of the face, wheeze, and if severe, hypotension. Allergic responses are not common in the recovery room, but may be serious when they do occur. The most severe manifestation of allergy is anaphylaxis.

Types of allergic response

There are three types of allergic response: immediate, intermediate and late.

Immediate response

Onset 0–1 hour: anaphylaxis and anaphylactoid response are the most severe. They present with hypotension, laryngeal oedema causing stridor or hoarse voice, wheezing, urticaria and hypotension.

An immediate allergic response
is a medical emergency.

Intermediate response

Onset 1–72 hours: urticaria, angio-oedema, laryngeal oedema with stridor, and wheezing.

Stridor is an emergency.

Late response

Onset after 72 hours: morbilliform rash, haemolytic anaemia, thrombocytopenia, neutropenia, and interstitial nephritis. Variations of this late response are called the Stevens–Johnson syndrome, and serum sickness.

How to avoid problems

Many drugs cause allergic responses including antibiotics, radio-contrast media and muscle relaxants. Even reactions to chlorhexidine are increasingly being reported.

Give intravenous drugs cautiously and slowly. Watch the patient's face and breathing. If the patient gasps or coughs this may forewarn of a developing allergic response. Although this sign is not present on every occasion, it is a useful warning. If there is any hypotension or wheezing after a patient has received a drug then consider anaphylaxis. If this happens notify the anaesthetist.

Many drugs given intravenously cause a red flare to run up the vein. This is usually just a local reaction caused by histamine release. If the patient develops a motley or hive-like rash then consider allergy.

Penicillin allergy

Many patients report they are allergic to penicillins. The actual prevalence is difficult to establish, but deaths from penicillin allergy are rare.

Patients' reports of penicillin allergy are unreliable, and usually arise from some vaguely remembered incident in the past. Often it was simply an unpleasant reaction, such as pain at the site of the injection, or nausea, or feeling faint or bowel upsets. This of course is not allergy, but from then on the patient is labelled 'allergic to penicillin', which may unnecessarily deprive them of this life-saving group of drugs. One in twenty patients who are truly allergic to penicillin, are also allergic to cephalosporins.

Latex allergy

Latex allergy is a major occupational health problem among exposed people. Allergy to natural rubber latex (NRL), commonly referred to as latex, was an uncommon occurrence before 1980. Since then latex allergy has become a major occupational health problem to those who work in hospitals.

Latex is ubiquitous in the domestic and hospital environment. In hospitals latex is found in gloves, infusion ports on intravenous sets, caps on drug vials, mattress covers—the list is long, varied and seemingly endless.

It affects up to 10 per cent of exposed workers and about 2.5 per cent of the general population. The symptoms of latex allergy range from mild local skin erythema after wearing latex gloves, through the range of reactions of urticaria, conjunctivitis, angio-oedema, and asthma, to a full-blown anaphylactic reaction.

Sensitized workers must have a safe environment. Non-sensitized people should use low-allergen powdered gloves, or better still use only powder-free latex gloves or gloves made from non-latex material.

It is important your recovery room and operating theatres have a carefully researched protocol on how to manage patients and staff allergic to latex. Establish a database of known latex-free products, and keep a stock of these in the operating theatre suite.

How to manage patients with latex allergy

- Clearly identify patients and staff with latex allergies.
- Remove all latex products from the vicinity of affected patients.
- Use only latex-free products.
- Tightly enclose equipment known to contain latex with plastic sheeting.
- Have a tray with suitable drugs available to treat any reaction should it occur.
- Report a reaction if it occurs. There should be a special form for this.

Delayed emergence

Some patients take a long time to fully emerge from their anaesthetics. There are many reasons for this; most are benign, but a few are serious (for some practical points about delayed emergence see Box 10.1).

Box 10.1 **Practical points about delayed emergence**

1. Everyone who is not brain damaged, will wake up—eventually.
2. The fewer drugs you use to achieve this, the safer it is for the patient.
3. Never use painful stimuli to rouse the patient, because they are not asleep, they are in a coma.
4. Nerve stimulators hurt. Do not use them on conscious patients.

Be aware that children having a TIVA anaesthetic may have a delayed emergence.

Why patients have postoperative apnoea

Hyperventilation-induced apnoea

The residual effects of intraoperative opioids, volatile agents and sedatives (such as midazolam) can all suppress patients' ventilation, but the commonest cause of post-operative apnoea is the inadvertent hyperventilation of the patient during the anaesthetic. Volatile agents raise the *apnoeic threshold*; this means that patients' medullary respiratory centres do not respond to rising arterial pressures of carbon dioxide ($PaCO_2$).

To treat hyperventilation-induced apnoea the anaesthetist may simply ventilate the patient at a lower tidal volume until their $PaCO_2$ increases enough to stimulate breathing again. This may take 15 to 20 minutes. Never leave the patient apnoeic, because they may become hypoxic. The brain, having little capacity to buffer abrupt pH changes, will be affected by a rapidly rising $PaCO_2$.

How much oxygen is too much oxygen? A recent meta-analysis shows significantly higher mortality with excessive use of high-flow oxygen in compromised patients.[1]

Hypothermia

Hypothermia increases the effects of the volatile agents, antagonizes the reversal of muscle relaxants, and delays drug *metabolism*.

Hypercapnoea

In a hypoventilating patient as the $PaCO_2$ rises above 70 mmHg (9.21 kPa) the patient becomes increasingly comatose.

Prolonged action of other drugs

Some patients are very sensitive to anaesthetic drugs. If the patient is cold, or has liver or renal disease, they will be slow to metabolize or excrete anaesthetic drugs.

Patients should progressively lighten from their anaesthetic in an orderly sequence. Look at the patient's eyes. Initially their pupils will not react to light and be about 2 mm in diameter. They may be eccentrically set in the iris. Next the pupils will start to react to light. Then the direction of gaze becomes divergent, and finally just before the patient wakes, the pupils dilate slightly (Figure 10.1). The process may take anywhere from a few minutes to 45 minutes or so. If the progress stops, then consider the more serious causes of delayed emergence.

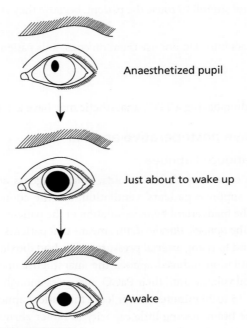

Anaesthetized pupil

Just about to wake up

Awake

Figure 10.1 Eyes' signs on emergence.

Check the history for drug interactions that may delay emergence; for instance, erythromycin prolongs the effect of midazolam for many hours; droperidol prolongs the effect of benzodiazepines (especially diazepam).

Naloxone rapidly reverses the effects of opioids. Proceed cautiously because you may well precipitate agonizing pain. Start with a dose of 1.5 micrograms/kg and repeat it in 2 minutes if necessary. Naloxone works for about 30 minutes. Once it wears off the remaining opioid may re-exert its respiratory depressant effects.

Benzodiazepines

Benzodiazepines have varying *half-lives*. The effect of diazepam 10 mg lasts as long in hours as the patient's age in years, so for an 80-year-old the diazepam would still affect their mental processing 80 hours after the dose. This does not necessarily mean the patient is sedated, but it certainly means their conditioned reflexes are affected to the extent that they should not drive a car. Smaller doses are cleared more quickly.

Midazolam is cleared ten times faster than diazepam. Midazolam has an elimination half-life of 1 to 3 hours. Men metabolize it more slowly than women, and the elderly, children, and adolescents metabolize it more slowly than other adults.

Flumazenil reverses benzodiazepines. It only works for 35–45 minutes, so it may need repeating, because most of the benzodiazepines, such as diazepam, have a longer action. Give flumazenil 3–5 micrograms/kg intravenously over 15 seconds. Be careful, because in susceptible people this drug may cause convulsions. Susceptible people include those with epilepsy, head injuries, cerebrovascular disease, or who are febrile.

Brain damage

A serious complication, and sometimes a cause of delayed emergence from anaesthesia, is neurological damage caused by hypoxia, stroke, fat or gas emboli, or intraoperative hypotension. Water overload after prostate surgery or uterine endoscopic procedures can cause coma or hemiparesis. Consider occult head injury or alcohol poisoning in trauma patients who are slow to wake up. A stroke following a carotid endarterectomy requires immediate re-operation.

How to tell if there is brain damage

If a comatose patient does not move one side of their body, or is rigid only on one side, has an asymmetrical face with their mouth drooping in one corner, or has a dilated or non-reacting pupil only on one side, then these lateralizing signs indicate brain damage. Seek help immediately. Occasionally you will need to give a painful stimulus to evoke a lateralizing sign. An effective way to this is to take the skin over patient's triceps muscle between your thumb and forefinger and squeeze firmly. This should evoke a withdrawal response. Do not rub your knuckles up and down their sternum, squeeze their ear, or press on their orbital ridge, because you will bruise your patient, and certainly cause their intracranial pressure to rise.

Lateralizing signs suggest
structural brain damage.

Other signs of possible brain damage are a change in the rate or pattern of breathing, especially if it becomes deep and sighing. A bilateral up-going plantar response is normal in patients emerging from anaesthesia, but if one toe goes up, while the other goes down, then you have a lateralizing sign.

Residual relaxant

Anaesthetists use neuromuscular blocking drugs to paralyse skeletal muscle so that the surgeon can get at the surgical site, and also to make it easier to ventilate patients. Deep anaesthesia achieves the same result, but also depresses the cardiac output.

The effects of muscle relaxants sometimes persist or recur in the recovery room. The best sign that patients' muscle relaxation is reversed adequately is their ability to lift their head from the pillow, and hold it up for 5 seconds (5-second head lift test). They must be able to do this before you discharge them from the recovery room. If you are concerned about residual relaxation, the straight leg lift, coughing and a firm handgrip (but only offer the patient two of your fingers otherwise you may be hurt) are all tests of recovered muscle power.

Although commonly used, asking patients to 'Stick out your tongue' is a useless test of muscle power, and of no help in assessing airway competence.

If patients are still partially paralysed their arms flop and jerk like a rag-doll when they try to move, they can look like 'a fish out of water' and they may complain of double vision. You will see tracheal tug as their larynx jerks downward every time they attempt to breathe in. You may see the strap muscles in their neck contract as they recruit them to breathe in. Fortunately, respiratory muscles are the last affected by muscle relaxants. Most patients can breathe adequately even though their skeletal muscles are floppy, and they are unable to cough effectively. Even if their oxygen saturation and respiration appear unaffected the patient is often very anxious.

If patients are struggling to breathe, or starting to panic, then support their breathing with a bag and mask, attach an oximeter and an ECG, and summon the anaesthetist.

Why muscle relaxants persist

There are many reasons why muscle relaxants fail to reverse properly. These include:

- over-dosage of relaxant drug;
- hypothermia;
- liver or renal disease delaying their excretion;
- hypokalaemia;
- concurrent use of certain antibiotics such as gentamicin or neomycin;
- intercurrent diseases affecting nerves and muscles such as myasthenia gravis, carcinomatous or alcoholic myopathy or motor neurone diseases.

What to do

Sugammadex is the drug of choice for the reversal of residual muscle relaxation for patients who have been paralysed with rocuronium. The anaesthetist may alternatively elect to use a half-dose of neostigmine 0.625 mg and atropine 0.3 mg intravenously. Before repeating the half-dose, consider the consequences. Excess neostigmine will potentiate the neuromuscular block, may disrupt bowel anastomoses, cause bronchorrhoea and bradycardia.

> *In the event of an emergency reintubation*
> *in the recovery room always use suxamethonium.*

Nerve stimulators do not help

Residual paralysis is not an emergency, but it can easily become one. If a patient is distressed, struggling to breathe or starts to become alarmed because of residual paralysis there is little point using nerve stimulators to diagnose the type of block. Safe treatment remains the same. Never allow the patient to struggle on. If a single small dose of neostigmine and atropine does not relieve the situation within 5 minutes, then the safest option is to sedate, re-intubate and ventilate the patient. The anaesthetist may elect to insert a laryngeal mask and use this to support the ventilation. Do not try to use additional doses of cholinesterase inhibitors of whatever type.

All muscle relaxants wear off eventually, and most within an hour. It does not matter what agent is causing the residual paralysis. We have encountered respiratory arrests, and some fatalities, where this rule has been circumvented. Residual paralysis is not the time 'to wait and see' what happens.

Plasma cholinesterase deficiency or 'sux apnoea'

Occasionally, a short-acting muscle relaxant, suxamethonium, causes prolonged relaxation. This phenomenon is colloquially known as *sux apnoea*. Patients may come to the recovery room needing a short spell on a ventilator.

Normally, a circulating enzyme called *plasma cholinesterase* (once called pseudocholinesterase), breaks down suxamethonium within 3–5 minutes. In people with a congenital or acquired *plasma cholinesterase deficiency*, suxamethonium may continue to act from between 10 minutes to an hour or more. In this case the only option is to sedate, re-intubate and ventilate the patient until the suxamethonium wears off. No drugs safely reverse this sort of block.

Emergence delirium and confusion

As they emerge from anaesthesia about 5 per cent of patients become agitated and bewildered (see Box 10.2). If they become combative they will need restraint (Box 10.3). This phenomenon is called *emergence delirium*. It tends to occur in younger patients, drug or alcohol abusers and especially where the patient was anxious before surgery. Patients seem not to know where they are, or what is going on around them, and are unable to concentrate sufficiently to obey simple commands. Usually the delirium settles within a minute or two as their conscious state improves. If it does not resolve quickly then eliminate other causes for delirium, especially hypoxia or hypoglycaemia because these will quickly cause serious harm.

Box 10.2 **Delirium**

1. If the patients have clouded consciousness, but are not excitable and they know where they are, then consider hypothermia, hypercarbia, or psychoactive drugs used during the anaesthetics.

2. If patients are excitable and agitated, and do not know where they are, then consider the early stages of hypoxia, or hypoglycaemia.

3. Children and those who were anxious or agitated before surgery are tenfold more likely to have emergence delirium.

4. Review the anaesthetic notes for hints about the cause: psychoactive drugs used during or before the operation, periods of hypotension, or gas or fat embolism.

5. Occasionally midazolam or other benzodiazepines can cause paradoxical excitement. This is reversed with flumazenil.

6. Pain is a potent cause of delirium in semi-comatose patients.

The principal causes of delirium are:

- residual effects of anaesthetic drugs during emergence;
- intraoperative complications;
- pre-existing confusional states;
- hypoxia;
- hypoglycaemia;
- pain;
- awareness during the anaesthetic.

Why emergence delirium occurs

The neurophysiology involved in emergence delirium is not fully understood. It probably occurs because various parts of the brain emerge from anaesthesia at different rates. For example, delirium occurs when the cortex 'wakes up' before the frontal lobes are able to moderate its behaviour. It is certainly worse if the patient has received additional psychoactive drugs such as hyoscine, atropine, ketamine or a phenothiazine (such as prochlorperazine used as an anti-emetic).

Alcoholics sometimes wake in a dream-like state. They may sit up, peer around and yet not respond when spoken to. If you forcibly try to restrain them, take care, because they may lash out. Guide them to lie down.

Emergence delirium is common after nasal surgery, especially if it is cosmetic surgery. Patients are distressed to wake and find their noses blocked by packs.

Emergence delirium in children is common, affecting approximately 13 per cent of those under the age of 15 years. If babies or toddlers go to sleep crying, they often wake crying. Poor intraoperative pain control is probably another major factor causing delirium. Children aged 2 to 5 years may wake agitated, combative and inconsolable.

Prevention of emergence delirium requires accurate identification of those patients at high risk of developing it, followed by a coordinated prevention and treatment effort carried out by the whole perioperative team including play therapists.

Box 10.3 **The violent patient**

Occasionally a patient will warn you they have become violent while emerging from previous anaesthetics. Take their warning seriously. They may become a danger to themselves or staff. Sometimes they rip out their drips and become combative. If you have no intravenous access, then give ketamine 1.5 mg/kg into any muscle mass you can find. It will rapidly bring the patient under control, but you will now have a fully anaesthetized patient to care for. Paradoxically benzodiazepines, instead of sedating these patients, make some of them more aggressive. If you cannot manage the patient you should call for help before anyone is hurt.

Intraoperative complications

Intraoperative complications include air or particulate embolism, cerebral ischaemia, intracranial haemorrhage, hypoxic encephalopathy, or hypotension. These complications may cause delirium, but are far more likely to present because 'the patient won't wake up'.

Pre-existing confusional states

If a patient has dementia, or a cognitive disorder, before their anaesthetic then it is not surprising that they are confused afterwards. Never simply assume that their cognitive disorder is the sole reason for their delirium. They are as much at risk of other causes of delirium as any patient.

Hypoxia

Severe hypoxia or hypoglycaemia causes irreversible brain damage within minutes. Suspect impending hypoxia if the pulse oximeter reading is 94 per cent or less. Give oxygen; review the patient's record to identify risk factors for hypoxia.

If, during the anaesthetic, the patient has had a transient hypoxic episode, such as a period of hypotension, then they may well wake up confused even if they are not hypoxic when the delirium is first recognized.

The cause of cerebral hypoxia can be subtle. Hypoxia can involve one or more of a combination of factors including inadequate inspired oxygen, airway or lung disease, anaemia, and cardiac failure. Each additional factor amplifies the effect to aggravate hypoxia; for example, anaemia amplifies hypoxia caused by lung disease.

Hypoglycaemia

As with hypoxia, hypoglycaemia can cause brain damage in minutes. Review the patient's record to establish risk factors for hypoglycaemia, check their blood glucose levels with a portable glucose meter, and get help. Hypoglycaemia is a particular risk in alcoholics who have fasted, and more predictably in diabetics receiving insulin.

Pain

While emerging from anaesthesia pain or especially discomfort from a full bladder makes patients extremely restless.

What to do for emergence delirium

- Give 100% oxygen.
- Reassure and orient patients as to where they are, and what has happened.
- Eliminate hypoxia and hypoglycaemia.
- Gently restrain the patient lest they fall from the trolley and hurt themselves.
- Notify the anaesthetist, who may give clonidine, propofol or a short-acting benzodiazepine.

Crying patients

Occasionally patients sob after emerging from their anaesthetic, particularly if they have been given propofol. Often they do not know why they are crying. It does not necessarily mean they are in pain.

Unpremedicated patients, and those anaesthetized for short procedures, are more likely to cry, especially if the procedure is for a sad reason such as a termination of pregnancy. Patients with anxiety or depression are more likely to cry as well, as are children and elderly demented patients. Sit with them; hold their hand. Do not try to comfort them with reassurances. Crying is a useful natural tranquillizer and a good way of resolving emotional stress. Others who may weep are those who have had mastectomies, lost a limb, or were involved in accidents.

Awareness

Some people are more resistant to the effects of anaesthetic drugs, and while paralysed with muscle relaxants and unable to move, may be consciously aware during their operation. Postoperatively, these patients are often upset and crying and restless. Awareness is more common in women having Caesarean sections under general anaesthesia, the very ill, trauma surgery, and during open-heart surgery. The incidence of recall is estimated to be about 0.5 per cent. Even under seemingly adequate general anaesthesia memories can be laid down, and the patient may subconsciously remember what has gone on. Hearing is the last modality lost. The experience may range from merely a fleeting impression of voices, through to the horrendous calamity of being completely conscious, in agony and unable to move or tell anyone about it. Those who experience awareness also range from those who are mildly interested, and not at all upset by the incident, through to those who develop post-traumatic stress disorder (PTSD). This is especially likely if the patient was in pain.

Post-traumatic stress disorder is characterized by flashbacks. These are like emotional malaria with intrusive memories, which recur again and again when the person is awake, or are relived in their nightmares. It may be all so awful that the patients hide it in a dark corner of their mind, and forget about it; but they become changed people: irritable, anxious, jumpy, depressed, and constantly on their guard. These patients need debriefing over many sessions with a psychiatrist—this is not a job for amateurs.

Explicit awareness

Explicit awareness occurs where the patient is consciously aware of what went on during surgery. They may or may not have felt pain.

Implicit awareness

Implicit awareness is more common. There are vague memories, but they are jumbled. This is more likely in the very old, the very ill, those undergoing emergency surgery, and especially during Caesarean section under general anaesthetic where the incidence can be as high as 3 per cent.

Pseudo-awareness

It is common for patients to recall wearing an oxygen mask in recovery room. If they have not been forewarned of this, some interpret this event as awareness. Some have even sued. It is always prudent to tell patients several times that their surgery is over, everything went well, and not to take off their oxygen mask because they might get a headache.

What to do

- Recognize that how you handle your patient may determine whether or not they are affected for years to come. This is a potent cause of a prolonged Stage 3 recovery.
- Reassure and comfort your patient but never negate the claims.
- Empathize with the patient, acknowledge their feelings and reflect them back to the frightened person. If it is appropriate, hold their hand. Allow them to cry.
- Notify the anaesthetist.

- Record your observations in the patient's unit record—what you see, hear and measure—but not your opinions.

Headache

About 30 per cent of women get postoperative headaches after surgery, but men are less often affected. Many factors contribute to postoperative headache including dehydration from excessive fasting, nuchal spasm (especially in patients who get tension headaches), and caffeine withdrawal. Ondansetron, often given during anaesthesia, also causes headaches. Place a cool wet towel on their forehead, and keep bright lights out of their eyes. Start with simple analgesics such as paracetamol. You may occasionally need to resort to pethidine, but avoid morphine because it tends to make headaches worse.

What are the serious causes of headaches?

Postdural puncture headaches occur after the dura mater is punctured with a spinal or epidural anaesthetic. The headache is exacerbated when the patient sits up, and relieved when they lie down. The patient may need a blood patch to relieve it.

Severe hypertension may cause headache, photophobia, vomiting, visual disturbance and clouding of consciousness. This malignant hypertension must be treated early before it causes a haemorrhagic stroke. Malignant hypertension may occur abruptly when the blood pressure exceeds 220/120 mmHg.

Water intoxication after urological surgery or hysteroscopy causes cerebral oedema, which presents with a headache.

Extravasation and arterial injections

Extravasation

Extravasation occurs when, during infusion, intravenous fluid leaks from the vein into the surrounding tissues. Some drugs are highly toxic to tissues and may cause horrific tissue damage, killing muscle, skin, tendon and nerves and requiring disfiguring and destructive debridement. Toxic drugs include dopamine, adrenaline, 50 per cent glucose, sodium bicarbonate, calcium chloride, potassium chloride, chemotherapeutic agents and some antibiotics.

The amount of damage depends on the type of drug, the amount extravasated, and how quickly it is recognized. Often the tissue damage is not immediately obvious, and can take days or even longer to become apparent.

Those most at risk are the elderly with delicate skin and fragile veins. Patients who are emerging from anaesthesia may not report pain before substantial damage occurs.

Where there is pain there is tissue damage.

Extravasation is easier to prevent than treat. If you are about to infuse something which could cause tissue damage, then it is prudent to set up the new infusion at a fresh site in a different vein. Give drug infusions into the largest possible vein. Avoid siting a cannula in the back of the hand, or a vein crossing a joint. Use clear plastic dressings so you can see the puncture site and surrounding skin. Do not cover the site with bandages.

Replace painful drips.

How to tell if the drip has tissued

Colloquially, extravasation has occurred when the drip has 'tissued'.
One or more of the following occur:

- the patient complains of pain over the drip site or up the vein;
- the infusion begins to run slowly;
- you cannot aspirate blood from the cannula;
- the tissues around the cannula start to swell.

If you press on the vein a few centimetres above the cannula and the drip does not slow or stop, then it is probable that the fluid is running into the tissues. Another test is to place one finger on either side of the tip of the cannula and press gently down on the tissues. If the drip slows or stops, then chances are the drip has tissued.

What to do about extravasation

- Stop the infusion immediately.
- Leave the cannula in place.
- Aspirate as much of the drug or fluid as possible.
- Outline the affected area with an indelible marking pen.
- Apply a warm compress on the site. This may not help prevent tissue damage, but it is comforting to the patient.
- Elevate the limb and notify the anaesthetist.
- Make clear and careful notes in the patient's record.

When to use specific interventions

It is best to use the following techniques as early as possible, but they can be used with decreasing effect up to 12 hours later.

For substances that cause tissue damage with increasing concentrations, hyaluronidase (an enzyme) reduces the extent of tissue damage following extravasation of parenteral nutrition solutions, concentrated glucose solutions, electrolyte infusions, antibiotics, aminophylline, mannitol and chemotherapeutic agents. Some anaesthetists dilute hyaluronidase to 15 units/ml and inject 1 ml of the solution through the catheter or sometimes subcutaneously around the site.

Extravasation of a vasoconstrictive agent, such as dopamine, dobutamine, adrenaline, or noradrenaline, can cause severe ischaemic tissue damage. Phentolamine, an alpha-adrenergic antagonist, reduces both arterial and venous vasospasm. Inject a dose of 10 mg in 5 ml of 0.9 per cent saline through the catheter or subcutaneously around the site.

Inadvertent intra-arterial injection

Whenever you give an intravenous injection, always check that bright red blood does not pulse back into the needle. Accidental injection of a substance into an artery usually occurs when intravenous injections are attempted in the antecubital fossa, but may occur anywhere, even on the back of the hand. In almost every case the patient immediately reports intense pain in their fingers or a site distal to the injection, and many will report soon thereafter sensory disturbances such as tingling, burning or paraesthesia. The consequences can be catastrophic, but it may take hours and sometimes up to a week or more before the full extent of the tissue damage becomes apparent. Within the first 2 hours you may see nail bed pallor and decreased capillary refill in the fingertips.[2]

What to do

- Stop the injection.
- Keep the arterial line in place.
- Aspirate, flush and inject procaine 0.1 ml/kg into the arterial line.
- Start a slow intravenous infusion of 0.9% saline.
- Give pain relief if necessary.
- Notify the anaesthetist.
- Seek the advice of a vascular surgeon.

Further steps

- Stellate or brachial plexus blocks may help.
- Phentolamine 1 mg diluted to 10 ml in 0.9% saline injected into the artery over 10 minutes is useful to relieve vasospasm. Papaverine with heparin has been used successfully but it is not known whether the eventual outcome is changed.

Eyes and pupils

Unconscious patients do not blink. It only takes a few moments for ulcers to form once the cornea dries out. Keep their eyes closed. Use a lubricating ointment such as methylcellulose to protect them. Do not use chloramphenicol ointment because of the slight risk of serious bone marrow depression. Recent evidence suggests that placing polyethylene sheeting (Gladwrap®) over the eyes is more effective than lubricating drops or gels.

The patient may complain of sore gritty eyes if they have been open during the operation. In this case, make a note in the record whether their eyes were taped shut during the procedure. If you are concerned then use fluorescein stain to reveal corneal or scleral damage. Irrigate the eye with saline, tape it shut, and consult an ophthalmologist.

When plaster of Paris is used to splint fractured noses, fragments easily enter the eye. Gently wash these out with 0.9 per cent saline.

Pupils

Dilated pupils occur with:

◆ hypoxia;

◆ severe head injury—this sign signals a poor prognosis;

◆ homatropine, used in eye surgery to dilate pupils.

   Pinpoint pupils occur with:

◆ pilocarpine eye drops used to treat glaucoma;

◆ *narcotic* overdose;

◆ pontine (brainstem) haemorrhage.

An oval pupil may indicate early brainstem compression. A fixed unilateral dilated pupil indicates severe brainstem compression. If this develops after neurosurgery, notify the neurosurgeon and the anaesthetist immediately.

A unilateral constricted pupil on the affected side occurs in Horner's syndrome. This occurs when the cervical sympathetic nerves are paralysed after surgery on the neck or thorax, or brachial plexus blocks.

Irregular pupils occur for a few minutes when the patient is emerging from a general anaesthetic where volatile agents were used. If you test the patient's plantar reflexes at this time, you will find they are up-going. This phenomenon lasts only about 10 minutes.

Deafness

Patients who are deaf also have surgery and come to the recovery room. They will have a close friend or relative hovering close by and as soon as practical allow that person to join the patient. They will interpret the patient's wishes and problems and guide your treatment.[3] Deaf patients need to be reassured that their deafness will not jeopardize their care.

Hiccups

Hiccups frequently occur after laparoscopy, or more rarely after open abdominal procedures where something is irritating the diaphragm. Usually patients respond to gently stimulating their oral pharynx with a soft sucker. If hiccups persist they usually disappear with a low dose of metoclopramide, or ephedrine. Tell the surgeon about persistent hiccups, because it may indicate blood accumulating under the diaphragm.

Nerve injuries are the commonest reason for patients taking legal action against their anaesthetists. Nerve injury is more common in diabetics, smokers, alcoholics and those with disseminated cancer, possibly because these patients are already susceptible to peripheral neuropathies. Nerve damage is usually caused by improperly positioning the patient on the operating table or the recovery room trolley. Sometimes, even with the most scrupulous care, injuries still occur. The physiological reason for this remains a mystery.

In the recovery room the patient may complain of numbness or tingling, or loss of power in a limb. Notify the anaesthetist immediately should you encounter this problem. Record this problem in the patient's notes so that it can be monitored on the ward.

Nerve injuries

Brachial plexus

Brachial plexus damage causes weakness in the hand with wrist drop. Brachial plexus nerve blocks are the commonest cause of plexus damage in the operating theatre. They may occur if the head is rotated in the opposite direction to the arm that is adducted on the operating table's arm board. About 20 per cent of brachial plexus injuries occur when the arm is dropped while moving a comatose patient where the sudden jolt stretches and tears the plexus. This can occur in the recovery room if the patient's arm falls off the trolley.

Ulnar nerve

Damage to the ulnar nerve causes numbness along the ulnar side of the arm and the hand. It is the commonest problem, and five times more likely to occur in men than women. It usually occurs in the arm that was adducted on the arm board away from the operating table. The ulnar nerve can be damaged in the medial superficial groove at the elbow (the 'funny bone') during transport to, or in the recovery room. Check that the patient's elbow is not resting against anything that could damage it, such as the trolley's cot sides, and pad it if necessary.

Median nerve

The median nerve is prone to damage where intravenous injections of drugs are attempted in the antecubital fossa. It causes numbness in the palm of the hand and weakness of the fingers.

Common peroneal nerve

The common peroneal nerve can be damaged if it is compressed against the head of the fibula in the lithotomy position when stirrups are used during surgery. The patient develops foot drop and paraesthesia in the lower leg. This may present in the recovery room.

Facial nerve

Damage to the facial nerve occurs if it is crushed against the mandible. This can happen when you are trying to maintain a difficult airway. The facial nerve passes through that little notch you can feel if you run your finger along the bony edge of the mandible just in front of the angle of the jaw.

Optic nerve

Hypotension or increased intraocular pressure may jeopardize blood flow to the retina. Patients most at risk are those with glaucoma who have either been hypotensive during surgery, or where a facemask has inadvertently pressed on their eyeball. This may occur when you are ventilating a patient with a bag and mask.

Shaking, shivering and rigidity

Shaking and *shivering* are quite different phenomenon. Shivering is a reflex response to cold. Treat this by warming your patient (Figure 10.2). In contrast shaking is a central nervous system response to unmodulated neural inputs into the brainstem and tectum. Usually this is triggered by an excessive adrenergic stimulus, such as we might experience after a big fright. About 35 per cent of patients shiver or shake after a general anaesthetic, but fewer do after spinal or epidural blockade.

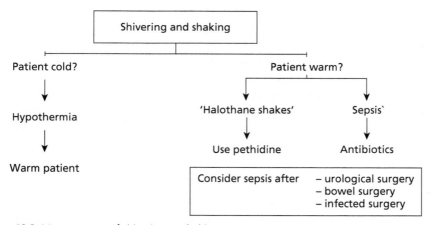

Figure 10.2 Management of shivering or shaking.

Shaking is worse where higher levels of adrenaline are circulating such as in the young, after long general anaesthetics; where the patient has breathed spontaneously for longer than 30 minutes on a volatile agent; if analgesia has been inadequate; or they have been hyperventilated during the procedure. This usually resolves within a few minutes as their circulating adrenaline levels declines. The shakes are accompanied by vasoconstriction, goose-bumps (*piloerection*), clonus, increased spike activity on an electroencephalograph (EEG), increased oxygen consumption and a rise in intra-ocular pressure.

Oxygen requirements increase up to sevenfold with shivering and shaking. Those with cardiopulmonary disease may become severely hypoxic and suffer the consequences of myocardial ischaemia, arrhythmias, and even a mild to moderate lactic acidosis.

What to do

◆ Take care to prevent patients hurting themselves.

◆ Protect their airway.

◆ Give oxygen.

◆ A small dose of intravenous pethidine 25 mg usually stops the shaking immediately. It is effective in more than 75 per cent of cases, but if it fails, and the shaking continues to cause problems, such as after delicate plastic surgery, then use doxapram 0.25 mg/kg intravenously.

Shaking after 'dirty' surgery

Shaking (rigor) is an early sign of a septic shower. Bacteria *endotoxins* enter the circulation when an abscess is drained, or during urological surgery. They cause tissue and white blood cells to release chemical distress signals called *cytokines* to alert the body to the invasion. One of the body's first-line responses is to raise the body temperature in an attempt to prevent the bacteria replicating. Alerted by cytokines, the hypothalamus signals the adrenal medulla to produce adrenaline, and the thermoregulatory centre to increase body temperature. The consequent rigors increase body temperature, while vigorous muscle activity increases oxygen consumption severalfold.

Start oxygen therapy in anticipation of the increased metabolic rate, and take blood cultures. During surgery showers of bacteria can enter the blood that may progress to septicaemia within a few hours. When surgery involves a potentially septic field then prophylactic antibiotics help prevent this complication.

Rigidity

Patients sometimes pass through a phase of transient muscle rigidity when emerging from their anaesthetic. They may clench their teeth tightly. This phenomenon of trismus can be dangerous because patients may catch their tongue between their teeth with the risk of partially amputating it; dislodge expensive dental caps, crowns and bridges; or patients may obstruct their airway.

Keep patients' lips, and tongues out of the
way of their teeth until they wake up.

Guedel airways have a metal flange to prevent the lumen being crushed. You can make patients open their mouths by inserting a soft catheter through their nose until it touches the posterior wall of the nasopharynx. This usually makes them shake their heads from side to side, grimace and then open their mouths.

Anti-emetics can cause the extrapyramidal syndrome with rigidity, dystonia and nystagmus. It is more common in children, young adults, and the debilitated elderly. The incidence is about 0.3 per cent, and a quarter of these occur after the first dose. The culprit drugs include prochlorperazine, metoclopramide, and droperidol. The symptoms can be alarming; the patient becomes rigid, unable to move, their eyes are flickering from side to side and they can only speak through clenched teeth. This rigidity responds rapidly to benzatropine 1 mg IV. You may need to repeat the dose in 10 minutes.

> *Persistent rigidity is a warning sign*
> *of malignant hyperthermia.*

Skin, nails, hair and joints

Bruising

If you do not apply firm pressure to a puncture wound after you withdraw the needle the patient will get a bruise. Venipunctures stop bleeding after one minute of firm pressure. Do not merely tape a piece of cotton wool over the site and assume the job is done. Underneath the cotton wool a hidden painful haematoma might develop.

After arterial punctures you must press firmly on the site for at least 5 minutes, timed by the clock. To be sure there is no bruising or swelling check the site again in 5 minutes' time.

Pallor

Pallor warns that an activated sympathetic nervous system is causing cutaneous vasoconstriction. The main reasons for this noradrenergic response are hypoxia, shock, bleeding, pain, hypoglycaemia, angina, and nausea. Other causes include anaemia and drugs such as pethidine, oxytocin, vasopressin and desmopressin.

Pressure areas

Pressure injury is a localized area of tissue damage caused by direct sustained pressure on the skin and underlying tissue. Sometimes they are called pressure sores, pressure ulcers or bed sores. Pressure injuries develop very quickly, progress rapidly and are difficult to heal.

Sustained pressure cuts off the circulation to vulnerable tissue. Normal skin can withstand about 30 minutes of moderate pressure without long-lasting damage, but if sustained over a long period it causes localized ischaemia and tissue death.

Initially stage 1 pressure injury appears as a persistent area of red warm inflamed skin, or in people with darker skin, appears to have a blue or purple hue. At this stage the injury quickly resolves. The next, stage 2, presents with a breach in the skin, an open sore that gets infected easily and is slow to heal. The final stage 3 injuries are deep necrotic ulcers with a large amount of underlying tissue damage.

Postoperative pressure sores are a major cause of postoperative morbidity and huge economic burden to health services. Timely intervention in the recovery room can prevent much morbidity later in the ward.

Those at greater risk of pressure injury are the elderly with their fragile thin skin, those with malnutrition or recent weight loss, the cachectic, and those patients with connective tissue diseases such as rheumatoid arthritis. It also affects people with vascular disease (especially smokers) and those who cannot move easily such as quadriplegics. Patients who are longer than an hour on the operating table are at higher risk.

The mattresses on most operating tables are firm and flat so that a patient's body weight is not evenly distributed, and some points such as the skin over the sacrum, hips, or heels, carry more than their fair share of weight. It does not take long for the skin over these pressure areas to become ischaemic: tissue death follows and then pressure ulcers become inevitable.

When patients come to the recovery room after a long operation, examine their pressure areas: their sacrum, heels, shoulder blades and thoracic spine. These are all areas which may have received excessive pressure. Also check tourniquet and blood pressure cuff sites, and the sites where the diathermy plate has been attached. If the erythematous skin on a pressure blanches when you press on it, then the skin is unlikely to break down, but if it is does not blanch or worse still is white, then expect an ulcer to form. Do not massage the area, because you will increase the risk of damage.

Even slight adjustments in the patient's position give some relief of pressure on the area. Once the patient is settled in the recovery room, alter their position to take the weight off their pressure areas. Moist skin is more at risk than dry skin so make sure the affected skin is clean and dry. If the patient is incontinent consider inserting a catheter to protect the skin.

The principle behind protecting pressure points is to distribute the pressure over as wide an area as possible. Gel pads are very effective, but rolled towels and foam pads are much less so.

Skin can also be damaged by friction or shearing forces. It is easy to tear or bruise elderly patients' skin. Be careful not to drag elderly patients across their bed sheets, because the friction may damage their skin. Be careful too when removing adhesive surgical tape. Ease it off; otherwise you may rip the skin.

Your hospital should have protocols for identifying patients at risk of pressure injury, and educating staff and patients, and management plans.

Shoulder tip pain

Shoulder tip pain is likely to occur after laparoscopic procedures. If the diaphragm has been irritated by carbon dioxide used to inflate the peritoneal cavity during laparoscopy then the pain will be referred to the shoulder tip. More ominously, shoulder tip can occur after the perforation of the bladder, bowel or uterus during endoscopic procedures. Occasionally it is a sign of angina.

Sit the patient up. Try a warm pack. Give NSAIDs if appropriate. Give reassurance, this pain usually settles down. If you are worried that something more ominous is occurring do an ECG and ask your anaesthetist to examine the patient with you.

Sweating

Sweating is sometimes called *diaphoresis*. Sweating, especially when associated with pallor, is a sign that something is very seriously wrong. It is associated with hypoxia, hypotension, hypoglycaemia, and cardiac failure, overt or silent myocardial ischaemia or if the patient is nauseated. Malignant hyperpyrexia can present with sweating in the recovery room after short procedures so stay alert to this possibility.

Management

♦ Give oxygen by mask and attach a pulse oximeter.

♦ Check the vital signs: pulse rate and rhythm, blood pressure, perfusion status and tympanic membrane (or rectal) temperature.

♦ Check the blood glucose levels.

♦ Check for chest discomfort.

♦ Is the patient able to take a deep breath comfortably?

♦ Notify the anaesthetist.

Fingernails

If a patient with long fingernails rests them on her chest, the nails quickly damage the skin.

Hair

Coagulated dry blood occasionally remains on the hair after head and neck surgery. Dried blood is difficult to get out, and putrefies if left. Wash and comb the hair with aqueous cetrimide being careful not to get it in the patient's eyes. Rinse with ample water.

Mouth and airway

Hoarse voice

A hoarse or croaky voice is likely in patients who were intubated, but it usually resolves over the next couple of hours. Following thyroidectomy it may be a sign of recurrent laryngeal nerve damage; in this case notify the surgeon. Characteristically the patient will not be able to say 'eeeee' in a high-pitched squeak.

Infants and children with a hoarse voice are at risk of developing laryngeal oedema an obstruction in a few hours' time. They must never be sent home, but admitted and observed carefully for the development of stridor, they could be developing Horner's syndrome.

Teeth

Damaged teeth are a common reason for patients taking legal action against their anaesthetists. Many patients' teeth are in poor repair with caries, and especially gum disease, while prolonged illness makes teeth fragile and brittle. Teeth can be chipped or dislodged during intubation, or when the patient develops masseter spasm (trismus) in the recovery room. Before placing an oropharyngeal airway check their teeth are stable enough to withstand biting on the airway. Move the airway to one side to avoid precarious teeth. Some recovery rooms stock special mouth guards to protect teeth. Make a note in the patient's record if you find loose, chipped, or other damage to teeth.

Thirst and dry mouth

One of patients' most vivid memories is their dry mouth and thirst in recovery room. They forget the pain, but remember their thirst. Dry mouths can make patients restless. Give them small sips of water, or ice (frozen grape juice is especially appreciated) or wet gauze to suck. Glycerine-based lip salves dehydrate the epithelium, causing painful cracks later.

Do not use glycerine-based lip salves.

After minor day surgery patients are often given something to drink and eat before leaving the hospital. There should be protocols in place to guide you for the timing of this.

Sore throat

Postoperative sore throat, hoarseness and cough are common problems in patients who have been intubated. If asked, about half of the patients complain of a sore throat. A recent Canadian study indicates that preoperative intravenous administration of dexamethasone alleviates postoperative sore throat more effectively than non-analgesic methods such as lubrication of the endotracheal tube.[4] The causes of postoperative sore throat are dry anaesthetic gases, which desiccate the mucosa; damage during intubation; pharyngeal packs; insertion of nasogastric tube after bronchoscopy. A few sips of cold water and reassurance that their sore throat will improve within 24 hours is usually all the treatment they need.

Urinary retention

A full bladder causes restlessness in a patient emerging from a general anaesthetic. Opioids tighten the bladder's vesical sphincter, while relaxing its detrusor muscle. They make it difficult for older men to know when their bladder is full, and then to pass urine. Patience, encouragement, privacy and perhaps the sound of running water help overcome the problem. A small dose of naloxone is also worth trying.

Patients under spinal or epidural anaesthesia cannot pass urine, because they do not know their bladder is full; and even if they did, they cannot voluntarily contract their muscles to empty it. Serious future bladder and continence problems occur if the bladder becomes over-distended. Aim to suspect, detect, and treat it early. Once the bladder extends above the pelvic brim it is severely damaged; in this case you will feel a bladder as a small firm dome just over the symphysis pubis. Bladder ultrasound is useful if it is available. Volumes estimated by ultrasound have good correlation to measured volumes. If the patient retains more than 600 cc and the patient cannot void then the bladder should be emptied by catheterization.

If urinary retention is likely, the surgeons will insert a catheter while the patient is in the operating theatre. In contrast, some orthopaedic surgeons are reluctant to catheterize patients with joint replacements, because they fear a urinary super-infection may migrate to the operation site. In this case, the surgeon may allow you to pass a catheter, empty the bladder and then withdraw the catheter under antibiotic cover.

Ocular injury

There is an increased risk of ocular injury following long, extensive spine surgery. It is important to be aware of this and check for it in the recovery room.[5]

Environmental responsibility

Climate change has been named the number 1 public health threat of the 21st century. Modern health care produces significant amounts of national greenhouse gas (GHG) emissions (10% in the USA, 7% in Australia, 5% in England from the NHS and 4% in Canada) with a combined release of 748 million metric tons of carbon dioxide equivalents annually.[6] It is the duty of the health care practitioner to not only care for patients but also to protect public health from health care pollution. Inhaled anaesthetic gases are strong GHGs, hundreds to thousands of times more potent than carbon dioxide. They are measurably accumulating in the atmosphere and account for 5% of a health care facility's carbon footprint. The global warming potentials of inhaled anaesthetics are 4 times greater than that of total intravenous anaesthesia (TIVA) with propofol. Nitrous oxide also causes ozone depletion. TIVA has the additional advantages of reduced postoperative delirium, reduced postoperative nausea and vomiting and smoother emergence as well as reducing the potential hazards of occupational exposure of teratogenic anaesthetic gases to staff (particularly in developing countries where scavenging systems are less common and nitrous oxide use is high).

References

1. **Chu DK**, *et al.* (2018) Too much oxygen is harmful. *Lancet*. Apr 28.
2. **Sen A, Chini E, Brown MJ**, *et al.* (2005) Complication after unintentional intra-arterial injection of drugs. *Mayo Clinic Proceedings* **80**(6):783–795.
3. **Middleton A, Niruban A**, *et al.* (2010) Communicating in a healthcare setting with people who have hearing loss. *British Medical Journal* **341**:c4672.
4. **Kuriyama A, Maeda H** (2019) Preoperative intravenous dexamethasone prevents tracheal intubation related sore-throat in adult surgical patients: a systematic review and meta-analysis. *Canadian Journal of Anesthesia* **66**:562–575.
5. **Hofer R, Evans K**, *et al.* (2019) Ocular injury during spine surgery. *Canadian Journal of Anesthesia* **66**:772–780.
6. **Sherman JD, Barrick B** (2019) Total intravenous anesthetic versus inhaled anesthetic: pick your poison. *Anesthesia and Analgesia* **128**(1):13–15.

Further Reading

Romero MR, Krumbach B, *et al.* (2011) EBP guidelines on corneal abrasion management in the PACU. *Journal of PeriAnesthesia Nursing* **26**(3):194–195.

Chapter 11

Pharmacology

Introduction

Pharmacology is the study of the uses, modes of action and effects of drugs. To administer drugs confidently in the recovery room staff need to understand how they work, and how they interact with anaesthetic agents and other drugs.

Most drugs given in the recovery room are administered intravenously. Once given drugs act rapidly, and they cannot be retrieved if something untoward should happen. Unless recovery room staff have a basic knowledge of pharmacology it is easy to harm patients. Never give a drug unless you understand what the likely effects are, and what to do if there is an abnormal reaction.

Drugs are substances given intentionally either to enhance, or to suppress normal physiological activities of the body with the aim of achieving a beneficial effect. Drugs cannot force a cell do something it normally would not do, for instance drugs cannot make nerve cells contract or muscle cells secrete thyroxine.

Surgical and anaesthetic stresses unmask many medical problems, some of which you will need to treat urgently. It is prudent to keep a wide range of drugs in the recovery room to treat pain, and medical emergencies.

Problems with drugs

- the incorrect dose is used;
- interactions with other drugs;
- adverse drug reactions;
- allergic responses.

Ignorance about drugs can be lethal.
If you are in any doubt...ask someone!

The potential for adverse effects

Many elderly patients do not take their medication either regularly or appropriately, and toxicity is common. Older people lose weight. They may be taking an inappropriate dose of drug prescribed years earlier. Many patients are taking non-prescribed complementary and alternative medicines (CAMs), which they have concealed from their doctors. Some of these, such as St John's wort, ephedra, and garlic concentrate, are potent drugs in their own right, and far from harmless.

Some patients are taking medication that may interact adversely with drugs used in the recovery room. The most potentially serious of these are psychoactive drugs such as selective serotonin reuptake inhibitors (SSRIs), *tricyclic antidepressants*, and *mono-amine oxidase inhibitors* (MAOIs), which can have lethal interactions with pethidine and tramadol. Patients occasionally and inadvertently present for major surgery still taking aspirin, warfarin, clopidogrel or other anticoagulants.

Drugs are often chemically incompatible with each other, and strange things happen if you mix them, or dilute them with the wrong fluid. Most, but not all, drugs are stable in 0.9 per cent saline or 5 per cent glucose. Do not add drugs to blood, blood products, fat emulsions, parenteral nutrition fluids, or albumin solutions and plasma expanders. Read and follow the manufacturer's instructions, or check with your hospital's pharmacist if you are in doubt about how to use a drug. Paste into a book the detailed instructions, which come in the drug packages, to use as a reference. Although drug information is available on the internet it is still useful to keep a good pharmacology reference book in your recovery room.

Drugs to keep in the recovery room

You may need to treat the problems listed in Table 11.1, so keep the appropriate drugs close by.

Table 11.1 Recovery room emergencies

Adrenal crises	Allergic reactions
Anaphylaxis	Bronchospasm
Cardiac arrest	Cardiac arrhythmias
Cardiac failure	Coagulopathies
Hypertension	Hypoglycaemia
Hypotension	Pulmonary oedema
Raised intracranial pressure	Residual paralysis
Respiratory depression	Seizures
Uterine atony	Violent patients

Prepare protocols about how to treat each of these crises including the drug doses, and importantly what to do next if what you have just done did not work. Some recovery rooms keep all the necessary drugs to treat a particular crisis in dedicated boxes; for instance, a 'Residual Paralysis' box might contain atropine, glycopyrronium bromide, neostigmine, physostigmine and diazepam, and a 'Violent Patient' box might contain haloperidol, diazepam, midazolam, and ketamine (which works almost immediately when injected into any accessible muscle).

Store drugs safely

Even though recovery rooms are areas of restricted access, drugs must be stored safely. Opioids and other scheduled drugs of addiction or dependence must be kept in an appropriate locked cupboard. A box with drugs that may be needed in an emergency should be stored on or close to an *emergency trolley*. Other drugs can be stored in alphabetical order on shelves in a cupboard, which is easily closed and locked when the room is unattended.

Generic names

In 2004, drug regulatory authorities in the UK and Europe changed the generic names of many drugs to conform to a uniform standard coordinated by the World Health Organization. For the most part this meant abandoning the British Approved Names (BAN) and following the terminology used in the US. European and UK legislation requires the packaging, labelling and prescribing of drugs to follow recommended International Non-Proprietary Names (rINNs). Australia and New Zealand regulatory authorities are finalizing an agreement to conform to the new standards.

In line with the Medicine Commission's (UK) advice, the terms *adrenaline* and *noradrenaline* are being retained rather than the USA's epinephrine and norepinephrine and pethidine has not been changed to the US name meperidine.

Syringe labelling

The International Colour Code for syringe labelling is widely used (Table 11.2). Beware of administering drugs from unlabelled syringes. Draw up a new ampoule if you are unsure.

Table 11.2 Syringe labels

Agent	Colour of label
Anticholinergic agents	Green
Hypnotics, e.g. midazolam	Orange
Induction agents	Yellow
Local anaesthetics	Grey
Muscle relaxants	Warm red
Narcotics	Blue
Vasopressors	Violet
Other agents	White

Pharmacokinetics

Pharmacokinetics is the study of drug absorption, distribution, metabolism, and excretion. Pharmacodynamics is the study of the effects of drugs, whether these are wanted (*therapeutic*) or unwanted and harmful (*side-effects*).

Absorption

In the recovery room most drugs are injected intravenously where they are quickly carried to every tissue in the body. Sometimes drugs are given intramuscularly, where they are absorbed and released slowly into the bloodstream. Most oral drugs pass through the liver, which may modify them, before they reach the general circulation.

Distribution

Once the drug reaches the circulation it is distributed to the organs and tissues. Cardiac failure slows the distribution of drugs. Some drugs soak into the tissues (especially fat or muscle tissue). Only a small amount of drug remains in the bloodstream, and its concentration is low. If you measure the concentration of drug in the blood it usually appears to be diluted in a larger volume than you would otherwise expect. This calculated volume, which may vary from a few litres to many hundreds of litres, is called the *volume of distribution*.

Following an appropriate loading dose; repeated smaller amounts will maintain the drug at a *therapeutic level*. The dose of drug needed to keep a constant therapeutic level is called the *maintenance dose*. To sustain a clinical effect the drug must be given at the same rate at which the body eliminates the drug (Figure 11.1).

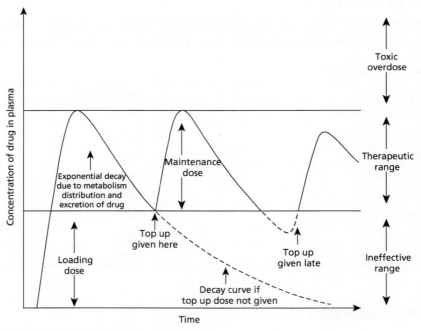

Figure 11.1 Exponential decay of drugs in blood.

Elimination and excretion

Once a drug is distributed the body immediately starts eliminating it by:

+ metabolizing it in the liver;

+ excreting it through the kidneys;

+ using *enzymes* to break it down;

+ storing it;

+ or a combination of two or more of the above.

Some drugs are eliminated from the body in a minute or two (such as remifentanil and suxamethonium), while others take months (such as amiodarone). The time taken to eliminate half the given dose is called the *elimination half-life*. The *context-sensitive half-life* is the time it takes for the clinical effects of the drug to fall below its therapeutic range.

Pharmacokinetics describes how the body handles the drug.
Pharmacodynamics describes what the drug does to
the body.

Pharmacodynamics

Once the drug reaches its site of action it causes an effect. Most drugs act on special structures called *receptors*, either on the cell membrane, or within the cell, while others alter cellular *metabolism* in other ways. The drug's effect depends on how much is given. All drugs are *toxic* if given in too great a dose, and ineffective if the dose is too small. The right dose is called the *therapeutic dose*. With many drugs it is necessary to give enough to build up the concentration to a level that will achieve the desired effect. The dose of drug needed to do this is called the *loading dose*. The dose range between the ineffective dose and the toxic dose is called the *therapeutic margin*. Safe drugs have a wide therapeutic margin.

A drug's *potency* is the amount you need to give to achieve the desired effect. For instance, one-thousandth of the amount of fentanyl is required to achieve the same level of analgesia as pethidine. Fentanyl is 1000 times more potent than pethidine.

Sometimes, despite a therapeutic level of a drug in the blood, the clinical effect begins to wear off. This phenomenon is called *tachyphylaxis* if it occurs over minutes or hours and *tolerance* if it occurs over days or weeks.

What factors alter the behaviour of drugs?

Clinical factors affecting the pharmacokinetics and pharmacodynamics of a drug given in the recovery room:

+ cardiac failure delays their distribution;

+ bleeding or shock alters their distribution;

♦ interaction with residual anaesthetic drugs;

♦ hypothermia delays drug metabolism and elimination.

In people with cardiac failure, give intravenous drugs twice as slowly as you would in a normal patient and monitor its effects as you do so. If you give intramuscular or subcutaneous injections to patients who are shocked, or have a poor perfusion status, the drugs will stay in the tissues waiting to be absorbed when the blood supply is restored. If the patient has received opioids during their anaesthetic, their tissues will already be partly saturated with the drug, so they may need a smaller dose when in the recovery room.

Drug doses

Drug doses are calculated on *ideal body weight* (IBW). For patients over 150 cm in height this equates to:

$$\text{IBW (kg)} = \text{height (cm)} - 100 \text{ (for men)}$$
$$= \text{height (cm)} - 105 \text{ (for women)}$$

For example, a man who is 184 cm tall would have an IBW of 184–100 = 84 kg.

If a patient weighs less than their ideal body weight, then the dose is calculated on their actual weight. In patients less than 150 cm tall, the drug doses are calculated in the same way as they are for children.

Drugs and the elderly

The elderly, with their multiple ills, are often taking many drugs, and frequently over-the-counter 'alternative' therapies as well. This increases the chance of drug interactions and unwanted effects. An elderly patient taking more than seven medications has a high chance of having drug conflicts, or taking inappropriate medication, or taking medication inappropriately.

Failure to adjust drug doses appropriately is the most important reason that the elderly have more adverse drug reactions than younger people.

Of all the factors that affect the behaviour of drugs in the aged, the most important is the decline in renal function that occurs with age. This delays the excretion of drugs and their active metabolites and prolongs their effects.

One of the reasons that an elderly person needs proportionally smaller doses of drugs is that their body contains more fat and less muscle than a younger person. Fat tissue contains about 10 per cent water; in contrast muscle is 60 per cent water. This means older people have less body water than young people, so that the same dose of a water-soluble drug is more concentrated in the elderly.

In the elderly drugs take longer to reach their target, because their cardiac output is lower and their circulation time is slower. The onset of fast-acting drugs is delayed; for instance, in the elderly intravenous naloxone may take 3 or more minutes to work, whereas in a young person the effect would be seen in less than 90 seconds. It is easy to give an overdose of fast-acting drugs if this point is not understood.

When using drugs in the elderly,
give half as much, twice as slowly.

The elderly cool down quickly on the operating tables. Hypothermia delays the metabolism and excretion of many drugs. This becomes an important cause of adverse drug reactions if operations last more than an hour. Bleeding associated with aspirin and other NSAIDs is more common in the elderly, and the consequences are more severe. The risk of postoperative bleeding is accentuated further if SSRIs are taken concurrently with aspirin, or anticoagulants.

Chronic benzodiazepine use

Some older patients have been taking one or more of the *benzodiazepine* drugs for many years. If a benzodiazepine is abruptly withdrawn in these patients it can cause *withdrawal syndrome*: acute unease, agitation, or even convulsions. Long-acting benzodiazepines, such as diazepam, nitrazepam and oxazepam, tend to cause problems some days after withdrawing the drugs, but the shorter-acting ones, such as temazepam or flunitrazepam, may cause symptoms within a day or so, and consequently problems may arise in the recovery room. Agitation in benzodiazepine-dependent patients settles quickly with a small dose of diazepam. The problem of their dependence on benzodiazepines can be addressed later.

Delayed respiratory depression

Fentanyl is a short-acting intravenous opioid analgesic often used during anaesthesia. It is extremely potent and may cause delayed and profound respiratory depression. The typical story is that of an elderly female patient, following a minor procedure such as a colonoscopy. She is awake and alert in the recovery room with no signs of respiratory depression. She returns to the ward, chats to the nurses, and is found an hour or two later—dead.

Fentanyl has a peculiar double camel-hump (biphasic) decay curve. When it is first injected most of it binds to skeletal muscle cells. In the recovery room the elderly woman is awake, but not moving much. The liver rapidly breaks down and inactivates any circulating fentanyl, and there is no sign of respiratory depression.

Then back in the ward, when she starts to move her limbs again, the increased muscle blood flow washes the bound fentanyl back into her circulation. Fentanyl is not very sedating but her breathing slows. Sleep dramatically increases the ventilatory depressant effects of the opioids. She dozes off, stops breathing, and silently dies. Warn the ward staff to watch for slow or shallow respiration when patients over the age of 70 years have received more than 75 micrograms of fentanyl.

Drugs and the obese

To avoid overdosing your obese patients calculate their drug doses on their estimated ideal body weight and not their actual weight. If you are giving drugs intramuscularly you may have to use special long needles to make sure they reach the muscle, and you are not injecting into poorly perfused fat tissue.

Drugs and children

Children under the age of 12 years do not respond to drugs in the same way that small adults of the same weight do. For this reason it is better to calculate children's drug doses on their body surface area; but it is still common practice to give drugs based on their body weight. As children in industrialized nations become fatter, there is the risk of a child receiving a greater than appropriate dose. If a child is under 15 years of age or 150 cm tall and weighs more than 50 kg then prescribe drugs according to their age and ideal body weight.

Preventing slips and mishaps

There are hundreds of drugs on the market: all have side-effects, and all interact with one or more other drugs. Most adverse events with drugs occur because staff do not fully understand the pharmacology of the drugs they are using.

All drugs are potentially hazardous.

Common slips include:

◆ wrong drug;
◆ wrong dose;
◆ wrong dosing interval;
◆ failing to anticipate predictable drug interactions;
◆ using trade names to prescribe drugs, instead of generic names.

Always use generic names, when discussing a drug.

Common mishaps include:

◆ adverse reactions;
◆ unpredictable or rare drug interactions;
◆ allergic reactions.

Drug interactions

Drug interactions occur when two or more drugs given concurrently result in increasing the effects (*synergism*), decreasing the effects (*antagonism*) or produce *adverse effects*. Drug interactions can be expected, predictable or obscure.

Expected interactions occur if two or more drugs are given that have the same effect or act on the same receptors. For instance, diazepam and midazolam will potentiate each other to produce additive sedation; while metoclopramide will antagonize dopamine used to support blood pressure.

Predictable interactions occur when two drugs are eliminated by the same pathway, produce similar clinical effects, or block a compensatory response. For example, volatile agents slow the breakdown of ketamine because volatile agents reduce liver blood flow. NSAIDs and warfarin exacerbates bleeding, and erythromycin or ketoconazole prolongs the action of midazolam by many hours.

Obscure interactions occur when the mechanism of the interaction is not well described. For example, low molecular-weight heparins can cause hyperkalaemia in patients taking *angiotensin-converting enzyme (ACE) inhibitors*, and droperidol can cause a fatal enceph-alopathy when given to patients taking lithium.

Gentamicin inactivates penicillin

Solutions containing penicillin chemically inactivate gentamicin. For this reason, do not combine gentamicin and penicillin in intravenous injections or infusions. The problem is especially likely in patients with renal failure, because they maintain a high level of peni-cillin for a longer time. If you are using both gentamicin and penicillin in patients with chronic kidney disease, then separate the infusion of each drug by at least 3 hours.

Always give gentamicin and penicillin separately.

Adverse events

An adverse drug reaction occurs when a drug, given in normal doses and at normal intervals, has an unintended effect. The effects can be life threatening (anaphylaxis), debilitating (prolonged vomiting), irritating (itchy rash), or merely annoying (sedation).

Adverse drugs reactions are more likely in the elderly, the sick and the frail. Because of their smaller size, and different distribution of body fat, women are more susceptible to mishaps than men. Higher doses of drugs are more likely to cause problems than lower doses. There are marked genetic differences in the way some people metabolize and excrete drugs; for instance Asians tend to be more susceptible to respiratory depression when given opioids than Caucasians. About one person in eight of Caucasian descent cannot metabolize codeine to its active forms, and so derive no benefit from it.

How to avoid problems

- Always use a drug's generic name.
- Do not use a drug unless there is a clear reason to do so.
- Never use a drug unless you know its effects, the dose and what can go wrong.
- Check the patient's record to know what drugs are already in the patient's system. Also check for over-the-counter complementary and alternative medications (herbal remedies).
- Check if a drug is suitable before giving it to a pregnant or breastfeeding patient.
- Never accept an illegible, altered or doubtful order for drugs.
- Discourage telephone orders for drugs.
- Check the patient's record and allergy bracelet before giving a drug.

- Check the drug, its dose, and the route of administration with a second person.
- Many slips occur because staff misread orders (illegible handwriting contributes too). For example:
  - *Correct:* insulin 40 units, morphine 5 mg;
  - *Incorrect:* insulin 40 u, morphine 5.0 mg.
- Query a prescription if it is difficult to read, or you have any doubt at all about the way it should be given.
- Give intravenous drugs slowly while monitoring the patient for adverse reactions.
- Reduce the dose in the elderly and frail.
- Obese patients do not need larger doses of drugs. Calculate the dose of most drugs on the patient's ideal body weight.

Anaesthetic drugs

Anaesthesia is derived from the Greek and means 'without feeling'. The history of anaesthesia is colourful, poignant and racy. In April 1857 Queen Victoria, courageously, and to demonstrate a point, because she certainly did not need an anaesthetic, gave birth to her eighth child (Leopold) under chloroform anaesthetic. The method of *chloroform à la reine* soundly rebuffed those people who believed the biblical injunction 'in sorrow shall thou bring forth children',[1] and was a big step towards making anaesthesia acceptable for surgical procedures.

Anaesthesia has three aims: to prevent the patient experiencing pain, to keep the patient safe from harm, and to provide the surgeon with the best possible operating conditions.

Anaesthetists use a variety of drugs, to induce *coma*, maintain it, and then reverse it at the end of the operation. Anaesthesia consists of three components: coma, muscle relaxation, and abolition of unwanted *reflexes*. Using drugs the anaesthetist can vary each these three components quite independently of each other.

Analgesia is omitted from this triad, because deeply comatose patients do not respond to pain, and in the lightly comatose pain causes unwanted reflex response. Furthermore the accepted definitions of pain do not allow the patient to be 'unaware' of it.

Induction

Coma is usually induced with propofol. The effects of this drug last for a few minutes. During this period the patient may be intubated using a short-acting muscle relaxant, or stabilized while spontaneously breathing on a volatile agent.

Maintenance

Coma is maintained with:

- a volatile halogenated hydrocarbon such as isoflurane, sevoflurane, or desflurane; or
- continuous intravenous anaesthesia with propofol.

Muscle relaxation is achieved with:

- short-acting muscle relaxants such as suxamethonium, and mivacurium;
- longer-acting muscle relaxants such as vecuronium, atracurium and rocuronium.

Unwanted reflex responses are managed with a variety of drugs according to need. For instance a fentanyl and propofol induction often causes *bradycardia*, which responds to atropine. Good analgesia modifies unwanted reflexes.

Analgesia is achieved with:

- opioids such as morphine, fentanyl, alfentanil, and remifentanil;
- ketamine;
- nitrous oxide.

Anxiolysis and sedation is achieved using midazolam, this is often given at the time of induction with fentanyl. If it is given before the beginning of the anaesthetic, in the holding bay, the patient must not be left alone as a small dose of midazolam can have a profoundly sedating effect in some patients. Midazolam is a very useful drug for patients having colonoscopies. A small dose up to 3 mg is appropriate. Larger doses can have unpredictable effects.

Dexmedetomidine[2] is also used for procedural sedation as well as sedation before awake fibre-optic intubation. Dexmedetomidine lowers the blood pressure and causes bradycardia. These side-effects are unlikely to cause problems in recovery room. Dexmedetomidine has a very short half-life of 6 minutes and it does not cause respiratory depression.

Emergence

At the end of the anaesthetic the anaesthetist may reverse the effects of:

- muscle relaxants with neostigmine or sugammadex;
- opioid-induced respiratory depression with naloxone;
- sedative effects of midazolam with flumazenil;
- usually the anaesthetist prefers to select the drugs in such a way that they have worn off by the end of the anaesthetic.

References

1. *Holy Bible*, King James Version, Genesis 3:16.
2. **Carollo DS** (2008) Dexmedetomidine: a review of clinical applications. *Current Opinion in Anaesthesiology* **21**:457–461.

Chapter 12

Mothers and babies

Pregnancy

Pregnant women come to the operating theatre for the usual elective and emergency operations, as well as those specific to their pregnancy. They present special challenges for those who look after them in the recovery room because their physiology is altered from the non-pregnant state.

Physiological changes during pregnancy

As pregnancy progresses the women's physiology:

- is affected by hormonal changes—principally involving progesterone;
- adapts to accommodate the mechanical effects of an enlarging uterus;
- adjusts to the increasing metabolic demands of a growing foetus;
- compensates for the low-pressure arteriovenous shunt in the placenta; and
- simultaneously prepares her for birth.

Changes in the cardiovascular system

Under the effects of progesterone in early pregnancy, the arterioles dilate decreasing peripheral vascular resistance. Having less *resistance* to push against, the heart needs to increase its output by 30 per cent merely to maintain the blood pressure. As pregnancy progresses the cardiac output increases by 30 per cent from about 4.5 L/min to about 6 L/min by the 17th week. The increase in stroke volume accounts for 40 per cent of the increase in cardiac output, while the remainder is due to a rise in pulse rate of about 15 beats/min. Because of the decreased peripheral vascular resistance the diastolic blood pressure falls, but the increase in cardiac output allows the systolic pressure to remain almost unchanged. Mean blood pressure is lowest at mid term and rises towards the non-pregnant level as the 37th week approaches.

Blood volume increases by 40 per cent, reaching a peak at 37 weeks. Pregnant women have a relative anaemia because the red cells are diluted in the increased blood volume, however they actually have a greater mass of red cells. Non-pregnant women have haematocrit of 40–45 per cent; and during pregnancy this drops to about 35 per cent. Because of this dilution the blood viscosity is lower, and blood flows more easily through the microcirculation. These physiological adaptations mean that any alteration in cardiac output or peripheral vascular resistance will cause larger changes in blood pressure than in non-pregnant women. Despite this adaptation, blood loss is better tolerated by the mother but it may be fatal for the foetus.

Supine hypotensive syndrome

About 11 per cent of pregnant patients who lie on their backs experience a fall in blood pressure of up to 30 mmHg. This supine hypotensive syndrome is caused by the pregnant uterus pressing on pelvic veins and reducing blood flow back to the heart. If a pregnant woman feels uncomfortable lying on her back, gently tilt her to her left side. The hypotension may be severe enough to cause foetal hypoxia and loss of consciousness of the mother.

What to do?
Fluid, ephedrine, call for help

Changes in the respiratory system

As the uterus grows larger, the work of breathing increases. Both mother and foetus need extra oxygen. Higher levels of the *hormones* progesterone and oestrogen stimulate the mother to breathe more deeply.

As the enlarging pregnant uterus pushes up the diaphragm, the lungs' functional residual capacity decreases. By full term the functional residual capacity is reduced so much that perfectly healthy women feel breathless at times. This is aggravated if the woman has an epidural during labour. As the abdominal muscles relax under the epidural the abdominal contents push the diaphragm up even further. Any increased demands for oxygen, such as shivering or severe agitation, will rapidly cause hypoxaemia that could compromise the foetus.

Changes in gastrointestinal function

As the uterus enlarges it pushes up the stomach, displacing the oesophageal sphincter and allowing reflux gastro-oesophageal contents to cause heart burn. Gastric emptying is delayed. After 24 weeks all pregnant patients coming to surgery should be treated as though they have a 'full stomach'. Nausea and vomiting are common. Because gastric emptying is slow it takes longer for drugs to reach the small intestine delaying the onset of drugs absorbed there, such as paracetamol. Opioids, such as pethidine, further delay gastrointestinal emptying.

Kidneys work more efficiently

Renal blood flow and the glomerular filtration rate increase with the rise in cardiac output. This enhances excretion, secretion and reabsorption of substances during pregnancy. Wastes are eliminated more efficiently so that plasma and creatinine concentrations decrease by almost half. Rising aldosterone secretion increases the reabsorption of water and sodium. Tissues tend to become oedematous as pregnancy progresses.

Blood coagulation increases

Pregnant women are specially adapted so that they do not bleed excessively after delivery. Although the mother's blood has a lower viscosity, it clots more easily. Deep vein thrombosis is always a risk. Fit graduated elastic stockings before surgery, or use sequential compression devices (SCD) and encourage leg exercises in recovery room. Heparin does not cross the placenta and is safe during pregnancy. Warfarin should not be used in pregnant patients as it causes fatal foetal abnormalities if used in during the first trimester, and may contribute to bleeding if used within a month of term. In some cases the postoperative use of enoxaparin should be considered.

Surgery for obstetric conditions

Surgery in obstetric patients can be usefully grouped as follows:

- before 24 weeks of gestation;
- between 24 and 30 weeks of gestation;
- after 30 weeks of gestation.

Before the 24th week

Before 24 weeks the most common operations are dilatation and curettage (D&C), cerclage, and surgery for *ectopic pregnancy* and termination of pregnancy.

Dilatation and curettage

D&Cs are performed for spontaneous, missed, or incomplete miscarriages. No attempt is made to save the foetus. Blood loss is sometimes enormous, especially if the pregnancy has progressed beyond the 12th week. Resuscitation for bleeding may begin before the patient reaches the operating theatre.

After their admission to the recovery room watch for any vaginal bleeding. This is usually treated with ergometrine, carboprost, or misoprostol. If these drugs cause nausea, give an antiemetic such as cyclizine, metoclopramide or ondansetron. These women are distressed by the loss of their baby. If practical allow her partner or mother to come and sit with her.

Box 12.1 **Tocolysis**

Tocolytics are drugs used to suppress premature labour. For example, the calcium channel blocker nifedipine is sometimes combined with the beta agonist, salbutamol, (this combination is highly likely to cause hypotension). These drugs are required initially to gain control of the contractions. The patient is then given steroids. Tocolytics are not used in cases of placental abruption, chorioamnionitis or where there is foetal death *in utero*, or after the 34th week of pregnancy.

Cerclage

Cervical incompetence, with threatened abortion, is the final common pathway of chorioamnionitis and placental abruption. A cervical stitch (Shirodkar), to close the cervix, is inserted in an attempt to forestall the threatened miscarriage. It is also used for women who repeatedly abort during the second trimester. This operation is sometimes called cerclage.

If the woman starts to bleed in the recovery room, it indicates she is either bleeding from the suture line, or is losing the foetus. Notify the obstetrician immediately. Either salbutamol or nifedipine is used to slow premature labour. Once the situation is under control the patient will be given steroids.

Painful uterine contractions often occur after cerclage. These do not necessarily indicate premature labour, but they will worry the patient. Tocolysis is now routinely used during and after the procedure, and will be continued in the recovery room (see Box 12.1). As a precaution against possible sepsis, make sure antibiotics have been given before the woman leaves the recovery room.

Ectopic pregnancy

An *ectopic pregnancy* is one that has formed outside the uterus, usually in the Fallopian tube. After about 10 weeks from conception the enlarging foetus ruptures the Fallopian tube causing bleeding. This is an emergency with a potentially massive blood loss. Usually surgeons excise the Fallopian tube, but if they decide to repair the tube, the procedure can take some hours.

In recovery room the patient may be cold, and anxious. Record her temperature, and warm her with a BairHugger™. The anaesthetist will order her intravenous fluids, which may include blood transfusion. Always use a blood warmer for these fluids. Take blood samples for full blood count (FBC) or make sure the ward have instructions to do this.

Termination of pregnancy

The surgical procedure is similar to D&C. The women's emotional response to having their pregnancy terminated ranges from relief, to heart-rending grief. Occasionally they are in a lot of pain, which responds to incremental doses of 20 mg of opioids plus simple analgesia. If the termination occurs after the 12th week, the patient may require an oxytocin infusion to prevent bleeding. The usual dose of oxytocin is 30 units in 500 ml of 0.9 per cent normal saline given at 85 ml/hour. Attach this as a side arm to the main intravenous infusion.

Watch for vaginal blood loss. If the woman soaks more than one perineal pad then notify the obstetrician.

From the 24th to the 30th week

From the 20th week to 26th week is the optimum time for doing unavoidable gynaecological surgery.

Between the 24th and 30th week the likely reasons for surgery are:

- antepartum haemorrhage;
- severe early onset pre-eclampsia requiring urgent delivery by Caesarean section;
- premature labour with breech or twin pregnancy facing unavoidable delivery.

Antepartum haemorrhage

Keep a close watch on the vaginal pads, and the bed sheet below the woman's buttocks for excessive blood loss. Notify the obstetrician if the blood loss continues or you need to replace one or two pads.

Monitor

Blood pressure, pulse rate, ECG, oximetry, urine output, perfusion status, and external blood loss. Watch for trends.

Laboratory

Haemoglobin, packed cell volume, platelet count, aPPT, international normalized ratio (INR), fibrinogen and fibrinogen degradation products. Cross-match four units of blood and notify the haematologist on duty.

Suspect disseminated intravascular coagulation (DIC) if:

- the platelet count is less than 70 000 /mm^3;
- there is increased INR or partial thromboplastin time (aPPT);
- the fibrinogen levels are less than 1.5 g/L;
- there are increased levels of fibrin degradation products.

Make sure the patient has a wide-bore needle in both arms, capable of conveying freely flowing infusions. Should DIC occur, then be prepared to give a massive blood transfusion. These patients are highly anxious; it is probable their baby has died, so they need a lot of comfort and emotional support.

From 30 weeks to term

Pre-eclampsia

Pre-eclampsia is a serious condition which can develop during pregnancy. It is associated with hypertension, proteinuria and fluid retention causing oedema. Complications can lead to death from cerebral haemorrhage, pulmonary oedema, gastric aspiration, and hepatorenal failure. Although delivery of the foetus usually terminates the disease it does not always. In some cases it may take up to 6 weeks to resolve completely.

In severe, early onset pre-eclampsia some form of coagulopathy is almost always present. It most commonly presents with thrombocytopenia with a platelet count less than 100 000 /mm^3. Pre-eclamptic women behave as if they are volume depleted with an excess noradrenergic drive pushing up their blood pressures. Their decreased blood volume is associated with decreased renal blood flow. This may progress to renal failure. Monitor the urine output closely in recovery room.

Before coming to the operating theatre the patient may be stabilized on an intravenous infusion of magnesium sulfate. Magnesium suppresses convulsions, controls hypertension, stabilizes cardiac rhythm, and improves renal blood flow. The usual infusion rate is about 1.5 mg/kg/hr. Other drugs including hydralazine, labetalol and methyldopa are also used to control the blood pressure and also phenytoin, and diazepam as the risk of convulsions is high. Make sure you have detailed written protocols about how to care for these infusions.

In the recovery room woman with pre-eclampsia should be kept very quiet. Avoid bright lights. Seizures can be stimulated by noise or light. Cautious use of fluids must be observed in these patients and careful records kept as they can easily go into pulmonary oedema if too much fluid is given.

Vomiting remains a grave risk, even after a spinal or epidural anaesthetic for Caesarean section. Because magnesium sulfate is sedating, the women will be drowsy, and remain at risk of aspiration pneumonitis. Never turn your back on these women, because they can quickly get into difficulties. Nurse them on their side and not on their back. Make sure you know how to tip the trolley head down.

Usually there is a urinary catheter in place. Note the urine output every 30 minutes, and report if it falls below 30 ml/hr. Monitor her blood pressure every 5 minutes for the first 30 minutes. If she has had a Caesarean section watch for excessive vaginal bleeding (more than one soaked pad or ooze from the suture line).

Eclampsia

Haemolysis, Elevated Liver enzymes and a Low Platelet count constitutes the *HELLP syndrome*. This indicates that pre-eclampsia is progressing towards eclampsia. A diastolic pressure greater than 110 mmHg needs immediate treatment with labetalol or hydralazine or nifedipine.

Patients who have a seizure or who lose consciousness have progressed from pre-eclampsia to eclampsia. Women who already show signs of toxaemia, such as hypertension, proteinuria, oedema, hyperreflexia, muscle twitching, headache, proteinuria, or thrombocytopenia may deteriorate in the recovery room. These women need close monitoring for at least 48 hours, and preferably longer. If they do have a fit while they are in recovery room call for help immediately and remember ABC.

> *Delivering the foetus is not the terminating event*
> *in eclampsia—or pre-eclampsia.*

If the woman starts to wheeze, then suspect encroaching pulmonary oedema. This is usually caused by over-enthusiastic fluid replacement, or less commonly by cardiac failure. An oxytocin infusion will aggravate the problem because it raises pulmonary artery pressures pushing fluid into alveoli. If carboprost, ergometrine or misoprostol have been given this will become an even bigger problem. The best sign of impending *pulmonary oedema* is an increasing respiratory rate, and feeling of shortness of breath. A chest X-ray will confirm the diagnosis.

Check that anticonvulsant drugs have been ordered before she leaves the recovery room. All pre-eclamptic patients must go to a supervised area such as labour ward or high dependency unit (HDU) for at least 24 hours post-delivery.

Premature labour

If the mother comes into labour before her due date, whether it is a single or multiple birth, she may well be anxious about the smallness and vulnerability of her baby or babies. Be supportive and reassure her where it is appropriate.

Often the woman will have been receiving *tocolytic therapy*, such as nifedipine or salbutamol, before her delivery. Nifedipine increases the risk of postpartum haemorrhage and hypotension. If she starts to bleed the loss can become overwhelming—be prepared for a *massive blood transfusion.*

The mother will also be receiving steroids to help prevent the baby developing *neonatal respiratory distress syndrome.*

Obstructed labour

Patients in obstructed labour are often well behind in fluid replacement. During their fruitless labour large fluid losses are caused by: hyperventilation, sweating, nausea, vomiting, and the inability to retain fluids by mouth. Furthermore, and especially in remote regions, the woman may have been like this for many hours. By the time they come to the recovery room these fluid deficits should be corrected. Check the fluid balance chart. The patient must have a urinary catheter, and it is important that her urine output is at least 60 ml/hr. The urine output is an excellent guide to fluid status.

Caesarean section

Traditionally Caesarean sections are only performed to deliver a baby who would otherwise be in jeopardy, or because the mother has an intercurrent medical or physical problem that makes it impossible to deliver her child safely. Increasingly, Caesarean sections are performed in otherwise healthy women who are capable of normal vaginal delivery, for reasons of convenience, or fear of medical litigation. Both the mother and baby undergo huge physiological changes in the first few hours after delivery. For this reason they need one-on-one nursing care over this period.

Common intercurrent morbidities in the mother include obesity, diabetes, asthma and anaemia. Lifestyle illnesses such as drug or alcohol and nicotine addiction affect both mother and baby. Sometimes religious beliefs or social pressure impinge on the care of the woman: for instance, blood transfusion in a Jehovah's Witness patient who refuses blood transfusion.

Let the mother have the baby as soon as safely possible. Position the mother on her left side with the baby beside her. You may need to give psychological support to the woman or her partner, especially as the normal maternal–child bonding process may have been circumvented.

*Watch the baby carefully
and monitor him or her continually.*

Monitor

Monitor perfusion status including pulse, blood pressure, oximetry, and urine output. Feel the uterine fundus; it should feel like a large orange just below the umbilicus. If it feels soft, like a loaf of bread, tell the obstetrician. A soft doughy uterus is likely to bleed later. Clots may prevent the uterus contracting. Ask the obstetrician to review the patient urgently. An atonic uterus is the main cause of postpartum haemorrhage.

Check that the indwelling catheter is patent: a full bladder prevents the uterus from contracting. Check that the intravenous line runs freely. Oxytocin is given to contract the uterus after delivery. Check for bleeding into the perineal pad, and look for pooling under the patient's buttocks. The normal vaginal blood loss is about 100 ml, or one saturated vaginal pad. If the blood loss exceeds this then tell the obstetrician.

If the patient continues to bleed from her vagina she may require an oxytocin infusion. Oxytocin 30 units is added to 500 ml of saline given at a rate of 85 ml/hr.

Record the blood pressure every 5 minutes for the first 30 minutes, and then every 10 minutes. Watch the trends. If the pulse rate exceeds 100 beats/min, or the systolic blood pressure falls below 100 mmHg, then assume the patient is bleeding. If bleeding persists the patient will need to return to the operating theatre to be examined under anaesthetic to see whether the bleeding is coming from the uterus (retained products) or a torn cervix.

Shivering after regional anaesthesia

Shivering postoperatively after regional anaesthesia is a common problem in the recovery room. Pethidine IV 25mg has been shown to be useful for reducing the incidence of shivering. Other agents such as giving dexmedetomidine intraoperatively are being evaluated but the evidence is inconclusive and cannot yet be recommended routinely.

Caring for the baby

'At-risk' babies are usually taken straight to the neonatal nursery. The babies who come with their mother to the recovery room are usually well, but remain vulnerable. They get cold easily. Keep them wrapped warmly. Often the mother is drowsy even if she has had had a spinal anaesthetic. She will find it difficult to care for the baby by herself. Let her hold her baby, and allow her to breastfeed once your initial observations are completed. The father will enjoy holding the baby but remember he cannot monitor it. You must watch that the baby remains pink, lively and warm.

Prolonged labour

If the labour has been long the woman's pain relief might include epidural infusions of local anaesthetics and diluted opioids. Her requirements for continuing postoperative pain relief and the liveliness of her newborn child will be affected by this preoperative medication. Continuing pain relief after the Caesarean section is not really a problem in recovery room. Make sure adequate prescriptions have been written for the ward.

*Never turn your back on the parents holding a
newborn baby in recovery room.*

Breech deliveries

Premature breech presentations and footling presentations often have a Caesarean section. With a vaginal breech delivery there may have been a period of great urgency, which the mother interprets as panic. If she was given an urgent general anaesthetic without much preliminary explanation, she might wake in a state of extreme anxiety. Have all the information about the baby ready to discuss with her. If the baby is unwell it is the obstetrician's duty to explain what has happened. Do not attempt this yourself.

Uterine muscle stimulants

Oxytocin is given to contract the uterus after delivery. Carbetocin[1] is an oxytocin agonist, 100 micrograms can be given instead of 5 international units of oxytocin and its effect is longer lasting. Carbetocin is associated with a reduced use of additional oxytocins. It is unclear whether this may reduce rates of haemorrhage and blood transfusions.

If the obstetrician requests an infusion to follow delivery of the baby this normally contains 30 units in 500 ml of 0.9 per cent saline. The usual rate is about 85 ml/hr. Oxytocin can sometimes drop the blood pressure because it reduces peripheral resistance, so check the blood pressure every 5 minutes. An alternative dilution is 40 units in 1 litre of fluid run at 166 ml/hr. This gives a lot of extra fluid and is not a better option.

Sometimes, intravenous ergometrine 5–10 mg is given to help contract the uterus. This causes nausea or vomiting. Always give an anti-emetic when you give ergometrine.

Carboprost is sometimes used for postpartum haemorrhage that does not respond to ergometrine. This must be given by deep intramuscular injection, and it may have unpleasant side-effects such as bronchospasm, nausea, vomiting, diarrhoea and flushing. Excessive doses have caused uterine rupture. Check the dose with another member of staff before giving it.

Primary postpartum haemorrhage

One of the most common causes of maternal death is inadequately managed postpartum haemorrhage.[2] Primary postpartum haemorrhage is where more than 500 ml of blood is lost within the first 24 hours after delivery. One reason is retained products of conception (a stray piece of placenta). In the absence of a coagulopathy, the empty contracted uterus should not bleed. If the woman is receiving blood when they arrive in the recovery room, then warm the intravenous fluids. Intra-arterial monitoring and a central line may be needed. The patient may require intensive care unit (ICU) care once stabilized.

Other postoperative problems

Other postoperative problems that may arise are: air embolism, aspiration pneumonitis, amniotic fluid embolism, and post-spinal headache and DIC.

Air embolism

Air emboli occur surprisingly often during Caesarean section. These small emboli seldom do harm, but may account for the feelings of alarm and restlessness that occur in patients having Caesarean sections under regional blockade. Occasionally air embolism is sufficient to cause hypotension, breathlessness and chest pain, which persists into the recovery room.

Aspiration pneumonitis

All pregnant patients are at risk of aspiration pneumonitis (Mendelson's syndrome). This is particularly fulminant and often fatal in obstetric patients. Following general anaesthesia, the anaesthetist will personally supervise her care until the woman is fully awake and has competent reflexes. Patients who have had their operation under spinal or epidural blockade are also at risk of aspiration, especially if they become hypotensive, which causes nausea, or they are sedated.

If aspiration has occurred in the operating theatre, the patient will remain intubated, and be transferred to intensive care for continuing management. In a fully resourced unit the woman will be given a trial without intubation and ventilation. This has the advantage that she will be able to deep breathe and cough on her own. She will require high oxygen flows, and if she cannot maintain her oxygen saturations above 90 per cent or develops a tachycardia or signs of hypoxia she will require intubation and ventilation. Steroids, bronchial lavage, and prophylactic antibiotics are no longer warranted in the early stages of aspiration pneumonitis. If lumps of food have been vomited then she may need a bronchoscopy to remove the foreign material. Chest X-ray changes do not show up for several hours. Young healthy people usually make a full recovery from aspiration pneumonia, especially if they have been premedicated with antacids. Do not blame yourself or your colleagues if you are present when aspiration occurs while you are looking after the patient.

Amniotic fluid embolism

Amniotic fluid embolism is fortunately an uncommon complication of labour and Caesarean section. It occurs when amniotic fluid enters the circulation, and is more severe if the foetus has been distressed *in utero* and produces meconium to soil the fluid. The incidence of amniotic embolism is thought to be about 1:50 000 deliveries. It is characterized by sudden collapse at the time of delivery, hypotension, cyanosis, DIC and continuing haemorrhage. There are no specific tests available to confirm the diagnosis, even though foetal cells can sometimes be isolated from the mother's blood. The patient will require ventilation in the intensive care unit with inotrope support of her blood pressure, antibiotics and management of the coagulopathy. The mortality exceeds 80 per cent.

Post-spinal headache

Post-spinal headache occurs in about 1–2 per cent of patients who have had either an epidural or a spinal anaesthetic. Excessive cerebrospinal fluid leaks into the *epidural space* causing traction on the meninges in the brain. This produces a fearful headache which is exacerbated by sitting or standing. Using pencil point spinal needles lessens the risk. Good hydration helps prevent spinal headache and eases the symptoms if they occur. Most patients will require a blood patch. See page 145.

Incidental surgery in pregnant women

Pregnant patients sometimes require surgery during their pregnancy for non-obstetric reasons. Appendicectomy is the most common emergency operation during pregnancy, and usually erupts in the third trimester.

Less common operations are cholecystectomy, ovarian cystectomy, and a procedure for strangulated haemorrhoids. If they are elective operations then they are usually performed between the 14th and 24th week of gestation. Since the women are mostly young, fit and otherwise healthy their recovery should be straightforward, however they remain at risk of aspiration.

Nurse the patient on their side to reduce the risk of aspiration. Give supplemental oxygen by mask to prevent hypoxaemia affecting either the mother or her foetus. Make sure that any drugs you give are safe in pregnant patients.

Laparoscopic surgery

Carbon dioxide insufflated during laparoscopic cholecystectomy can cause problems. Carbon dioxide embolism is more likely during pregnancy because of the increased vascularity of the vessels in her abdomen. Carbon dioxide causes capillaries to dilate increasing the risk of postoperative ooze into the peritoneal cavity.

Following appendicectomy, systemic sepsis may be a great risk to the baby. Women having an appendicectomy will need prophylactic antibiotics; usually with a combination of a cephalosporin and metronidazole.

Major surgery

If the woman is having major surgery then consult the labour ward staff about monitoring the foetus to detect signs of foetal distress such as bradycardia or persistent tachycardia. Usually the labour ward staff will come to the recovery room to help you with this.

If foetal distress occurs then do everything possible to improve uterine perfusion and foetal oxygenation. Keep the mother on her left side, give supplemental oxygen, and ensure the maternal perfusion status is optimal—her skin is warm and her urine output exceeds 60 ml/hr. Give IV fluids to restore vascular volume.

It is good practice to check the maternal blood glucose levels in pregnant women in the recovery room because surgery increases the levels of stress *hormones*, to cause hyperglycaemia.

Should a pregnant patient need an X-ray in the recovery room, then shield her uterus and her baby from stray X-rays.

Ask the ward nurses to check the foetal heart once they have the patient back in the ward. If everything is fine with the baby this will reassure the mother.

Options for pain relief

After surgery

Pain relief after surgery during pregnancy is managed in the same manner as pain relief after surgery in patients who are not pregnant.

Opioids

Morphine and diamorphine are cleared very quickly in labour and the concentration of morphine in the newborn is almost undetectable. Pethidine has traditionally been described as the safest opioid in obstetrics but this has never been substantiated by controlled trials. Many studies suggest that pethidine is no better, and sometimes is worse than other narcotics. Placental cord concentrations of pethidine reach two-thirds of the concentration in the mother's blood.

After Caesarean section

Most mothers are not overly concerned by pain after Caesarean section and they are distracted by their babies. If they have been given opioids as part of their anaesthetic these may still be effective.

Frequently a small dose of fentanyl is added to the spinal anaesthetic to provide analgesia that lasts a few hours after the block wears off. Adding morphine to spinal anaesthesia provides long-lasting postoperative analgesia but can cause an annoying itch. After receiving spinal morphine, the mother's respiratory rate needs monitoring when she returns to the ward.

*Patients who have had spinal
morphine need close monitoring*

Many obstetric units routinely give paracetamol intravenously in theatre, or orally in the recovery room. Long-acting oral morphine is useful and can be supplemented with small doses of a short-acting opioid like Sevredol® morphine sulfate for breakthrough pain. Patient-controlled anaesthesia (PCA) is favoured by some units. If so, then PCA should be started before the effects of the spinal anaesthetic wear off. Before considering

PCA remember that most women prefer to be free of all drips and catheters as soon as possible so that they can care for their babies.

Make sure the pain relief to follow the spinal anaesthetic is given while you are still in charge of the patient. It is extremely distressing for a patient to have spinal block wear off before another analgesic regime has been established.

References

1. Attilakos G, Psaroudakis D, *et al.* (2010) Carbetocin versus oxytocin. *BJOG: An International Journal of Obstetrics and Gynaecology* **117**(8):929–36.
2. Kayem G, Kurinczuk JJ, *et al.* (2011) Specific second-line therapies for postpartum haemorrhage. *BJOG: An International Journal of Obstetrics and Gynaecology* **118**(7):856–64.

Further Reading

Royal College of Obstetricians and Gynaecologists (2011) *Prevention and Management of Postpartum Haemorrhage.* Green-top Guideline No. 52. London: Royal College of Obstetricians and Gynaecologists.

Chapter 13

Paediatrics

Introduction

Children and babies frequently have operations and come to the recovery room. In the recovery room cardiac arrest and emergencies are three times more common in children than in adults. Children's anatomy and physiology is not similar to that of a scaled-down adult; they pose special problems.

Most complications are caused by laryngospasm following difficult intubation, or an overdose of anaesthetic drugs. Infants under the age of 1 month are at greatest risk because they are more likely to have major surgery, and tend to be sicker than older children.

For the purposes of this book:

+ premature babies are those born before the 37th week from conception (see Box 13.1);

+ neonates are babies born within 44 weeks from the date of conception;

+ infants are under the age of 1 year;

Box 13.1 Prematurity

The age of premature babies is calculated in post-conceptual weeks. A baby born at 28 weeks and now 4 weeks old, is 32 weeks post-conception.

Premature babies are less able to maintain their body temperature, swallow, suck or even breathe properly. Asphyxia during birth predisposes them to brain damage. If they are given 100 per cent oxygen they are at risk of developing retinopathy of prematurity (ROP). They are also at risk of intraventricular haemorrhage, respiratory distress syndrome, bronchopulmonary dysplasia, anaemia, and apnoeic episodes. They may have a patent ductus arteriosus and are at risk of necrotizing colitis.

Premature babies normally consume oxygen at about 8 ml/kg/min (compared with a full-term baby's 7 ml and an adult's 3.5 ml). Their respiratory rate can be as high as 60 breaths/min with tidal volumes of 110–160 ml/kg/min.

Compared with full-term babies, premature babies are more sensitive to anaesthetic agents. The volatile anaesthetics prevent their heart rate from increasing and their baroreceptors and chemoreceptors do not trigger responses, so they do not compensate for hypoxia or failing perfusion. They are also particularly intolerant to hypothermia.

- babies include neonates and infants;
- children are aged 1 year to 12 years;
- adolescents are between the age of 13 and 16 years.

Neonates and infants

Neonates have a high metabolic rate; their oxygen consumption is about 7 ml/kg/min, which is twice that of an adult's 3.5 ml/kg/min and is the reason why they desaturate more rapidly than an adult.

The dead space volume of the neonatal airways is proportionally the same as an adult's so they must breathe twice as quickly to meet their high oxygen demands. Children become hypoxic and cyanosed rapidly.

*Neonates cannot alter their volumes
so they alter their rates instead.*

Although neonates, and to a lesser degree infants, have pliant chest walls, their lungs are stiffer than those of an adult's. The alveoli are thicker walled, and events such as pneumonia or neonatal respiratory distress syndrome make their lungs even stiffer. They only use their diaphragms to draw air into their lungs. They compensate for this by having a high respiratory rate (about 32 breaths/min).

When neonates breathe in, instead of their lungs filling fully with air, their chest walls tend to cave in. This results in a reduced amount of air entering their lungs. At the end of expiration there is proportionately less air left in their lungs than in an adult. This means that neonates do not have a big reservoir of air (*functional residual capacity*) left in their lungs at the end of expiration, and without this store they become hypoxic quickly. After an anaesthetic, babies' muscles are sometimes too fatigued to breathe. Babies should be completely awake before the anaesthetist leaves them.[1]

*While the hearts of babies and children are relatively
resistant to hypoxia, their brains are not.*

Airway obstruction

Neonates breathe through their noses, and their narrow nasal passages are easily blocked by nasal secretions.

Factors contributing to an obstructed airway in neonates and infants are:

- large heads, short necks and prominent occiputs;
- big floppy tongues;
- large tonsils and adenoids;
- a large stiff epiglottis;
- a high larynx, with a small opening which is prone to oedema if it is traumatized or the infant is over-hydrated; the narrowest part of a child's airway is at the cricoid cartilage;

• the ribs are flexible making forceful coughing difficult;

• neonates and infants less than 2–3 months old cannot breathe through their mouths.

Airway problems seen in the first postoperative hour include:

• airway obstruction caused by the tongue obstructing the nasal pharynx;

• laryngeal spasm;

• croup following extubation;

• respiratory depression;

• aspiration;

• apnoea.

Signs of an obstructed airway in an infant or child are:

• supracostal, intercostal and subcostal retraction;

• inspiratory stridor or crowing;

• nasal flaring;

• decreased or absent breath sounds.

Since neonates and younger babies cannot increase their tidal volume to increase their minute volume they need to increase their respiratory rate.

If a spontaneously breathing baby cannot sustain a PaO_2 greater than 60 mmHg (7.89 kPa) or a $PaCO_2$ less than 60 mmHg (7.89 kPa) it should be re-intubated. Intubation in babies is not difficult. An emergency tracheostomy is almost never required.

Foreign body aspiration

Foreign body aspiration (FBA) presents with an abrupt onset of coughing or respiratory distress, using every available muscle to breathe. It occurs if a child has inhaled something through the larynx into the lower airway. Give oxygen and call for help.

If the aspiration is severe the child is unable to make much sound, unable to breathe, becomes cyanosed quickly and loses consciousness. Establish an airway and start *basic life support* (BLS).[2]

Apnoea in the newborn

Neonates commonly stop breathing after having a general anaesthetic. This *apnoea* becomes serious if it lasts longer than 15 seconds, severe if the pulse oximeter reveals desaturation, and critical if associated with bradycardia, cyanosis or pallor.

Infants born prematurely, or those babies with a history of respiratory distress syndrome or bronchopulmonary dysplasia, are susceptible to apnoea following even short general anaesthetics. Their susceptibility to apnoea persists for the first 6 months of life, and can occur up to 12 hours after surgery. It is more common if muscle relaxants were used. For these reasons, all infants who have been premature babies and all infants who are less than 3 months old (52 post-conceptual weeks) are unsuitable for day case surgery. They need hospital admission and respiratory monitoring for the first 24 hours. Monitor infants of less than 45 post-conceptual weeks for 18 hours post anaesthesia. Monitor all infants under 6 months of age (64 post-conceptual weeks) with a pulse oximeter, and if possible a respiratory monitor for at least two hours postoperatively.

Factors contributing to episodes of apnoea in the recovery room are:

- immaturity of the central nervous respiratory control centres;
- depression of the chemoreceptor response to hypoxia by residual anaesthetic agents; and
- residual effects of muscle relaxants.

Pneumothorax in infants

Pneumothorax, where air escapes from the lungs into the pleural cavity, is not uncommon. It occurs if their little lungs are over-inflated, and can easily happen if the baby coughs during intubation or extubation. Physical signs, such as an absence of breath sounds, are difficult to detect, but the heart's apex beat may be displaced as the mediastinum shifts. Shine a light through the chest wall from behind and you may see the outline of the collapsed lung. Cyanosis and bradycardia are late signs. If a baby's oxygen saturation suddenly deteriorates, or their respiratory rate rises, think of pneumothorax. Always keep the necessary equipment to drain a pneumothorax sterilized and ready.

Children

Prevent airway obstruction, caused by the tongue falling back into the pharynx, by routinely nursing children on their sides. If this fails gently extend the head to relieve the obstruction. Call for help now. If the obstruction is still not relieved then insert a nasal airway. Nasal airways are better than oral airways in children because they are less likely to stimulate gagging, vomiting or laryngospasm. Give 100 per cent oxygen until the airway is completely clear. Use gentle suction, and if this is not successful have a proper look at the pharynx with a laryngoscope.

Keep nasal airways available
when recovering children.

Laryngeal spasm

Stimulation of the pharynx causes a *reflex* contraction of the intrinsic muscles of the larynx. This *laryngeal spasm* may tightly close the glottis so that no air can pass. The sound you will occasionally hear is stridor. Stridor means that the airway is not completely blocked.

Laryngeal spasm is the body's emergency response to prevent foreign material entering the lower respiratory tract. Spasm can be triggered by mucus, blood or other material in the pharynx and sometimes merely by suction of the upper airway. Be gentle when using a sucker.

The incidence of laryngeal spasm is higher in children under the age of 9 years and reaches a maximum between the ages of 1–3 months. Patients with Down's syndrome are particularly susceptible to laryngeal spasm. The problem is more likely to occur if the child has a respiratory tract infection. Laryngeal spasm is a frightening event. It may not resolve spontaneously until the child has become deeply and dangerously hypoxic. Seek help early.

Initial management of laryngospasm

- Give oxygen by mask.
- Call for help.
- Fetch the emergency paediatric trolley.
- Attach a pulse oximeter.
- Attach an ECG monitor.

Then attempt to relieve the spasm by firm pressing behind the angles of the jaw to lift it forward. Try ventilating the child using firm *positive pressure* from a mask. This may fail. Attempts to strenuously ventilate the patient by forcing air into the pharynx can worsen the obstruction.

Further management of laryngospasm

If the initial measures fail to relieve the obstruction within 30 seconds a dose of 1 per cent lidocaine 1.5 mg/kg intravenously usually resolves the spasm. If lidocaine is unsuccessful the anaesthetist should give suxamethonium 0.5 mg/kg intravenously together with atropine 20 micrograms/kg and then '*bag and mask*' the patient until the situation is assessed. The patient may need intubation for a short spell.

Acute *pulmonary oedema* is an uncommon complication of laryngospasm. It is probably caused by the violent swings in intrathoracic pressure generated as the child struggles to breathe sufficiently to overcome the obstruction.

How to manage stridor

Sit the child up, summon help, give oxygen, and get ready to give humidified oxygen and nebulized adrenaline. To prepare the adrenaline for the nebulizer, take 2 ml of 1:1000 solution of adrenaline and make it up to a total of 5 ml in 0.9 per cent saline. Put it into the nebulizer's reservoir and give it using a flow rate of oxygen of 5 L/min.

Adrenaline reduces the oedema by causing vasoconstriction in the inflamed mucosa. The effects are short-lived, lasting about 2 hours. Children undergoing day case surgery who experience stridor postoperatively should be admitted as an inpatient overnight for observation.

Always get an expert to assess the child. A child with severe airway obstruction may look reassuringly pink on supplemental oxygen with satisfactory pulse oximeter readings, but be gravely hypoventilating and in danger of totally obstructing their airway.

Stridor means airway obstruction; treat it immediately. It is a dangerous waste of time to confirm the obstruction with lateral cervical X-rays.

The anaesthetist may need to re-intubate the child. Prepare a range of endotracheal tube sizes because children with stridor need a smaller tube diameter than their normal size.

Croup

A hoarse voice, or a barking cough are signs of developing croup. These signs tend to resolve spontaneously. Croup usually occurs because the delicate mucosal lining of the trachea is irritated by the endotracheal tube and becomes oedematous. Croup is caused by oedema partially closing the airway just below the larynx. It occurs in about four per cent of children who have been intubated. Oedema fluid easily accumulates in the loose submucosal tissue, where the cricoid cartilage forms a complete ring around the trachea.

Infants are more susceptible than older children, because they have a smaller larynx (4 mm in diameter compared with 8 mm in an adult) so that an equivalent amount of oedema reduces the diameter of the trachea by a proportionally greater amount (Figure 13.1). Rarely the cough progresses to stridor, a far more serious problem, heralding complete airway obstruction and respiratory arrest. The signs of croup or stridor usually occur within the first hour after extubation but it can be much later.

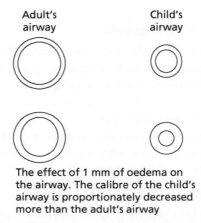

Adult's airway   Child's airway

The effect of 1 mm of oedema on the airway. The calibre of the child's airway is proportionately decreased more than the adult's airway

Figure 13.1 The effect of one millimetre of oedema on the cross-sectional area of an adult's and a child's bronchus.

When to get help

Get help immediately if there is stridor or you can see signs of increased work of breathing with rib and subcostal retraction, or if the child is unsettled, worried or restless. Anaphylaxis may also present with stridor, wheeze and an urticarial rash. Later the face and tongue swell. See page 332.

Respiratory depression

As a rough guide the normal respiratory rate in children is

$$24 - \frac{age}{2}$$

If the child's respiratory rate is less than this (see Box 13.2), or their breathing is weak and shallow then they have respiratory depression. Children recover quickly and predictably from muscle relaxants so look for other reasons for the respiratory depression. Infants pulling their legs up when they cry are unlikely to have residual muscle relaxation causing their respiratory depression. Older children should be able to lift their heads from the pillow.

Box 13.2 **Assisted ventilation in infants < 10 kg**

Aim for:

- respiratory rate 30–40 breaths per minute;
- inflation pressure of up to 25 cm H_2O;
- fresh gas flows of 4 L/min;
- positive end expiratory pressures of 5 cm H_2O.

When to worry

Get help immediately if the child:

- is anxious, unsettled or restless;
- has an oximeter reading < 95%;
- is fatigued, listless or their conscious state is deteriorating;
- appears to be working hard to breathe.

Other reasons for residual muscle paralysis following relaxant anaesthesia are hypothermia, hypocalcaemia or acidosis. Under these circumstances the anaesthetist should not hesitate to re-intubate the infant and transfer him to intensive care for observation and monitoring.

Opioids also contribute to respiratory depression. They may need naloxone 4 micrograms/kg to reverse the effects of the opioids. Naloxone only lasts for 30–40 minutes and when it wears off the respiratory depression may recur.

Fentanyl is very slowly metabolized in babies and should not be used in the recovery room.

Aspiration

Suspect aspiration if a child suddenly develops a wheeze or a cough. Infants are susceptible to aspiration because they have a short oesophagus, their cough *reflex* is not well developed and their laryngeal competence is decreased for 6–8 hours following extubation.

Endotracheal intubation

Table 13.1 and the following equations will assist with selecting the correct endotracheal tube size should this be required.

Table 13.1 Endotracheal tube sizes

Age	Weight (kg)	Tube size (mm)	Length to tip (cm)
Neonate	3.5	3.0	8.5
2 months	5	3.5	9
6 months	8	4.0	10
1 year	10	4.0	11

Endotracheal tube specifications

For children older than 1 year:

$$\text{Tube size} = \frac{\text{age(yr)} + 4}{4}$$

$$\text{Tube length} = \frac{\text{age (yr)} + 12}{2}$$

Salivary gland enlargement

Sometimes acute engorgement of the parotid, submaxillary or sublingual glands occurs during anaesthesia and persists in the recovery room. The face appears to be bloated, as if the child has mumps, and the glands are felt as firm masses. The problem usually subsides with an hour and is not dangerous unless it causes airway obstruction.

Cardiovascular physiology

Pulse rates

The cardiac muscles of a neonate contract less forcibly than older children, and the heart is also stiffer. This means that if neonates need to raise their cardiac output, they must increase their heart rate.

As soon as babies are settled check their notes to find out their preoperative baseline pulse rate, pulse rates vary widely from baby to baby. The pulse rate is an excellent guide to their physical progress in recovery room. A return to the preoperative pulse rate is a happy sign that all is well (Table 13.2).

Bradycardias

The cardiac output in children is rate-dependent, and as a result a bradycardia causes hypotension. The sympathetic innervation of the heart is not as well developed as the parasympathetic, making babies prone to bradycardia. They do not tolerate bradycardia well; for instance, apnoea and bradycardia may follow suctioning the pharynx and this can quickly cause severe hypoxaemia.

A child's heart is relatively resistant to hypoxia, so that by the time hypoxia is severe enough to cause a bradycardia cardiac arrest is near and brain damage has already occurred.

> *Bradycardia causing hypoxia in children*
> *is a grave sign.*

Ensure a clear airway and oxygenate the child while preparing to give atropine. Use a close-fitting face mask and insert a suitable Guedel airway. Use positive pressure ventilation. Short, small, frequent breaths are best. Uncover the baby's chest and observe the results of your ventilation. Notify the anaesthetist and call for help. Atropine alone without oxygenation is not effective. If bradycardia does not respond quickly then commence the advanced life support protocol with cardiac massage and prepare to give adrenaline.

Table 13.2 Normal paediatric heart rates and blood volumes

Newborn and young babies	Older babies and toddlers	Pre-school children	School children
Pulse (P): 110–160 beats per minute Tachycardia (T): over 180 beats per minute	P: 110–160 beats per minute T: over 160 beats per minute	P: 110–160 beats per minute T: over 160 beats per minute	P: 80–120 beats per minute T: over 120 beats per minute
Systolic blood pressure (SBP): variable, but range 50–85 mmHg	SBP: 80–95 mmHg	SBP: 80–100 mmHg	SBP: 90–110 mmHg

Tachycardia

Children often have a high resting pulse rate. Look in the notes to find the preoperative rate and use this as a guide. A child in the recovery room with a tachycardia may be either in pain or hypovolaemic. Suspect hypovolaemia if the child has cool hands and poor capillary return in the fingernail beds.

Attach an ECG. Tachyarrhythmias are uncommon in children, but if they do occur it is usually a narrow complex *supraventricular tachycardia* (SVT). The anaesthetist may choose to treat this with either vagal stimulation, or if that fails, with intravenous adenosine 0.05 mg/kg up to 0.25 mg/kg.

Transient viral myocarditis in the first few weeks following a respiratory infection occasionally occurs in children. Usually the irregular pulse is not noticed by the parents and resolves without incident, but if the child has an operation during this period they may develop a supraventricular tachycardia in the recovery room. An ECG with looping ST segments in all leads adds weight to the diagnosis.

Hypertension

Acute hypertension in a child is unusual. It may reflect over-enthusiastic fluidreplacement, and is more common in children with pre-existing kidney disease.

Fluids in children

By the age of 3 years the volume of body water has decreased from 80 per cent of body weight at birth to the adult value of about 60 per cent. Of this, a third of the volume is in the extracellular space and two-thirds is in the intracellular compartment. The extracellular compartment is further divided into interstitial fluid (lying between the cells), and intravascular fluid (*plasma*). When fluid is lost from the body it initially comes from the smallest of the compartments—the plasma.

Why give fluids?

Intravenous fluids are given for four reasons: maintenance, replacement of losses, resuscitation, and as a vehicle for intravenous drugs.

When to give fluids

Most well children undergoing minor surgery do not need intravenous fluids when they return to the ward. Conversely, those having major or prolonged surgery where continuing losses are anticipated, or where the child is unable to take oral fluids for some time will need intravenous replacement and maintenance fluids.

Hypovolaemic children, or those that are shocked will be resuscitated either before surgery, or while they are in the operating theatre. Sometimes resuscitation needs to continue in the recovery room.

What sorts of fluid are available?

Isotonic crystalloid solutions contain the same concentration of ions as blood, and so they exert the same osmotic pressure. Examples of isotonic fluids include: 0.9 per cent normal saline, Hartmann's solution (Ringer's lactate) and Plasma-Lyte®. Plasma-Lyte® is the most appropriate fluid to give in the recovery room.[3] *Third space fluid* in the gut is an isotonic fluid with small variations in potassium and other ions.

Hypotonic fluids contain fewer ions than are present in the blood, and so exert a lower osmotic pressure. This means that when you give a hypotonic fluid, water floods into cells everywhere until the osmotic balance is re-established. Examples of hypotonic fluids are 5 per cent glucose in water, and 4.5 per cent glucose and 1/5 normal saline. These fluids are used to replace water lost in dehydration. This problem is very unlikely to occur in recovery room.

What fluids to give

The choice of intravenous fluid depends on the cause of the problem, and usually replaces what was lost. Heavily bleeding patients need blood. Gastrointestinal loss is replaced with isotonic crystalloid solutions, preferably Hartmann's solution or Plasma-Lyte®. For simple dehydration, where a child has been fasting and has not been drinking water, then 4.5 per cent glucose and 0.18 per cent normal saline is still used.

On admitting the child to recovery room

As soon as practical after the child has been admitted to the recovery room check what fluids were given in theatre. A baby of up to 15 kg should have received approximately 20 ml/kg. Children weighing from 15–30 kg need approximately 15 ml/kg and older children 10 ml/kg.

Hypovolaemia

Acute reduction in plasma volume is called hypovolaemia, and unless treated rapidly progresses to shock. Bleeding and loss of fluid into the gut are the commonest causes of postoperative hypovolaemia.

Hypovolaemia is a grave threat to neonates and infants. An adult can lose 10 per cent of their blood volume without noticeable effect; in a neonate a 10 per cent loss of blood volume is life threatening. A 2.5 kg neonate, with a normal blood volume of about 250 ml is severely shocked by a blood loss of only 20–25 ml, which is the amount of blood absorbed on one small well-soaked gauze square.

A loss of surprisingly little fluid from *plasma* activates physiological compensatory mechanisms. These include neuroendocrine responses that cause the kidney to retain sodium and water, vasoconstriction and a tachycardia. In effect children go white or mottled, have a fast heart rate, cool hands, and low urine output. Hypotension is a late and serious sign of hypovolaemia. For most purposes you can estimate a child's normal blood pressure to be 80 + (age in years × 2) mmHg.

Young infants may not develop a tachycardia. If the fluid loss has been slow the baby may also have a sunken fontanelle.

> *Do not be afraid to give fluids to neonates,*
> *hypovolaemia is a greater threat than fluid overload.*

Capillary refill time

Capillary refill time is a useful and easy test to determine whether the child is mounting a neuroendocrine response to hypovolaemia. Press on the child's sternum or finger for 5 seconds, remove the pressure and then time how long it takes for the white blanche mark to fade. In normally hydrated children this should be less than 3 seconds. If it takes longer than that then assume the child is hypovolaemic and prepare to give intravenous fluids.

If hypovolaemia is suspected check the drains and catheters for continuing loss. Check the haemoglobin (or haematocrit) and prepare to cross-match blood.

How much fluid to treat hypovolaemia?

First give 20 ml/kg of Plasma-Lyte® or Hartmann's solution, and repeat it as necessary if the capillary refill time is more than 3 seconds. If you need to repeat it more than once then seek advice from the anaesthetist.

How to calculate fluid deficit

A child's fluid deficit is calculated from an estimation of their fluid deficit expressed as a percentage of body weight (not their body water). For example, a child weighing 10 kg who is estimated to be 5 per cent dehydrated has an isotonic fluid deficit of 500 ml.

Ongoing losses from drains are measured and then replaced with a similar fluid. For instance, blood is replaced with blood, and gastrointestinal losses with Plasma-Lyte® or Hartmann's solution.

4.5 per cent glucose and 0.18 per cent normal saline is NOT
an appropriate fluid for unwell children.

Shock

Shock is a clinical diagnosis based on a set of symptoms and signs that occur when the circulation is insufficient to meet the metabolic demands of the tissues and to remove their waste products. The biochemical marker of shock is lactic acid produced by hypoxic tissues.

Delivering oxygen to the tissues depends on a chain of events: the heart pumps oxygen and nutrients dissolved in the blood through a series of vessels to the tissues where they are used. The type of shock depends on where this chain of events is disrupted. *Cardiogenic* shock occurs when the pump fails. *Haemorrhagic* or hypovolaemic shock occurs when there is not enough blood or body fluids. If the normal vascular tone is lost, the *resistance* vessels (arterioles) dilate causing the blood pressure to fall. This loss of peripheral resistance can be caused by tissue factors (anaphylaxis or toxins). Septic shock disrupts all three links in the chain: the heart, body fluids, and the vessels.

Diagnose shock early,
and treat it vigorously.

Shock is a progressive phenomenon, but roughly falls into three phases: compensated, uncompensated, and irreversible. Compensated shock presents with oliguria, tachycardia and poor capillary return time, uncompensated shock occurs when the blood pressure falls and the pulse rate drops, and irreversible shock is a post-mortem diagnosis where the organ damage is so severe that recovery is impossible.

Haemorrhagic shock

Diagnosis

If the child looks pale check the pulse rate and compare it to the preoperative rate. If possible check the urine output (Figure 13.2).

The volume should be greater than 2 ml/kg/hr. Check the blood pressure. If you do not have a small enough cuff let the pulse pressure guide you. If you cannot feel a radial pulse, try for the brachial, then the axillary. Hypotension in older children is a disastrously late

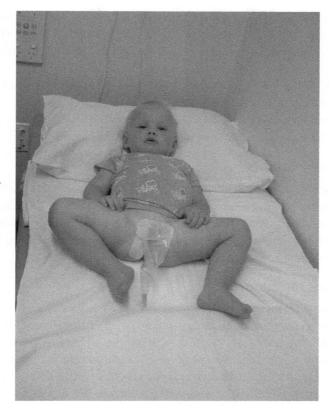

Figure 13.2 Urine collection in an infant.

sign of hypovolaemia. If it does occur it begins with a falling systolic pressure, rising diastolic pressure and a muffled apex beat when you listen with a stethoscope.

Management

+ Give high flows of oxygen with a face mask.
+ Lay the child flat and lift the legs on to a pillow. Do not tip the child head down.
+ Call for help.
+ Prepare to give fluids rapidly. Ideally, this requires two short wide-bore cannulae, one in each cubital fossa.
+ Prepare to take blood for full blood count, electrolytes and urea, glucose, and cross-matching.
+ Give blood; use either cross-matched or rhesus negative type-specific blood.
+ Look for a source of bleeding.
+ If sepsis is thought to be a possibility then collect blood for culture.

Give a fluid bolus of 20 ml/kg through a blood warmer of isotonic crystalloid and then recheck the capillary refill, pulse rate, and blood pressure. Suitable crystalloids are Plasma-Lyte®, Hartmann's solution or 0.9 per cent saline. Do not give glucose-containing solutions.

Then check the capillary return time. If it is longer than 3 seconds then repeat the dose of 20 ml/kg of isotonic crystalloid.

If further boluses are required, then use blood: either low antibody-titre O negative, or type-specific blood, or if there is time fully cross-matched blood.

Transfusion in infants

Blood volume is higher in the neonate, 90–100 ml/kg compared with the 70–80 ml/kg in the adult. When replacing blood give it to the nearest 10 ml above the estimated loss. For example, if the estimated blood loss is 35 ml, then give 40 ml. It is safer to slightly overload neonates and infants than to have them plasma volume deplete. While you are waiting for the blood prime your blood giving set and line with normal saline.

Intraosseous injection

Finding a vein can sometimes be a problem in shocked children. Rather than attempting saphenous vein cut downs, the anaesthetist may site an intraosseous needle (Figure 13.3). This approach is life-saving and under used. It has two advantages: bone marrow can be collected for haemoglobin and electrolytes (but not glucose concentrations), and it is possible to run fluids in rapidly. If children are conscious they will need a local anaesthetic. It is a strictly sterile procedure. Stop the infusion once intravenous access has been established.

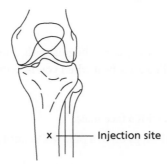

x ———— Injection site

Figure 13.3 Tibial site for intraosseous injection.

Fluid replacement

Normal maintenance fluids are fluids given to otherwise well children who are not taking any fluids by mouth. Normal fluid maintenance replacement should not exceed 2400 ml per day.

The volume of maintenance fluid replaces the normal urine output and insensible losses (sweat, loss through the lungs and in the stools). As children grow older, they require proportionately less fluid (see Table 13.3).

Table 13.3 Calculating the volume of maintenance fluid

Weights in kg	ml per day	ml per hour
3–10	100 × weight (kg)	4 × weight (kg)
10–20	1000 + (50 × (wt – 10))	40 + (2 × (wt –10))
> 20	1500 + (20 × (wt – 20))	60 + (1 × (wt –10))

For instance:

An 8 kg baby needs:

$$100 \times 8 = 800 \text{ ml per day}$$

$$4 \times 8 = 32 \text{ ml per hour}$$

An 18 kg baby needs:

$$1000 + (50 \times (18 - 10)) = 1400 \text{ ml per day}$$

$$40 + (2 \times (8 - 10)) = 46 \text{ ml per hour}$$

A 30 kg child needs:

$$1500 + (20 \times (30 - 20)) = 1700 \text{ ml per day}$$

$$60 + (1 \times (30 - 10) = 70 \text{ ml per hour}$$

Which fluid to use

For otherwise well children use 0.45 per cent sodium chloride with 5 per cent glucose and add 20 mmol/L of potassium chloride (KCl).

Do not use this solution if the:

• serum potassium is elevated beyond 4.5 mmol/L;
• serum sodium is less than 136 mmol/L;
• child is hypovolaemic or shocked;
• child is dehydrated.

Problems with glucose solutions

Do not use 5 per cent glucose for replacement or maintenance fluids. Even a small rise in blood glucose to 8 mmol/L can cause an osmotic diuresis leading to excessive extracellular fluid loss. If you use 5 per cent glucose to replace isotonic fluid lost during surgery the infant's serum sodium concentration will fall, and water will move into the cells. This shift may cause cerebral oedema in which case the infant develops signs of irritability, restlessness, a mew-like cry, drowsiness, vomiting and in severe cases, convulsions.

Kidneys

For the first 2 years of life blood flow through the kidneys, and consequently the glomerular filtration rate is proportionally lower than in an older child. Until about the age of 8 months, the kidney tubules are unable to excrete a large sodium or water load, which is the reason that in infants the maintenance fluid of choice is 4.5 per cent glucose and 0.18 per cent normal saline.

In children oliguria is considered to be a urine output of less than 1 ml/kg/hr. Once fluids are replaced the oliguria that accompanies hypovolaemia usually resolves. If oliguria persists the paediatrician or anaesthetist may use a diuretic and support the circulation with an inotrope.

Central nervous system

Intracranial haemorrhage

The cerebral vessels in the premature baby are fragile and thin-walled. If neonates are circumcised or intubated without adequate anaesthesia their blood pressure will surge abruptly. This may rupture intracranial, especially intraventricular, vessels. If a neonate's conscious state deteriorates for no obvious reason in the recovery room consider this possibility.

Blood–brain barrier

In neonates the blood–brain barrier is not yet fully functional. This means that drugs such as antibiotics and opioids cross the blood–brain barrier more readily, which prolongs their action. Bilirubin too can cross the blood–brain barrier and cause kernicterus in babies with blood group ABO or rhesus incompatibility with their mother.

Emergence phenomena

Otherwise healthy children are often restless and agitated after anaesthesia, especially children who have had their entire anaesthetic with sevoflurane. Propofol used as TIVA reduces the incidence of emergence agitation.[4] The pathophysiology is incompletely understood, however inflammation, poorly controlled pain and delirium inducing drugs appear to be risk factors in its appearance. Most anaesthetists will use methods to reduce the possibility of postoperative delirium in identified at-risk patients. These include giving a sedative pre-med, giving a small dose of propofol prior to extubation and treating intra-operative pain well.[4] Other drugs such as dexmedetomidine have also been shown to be useful in reducing the incidence of postoperative agitation and delirium. Giving ondansetron to an agitated child is ineffective.[5] A small dose of ketamine is sometimes helpful.

Never turn your back on a child.
They get into trouble quickly.

Liver

In neonates and young infants the liver enzymes are not fully functional and cannot easily breakdown many drugs. Opioids, for example, have a longer action. Consequently they should be used in small doses, and the dosing interval should be longer.

Metabolism

Glucose

Babies' immature livers do not store much glycogen. Glycogen can be quickly mobilized into glucose that is essential for the brain's *metabolism*, and without it brain damage occurs quickly.

Hypoglycaemia is common in the stressed neonate, especially if it has had a period of prolonged fasting, or becomes stressed by hypovolaemia, pain or hypothermia. Children most at risk are those weighing less than 15 kg.

Hypoglycaemia is defined as a blood glucose of less than 2.2 mmol/L, at a level of 1.7 mmol/L permanent brain damage is imminent. It is difficult to diagnose as signs and symptoms vary. It usually presents as muscle twitching, an *obtunded mental state*, convulsions or just a reluctance to breathe.

It is far better to predict and then prevent hypoglycaemia than to wait until signs appear with the risk of brain damage. Accordingly measure the blood sugar concentrations of stressed babies as soon as they are admitted to the recovery room.

Use an infusion of 10 per cent glucose to prevent hypoglycaemia.

An increasingly drowsy infant may be hypothermic

Thermoregulation

Hypothermia

Babies and infants have a large surface area when compared to their volume. This means that heat is lost proportionately more quickly than in adult. Under about the age of 6 months infants do not sweat, neither do they shiver nor vasoconstrict in response to cold. Neonates lose heat even more rapidly because they have little subcutaneous fat to insulate them.

During anaesthesia heat is lost predominately by radiation, but also by conduction, convection and evaporation. Considerable amounts of heat can be conducted to cold mattresses and blankets.

Hypothermia causes respiratory depression, decreased cardiac output, tissue hypoperfusion and lactic acidosis, increases the risk of infection, decreases the breakdown of drugs and decreases platelet function. Hypothermia is the most common reason for blood failing to clot.

Special brown fat is located between the scapulae, in the mediastinum and around the kidneys. It comprises about 4 per cent of a neonate's body weight. As a once-only response, babies can metabolize brown fat to provide heat energy should they become cold, but this requires a plentiful supply of oxygen. Brown fat can, at the best, only provide energy for a few hours. Once the brown fat is metabolized it is not replaced.

The optimal ambient temperature (neutral thermal environment) to prevent heat loss is 35°C for premature infants, 32°C for neonates, 30°C for infants and children, 28°C for adolescents and adults.

Hypothermia causes profound problems for babies. Unless they were well wrapped or under special lights in theatre nearly all have cooled to a certain extent by the time they come to the recovery room.

Measure the temperature of a baby
as soon as possible after arrival in recovery room.

Babies are often cool when they come to the recovery room. Keep small infants warm. Cover their heads with a woollen or gamgee hat, infants lose heat through their bald heads quickly. Ideally they should go straight into an incubator after surgery. Their oxygen requirement is high; so make sure that 28 per cent oxygen flows into the incubator.

Anaesthesia makes small infants drowsy postoperatively. If the infant becomes lethargic and floppy and their respiration and pulse rate are slow, assist their breathing with a Cardiff ™ or small Ambu Bag™ and summon someone to help you. Warm the baby and check their blood sugar.

Hyperthermia

Hyperthermia can occur. Babies do not sweat, instead they simply vasodilate and go red. Consider the following causes:

- an overdose of atropine—the baby will have a rapid pulse > 150 beats/min;
- an infection;
- CO_2 retention;
- malignant hyperthermia.

Pharmacology

Children under 12 years do not respond to drugs in the same way as small adults; this particularly applies to neonates. Children's doses may be calculated from adult doses by body weight, or more reliably, by body surface area. The upper outer lateral aspect of the thigh is the only safe intramuscular injection site in children.

Box 13.3 **Ideal body weight in children**

A well-nourished child's approximate ideal weight:

Age less than 9 years: weight in kg = (2 × age) + 9

Age more than 9 years: weight in kg = age × 3

$$\text{Approximate dose for a child} = \frac{\text{Surface area of child (m}^2) + \text{adult dose}}{1.8}$$

Keep a weight-for-age nomogram available in case you do not know the child's weight. Having determined the correct dose of a drug you may need to convert this into millilitres of drug as supplied by the maker. Under a stressful situation it is easy to make mistakes. So make up charts to convert directly from body weight to millilitres of solution and tie the charts to your paediatric resuscitation trolley.

Calculate drug doses from an ideal weight based on height and age (Box 13.3). If you need to calculate doses on weight alone, never give more than you would to a 50 kg patient. Be careful of sedatives, which may cause hallucinations; also anti-emetics, which can cause dystonic reactions.

It is better to use a table such as Table 13.4 to calculate approximate drug doses. Even the use of this table does not ensure safety because some drugs, such as aminophylline, have a small margin between the therapeutic dose and the toxic dose. If you have any doubts about the safety of a drug, or how to use it in children, consult the literature, the internet or a paediatric specialist. Be especially cautious and give drugs slowly to babies in their first 30 days of life.

Pain relief

How to assess pain

Children waking from anaesthesia are often distressed, frightened, disoriented and in pain. Small children quickly respond to the warmth of a cuddle. It may not be possible to pick the child up but touch is very reassuring. A toddler out of his routine is anxious and upset; but a toddler out of his routine, and in pain, is inconsolable and very, very angry.

Ideally pain relief should be established in theatre or even preoperatively. Depending on the site of the surgery a combination of regional techniques such as caudals; with opioids and/or paracetamol suppositories can be used to suit most circumstances. Never let a baby or child cry in pain. Incremental small doses of opioids, especially pethidine, are ideal for quickly settling small patients. Paracetamol suppositories are less reliable. Intravenous paracetamol can be given; the dose is 15 mg/kg. Do not use aspirin in children, because it may cause Reye's syndrome (see Box 13.4).

Table 13.4 Paediatric drug doses

Age	Average body weight (kg)	Percentage of adult dose
Neonate*	3.5	12.5
1 month*	4.2	14.5
3 months*	6	18
6 months	8	22
1 year	10	25
2 years	13	28
3 years	14	33
4 years	16	35
5 years	18	40
6 years	20	45
7 years	22	50
8 years	25	54
9 years	28	60
10 years	30	66
11 years	35	70
12 years	40	75
13 years	43	80
14 years	50	100

*Applies to full term but not to premature infants.

Box 13.4 **Reye's syndrome**

Reye's syndrome is a very rare fulminating encephalopathy associated with liver failure that occurs in children. It follows after an acute viral illness, and is thought to be aggravated by aspirin. The child becomes drowsy, confused, ataxic and starts to vomit. He may bleed. Reye's syndrome has a high mortality. Do not use aspirin in children or adolescents.

Babies

Postoperatively it is sometimes difficult to tell whether babies are crying because they are in pain, or simply because they are hungry. As soon as possible allow babies to feed. Milk has a calming effect because it releases endogenous opioids, and is unlikely to cause any harm.

Diazepam suppositories 0.1 mg/kg are sometimes used to relax the painful adductor spasms that occur when babies have plaster splints applied.

Morphine and pethidine are effective analgesics for children, but the onset of action of pethidine is quicker than morphine. Titrate the initial doses of these drugs to achieve the desired effect.

Opioids are metabolized in the liver. Pethidine has pharmacologically active metabolites and occasionally these cause twitching and even seizure; especially if doses are repeated.

All the side-effects of opioids seen in adults also occur in children. Up to the age of 3 months the duration of action of opioids is unpredictable. Fentanyl in neonates or babies is metabolized slowly and unpredictably giving it a long action. It can readily cause respiratory depression and excessive sedation. Avoid all opioids in babies after neurosurgery.

Providing the child can be monitored closely in a special care unit, continuous morphine infusions are useful after major surgery. The loading dose is 0.1 mg/kg before the end of surgery then 0.5 mg/kg added to 500 ml of Hartmann's solution and given via an infusion pump or burette at 10–40 ml/hr.

Continuous epidural, with or without opioids, can be used successfully if the child is going to a supervised area, such as intensive care. Use 0.5 ml/kg of 0.25 per cent bupivacaine and infuse at a rate of 0.1–0.15 ml/kg/hr.

Vomiting

Although children frequently vomit after anaesthesia they are not usually distressed. Clean the mouth and pharynx carefully and allow the child to sit up. Since most children only vomit once, use anti-emetics cautiously because they can cause severe dystonic reactions. Severe or intractable vomiting occurs in about 2 per cent of children postoperatively.

Using intraoperative non-steroidal anti-inflammatories (NSAIDs) instead of opioids for analgesia reduces the incidence of postoperative vomiting. If children are vomiting do not remove the intravenous line. Use either 0.9 per cent saline or Hartmann's solution while children are vomiting to avoid electrolyte imbalance; do not use 5 per cent glucose.

Children who are older than 18 months and have uncontrolled postoperative vomiting may need rescue therapy. Use granisetron 40 micrograms/kg or ondansetron. If they are vomiting because they have swallowed blood (i.e. after tonsillectomy), give them simethicone.

Dystonia

Anti-emetics can cause dystonic reactions in children. Dystonia causes the child to become stiff, with their arms held rigidly at their sides, their neck extended and their teeth clenched. Extra-orbital muscle spasm causes upward and outward deviation of the eyes.

Another name for the side-effect of dystonia is the extrapyramidal syndrome. Although alarming and uncomfortable the effect is reversed with benzatropine) as a 0.02 mg/kg bolus given intravenously.

Psychological aspects

Infants

Infants under the age of 6 months of age are not usually upset when separated from their mother, and readily accept comfort from a stranger (Figure 13.4).

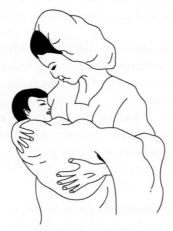

Figure 13.4 Cuddle crying children.

Younger children

Children up to the ages of 4 or 5 years are upset when separated from their mother and disturbed by unfamiliar faces and surroundings. It is difficult to comfort or reason with children of this age, especially when they are crying or distressed. Children are comforted by seeing their mothers as they emerge from their anaesthetic and staff are more accepting of the mother's presence. Children are extremely perceptive and readily detect anxiety in their parents. Thoroughly brief the mother on what to expect beforehand so that she does not convey her anxiety to the child.

Older children

School-aged children are more frightened of the prospect of being disfigured by the surgery than the possibility of pain. They are more easily reassured by strangers, and not so disoriented by unfamiliar places.

Adolescents

Adolescents are shy about their bodies, keep them well covered and do not embarrass them. They tend to fear going to sleep for their surgery, or dying during the procedure. They are not so worried by pain, but they do fear losing control of themselves or their surroundings.

Teenagers and young adult patients can become restless while waking up. They roll about and may try to climb off the trolley before they can be reasoned with. Make sure the trolley sides are raised and there is a strong person to help restrain the patient. Secure the intravenous lines, nasogastric tubes and other drains, otherwise they may be pulled out during this restless phase.

When emerging from any of the volatile agents, younger patients sometimes develop muscle rigidity and experience violent shaking. This muscle activity uses a lot of energy, and consequently a lot of oxygen, so try and keep their oxygen masks on and cover them with warm blankets.

From their early teenage years through young adulthood, many patients seem surprisingly resistant to sedative and analgesic drugs. An alarmed young person diverts most of his blood supply to his muscles (a part of the flight response). When drugs are given intravenously they are more likely to be pumped to their muscles rather than their brain.

Cardiac arrest

Cardiac arrest in children is usually caused by lack of oxygen to the heart. The principal causes of cardiac arrest in children in the recovery room are hypoxia caused by respiratory obstruction and haemorrhage.

Children under the age of 1 year are most at risk. There is less time to respond to apnoea in children because they become hypoxic so quickly. Children nearly always have asystole or bradycardia as the initial rhythm.

Cardiac arrest is usually preceded by:

- respiratory distress with tachypnoea, cyanosis, distress and decreased breath sounds;
- tachycardia, bradycardia;
- hypotension or reduced pulse volume;
- poor perfusion with tachycardia, poor capillary return, cool or mottled peripheries;
- deterioration in conscious state;
- flaccidity.

The presence of any one of these signs needs urgent resuscitation. Summon help immediately.

The most common arrhythmias are severe bradycardia, pulseless electrical activity or asystole; all of which have a bad outcome. Ventricular arrhythmias such as ventricular fibrillation and ventricular tachycardias usually only occur in children with pre-existing cardiac disease.

How to recognize cardiac arrest

You cannot feel either the brachial pulse or the apex beat; or the pulse rate is less than 60 beats/min; or you are not sure.

Then immediately:

+ Call for help.
+ Stimulate the child and assess the result.
+ Then start the ABC of resuscitation.

A = Airway

Position the head in a neutral position (for children aged less than 1 year), or the *sniffing position* (for older children).

Open the airway with head tilt, chin lift and a jaw thrust.

Insert an oropharyngeal airway.

B = Breathing

If the child is not breathing immediately start assisted ventilation. Use the correct sized resuscitating bag: for an infant under 2 years use a 500 ml bag; for older children use an adult 1500 ml bag. Use an appropriate-sized mask which should not overlap the chin and gives a good airtight seal. Use an oxygen flow rate of 15 L/min and attach a reservoir bag to give 100 per cent oxygen. If necessary, clear the mouth and pharynx with a Yankauer sucker. Ventilate to produce a normal rise and fall of the chest. The recommended ventilation rate is 10 breaths/min. Do not over-inflate the chest, because there is a risk of causing a pneumothorax. The anaesthetist may decide to intubate the child. Once circulation is restored, ventilate the child at a range of 12–20 breaths/min to achieve a normal PCO_2, and monitor expired CO_2.

C = Circulation

If there are no signs of circulation, or if the pulse is less than 60/min or you are not sure then commence external cardiac compression. Attach an ECG to determine the cardiac rhythm.

Cardiac massage

When performing cardiac massage remember the heart is positioned under the lower third of the sternum in children. Place the index finger of the lower hand just under the line between the nipples. The area of compression is at the junction between the middle and ring finger (Figure 13.5). Compress the heart with either two fingers or the heel of your hand depending on the size of the child use about 100 compressions per minute. You get the number about right by singing (silently) to the beat of 'Happy birthday to you' at normal speed (but don't pause at the end of each line).

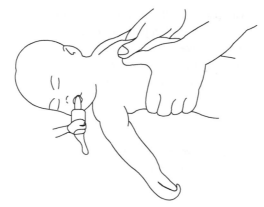

Figure 13.5 Position of thumbs on baby's chest for cardiac massage.

Important points

- Do not stop cardiac compression except for defibrillation.
- Compress the sternum to about one-third the depth of the chest.
- For infants use two fingers.
- For neonates, the best technique is the two-hand hold. Grasp the baby with both hands to encircle their thorax and with your thumbs pointing to the baby's head. Now compress the lower third of the sternum.
- During cardiac massage do not stop to check the pulse unless the ECG is showing an organized rhythm.
- After DC shock, continue cardiopulmonary resuscitation (CPR) for 2 minutes before stopping to check the pulse.

The brachial pulse is easier to feel in chubby children than the carotid. Neonates, infants and small children have short necks. Do not hyperextend the neck, just lift the head forward a little into a neutral position. Insert a Guedel airway, use an appropriate-sized mask, and ventilate at a rate of 40–60 breaths per minute with puffs of 100 per cent oxygen.

Cardioversion

Cardioversion should be done with a single 4 joule/kg shock. Repeated shocks damage the myocardium. Use appropriate-sized paediatric paddles. This is 4.5 cm for infants weighing less than 10 kg and 8 cm for older children. If necessary, you can use the larger 8 cm paddles by placing them on the chest and back. The entire surface of the paddle must contact the chest wall over its entire surface area.

Unlike adults, cardioversion is rarely needed in children. The most common tachyarrhythmia in children is paroxysmal supraventricular tachycardia. This comes on abruptly with a rate exceeding 220 beats/min. Other reasons for cardioversion are pulseless electrical activity (PEA), *ventricular fibrillation* (VF) and *ventricular tachycardia* (VT). Adult defibrillators can be used in patients aged 8 years or older.

Most modern defibrillators have a preset maximum dose of 80 joules when the paediatric paddles are connected. Remember that small babies who have been stressed or starved are at risk from hypoglycaemia and need their blood glucose levels assessed following cardioversion.

Drugs

The dose of adrenaline is 10 micrograms/kg for each dose. Drugs should be given intravenously or by the intraosseous route, and only as a last resort down the endotracheal tube.

When to stop?

The outcome of paediatric cardiac arrest is poor. Failure to achieve a return to spontaneous respiration after 15 minutes has a dismal outcome. The exceptions for this are arrests associated with hypothermia, hyperkalaemia, and bupivacaine toxicity. If in doubt consult a paediatrician for advice.

References

1. **Bould MD, Sury RJ** (2011) Defining awakening from anesthesia in neonates: a consensus study. *Pediatric Anesthesia* **21**:359–363.
2. **Allan R, de Caen ME,** *et al.* (2010) Paediatric basic and advanced life support. *Resuscitation* **81**(1):e213–e259.
3. **Houghton J, Wilton N** (2011) Choice of isotonic perioperative fluid in children. *Anaesthesia & Analgesia* **112**(1):246–247.
4. **Key KL, Rich C,** *et al.* (2010) Use of propofol and emergence agitation in children. *AANA Journal* **78**(6):468–473.
5. **Hosten T Ozgun M,** *et al.* (2011) Ondansetron does not modify emergence agitation in children. *Anesthesia and Intensive Care* **39**(4):640–645.

Chapter 14

The elderly patient

Introduction

As we grow older, our bodies change. They adapt to the physiological needs of that time in our lives. We need to take into account each patient's physical fitness, intercurrent medical problems, psychological state, and the medication they are taking as well as the type of surgery and anaesthetic they have undergone.

Old age

> *Old age is a process;*
> *not a disease*

In industrialized countries the population is ageing. *Elderly* people are defined as those over the age of 65 years, while the *aged* is a subgroup of those over 85 years. Old age in itself is not a disease, but old people inherit the residual effects of past and continuing illnesses while undergoing a progressive decline of organ function.

Not everyone ages at the same rate. Physiological age varies enormously with chronological age. Some individuals are decrepit in their early 60s, while others are sprightly and active into their late 80s. It can be difficult to assess the physical condition of elderly patients, because their mobility is limited by the pain and stiffness of arthritis.

Often chronic illness, undiagnosed disease, malnutrition, multiple pathology and particularly *polypharmacy* are unwelcome companions to the elderly. Older patients coming to surgery should write down a problem list of every symptom, both major and trivial, that troubles them. In the recovery room this problem list will enable you to see patterns emerging so that you can separate the effects of the ageing process from disease. For instance, elderly patients who cannot cough effectively may have chronic airway disease, in which case they might benefit from humidification or a BiPAP mask, or they may simply be physically weak, in which case gentle physiotherapy could help them cough up retained secretions. If they have low muscle mass they may still be affected by the residual effects of muscle relaxants.

It is helpful to have a list of all the patient's problems,[1] even the ones that seem trivial. It is difficult to make sensible decisions if you do not have access to all the facts.

How to predict problems in the elderly

Many factors predict problems that are likely to occur in the recovery room:

1. surgery lasting longer than 45 minutes;
2. poor cardiopulmonary function;
3. previous chronic illnesses;
4. medication;
5. dementia.

How function alters with age

We do not die quickly; we slowly degenerate over many years. As nerve cells and muscle cells everywhere inevitably die, they are not replaced with more muscle and nerve cells, but with collagen, amyloid and fat (see Box 14.1).

Box 14.1 **Collagen and elastin**

The scar tissue of ageing is *collagen*. *Elastin* is the elastic springy connective tissue found almost everywhere, especially in the walls of arteries and arterioles, the heart, lungs, joints, tendons. Its job is to return things to their original shape. A young person's skin is tight, but with ageing it becomes loose and saggy. As we age, elastin unravels, loses its springiness and converts to stiff unyielding *collagen*. Elastin allows young blood vessels to spring back if they are stretched. However, as elastin turns into collagen it loses its elasticity and becomes stiffer. If blood vessels do distend in the elderly, they stay dilated to eventually form aneurysms.

Age causes floppy lungs

All other things being equal, the elderly are as fit as the combined capacity of their heart and lung function allows them to be. The heart and lungs work together as a single *cardiopulmonary unit* supplying oxygen to the tissues and removing their metabolic waste.

Lungs in elderly people are less elastic, their chest walls are stiff, their respiratory muscles are weaker, the airways are floppy and collapse more easily, and the alveolar surface area is reduced. All this means that gas exchange is less efficient. The elderly become hypoxic more rapidly, are slower to respond to oxygen therapy, and cannot cough efficiently making sputum retention more likely.

Oxygen levels fall in the elderly

While breathing air the arterial PaO_2 falls with age from about 100 mmHg (13.3 kPa) in a fit young person, to about 80 mmHg (10.5 kPa) in an 80-year-old. Oxygen demands are highest as the patient first emerges from anaesthesia. Pain, coughing, hypertension or a tachycardia aggravates any hypoxia. Shivering or shaking can increase oxygen requirements sevenfold.

Diffusion hypoxia is a special problem unique to the recovery room. For about 10 minutes after the end of a general anaesthetic nitrous oxide seeps out of the blood into the lungs, displacing oxygen. You may see the patient's oxygen saturations decrease. Treat this with high flows of supplemental oxygen via a rebreathing mask. Notify the anaesthetist if the patient's saturations fall to 90 per cent.

Spinal and epidural anaesthesia may cause problems too because the vasodilatation caused by the regional block diverts blood to the lower limbs. With less peripheral *resistance* to push against, the heart needs to increase its force and rate of contraction to maintain the blood pressure. This increased work requires an increase in oxygen supply. If the heart does not receive enough oxygen, it becomes ischaemic and begins to fail.

How the heart ages

All forms of cardiac disease are more prevalent in the elderly. Circulation time is slower, and the vascular system more rigid. As the myofibrils in the heart die they are mostly replaced by collagen tissue. With fewer myofibrils and more collagen, the heart becomes stiffer (less compliant), and it cannot contract so forcibly. Consequently, it is no longer able to compensate quickly for sudden changes in blood pressure or blood volume.

Why joints are stiff

Old joints are stiff. Joints and tendons lose their ability to flex and absorb shocks as springy elastin converts to stiffer collagen. Older people cannot move easily because their tendons and ligaments no longer stretch to absorb the shock of impact. Be careful how you position them so that you do not injure their backs, hips, shoulders and knees. Be especially careful of moving patients who have had regional blocks, without warning pain ligaments and tendons are easily overstretched and torn. This is a potent cause of the backache which is so often reported after spinal and epidural anaesthesia, where the lumbar arch has not been supported properly in the operating theatre or afterwards in the recovery room.

Why skin is fragile

Old people's skin is thin and easily torn by simple things such as turning them over, or removing adhesive dressings. Be particularly careful if they have bruises or brown staining on their arms or legs—this is a sure sign of atrophied skin. The elderly are very susceptible to pressure sores and need cushioning under bony protuberances such as their sacrum and heels.

Age and malnutrition

Many elderly patients suffer from malnutrition, especially the lack of dietary protein and vitamins. Vitamin and mineral deficiency places them at risk of poor wound healing and low resistance to *nosocomial infection*.

The *aged* (people older than 85 years) are usually thin, and have little subcutaneous fat. Because of their wasted muscles they are weak and cannot cough effectively, or move quickly. They need help to sit up or roll on to their side.

The elderly lose heat quickly

Elderly people cannot rapidly increase their metabolic rate to compensate for heat loss, so that their temperature is likely to fall further on the operating table than younger people. Additionally, the aged have less insulating subcutaneous fat to prevent heat loss. Hypothermia delays the enzymatic degradation of drugs, prolonging their action.

How the kidneys decline

With ageing, kidney function declines. We lose about 1 per cent of our *nephrons* each year after we turn 30. By the age of 70 years less than 70 per cent of the nephrons are still working. This delays the excretion of many drugs.

The liver is robust

As the years pass the liver loses little function, and provided the blood supply to the liver is good, and the patient is not hypoxic, septic or hypothermic the elderly liver metabolizes drugs just as efficiently as a younger person. However, if the blood supply to the liver is reduced, or the liver is affected by disease, such as cardiac failure, or the patient has a high alcohol intake then drugs are not cleared as efficiently, which prolongs their effect.

The liver is sensitive to the amount of circulating endotoxins from bacteria in the bloodstream, and is particularly likely to be affected after bowel surgery. This effect is aggravated during abdominal surgery when blood flow to the liver decreases by about half. To prevent problems occurring later in the ward it is particularly important that these patients are kept well oxygenated, well perfused, and have no pain in the recovery room.

How drugs affect the elderly

The elderly are usually taking multiple medications, and frequently a few pharmacologically active herbal remedies as well. More than half those admitted to our hospitals are taking inappropriate drugs, have drug conflicts, or are not taking their medication consistently, or at the correct interval. This is a major cause of morbidity, and unless detected before surgery can cause problems in the recovery room. For example, NSAIDs are a common cause for acute postoperative oliguria, and garlic pills can cause bleeding.

A slow circulation time delays the onset of even fast-acting drugs such as naloxone. Naloxone may take 3 minutes or more to produce an effect in an older person, where in the younger patient it works within 90 seconds.

In general most drugs used during anaesthesia, and in the recovery room, initially have a more pronounced effect and last longer in the elderly than in the young. Most of the differences occur because an old person's physiology differs to that of a younger person.

Much of the body mass in a younger person is muscle with its high water content. In the elderly the bulk of their body mass is fat with its low water content. This means that the elderly have proportionately less water in which water-soluble drugs can dissolve, and proportionally more fat in which fat-soluble drugs can eventually disperse. In the elderly water-soluble drugs, such as the muscle relaxants, have less water in which to dissolve, and are therefore more concentrated.

Muscle relaxants

Although older people seem to need the same dose of muscle relaxant as younger people, the drugs take longer to act, and wear off more slowly. This can cause a problem in short procedures, because residual paralysis may persist into the recovery phase. Residual paralysis causes jerky movements, and patients who are unable to lift their head clear of the pillow for 5 seconds. Notify the anaesthetist if you encounter this problem.

NSAIDs

One dose in an acute situation probably won't cause a problem but NSAIDs[2] should be avoided for postoperative pain relief. They cause side effects in diabetes and those taking angiotensin-converting enzyme (ACE) inhibitors, angiotensin receptor blockers and furosemide.

Midazolam

In older people midazolam is dispersed widely, and its plasma concentration decreases slowly. The reason why equivalent plasma levels cause more sedation in the elderly is unclear. Flumazenil (a benzodiazepine receptor antagonist) reverses the effects of midazolam but the effect wears off after about 45 minutes, leaving any residual midazolam to re-exert its effects. There are occasional reports of sudden deaths, because recovery room staff did not realize that midazolam may cause cardiorespiratory depression later in the ward. This disaster is more likely if opioids have been used during or after the procedure.

Morphine

Opioids are well tolerated in the elderly,[3] however the effective dose may vary widely; a small dose of morphine can profoundly sedate one 80-year-old, while another similar 80-year-old may require a much higher dose to get adequate pain relief. The older brain is more susceptible to opioid-induced respiratory depression. As a general rule, elderly patients need small doses, and longer intervals between doses.

Fentanyl

The opioid fentanyl causes problems in the elderly. A proportion of an injected dose of fentanyl binds to skeletal muscle cell membranes. While the patient is not moving it stays there, but once the patient starts to move around, the muscle blood flow increases and the fentanyl is washed back into the circulation. This rush of fentanyl is probably the cause of the delayed respiratory depression sometimes seen many hours after the last dose.

In summary

Two useful questions to ask about the elderly, but particularly about the aged, are:

- Should I use half the normal dose and give it twice as slowly?
- Is this drug really necessary?

Confusion and postoperative delirium are common

Postoperative confusion is common. Although hypoxia is the principal culprit, sometimes it is simply poor eyesight or hearing problems that disorientate the patient. Despite their confusion elderly people have an accurate perception of pain, and discourtesy. Respect for their dignity helps reduce the feelings of alienation.

> *In the agitated and confused patient you must eliminate*
> *two killers: hypoxia and hypoglycaemia.*

Hypoxia is common. Acute hypoglycaemia is rare, however if it is not diagnosed and treated promptly it causes permanent brain damage. Those at risk include diabetics, especially those who are taking insulin, and alcoholics who, under certain circumstances, cannot manufacture glucose in their livers to maintain their blood glucose levels.

How to predict problems

Often there are signs of a developing acute brain syndrome in the recovery room that predict a full-blown *delirium* later in the ward. About 50 per cent of patients who fracture their femurs become confused postoperatively. As always hypoxia, in one of its many guises, is the prime suspect. Even though cardiopulmonary function may be adequate, if the patient has bled during the operation, the resulting anaemia will contribute to hypoxia. A blood transfusion does not necessarily prevent the problem. Stored blood picks up oxygen readily, but does not so easily download it to the tissues. It takes about 12–18 hours for the body to fully restore the oxygen-carrying ability of transfused blood. Merely because the oxygen saturation meter is reading 98 per cent does not mean that the tissues are taking up oxygen.

An older person, who has been hypoxic even for a minute or two, will suffer brain damage. They may take hours or days to recover, and they may never recover completely. It is far better to prevent confusion than to have to manage it.

Contributors to postoperative confusion include:

- pre-existing dementia;
- hypotension during the anaesthetic;
- anti-cholinergic medication such as atropine, and the phenothiazines;
- previous stroke or transient ischaemic attack;
- vascular disease including cerebrovascular or ischaemic heart disease;
- paradoxically, occasionally benzodiazepines aggravate confusion.

How to manage acute agitation and confusion

Patients with established dementia have operation and come to the recovery room. Do not assume they feel less pain, this is not true. It is difficult to treat and manage confusion, restlessness, agitation and aggression. Agitation is harmful. The accompanying surge of noradrenaline and adrenaline raises the heart rate and blood pressure, putting the patient at risk of myocardial ischaemia.

*You cannot drug a patient
into mental competence.*

Start by giving high concentrations of oxygen by mask. Orient your patient by telling them where they are, and why they are there. Attach an electrocardiograph machine (ECG). Check the patient's blood pressure, pulse rate and perfusion status. All this is far easier said than done. An agitated fearful patient is not likely to be cooperative. They will not tolerate a mask; they can rip out their lines and become aggressive. Notify the anaesthetist; and prepare to sedate the patient. Every anaesthetist has a recipe for such occasions, but a useful one contains a mixture of haloperidol and midazolam. Once order has been restored, you will have a patient with a clouded conscious state whose airway needs protection. Check their blood gases, and blood glucose levels. Make a plan for their ongoing management. This may require the help of the high dependency unit.

In order to maximize cognitive outcome in elderly patients, it is important to consider a first-do-no harm approach. This includes minimizing anaesthetic depth, limiting the duration of continuous anaesthesia, using regional anaesthesia with light or no sedation and considering anaesthesia along with the surgical intervention in determining the cost/benefit ratio of proceeding with surgery.[4]

How to communicate with the elderly

Deafness isolates older people from those around them. If a patient has a hearing aid, put it back as soon as they are conscious. Some recovery rooms have background music playing. Older patients with hearing aids find background noise distracting because it distorts how they hear voices. Turn the music off. Look at their faces when you speak to them. Speak slowly and clearly.

*Sensory impairment leads to frustration.
Frustration leads to withdrawal or anger.*

If older patients are in pain it is difficult for them to process new information. They are likely to forget what you have just said to them. A patient in pain will find it difficult to concentrate on what you are saying.

Age does not mean loss of intelligence, and older patients deeply resent being treated as child-like. Older patients find it easier to deal with one piece of information at a time. If you need to give instructions then present each point separately and make sure it is understood before moving on to the next point.

Respect cultural differences. Ethnicity, cultural beliefs and social norms affect patients' expectations. Remember that older people, even if born in the country, were raised in a different generation. They have different attitudes to privacy, modesty and communication. Many dislike being called by their first names, they have been taught to 'grin and bear' pain, not to 'worry other people', and the hospital staff 'know best'.

The disorientation of coming to hospital, the pain and discomfort, the time without food or fluids all contribute to disorientate elderly people. Sedatives have a serious effect on their memory. The effect can be insidious. For many hours, and even days after an anaesthetic the patient's ability to process and remember information is blunted. They may appear to have understood what you have just told them, but a few minutes later the whole conversation has become a hazy blur in their memory, or has disappeared completely. If there are important points that the patient should know then make this clear to the nurses from the ward so that they can write instructions down for the patient or to alert the patient's relatives.

Frailty

Recently there has been a lot of interest in frailty as a marker for morbidity and mortality in elderly surgical patients. Frailty has been established as an independent predictor of morbidity and mortality in elderly surgical patients. Frailty scores have been developed to predict this. Frailty is defined as a state of decreased physiological reserve. It gives a holistic sense of how a set of conditions affects a patient's level of function. Recent studies suggest that an intact autonomic nervous system confers lower perioperative mortality but that frail elderly develop 'homeostenosis' whereby the physiological response to stress is impaired.[5] Frailty is hence a useful tool to identify at-risk patients for optimization and targeted intervention prior to surgery.[6]

Dementia and advanced care directives

The elderly have greater incidences of dementia. Patients with dementia present for emergency and increasingly elective surgery. Fortunately recent guidelines have been published for the care of these patients.[7]

It is useful to ascertain a patient's wishes in regard to end-of-life care. Often a patient will have completed an advanced care directive. Check the notes for this or speak to the next-of-kin to see if it has been done. A useful website for further information on this subject is myValues.org.au.

References

1. **Catananti C, Gambassi G** (2010) Pain assessment in the elderly. *Surgical Oncology* **19**:140–148.
2. **Pratt N, Roughhead EE,** *et al.* (2010) Differential impact of NSAIDS. *Drugs and Aging* **27**:63–71.
3. **Coldrey JC, Upton RN,** *et al.* (2011) Advances in analgesia in the older patient. *Clinical Anaesthesiology* **25**:367–378.
4. **Cottrell JE, Hartung J** (2020) Anesthesia and cognitive outcome in elderly patients: a narrative viewpoint. *Journal of Neurosurgical Anesthesiology* **32**(1):9–17.
5. **James L, Levin M,** *et al.* (2019) Association of preoperative frailty with intraoperative hemodynamic instability and postoperative mortality. *Anesthesia and Analgesia* **128**:1279–85.
6. **Lee DJK,** *et al.* (2019) Frailty in surgical preoperative evaluation and postoperative recovery. *Current Geriatrics Reports* **8**(2):87–96.
7. **White S,** *et al.* (2019) Guidelines for the perioperative care of people with dementia: guidelines from the Association of Anaesthetists. *Anaesthesia* **74**(3):357–372.

Chapter 15

Respiratory physiology

Introduction

An exchange of gas occurs between the atmosphere and venous blood in the lungs. Pulmonary ventilation is the total exchange of gases and alveolar ventilation is the exchange of gas between the alveoli and the pulmonary capillaries.

Breathing

Breathing is a process where air containing oxygen is inspired into the lungs, and carbon dioxide laden air is expired. The thorax behaves like a closed box that alters in size and shape with each breath. On inspiration, the cavity of the thorax enlarges, and the elastic lungs expand to fill the space. On expiration, the thorax returns to its former size and air is expelled. Then there is a short pause before the process starts over again.

In forced, or deep, inspiration the accessory respiratory muscles of the neck and shoulder girdle are recruited to assist. Laboured breathing occurs when the patient is using their accessory muscle to assist each breath.

Never ignore laboured breathing. Find the cause.

In contrast, *expiration* relies on the springiness of the lungs to drive the air out again. It is a passive process. If the patient is using his accessory muscles in his neck or abdomen to breathe out then they probably have some form of airway obstruction.

There are two principal gases: oxygen (O_2) and carbon dioxide (CO_2). Cells use oxygen to gradually burn carbohydrate, fats and amino acids to produce energy. This process is called *oxidative metabolism*. The three terms *concentration, tension,* and *partial pressure,* all mean roughly the same thing. They are used to express how much of a particular gas is present in each litre of a mixture of gases.

Gases exert pressure, even when they are dissolved in fluids (for example, the bubbles in beer). PCO_2 is the shorthand for pressure of carbon dioxide; similarly PO_2 is the pressure exerted by oxygen. By convention we use the Pappenheimer notation to describe the physical state of gases and fluids in biology (see Box 15.1).

The term *fractional inspired concentration of oxygen* (FiO_2) is used to describe the concentration of oxygen in inspired air. Room air contains 21 per cent oxygen, and therefore the FiO_2 is 0.21. Using the FiO_2 we can calculate the pressure exerted by oxygen in a mixture of gases such as air. The Hudson mask most commonly used in the recovery room delivers an arterial FiO_2 of 0.36 (36 per cent oxygen) at a flow rate of 6 L/min.

For a healthy person breathing air (FiO_2 = 0.21) the normal arterial PaO_2 is about 100 mmHg (13.3 kPa). The PaO_2 declines with age and at 80 years is about 80 mmHg (10.5 kPa).

Giving patients supplemental oxygen raises their FiO_2. In a person with normal lungs as you increase their FiO_2, their PaO_2 rises roughly in proportion. If their FiO_2 doubles so will their PaO_2. However, in a patient with diseased lungs this does not occur.

Box 15.1 **Pappenheimer notation**

The Pappenheimer notation is a shorthand for describing gases in various situations.

1. Upper case 'P' applies to pressures, e.g. PO_2 = partial pressure of oxygen.
2. Upper case 'A' applies to gases, e.g. PAO_2 = partial pressure of oxygen in alveolar gas.
3. Lower case 'i' applies to inspired gas, e.g. FiO_2 = fractional inspired concentration of oxygen.
4. Lower case 'a' applies to gases dissolved in arterial blood, e.g. $PaCO_2$ = partial pressure of carbon dioxide in arterial blood.

Oxygen transport

Four steps ensure oxygen from the outside air reaches the mitochondria in the cells:

1. Breathing.
2. Gas transfer between the lungs and the blood.
3. Transport of oxygen in the blood to the tissues.
4. Oxygen diffusing to the mitochondria.

Humidification stops the airway drying out

As air is sucked through the upper airway, it is warmed and humidified. It then passes through a bottleneck in the larynx, and flows down either the left or right bronchi, and on through another 20 branches of airways, to reach the alveoli. Here oxygen diffuses into the blood, and carbon dioxide diffuses into the lungs.

Normal respiratory rate

The normal respiratory rate is 12–14 breaths/min. Each breath contains about 400 ml (*tidal volume*). About half the tidal volume reaches the alveoli where gas exchange occurs;

but the other half remains in the airways as *dead space volume* where no gas exchange is possible. If the tidal volume is less than the dead space volume carbon dioxide banks up in the alveoli and blood, causing the $PaCO_2$ to rise.

A rising respiratory rate is a useful sign, warning that the patient is becoming physiologically unstable. Once the rate reaches 18 breaths/min you should start looking for a cause.[1]

A rising respiratory rate?
Find the cause.

Functional residual capacity acts as an oxygen store

At the end of a quiet expiration about 3 litres of residual air remain in the lungs. This volume is called *the functional residual capacity* (FRC). The FRC acts as a small oxygen store that we draw on when we breathe out, talk, or hold our breath. If it were not for this residual air we would turn blue every time we breathed out, and pink when we breathed in. As we grow older our lungs lose their elasticity and become floppy and the FRC becomes larger. Neonates and infants have proportionally the same FRC as an adult, but because they use oxygen twice as fast as an adult they become hypoxic quickly once they stop breathing.

Less air is stored in the FRC during, and directly after general anaesthesia. When a person lies down their abdominal contents push their diaphragm up into the thorax. This partly collapses the bases of the lung. This is the physiological reason pregnant or very obese patients become breathless when lying on their backs.

Respiratory centres drive breathing

Respiratory centres in the brainstem regulate breathing. They act like a biological computer receiving input messages from the lungs and elsewhere, processing the signals and organizing an appropriate output response. This sequence is an example of a feedback control loop maintaining *homeostasis*.

Chemoreceptors sense oxygen and carbon dioxide tensions

Some of the inputs come from *chemoreceptors* in the aorta, carotid arteries and brainstem. When brainstem chemoreceptors detect a tiny increase in $PaCO_2$ levels, they stimulate the respiratory centres to make the patient 'breathe-up' deeply and quickly. This causes the person to 'blow-off' the carbon dioxide to restore a homeostatic equilibrium. We are all familiar with becoming short of breath when we run up a flight of stairs. All that extra muscular activity produces a lot of CO_2, which accumulates in our blood, and is sensed by brainstem chemoreceptors. To restore homeostasis the chemoreceptors stimulate our breathing to get rid of the excess CO_2.

In contrast, the chemoreceptors' sensitivity to a falling PO_2 is not good. In most people the arterial PaO_2 has to fall to at least 55 mmHg (7.24 kPa) before the carotid chemoreceptors make us breathe-up. In 10 per cent of people the chemoreceptors do not work at all.

Drugs depress chemoreceptors

Anaesthetic drugs depress *chemoreceptors*. Why is this important in the recovery room? If a patient has a general anaesthetic with volatile agents or receives an opioid we cannot depend on their normal reflexes to stimulate breathing. The reasons are: first, that opioids depress the brainstem chemoreceptor response to a rising $PaCO_2$ so the respiratory rate slows, and the tidal volume decreases. Second, the carotid body chemoreceptor response to hypoxaemia is abolished by even a tiny amount of residual volatile anaesthetic agent. These effects last for 6 hours or more after the end of anaesthesia.

Dyspnoea is a subjective feeling

Patient are said to be *dyspnoeic* when they feel short of breath. Dyspnoea is a sign that the patient is working hard to breathe. If your patient becomes dyspnoeic find the reason their work of breathing has increased. Anything impeding breathing (for example, asthma, a pneumothorax, or bronchospasm); or increasing the stiffness of the lung (for example, fibrotic lung disease, pneumonia, *pulmonary oedema*; or gas, fat, or air embolism) causes dyspnoea.

Reflexes guard the airway

Epithelial receptors guard the airway to stop foreign material becoming inhaled into the lungs. When stimulated these receptors cause sneezing, coughing, gagging, breath-holding or laryngospasm. Spraying the throat or airway with local anaesthetic abolishes the protective reflexes, consequently increasing the risk that the patient might aspirate material into their lower airway.

Gas transfer in the lungs

The surface area of the lung is about 70 square metres; about the size of a tennis court. Oxygen does not diffuse easily and needs this large surface area to move across the membranes separating the alveolus from the bloodstream (Figure 15.1). In contrast carbon dioxide diffuses easily, and only needs about a fifth of the area that oxygen requires. This is the reason that the arterial PaO_2 decreases in proportion to the area of damaged lung, while $PaCO_2$ does not start to rise until 75 per cent or more of the lung's membranes are severely damaged.

How shunting causes hypoxia

In a normal lung less than five per cent of the blood bypasses oxygenated alveoli. In contrast, in patients with pulmonary disease larger proportions of blood are *shunted* through the diseased lung so that blue deoxygenated blood emerges still blue at the venous end (Figure 15.2). The blue deoxygenated blood then mixes with red oxygenated blood in the pulmonary vein. The result is a *venous admixture*, which causes the overall PaO_2 to fall.

Why giving oxygen may not be effective

Paradoxically, the more severe the patient's lung disease, the less effective is supplemental oxygen in raising their PaO_2.

Consider the case of a person with a totally blocked right main bronchus but a normally aerated left lung. In this case, blood flowing through the right lung will not be oxygenated, while the blood flowing through the left lung is fully oxygenated. This creates a 50 per cent shunt and the arterial PaO_2 will be about 40 mmHg. Such a patient is severely hypoxaemic, so that even if you give them 100 per cent oxygen the PaO_2 will not increase by more than about 10 mmHg.

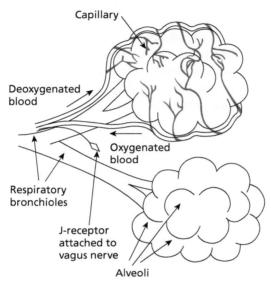

Figure 15.1 Two terminal respiratory units. Gas exchange takes place in the terminal respiratory unit (TRU). Ironed out flat they would cover an area of about 70 m². Each TRU is composed of a collection of 20–30 alveoli fed by an arteriole, encased by a capillary network and drained by small veins. Each TRU is polygonal in shape and about the size of a match-head. During surgery and anaesthesia TRU collapse and turn from pink to grey. If the fragile capillary network is damaged then the capillaries leak fluid into the spaces between the TRUs accumulating there to cause interstitial oedema. If fluid then leaks into the alveoli themselves it produces alveolar oedema. Near the junction of the TRUs and the bronchioles there are little strands of smooth muscle that act as stretch receptors called J-receptors. Fluid collecting in the lung's interstitial spaces stretches the J-receptors. They send an impulse up the vagus nerve to the brainstem respiratory centres, which in turn increase the rate and depth of breathing making the person feel breathless.

How atelectasis causes hypoxia

Surface tension tends to stick alveolar walls together. Normally, the alveoli secrete a natural detergent (*surfactant*) to overcome surface tension. During long anaesthetics the alveolar cells stop producing surfactant, and many alveoli collapse (*micro-atelectasis*). Blood now shunts past the collapsed alveoli causing PaO_2 to fall. In the recovery room once patients deep breathe and cough effectively they blast open collapsed alveoli.

How hypoventilation causes hypoxia

Measuring blood gases gives a good estimation of the carbon dioxide concentration in the alveoli. If a patient does not exchange enough tidal air into and out of their lungs then the concentration of CO_2 builds up in the alveoli, displacing oxygen to cause hypoxaemia. This is the reason patients who *hypoventilate* become hypoxic.

Carbon dioxide diffuses so easily across the alveolar–capillary membrane that a patient's arterial $PaCO_2$ is almost the same as their $PACO_2$ in their alveolar gas. The alveolar gas approximates to the end-tidal CO_2 measured with the carbon dioxide monitor.

According to *Dalton's law of partial pressures* the more carbon dioxide in the lungs, the less room there is for oxygen (and vice versa). Roughly, for every 10 mmHg rise in arterial $PaCO_2$, the PAO_2 in the lungs decreases by 10 mmHg.

Unlike carbon dioxide, oxygen is a poorly diffusible gas, so its concentration in arterial blood does not give a useful estimate of oxygen concentrations in the lungs.

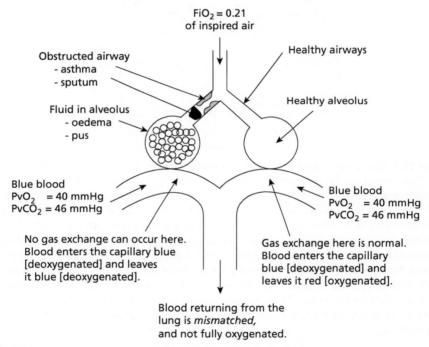

Figure 15.2 Why blood may not be fully oxygenated—shunt mechanisms.

Oxygen transport to the tissues

Once in the alveoli oxygen diffuses across the alveolar–capillary membrane into the red cells where it loosely binds to haemoglobin. The blood flow then carries oxygen to the tissues where it diffuses into the cells. Enormous amounts of oxygen are carried by haemoglobin inside the red cells. For example, 140 g/L of haemoglobin carries 195 ml of oxygen; in contrast only 3 ml of oxygen is dissolved the *plasma*.

At the arterial end of a capillary the PaO_2 is about 100 mmHg. As the red cell moves along the capillary it unloads oxygen and picks up carbon dioxide. On its journey the

PaO_2 progressively falls so that by the time it reaches the venous end of the capillary the Pv^-O_2 is only 40 mmHg.

There are four interlinked processes involved in supplying oxygen to the tissues:

1. Healthy lungs to ensure good gas exchange.
2 Good cardiac output to pump blood to the tissues.
3 Sufficient haemoglobin to carry the oxygen.
4 Metabolic factors affecting the shape of haemoglobin.

The ability of haemoglobin to carry oxygen to the tissues and then release it is reduced by metabolic factors such as hypothermia, disordered electrolytes in the blood, and particularly alkalosis (Table 15.1).

Table 15.1 Causes of tissue hypoxia

Disease	Hypoxia
Anaemia	Possible
Anaemia + cardiac failure	Probable
Anaemia + cardiac failure + lung disease	Certain
Anaemia + cardiac failure + lung disease + fever	May be lethal

Massive blood transfusions produce a *functional anaemia* that may cause hypoxia. Stored red cells, near their expiry date, pick up oxygen easily enough, but are reluctant to release it to the tissues. In effect the blood enters the tissues pink, and emerges pink at the other end.

Patients dying from septicaemia or severe shock have cells that are so deranged they cannot use oxygen even if it is delivered to them.

See Box 15.2 for information regarding oxygen and combustion.

Box 15.2 **Oxygen supports combustion**

Although oxygen itself does not burn, flammable material burns extremely vigorously in oxygen. Keep naked flames and sources of electrical sparks at least 2 metres away from an oxygen source.

Some patients are resistant to carbon dioxide

In a normal person a small rise in $PaCO_2$ vigorously stimulates breathing. Some patients with severe long-standing chronic obstructive airways disease have chronically raised $PaCO_2$. Their central chemoreceptors are no longer sensitive to changes in carbon dioxide tension. Instead their carotid chemoreceptors are responding to a PaO_2 less than 60 mmHg (7.89 kPa), and drive their respiration. These *blue bloaters* may stop breathing if given more than an FiO_2 of 0.28 (28 per cent oxygen). Blue bloaters are easy to recognize because they have *cor pulmonale*. They are plethoric, cyanosed and blue-faced, with oedematous (bloated) ankles, and they are breathless with minimal exercise. Using opioids in such a patient is a recipe for disaster, because they will stop breathing.

Never deprive blue bloaters of supplemental oxygen 'just in case they might stop breathing'. Watch them closely. If their respiratory effort fails, their $PaCO_2$ will rise even further. They will become drowsy, hypertensive and may sweat. Assist their breathing with a bag and mask. Ask your anaesthetist to help you. Treating persistent hypoventilation in blue bloaters is difficult. If you put them on a ventilator, they are difficult to wean. Many can be helped though an acute episode of *respiratory failure* with an intravenous infusion of the non-specific stimulant doxapram, but this is not always successful.

Terminology

Clinicians use special jargon when talking about respiratory medicine. The terms are not difficult to understand (see Box 15.3), but when used carelessly they can be confusing.

Box 15.3 **Terminology in respiratory medicine**

Symbols

- O_2 = oxygen;
- CO_2 = carbon dioxide;
- H_2O = water;
- PO_2 = partial pressure of oxygen;
- PaO_2 = partial pressure of oxygen in arterial blood;
- $PaCO_2$ = partial pressure of carbon dioxide in arterial blood;
- FiO_2 = fractional inspired content of oxygen;
- H^+ = hydrogen ion;
- $[H^+]$ = hydrogen ion concentration;
- pH = a logarithmic scale for measuring hydrogen activity;
- FRC = functional residual capacity.

Units

- cm H_2O = centimetres of water pressure;
- mmHg = millimetres of mercury pressure;
- kPa = kilopascals of pressure, for example: 7.60 mmHg = 1 kPa;
- 1.32 mmHg = 10 cm H_2O.

   In the UK and parts of Europe the kilopascal (kPa) is the preferred unit for measuring pressure, whereas in Australasia and the US they use mmHg.

Reference

1. **Parkes R** (2011) Rate of respiration: the forgotten vital sign. *Emergency Nurse* **19**(1):12–17.

Further Reading

British Thoracic Society (2010) Pleural Disease Guidelines 2010. *Thorax* **65**(2):1–176.

Chapter 16

The respiratory system

Introduction

As soon as your patient arrives in the recovery room and you have your routines in place put your hand on the patient's chest and count the respirations for one full minute. A healthy adult breathes at between 12 and 20 breaths per minute. Also note the depth of breathing as either shallow, normal or deep. Observe the accessory muscles. Is the patient using them? To breathe in? Or breathe out? Is the chest moving equally on both sides?

These observations are your baseline assessment. This minute you spend closely observing your patient will be valuable if there are subsequent changes.

Hypoxia

The events leading to hypoxia can start at any point between the patient's lips and their mitochondria.[1] On inspiration, oxygen-rich air flows along a series of airways into the lungs, where the oxygen enters the bloodstream. Here it is loaded on to haemoglobin in the red cells and pumped through the circulation to the tissues, finally diffusing into the cells where it is used. Weak points in this sequence are: the patency of the airways, the health of lungs, the quantity and quality of the haemoglobin, the adequacy of cardiac output, and various metabolic factors.

Above all you must make sure patients under your care do not become hypoxic. The onset of hypoxia is subtle, it is neither obvious nor predictable but quickly maims or kills. If you thoroughly understand how and why hypoxia occurs, and how to recognize it, then you are better equipped to prevent it.

The terms *hypoxia* and *hypoxaemia* mean different things. Hypoxia occurs when the tissues do not receive enough oxygen to meet their metabolic needs. The cells respond by temporarily switching to anaerobic metabolism, but the accumulating lactic acid soon poisons them. Brain tissue is irreversibly and quickly damaged by lack of oxygen. Hypoxaemia occurs when the arterial PaO_2 falls to 60 mmHg (7.89 kPa) or less.

Lactic acidosis is a sign
of tissue hypoxia.

Common causes of hypoxaemia

In the recovery room the most common reason for hypoxaemia is a mismatch of perfusion to under-aerated parts of the lung caused by small airway collapse during the anaesthetic.

Risk factors include older age, obstructive lung disease, obesity, raised intra-abdominal pressures (such as following laparoscopy) and immobility. Suspect if the patient is drowsy, has received intra-operative opioids, has pinpoint pupils, or cannot sustain a 5-second head lift.

Therapeutic targets

The pulse oximeter is a guardian of safety in the recovery room.

Aim for:

- oxygen saturations above 95% (equivalent to a PaO_2 > 80 mmHg 10.53 kPa);
- the ability to sit up, breathe deeply and cough effectively;
- respiratory rate between 12–14 breaths/min;
- tidal volume of 7 ml/kg or more;
- clear airways with no wheeze.

Clinical signs

Hypoxia presents with a progression of symptoms.

Early signs include:

- difficulty in concentrating;
- confusion, restlessness, and agitation;
- signs of adrenergic discharge: cool hands and feet, tachycardia;
- oxygen saturation falls below 90%;
- cyanosis.

Hypoxia is difficult to assess, at first it may give no signs,
and the absence of cyanosis does not exclude it.

Later signs include:

- pallor;
- ischaemic chest pain;
- ST segment depression on ECG;
- hypotension;
- sinus bradycardia;
- convulsions;
- nodal bradycardia;
- coma;
- death with an asystolic arrest.

There are many reasons for the earlier signs of hypoxia and it is easy to be misled and to miss the diagnosis (Figure 16.1).

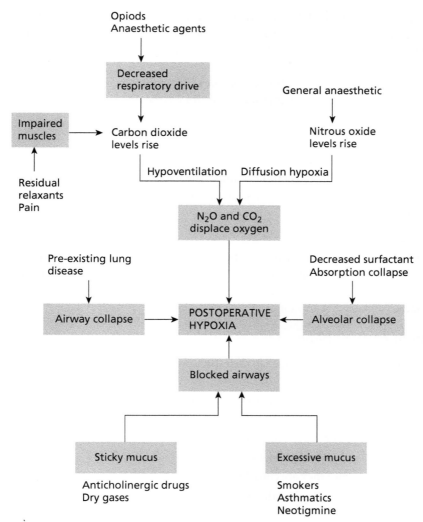

Figure 16.1 Causes of postoperative hypoxia.

The best sign of early hypoxia is the inability of the patient to concentrate.

Cyanosis

Cyanosis, with its bluish discolouration of the skin and mucous membranes, is an unreliable sign of hypoxia. It only occurs when more than 3 grams of deoxygenated haemoglobin is circulating. In normal people, this corresponds to a PaO_2 of about 50 mmHg (6.6 kPa), or a pulse oximeter reading less than 85 per cent.

Cyanosis depends on the amount of haemoglobin in the blood and may never appear in *anaemic* patients, and it may appear earlier in those with *polycythaemia*.

Cyanosis is difficult to detect in darker-skinned people. Check their nailbeds, the inside of their mouth, or inside the lower eyelid. The colour of their tongue is usually a good guide. Artificial light also makes it difficult to assess colour accurately.

Skin colour does not affect
the accuracy of an oximeter.

There are two types of cyanosis: *central cyanosis* and *peripheral cyanosis*.

Central cyanosis

Severe hypoxaemia causes central cyanosis. The patient will have blue lips, tongue and mucous membranes. If a patient has central cyanosis, they will also have peripheral cyanosis.

Peripheral cyanosis

Peripheral cyanosis presents with blue hands, feet and nailbeds. Poor peripheral circulation causes peripheral cyanosis (without central cyanosis). It may indicate the patient is cold, has venous congestion in the limb, or is shocked. Rare causes of cyanosis include methaemoglobinaemia and sulphaemoglobinaemia.

How to prevent hypoxia

- Give oxygen to patients during their transport from the operating theatre to the recovery room.
- As a minimum precaution give oxygen by mask at 6 L/min for at least 10 minutes after their anaesthetic.
- Nasal prongs do not give enough oxygen, and are useless in the recovery room as patients tend to breathe through their mouths.
- Sit patients up once they are conscious.
- Encourage them to deep breathe and cough.

How to manage hypoxia

Initially:

- Give 100% oxygen with a bag and mask.
- Call for help and summon the anaesthetist.
- Check the airway is clear, the patient is breathing, and air is going in and out of the chest.
- Attach standard monitoring: ECG, pulse oximeter, blood pressure cuff.
- Use a stethoscope to check that air entry is distributed to both lungs.
- Measure the expired CO_2 if you have the equipment but do not rely on this as a guide to the patient's well-being.

- Are patients breathing normally? If you are uncertain then use a respirometer to check their tidal and minute volumes. Their tidal volume should be greater than 5 ml/kg. If it is less than this, then support their breathing with a bag and mask and find a reason.

Later:

- Take arterial blood gases, check the haemoglobin levels, and order a chest X-ray.
- Further therapy could include intubation and the application of *positive end expiratory pressure* (PEEP) and the use of nitric oxide.

> *Hypoxia causes agitation and anxiety.*
> *Hypercarbia causes drowsiness and lethargy.*

Hints

- Treat hypoxaemia (oxygen saturations less than 92%) with high concentrations of oxygen.
- Treat hypoventilation (raised end-expired CO_2) by improving breathing.
- Monitor all patients with a pulse oximeter, but know its limitations.
- Assume that your patients are severely hypoxic if they are restless, agitated, confused or have a clouded conscious state.
- Eliminate the more serious causes of hypoxia: pneumothorax, cardiac tamponade, gas embolism, and anaphylaxis.
- Opioids may cause respiratory depression, which in the elderly may last for many hours.
- Send elderly patients to the ward on oxygen.
- Naloxone, an opioid antagonist, works for about 30–40 minutes, and may wear off before the effects of the opioid. You can prolong naloxone's action by 10–15 minutes if you give it intramuscularly.
- It is difficult to give oxygen to active children. Hold the mask in front of their face and use a high flow.

Hypoventilation

Hypercarbia occurs once the arterial $PaCO_2$ rises above 45 mmHg (5.92 kPa). Someone with hypercarbia is, by definition, hypoventilating. Clinicians prefer to use the term hypoventilation instead of hypercarbia. Hypoventilation may be acute or chronic (Table 16.1). *Chronic hypoventilation* occurs with severe chronic obstructive airways disease. A HCO_3^- of more than 30 mmol/L warns of chronic disease. As the patient's PCO_2 creeps up over time, the kidneys retain bicarbonate to keep the plasma pH normal.

Acute hypoventilation occurs commonly in the recovery room because patients' breathing is frequently depressed by opioids, or the incomplete reversal of muscle relaxants. This prevents carbon dioxide being washed out of their lungs. As their minute

Table 16.1 Signs of hypoventilation and hypoxia

Signs of hypoventilation	Signs of hypoxia
High PaCO$_2$	Low PaO$_2$
Drowsiness	Inability to concentrate and anxiety
Coma	Restlessness
Bounding pulse	Vasoconstriction cyanosis
Vasodilation	Hypertension and tachycardia
	Breathlessness
	Bradycardia
	Asystolic cardiac arrest
Treat by improving ventilation	Treat with oxygen

volume decreases, they develop a progressive respiratory acidosis and eventually become hypoxaemic. For this reason patients who have received an opioid need supplemental oxygen.

Clinical signs

Hypoventilation presents with a progression of signs:

- initially breathlessness (but not if the patient has received an opioid);
- tachycardia;
- hypertension;
- drowsiness;
- ventricular extrasystoles;
- flushing and cutaneous dilatation;
- coma.

In an otherwise healthy person, breathing air, hypercarbia causes hypoxaemia once the PaCO$_2$ exceeds 80 mmHg (10.53 kPa). If the patient is receiving supplemental oxygen hypercarbia is not lethal in itself until the PaCO$_2$ exceeds 120 mmHg (15.79 kPa).

How to manage hypoventilation

If a patient is not breathing deeply enough, or has a respiratory rate of less than 8 breaths a minute, then give oxygen while you assess the problem.

Is the respiratory centre depressed?

All opioids depress the rate and depth of breathing. Babies and the elderly can remain affected by the short-acting ones such as fentanyl after admission to the recovery room. Look for signs of opioid intoxication: pinpoint pupils, shallow breathing and pallor.

Patients affected by excessive opioids will take deep breaths and cough actively when you ask them to, but then resume their shallow breathing.

Are the respiratory muscles weak?

Residual paralysis from muscle relaxants may persist after the patient is admitted to the recovery room, but more insidiously it may return when the anticholinergic drug used to reverse the muscle relaxant in the operating theatre wears off. This takes about 30–40 minutes. Patients with residual paralysis move jerkily like a floppy rag doll. They are unable to lift their heads from the pillow and maintain this for 5 seconds. You can test peripheral muscle strength by asking patients to squeeze your fingers. Offer your forefinger and middle finger and ask them to squeeze them as hard as they can. If you are doubtful ask the anaesthetist's opinion. It is preferable to give an additional dose of reversal drug than use the nerve stimulator as this is painful in a conscious patient.

Airways obstruction

Airway obstruction can be total or partial. It can occur at any point between the lips or nose and the alveoli. The commonest points are in the oropharynx, or at the airway's narrowest point between the vocal cords in the larynx.

Anatomy of the airway

Figure 16.2 illustrates the anatomy of an airway. Simply placing the head on a pillow and extending the neck usually opens up an obstructed airway. The main cause of airway obstruction in recovery room is the tongue falling back into the pharynx. This is more likely to occur when the patient is lying flat.

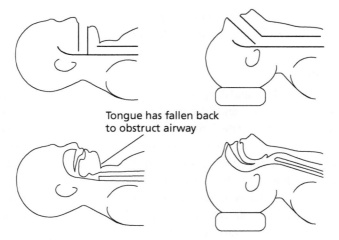

Tongue has fallen back
to obstruct airway

Figure 16.2 How to maintain an airway.

Neonates are obligate nose breathers. They cannot breathe through their mouths, so if their nose becomes blocked they will struggle for breath. Their whole chest may be drawn in by the respiratory effort.

Total airway obstruction

Total airway obstruction is silent and lethal. Simply because you can see the chest move up and down does not mean any air is going in or out. Seesaw breathing is a sign of a totally obstructed airway. While trying to breathe the patient's chest falls away as their abdomen rises, and vice versa. However, with ordinary breathing, both the abdomen and the chest wall rise and fall together.

Obstruction of an artificial airway

Patients awakening from anaesthesia often clench their jaws tightly shut (trismus). If their endotracheal tube or laryngeal mask happens to be between their teeth, they will bite down and occlude the lumen. Prevent this by inserting a Guedel airway or bite block alongside their endotracheal tube.

Stridor

Stridor is the crowing noise made by turbulent airflow as it is forced through a narrowing in the larynx or upper airway. Stridor trumpets disaster. Once the airflow through the larynx is narrow enough to cause stridor complete airway obstruction is not far off. Get help quickly.

Snoring is a form of stridor caused by soft tissues collapsing around the upper airway. Relieve it by extending the patient's head to open the airway or by inserting a nasopharyngeal tube.

*In the recovery room no one should be
allowed to snore.*

Laryngospasm

Laryngospasm is a common and dangerous sign that something is irritating the larynx or pharynx, and causing the true and false vocal cords to clamp shut.[2] Normally this reflex prevents food or fluid entering the lungs when we eat or drink. However, in the recovery room it becomes rapidly life threatening if not relieved. *Laryngospasm* is another cause of stridor. You will hear a harsh crowing noise as the patient tries to breathe in. A conscious patient who is struggling to breathe will panic.

Extubation sometimes triggers laryngospasm particularly in children, and is more likely if intubation has been difficult or traumatic. The risk of laryngospasm is increased in surgery involving the upper airway, e.g. dental and ENT.

Initial management

- Call for help. Hit the emergency bell.

- Give 100% oxygen by mask

- You will need two assistants. The first assistant to attach your standard monitors: ECG, oximeter, and measure the pulse rate and prepares to measure blood pressure. The second assistant to fetch the emergency trolley (cart) and prepares to draw up drugs for intubation.

- Inspect the patient's airway with a laryngoscope and suck out the pharynx, especially the nasopharynx and nose if they have had ENT surgery.

- Firmly thrust the patient's jaw forward with your fingers behind the angle of the mandible and pull firmly upwards. (Ask an anaesthetist to teach you this very useful manoeuvre.)

- Once you are sure the airway is clear, use a bag and mask to apply firm continuous *positive pressure* to relieve the spasm.

If this is unsuccessful:

- An intravenous bolus of 1.5 mg/kg lidocaine or a small dose of propofol (0.5mg/kg) often resolves the problem.

- If this fails then the only option is urgent intubation with suxamethonium to achieve rapid muscle relaxation and hence full opening of the vocal cords.

Other problems:

- Attempts to inflate the patient may cause the stomach to distend with gas. Once you have relieved the laryngospasm consider a nasogastric tube to deflate the stomach.

- *Pulmonary oedema* occasionally occurs in young people who try to inspire vigorously against a closed glottis. This is termed negative pressure pulmonary oedema.

Laryngeal oedema

Laryngeal function is disturbed for at least 4 hours after tracheal extubation. Keep patients who have been intubated under observation for this period. This precaution is especially important in children who have been intubated for day case surgery. Oedema in the upper airways occasionally follows extubation in children, and more frequently in neonates and infants. A small amount of reactive oedema will intrude on the narrow lumen rapidly occluding it.

Mild cases respond to warmed and humidified oxygen. However, it may be necessary to use nebulized adrenaline to shrink the mucosa. Take two 1 ml ampoules of 1:1000 adrenaline and make them up to 5 ml in 0.9 per cent saline. Give this by oxygen-driven nebulizer at a 5 L/min flow through a face mask. The effect lasts about 2 hours. Although this seems to be a big dose for a small child, it is most effective.

Other causes of *laryngeal oedema* occur with:

◆ thyroidectomy, carotid endarterectomy, or other operations on the neck;

◆ airway burns;

◆ trauma to the neck;

◆ subcutaneous surgical emphysema.

Vocal cord damage

Vocal cord paralysis or damage is a rare complication of surgery, it is easily diagnosed, because the patient is unable to say 'eeeee' in a high-pitched whine like a mosquito.

Vocal cord paralysis occurs if the laryngeal nerves are damaged during thyroid or major neck surgery. Unilateral vocal cord paresis presents as hoarseness in the recovery room but usually resolves over several weeks.

Bilateral vocal cord paralysis is serious. It presents with upper airway obstruction as soon as the patient is extubated but it does not respond to standard measures to control stridor. Applying firm continuous positive airway *pressure* with a bag and mask may temporarily overcome the obstruction. Laryngoscopy reveals motionless vocal cords lying slightly apart (adducted) and a narrow V-shaped aperture. The patient will need a tracheostomy.

Patients with rheumatoid arthritis or other connective tissue diseases have tenuous attachments where their laryngeal muscles insert into cartilage. The muscles easily tear off their insertions during intubation, or if the patient coughs on the endotracheal tube.

Cough

Coughing indicates irritation in the larynx or lower airway. This protective reflex so explosively expels material in the airway that the velocity of the ejected air exceeds the speed of sound. With paroxysms of coughing, patients may be unable to get their breath; they become distressed and turn purple in the face. The venous congestion aggravates bleeding in head and neck surgery, and can cause catastrophic bleeding following eye, ear or neurosurgery. The raised vascular pressures can cause retinal detachment. Coughing may contribute to cardiac arrhythmias and disrupt abdominal sutures; or in the elderly break their ribs (cough fractures).

A cough progressing to
stridor is life-threatening.

Frequently, coughing is a problem after rigid bronchoscopy or laryngeal surgery. Patients may not be able to get their breath between paroxysms and become cyanosed, hypoxic and distressed. Sit them up, and give high doses of humidified oxygen. Attach a pulse oximeter. Summon the anaesthetist. Listen to the chest with a stethoscope. A localized wheeze may suggest aspirated foreign material, usually into the right upper lobe posteriorly.

Nebulized lidocaine 1.5 mg/kg in 5 ml of saline will settle almost any cough. If not, then sedation and intubation allow time to appraise the situation.

Morphine is an effective cough suppressant. With excessive sputum production, it is unwise to suppress cough, because any accumulating sputum will block airways causing partial lung collapse.

Dyspnoea

Dyspnoea is a subjective feeling of breathlessness. In the recovery room dyspnoea is always a warning sign of something serious. Causes include: pneumothorax, cardiac failure myocardial ischaemia, anaphylaxis, aspiration and late in haemorrhagic shock. Patients with cardiac failure become uncomfortable if they attempt to lie flat; conversely shocked patients feel worse sitting up.

Sputum retention

Sputum retention is common in smokers and those with chronic bronchitis. Some people, especially those with severe emphysema, are unable to cough effectively enough to eject their sputum. Sputum sticking in their larynx may cause stridor. Humidified oxygen helps keep the sputum liquid enough to cough up.

Some elderly patients (especially those with brainstem ischaemia) lie there oblivious of the gurgle they make every time they breathe. Most of these patients have such poor laryngeal and pharyngeal protective reflexes that you can simply open their mouth, and with the aid of a laryngoscope and Magill forceps pass a soft plastic sucker down their trachea. Thoroughly pre-oxygenate them first. Do not distress them by persisting with suction if they do not cough.

Wheeze

Wheezing indicates irritation, inflammation or oedema of the bronchioles. As air passes along narrowed tubes it causes their walls to vibrate producing an audible sound like the reed vibrating in a clarinet. You will hear wheeze best if you listen near patients' mouths as they breathe out forcibly with their mouth wide open.

In the recovery room a developing wheeze is always potentially serious.

Causes of wheeze include aspiration, anaphylaxis, developing pulmonary oedema, and pulmonary embolism; but almost never asthma.

Consider any wheeze occurring within an hour of an offending stimulus to be anaphylaxis.

Aspiration

By far the most common cause of wheeze starting in the recovery room is aspiration of a small amount of material from the pharynx into the lower airway. This usually occurs shortly after extubation, especially if the patient is lying on their back. Immediately after the patient has aspirated the wheeze will be confined to one lung.

Anaphylaxis

Anaphylaxis may present with a generalized wheeze and a rash. Anaphylaxis usually presents a few minutes after some offending substance is given intravenously. Wheezing frequently precedes profound cardiovascular collapse. Call for help. See page 332 for more on anaphylaxis.

Gas embolism

Air or gas embolism is a worrying cause of wheeze. If a patient starts to wheeze abruptly, immediately check that the central venous catheter connection has not come apart.

Cardiac failure

Acute left ventricular failure with pulmonary oedema is often a result of fluid overload during or after the anaesthetic. Check the fluid balance sheet. If the patient has received more than 2 litres of fluid during their procedure then suspect pulmonary oedema. Other causes of acute pulmonary oedema include heart failure caused by acute myocardial infarction or ischaemia.

Cardiac failure or asthma?

Because wheeze is common to both conditions acute left ventricular failure is often confused with an acute asthmatic attack. It is extremely unlikely elderly patients will have their first acute asthma attack in the recovery room.

All wheezes are not asthma.

A chest X-ray helps diagnosis

A chest X-ray can help with the diagnosis of wheeze. At first, cardiac failure shows up as a generalized haziness on the film. Later this may coalesce into the classic bat's wing picture stretching out from the hilum of the lung. Aspiration shows nothing at first, and it may take several hours or more to develop a picture of localized haziness, especially in the right lower lobe. The chest X-ray after air or gas embolism may never show anything at all.

Difficult airways

Anticipate that you may have difficulty in maintaining an airway in patients with:

+ short or fat bull necks;
+ stiff necks;
+ prominent upper teeth;
+ underslung jaws;

- Down's syndrome;
- Turner's syndrome;
- patients who cannot open their mouths widely;
- previous cervical spine surgery;
- patients with rheumatoid arthritis show 20 per cent have cervical spine instability. It is possible to cause *subluxation* of the atlantooccipital joint when you extend the neck. This may sever the spinal cord, or damage their vertebral arteries; be gentle. Patients with rheumatoid arthritis often have temporo-mandibular joint (TMJ) stiffness and are unable to open their mouths widely;
- a forgotten throat pack after surgery on the upper airway;
- laryngeal oedema after neck surgery;
- tracheomalacia occurring after long-standing tracheal compression;
- a foreign body at any point in the airway.

Aspiration of foreign material

Aspiration of stomach contents into lungs is every anaesthetist's nightmare. Aspiration occurs if the laryngeal reflexes fail to prevent foreign material entering the trachea and lower airways. A flood of blood or gastric acid may kill the patient. Lesser degrees of aspiration cause a progression of stridor, wheeze, respiratory distress and partial or complete collapse of the lungs.

The foreign material can be:

- vomitus, gastric secretions, blood, pharyngeal secretions;
- a piece of tooth, a forgotten throat pack, a fragment of adenoid tissue or the top of your sucker.

If there is any evidence of aspiration the patient needs to be re-anaesthetized and the situation assessed with a rigid bronchoscope. Every recovery room needs the provision to do an urgent adult or paediatric bronchoscopy.

Any sedated patient is at risk of aspiration.

Aspiration pneumonitis

Depending on the amount and nature of the aspirated material, acute chemical aspiration pneumonitis may be fatal. This event is particularly fulminant and deadly in pregnant patients where it is termed Mendelson's syndrome (although the term is now used for all aspiration pneumonitis).

Many patients aspirate small quantities of fluid from their pharynx soon after they emerge from anaesthesia. The immediate consequences are few, but these small amounts probably contribute to postoperative chest infections in the elderly that surface a day or so later.

How to prevent aspiration pneumonitis

- Where possible, nurse each patient on their side until they are fully conscious.
- Treat all pregnant women as high-risk patients.
- Proper but not prolonged fasting preoperatively.
- Use prophylactic antacids 2–3 hours before surgery.

Suspect aspiration if the patent has vomited or regurgitated and then becomes wheezy, tachypnoeic, and coughs vigorously. They may desaturate as the wheeze develops. Usually, these initial symptoms resolve with humidification and bronchodilation, but the real trouble starts several hours later as the patient becomes progressively hypoxaemic, tachypnoeic and develops respiratory failure.

It is difficult to predict which patients are going to develop severe aspiration pneumonitis and respiratory failure. The aspiration of large volumes (>25 ml) is more serious than small volumes, particulate matter (such as milk curds) causes more problems than clear fluid, and acid aspiration is the most devastating event of all. Watch all patients suspected of aspiration very closely and if possible transfer them to a high dependency area, rather than a regular ward. They will need a follow-up X-ray a few hours after the event.

How to manage massive aspiration

Massive aspiration is an emergency. As with all emergencies, you will need three additional staff to help you. One person to monitor the vital signs, the second to prepare drips, drugs and fetch trolleys, and the third to summon the anaesthetist and be ready to run errands. Your job is to keep the patient alive by preserving their airway and ensuring oxygenation.

If an unconscious patient vomits or regurgitates then:

- immediately place the patient in the left lateral position with a 30° head-down tilt;
- suck out the pharynx including the nose;
- ventilate with 100% oxygen;
- get help to attach oximeter, and ECG;
- send for the anaesthetist;
- prepare to re-intubate the patient for bronchoscopy;
- expect bronchospasm, and prepare to treat it.

Later treatment may include:

- bronchoscopy to unblock airways and assess the damage;
- give salbutamol by aerosol, or intravenously if necessary;
- bronchial lavage is not recommended. It tends to spread the aspirated to unaffected parts of the lungs;
- steroids are contraindicated because they impair the immune response, and prevent localization of the inevitable infection;

- prophylactic antibiotics are not recommended at this early stage, because they select out the resistant bacteria;

- transfer to HDU or intensive care, but avoid ventilation if possible. Ventilation abolishes the vital ability to deep breathe and cough;

- antibiotic therapy when the principal (usually anaerobic) bacteria have declared themselves and the patient has developed a fever.

Pneumothorax

When air, which is normally confined to the lung, escapes into the pleural space and is trapped there it causes a *pneumothorax*.[2] Pneumothorax is usually accompanied by pleuritic pain that is so sharp and severe that the patient dare only to breathe in short shallow pants, and stops abruptly with a grunt when he feels pain. Other signs include an unexplained tachycardia, hypotension, wheeze, short sharp inspiratory movements, cyanosis and sometimes *surgical emphysema*.[3]

A pneumothorax may occur:

- during the insertion of intercostal, cervical, or supraclavicular brachial plexus blocks;

- during the insertion of a central venous line or pulmonary venous catheter;

- in patients with bullae in the lung (congenital or acquired with emphysema); Marfan's syndrome, chest trauma or rib fracture, and barotrauma;

- after thoracic surgery if the tubing on a chest drain becomes kinked or occluded in some way. If the drain tube stops bubbling exclude this cause first;

- following nephrectomy, where the pleura has been accidentally breached or a rib resected for easier surgical access;

- as a complication of laparoscopic surgery.

Diagnosis of pneumothorax

Breathlessness is accompanied by reduced movement on the affected side with diminished breath sounds. Call for a chest X-ray and have the patient as erect as possible for this. The diagnostic characteristic is displacement of the pleural line. If breathlessness is accompanied by severe tachypnoea, tachycardia and hypotension the patient may have a tension pneumothorax.

If the escaped air or gas collects under pressure it causes a tension pneumothorax. The collection of air progressively grows in size to squash the lungs, heart and major blood vessels. Blood vessels get kinked and the cardiac output falls. In the recovery room the patient may suddenly panic, collapse, go blue in the face and struggle to breathe, with almost undetectable pulses. Sometimes the neck veins will be grossly distended. The displaced heart and lungs push the trachea to the opposite side. No breath sounds can be heard on the affected side, and if you percuss the chest the note will be booming (similar to what you hear if you percuss a pillow). Listening with the stethoscope at the same time as the percussion improves your ability to diagnose a pneumothorax.

In neonates sometimes simply holding a bright light behind the chest will reveal the pneumothorax.

For information about performing a cricothyroid puncture see Box 16.1.

Box 16.1 **Cricothyroid puncture**

There are a number of commercially available tracheostomy sets which are designed for quick and easy insertion. However, in an emergency situation, where the patient is becoming cyanosed, or his conscious state is deteriorating, you may not have time to organize this. You may have to perform an acute cricothyroid puncture.

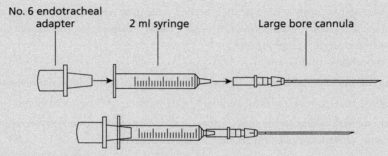

Figure 16.3 Improvised cricothyroid puncture set.

Take the largest bore intravenous cannula you have (preferably 10 G or bigger) and insert it through the cricothyroid membrane into the trachea. Attach the barrel of a 2 ml syringe into the needle and then jam a No. 8 endotracheal 15 mm adaptor into the barrel of the syringe. It will now be possible to attach the cannula to a self-inflating bag or T-piece to support the patient's oxygenation until a tracheostomy or other means of establishing an airway can be achieved. See Figures 16.3 and 16.4.

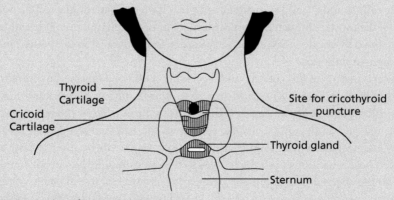

Figure 16.4 Location of cricothyroid puncture.

*A tension pneumothorax is
a medical emergency.*

Initial management

- call for help;
- sit patient up;
- give high concentrations of oxygen;
- attach pulse oximeter and ECG.

Further management

If the patient has collapsed with a suspected pneumothorax, and you are unsure what side is affected, then aspirate each side with 23 G needle through the second intercostal space in the mid-clavicular line on either side. If you freely aspirate air on one side then you will need to insert an intercostal catheter on that side. While preparing to insert the catheter push a 14 G cannula through the same spot you found free air when you aspirated. This will relieve the pneumothorax quickly.

For information about surgical emphysema see Box 16.2.

Box 16.2 **Surgical emphysema**

Surgical emphysema occurs when air or gas escapes into the tissues. There is a peculiar crackling feeling to the skin and subcutaneous tissues. The most likely cause is a breach in the pleura and a hole in the lung during operations on the neck, rib resection, kidney operations, trauma to the rib cage; and following external cardiac massage where ribs are fractured. It also occurs with distension and rupture of alveoli if the expiratory limb of the anaesthetic circuit or ventilator becomes obstructed. The gas tracks along the sheaths of the blood vessels to the hilum of the lung, from where it spreads to the neck and chest wall. Sometimes the crackling crepitations can be felt in the suprasternal notch. This is diagnostic of air in the mediastinum and may follow a ruptured bronchi, or mid-line trauma such as a stab wound.

Ventilators

Ventilators support the breathing of patients who are not able to breath for themselves. They are used on paralysed patients under anaesthesia, and in the intensive care unit to manage acute respiratory failure for whatever the cause. They are occasionally used in the recovery room where a patient does not reverse properly from their muscle relaxants.

About normal breathing

The normal respiratory rate is about 12 to 15 breaths/min. The active inspiratory phase takes about 1 second, the passive expiratory phase takes about 2 seconds, where air and the pause lasts for just under 2 seconds. The ebb and flow of air give a tidal volume of about 400 ml with each breath so that the normal minute volume is about 5 litres. Depending on the health of the lungs, it takes an intrathoracic negative pressure of minus 3 to minus 7 cm H_2O to suck the tidal volume into the lungs.

How a positive pressure ventilator works

Breathing in is easy

Ventilators impose intermittent positive pressure ventilation (IPPV) on the lungs; they blow them up like a balloon, and then pause to allow them to passively deflate. In normal lungs the pressure needed to inflate them is 7–15 ml H_2O.

Breathing out may be a problem

Air is forced out of the lungs by the springiness of the elastic tissue in the lung parenchyma. This works well in young people with healthy lungs, but ageing causes the lung elastin to degenerate into collagen. The young have compliant lungs, which when stretched behave like an elastic band. In contrast the elderly have non-compliant lungs that behave more like chewing gum. The result is that, in the elderly, more air remains in the lungs at the end of the expiration and their functional residual capacity is higher.

How ventilators work

Ventilators inflate the patient's lungs, and then allow time for expiration. They generate a *positive pressure*, then cycle from the inspiratory phase to the expiratory phase and back again. Older ventilators deliver a fixed volume of gas before cycling to the expiratory phase, and have controls to alter the volume, the timing or the pressure of gas delivered. Modern ventilators have a variety of modes to suit the lung functions of individual patients.

Other features include provision to: nebulize and humidify the gas; apply a sigh; adjust the inspiratory waveform; provide intermittent mandatory ventilation; allow the patient to trigger the switching mechanism; control of oxygen concentration and applying positive end-expiratory pressures (Figure 16.5). Safety features include alarms to warn if the preset conditions are not achieved, and safety release valves to prevent barotrauma. Ventilators also affect pulse pressure (see Box 16.3).

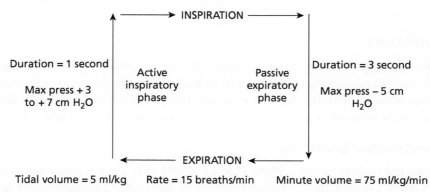

Figure 16.5 The respiratory cycle.

Ideal ventilators should be:

+ simple to operate;
+ easy to maintain;
+ compact;
+ robust;
+ portable;
+ economical to run.

Ventilators should be able to generate:

+ an inspiratory flow rate of 100 litres/min;
+ tidal volume between 50 and 1500 ml;
+ rates between 5 and 50 per minute;
+ variable inspiratory and expiratory ratios.

Box 16.3 **How ventilation affects pulse pressure**

The outcome of this pumping effect on the veins in the thorax is that the blood pressure rises on inspiration and falls on expiration. You can often see this if the patient has an arterial line. The reverse happens if the patient is breathing spontaneously; the pulse pressure falls on inspiration and rises on expiration (Figure 16.6).

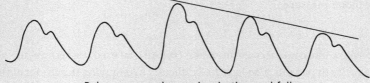

Pulse pressure rises on inspiration and falls
as pressure in the great veins decreases.

Figure 16.6 Pulse pressure rises on inspiration and falls as pressure in the great veins decreases.

This effect is more obvious if the patient's vascular volume is under-filled. So if you see this arterial wave pattern developing on the monitor suspect the patient vascular volume is depleted. You can confirm this by looking for the *postural drop* in their systolic blood pressure.

Maintain a normal $PaCO_2$ in a ventilated patient in the recovery room.

Typical ventilator settings

For an unconscious adult patient with normal lungs the usual settings are:

1. Respiratory rate = 14 breaths/min.
2. Inspiratory pressure = + 5 cm H_2O.
3. Inspiratory time = 1.2 seconds.

4. Expiratory time = 3.5 seconds.

5. Tidal volume = 8 ml/kg.

6. The sigh mechanism = 40 sighs an hour.

Positive end expiratory pressure

Positive end expiratory pressure (PEEP) improves oxygenation by recruiting alveoli that would otherwise not be aerated. This increases the surface area of the alveoli available for gas exchange and prevents *terminal respiratory units* collapsing at the end of expiration. PEEP keeps the intrathoracic pressure continually elevated. Typical pressures are between 4 and 10 cmH$_2$O.

Advantages of PEEP

PEEP keeps small airways open, especially the non-axial airways, which otherwise would be closed. It therefore reduces the lungs' dead space. PEEP increases the total available surface area of the respiratory units by opening up airways in the apex and mid-zones of the lung. The useful effects of PEEP rapidly disappear once the patient returns to spontaneous breathing. There is some evidence to show that patients with compromised lung functions are helped by SIGHs which stretch and open the remote alveoli, given intermittently during surgery have a beneficial effect for the patient in recovery room.[4]

Disadvantages of PEEP

PEEP increases the risk of barotrauma to lungs, and it causes cardiac output to fall and lowers the blood pressure.

BiPAP

Bi-level positive pressure airway pressure (BiPAP) is used to restore the functional residual capacity in patients who have had difficulty in emptying the air out of their lungs.

BiPAP is also used to treat high-pressure pulmonary oedema, and pneumonia. It can be used in recovery room to help patients with poor lung function regain appropriate spontaneous ventilation after a long operation. The patient wears a tight-fitting mask strapped over their mouth and nose. When the patient starts to breathe in, the device delivers an inspiratory positive airway pressure (IPAP) to help the patient achieve a larger tidal breath. When the patient finishes inspiration, the machine allows the patient to exhale passively with a little bit of back pressure support (PS) to splint the floppy airways open to the expiratory positive airway pressure (EPAP).

$$PS = PAP - IPAP$$

Most machines allow the patient to take a spontaneous breath in (assist mode), or they can be set to cycle in (control mode).

Normal settings are:

IPAP 5–10 cm H$_2$O

EPAP 3–5 cm H$_2$O

If the patient's oxygen saturations fail to improve then the settings are adjusted in 3–5 cm H_2O increments.

BiPAP is not easy to use. Most patients resist wearing the tight-fitting mask. Encourage them gently. It requires persistence to make BiPAP work effectively. If the patient's respiratory rate rises to 20 breaths/min or they start to use their accessory muscles to help them breathe, then it is time for the anaesthetist to reassess the situation.

Lung diseases

Asthma

Asthma is a chronic lung disease with reversible airway obstruction. It occurs when a usually trivial stimuli causes the bronchioles to become inflamed and oedematous. In some countries asthma affects up to 10 per cent of the population, and is particularly common in children. For most surgery the patient's peak flow rate (PFR) should not be less than 150 L/ sec, but for abdominal or thoracic surgery the PFR needs to be at least 220 L/sec.

In the recovery room, asthma usually does not cause problems, because volatile anaesthetic gases are superb bronchodilators. However it's still a possibility particularly if TIVA or regional anaesthesia have been used instead of volatile anaesthetic. If a non-asthmatic patient starts to wheeze then suspect aspiration, anaphylaxis or cardiac failure.

Wheezing in the recovery room?

Very unlikely to be asthma.
Look for another cause.

Because morphine can release histamine it may theoretically cause bronchoconstriction in asthmatics, but this does not seem to happen. On the other hand NSAIDs often aggravate bronchoconstriction and should not be used in asthmatics unless they tell you they have had them in the past without problems.

Chronic obstructive airways disease

Smoking is the main reason for chronic obstructive airways disease (COAD). In older people the usual reason is cigarettes and, in those under the age of 40 years, marijuana remains a suspect.

COAD ranges between two extremes. At one extreme is *emphysema*, where the lung's *parenchyma* is extensively damaged. The walls between the terminal respiratory units are destroyed forming large blebs in the lung where air gets trapped. In severe cases these patients are more comfortable breathing in short shallow breaths—the so-called pink *puffers*.[5]

At the other end of the range is *chronic bronchitis* where years of inflammation have destroyed the cartilage rings holding the bronchi open. Consequently airways become floppy and collapse. Moreover mucosal goblet cells proliferate producing large amounts of sputum.

With COAD and asthma the patient has no trouble breathing in, but because small airways collapse, getting the air out again is a problem. These patients (called *blue bloaters*) are more comfortable taking deep gulping breaths, and then blowing out through pursed lips which creates back pressure on the airways. The back pressure splints their floppy airways open allowing them to expire more fully. The closer the surgical incision is to the diaphragm, the greater the respiratory problems in the recovery room. Pain from upper abdominal or thoracic incision severely limits respiratory effort. Epidural analgesia gives optimal pain relief. In contrast, morphine depresses ventilation.

Patients with COAD are more comfortable, and have better gas exchange if they sit up in the recovery room. Give 35 per cent oxygen by mask and where possible humidify the inspired air. Encourage deep breathing and coughing. If patients find it difficult to breathe, become distressed or hypoxaemic then consider short-term respiratory support with continuous positive airway pressure (CPAP) or BiPAP masks. Arterial blood gases help decide about ongoing management.

Embolism to the lungs

Various materials can be carried in the blood stream to lodge in the lungs. This event can obstruct blood flow and cause an inflammatory response. The most common emboli are air, blood clots, fat and amniotic fluid.

Air embolism

Air embolism occurs when air, or some other gas, enters the circulation, usually through a vein. Air embolism causes the patient to collapse abruptly. In the recovery room, it usually occurs during the insertion, or accidental disconnection of a central venous line. About 100–200 ml of gas abruptly entering a vein is enough to cause a cardiac arrest. About 100 ml of air can be sucked through a 14-gauge needle in 1 second with a negative gradient of 5 cm H_2O. Despite these alarming facts, most air emboli are minor, and their effects transient.

Once a large bolus of air enters the right ventricle, it makes the blood froth. The churning mass of bubbles blocks blood flow to the lungs. Unable to achieve a cardiac output the patient suddenly becomes hypoxic, cyanosed, hypotensive, with a feeble pulse, tachycardia and engorged neck veins and has a cardiac arrest. You may hear the characteristic *mill-wheel murmur* if you listen over the posterior chest wall. The murmur sounds as if water is squelching around inside a Wellington boot.

Signs of less severe embolism are a strident dry cough, wheeze, chest pain and breathlessness. Detectable air embolism occurs during 11 per cent of Caesarean sections. Air enters the circulation when the surgeon is handling the uterus. If the patient is awake, she usually becomes breathless, alarmed, hypotensive and her oxygen saturations decline. The anaesthetist will notify the surgeon, and then manage the problem appropriately depending on its severity. However, the patient may still be alarmed and fearful when she returns to the recovery room. Her chest may still feel painful, if necessary a small dose of morphine usually helps her. Comforting reassurance from the nursing staff that her distress will pass quickly is a better option.

Gas embolism occurs quite frequently in the operating theatre. During laparoscopy carbon dioxide under pressure is used to inflate the peritoneum. Sometimes some of the gas enters the venous circulation and is carried to the right heart. Occasionally bubbles of gas pass through a patent foramen ovale or ventricular septal defect to enter the left ventricle and embolize to some distal vascular bed. Since 18 per cent of the cardiac output goes to the brain there is an 18 per cent chance of the gas bubble causing a stroke.

What to do first

In the recovery room most gas embolism occurs during the insertion of a central venous line, or if the line is accidentally disconnected allowing air to enter. Immediately stop further air entering the vein; if necessary put your finger over the hole where air is going in. Call for help. Give high concentrations of oxygen. Tip the patient into a 15° head-down position so that the hole is below the heart level. Do not put them in a steep head-down tilt, because you will jeopardize gas exchange in their lung.

Turn the patient on to their left side (*Durant's manoeuvre*). This manoeuvre may possibly lessen the amount of air entering the pulmonary arteries. Attempt to aspirate air from the central venous line (this is not usually fruitful). If you cannot feel the carotid pulse then treat the patient as a cardiac arrest. Some clinicians feel cardiac massage may help break up the froth. There are reports of extreme cases of air embolism have been treated successfully with direct large-bore needle aspiration of the right ventricle, cardio-pulmonary bypass, or thoracotomy.

What to do next

The patient needs high-flow oxygen for at least 6 hours to help wash the nitrogen out of their blood, and absorb the air from the bloodstream. Hyperbaric oxygen rapidly speeds this process, but it is not always available.

Fat embolism

Fat embolism syndrome (FES) is a major hazard affecting 10 per cent of patients who have had major bone trauma. FES occurs 12–72 hours after bones are broken either from trauma or with orthopaedic surgery. Broken or cut bone releases fat globules from the marrow into the circulation. Almost instantly, plasma lipases degrade the fat into fatty acids that are toxic to the cells lining the lung's capillaries. The damaged alveolar capillary membrane allows fluid to leak into the lung's interstitium and alveoli causing pulmonary oedema. To add to the disaster, the fat can trigger disseminated intravascular coagulation.

FES may present in the recovery room, especially in trauma cases admitted the previous day or after surgery such as on the tibia. As pulmonary oedema develops the patient becomes progressively breathless, and their oxygen saturation begins to fall. Damage to the capillaries in the brain allows fluid to leak out to cause cerebral oedema resulting in headache, confusion and eventually a deteriorating conscious state. Although not always present a good clinical sign are tiny pricks of purple petechiae on the patient's trunk, under their fingernails, and even in their retina.

Early stabilization of fractures and good resuscitation helps prevent this disaster. There is no specific treatment apart from preserving oxygenation. Mortality can reach 45 per cent in florid cases. Occasionally, FES also occurs after bone marrow transplantation and liposuction.

Thromboembolism

You are very unlikely to encounter a pulmonary thromboembolism (PE) in the recovery room. These are caused by blood clots, formed in the walls of the large veins of the legs or pelvis which break off and become lodged in the lungs. The patient immediately becomes very short of breath and frightened. Treatment involves oxygen, relief of bronchospasm and anticoagulation with heparin. Read about preventing deep vein thrombosis in Chapter 2, page 34.

References

1. **Ward DS, Karen SB**, *et al.* (2011) Hypoxia: developments in basic science, physiology and clinical studies. *Anaesthesia* **66**:19–26.
2. **Visvanathan T, Kluger MT**, *et al.* (2005) Crisis management during anaesthesia: laryngospasm. *Quality & Safety in Health Care* **14**:e3.
3. **MacDuff A, Arnold A**, *et al.* (2010) Management of spontaneous pneumothorax: British Thoracic Society Pleural Disease Guideline 2010. *Thorax* **65**(2):ii18–ii31.
4. **Tusman G, Böhm SH** (2010) Prevention and reversal of lung collapse during the intra-operative period. *Best Practice and Research Clinical Anaesthesiology* **24**:183–197.
5. **Kane B, Turkington PM**, *et al.* (2011) Rebound hypoxaemia after administration of oxygen. *British Medical Journal* **342**:d1557.

Chapter 17

Cardiovascular physiology

Introduction

The heart, circulatory system and the lungs work together as an integrated *cardiopulmonary unit*. The lungs transfer oxygen to the blood, and evict the waste carbon dioxide, while the heart pumps enough blood, at an appropriate pressure, through the circulation to deliver sufficient oxygen and nutrients to the tissues and organs, and to remove their metabolic waste products. The heart is a pump, it supplies blood to the organs at low pressures. If the heart is forced to pump blood at high pressures it will, sooner or later, fail.

Blood pressure oscillates. When the ventricles contract (*systole*) the blood pressure in the arteries rises, and as they relax (*diastole*) the pressure falls. The pressure at the peak of the pulse wave is the *systolic blood pressure*, and the trough is the *diastolic pressure*. The difference between the two pressures is called the *pulse pressure*.

> *In the recovery room adequate blood flow*
> *with good tissue perfusion, a clear conscious state*
> *and a good urine output, is more important*
> *than a high blood pressure.*

The heart consists of two *demand* pumps set in *series*. The right side of the heart is a low-pressure pump supplying the lungs. Simultaneously the left side of the heart, working as a high-pressure pump, feeds blood to the organs and muscles. Because they are set in series each pump feeds the other, and being demand pumps they adjust their output to the metabolic needs of the tissues. Sometimes the heart cannot keep up with the demands of the tissue for oxygen. This does not necessarily mean the heart is diseased. When you get puffed running up stairs, your heart is failing to meet the demands of your muscles: this is not heart disease. If you get puffed doing normal day-to-day activities then some sort of cardiopulmonary dysfunction is probable.

What is cardiac output?

Cardiac output is the volume of blood the heart pumps out every minute (Table 17.1). In a resting individual the normal heart rate is about 72 beats a minute. It ejects 70 ml of blood (*stroke-volume*) with each beat.

$$Cardiac\,output = heart\,rate \times stroke - volume$$

$$Thus\,the\,cardiac\,output = 72 \times 70 \approx 5000\,ml\,/\,min$$

Table 17.1 Where the cardiac output goes

Organ	Proportion of cardiac output
Heart	4%
Brain	15%
Kidneys	25%
Muscle	5–20% depending on demands
Liver	15–25% depending on proximity to a meal
The rest	15%

Role of heart rate

One might suspect that the faster the heart beats the more blood it pumps out. This is partly true, it depends on the age of the person. With exercise or increased demand an older person's stroke volume does not increase, consequently they compensate by increasing their heart rate instead. Similarly, neonates depend on their high heart rate to maintain cardiac output. In most adults, the heart becomes increasingly inefficient at rates above 130 beats per minute. In the recovery room, worry about an adult's heart rate if it exceeds 100 beats per minute. Always look for a cause of tachycardia.

Role of stroke volume

Healthy hearts can double their stroke volume with ease. In young people, this pump, a little larger than the size of your clenched fist, can increase its output to 20 L/min or more, however this ability declines with age and deteriorating physical fitness. Athletes often have stroke volumes exceeding 130 ml per beat (and so do severely obese people).

Three factors determine stroke volume:

1. Preload.
2. Myocardial contractility.
3. Afterload.

So that we can compare the cardiac output in people of different sizes it is standardized to a *cardiac index*; this is the cardiac output per square metre of body surface area, which at rest, is about 3 L/m^2.

Every time the ventricle contracts it ejects about half the blood it contains (*ejection fraction* of 50 per cent). Those with *systolic heart failure* have ejection fractions of 40 per cent or less. Ejection fractions are measured with transthoracic echocardiography.

Starling's law describes contractility

Over a hundred years ago two physiologists, Frank and Starling, noted that like an elastic band: 'The more the myocardial fibres are stretched during diastole, the more they will contract during subsequent systole, and therefore the more blood will be expelled'. This initial stretching is now called *preload*.

Cardiac preload

Within limits, the more cardiac myocytes are stretched (preload) the harder they contract. The myocytes, however, are damaged if they are overstretched. The preload on the ventricles is determined by how hard the atria needs to contract to fill (prime) the ventricles with blood.

Ventricular pump priming by atrial contraction contributes to 25 per cent of the cardiac output in a normal person, and over 50 per cent in patients with diastolic dysfunction. If a patient with diastolic failure develops atrial fibrillation, then their cardiac output may drop precipitously.

Cardiac contractility

Healthy muscles contract more forcibly than unhealthy ones. Many factors reduce the ability of ventricular muscle to contract forcibly; they include old age, hypertension, ischaemic heart disease, the long-term effects of chronic alcoholism, and there are many others.

Cardiac afterload

Blood pressure is a result of the balance between the volume of blood ejected with each beat (*stroke volume*), and the *resistance* the arterioles (*afterload*) impose on blood flowing through the systemic vascular bed.

If the arterioles dilate reducing afterload, then the blood pressure falls, and if they constrict, increasing the afterload, the blood pressure rises.

How blood pressure is controlled

A normal blood pressure in an adult is considered to range between 110–130 mmHg systolic, and 65–80 mmHg diastolic. It is kept within this range by a number of homeostatic feedback mechanisms (Figure 17.1). Patients coming to surgery with poorly controlled blood pressure are at a higher risk of adverse cardiac events in the recovery room.

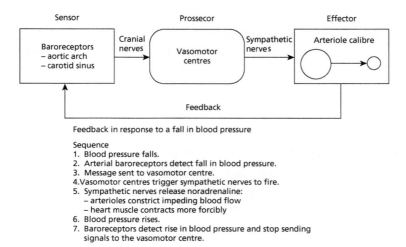

Sequence
1. Blood pressure falls.
2. Arterial baroreceptors detect fall in blood pressure.
3. Message sent to vasomotor centre.
4. Vasomotor centres trigger sympathetic nerves to fire.
5. Sympathetic nerves release noradrenaline:
   – arterioles constrict impeding blood flow
   – heart muscle contracts more forcibly
6. Blood pressure rises.
7. Baroreceptors detect rise in blood pressure and stop sending signals to the vasomotor centre.

Figure 17.1 Negative feedback control of blood pressure.

Homeostasis

Interlinked feedback control mechanisms stabilize the circulation. These include:

+ baroreceptors to sense pressure changes;
+ chemoreceptors to sense changes in the composition of the blood;
+ sensory nerves to carry the information to central processors;
+ processors in the central nervous system to coordinate these mechanisms;
+ effector nerve to instantly make adjustments;
+ hormones to maintain the changes over a long period.

Baroreceptors

Baroreceptors are special stretch receptors located in the walls of the veins, and arteries near the heart. There are two types of stretch receptors: *high-pressure baroreceptors* located in the arch of the aorta, and the carotid arteries; and *low-pressure baroreceptors* in the great veins and right atrium.

Baroreceptors sense changes in mean blood pressure, and instruct the autonomic nervous system to restore the blood pressure to an optimal level. General anaesthetics blunt baroreceptor function, particularly if the patient is also taking long-term vasodilator anti-hypertensive drugs. If a patient is taking ACE inhibitors or angiotensin receptor blockers, do not suddenly sit them up because their blood pressure will fall, and with it their cerebral perfusion. Should this occur they will feel nauseated, faint and may lose consciousness, and even have a seizure.

Neural regulation

If the arterial blood pressure falls, the fast-acting sympathetic nervous system, backed up by several slower-acting hormones, attempts to increase cardiac output and decrease the arteriolar calibre to restore the blood pressure.

Chemoreceptors

Chemoreceptors respond to chemical changes in the blood. One type of chemoreceptor located in the arch of the aorta and carotid bodies responds to hypoxia. Their job is to stimulate breathing should blood oxygen levels fall. They start firing vigorously once the PaO_2 falls below 60 mmHg (kPa = 7.89) or where the oxygen saturation is less than 90 per cent. Even tiny amounts of volatile anaesthetics blunt this response, and so for several hours after a general anaesthetic, the rate and depth of breathing may not increase if the patient becomes hypoxaemic.

The MET (Metabolic Exercise Tolerance) score

The heart must be able to attain and sustain the demands placed on it during the postoperative period. Instead of reporting a patient's cardiac function as 'poor', or 'good', or 'excellent' we now calibrate this with the MET

One MET is the amount of oxygen used each minute by a 70 kg man at rest (3.5 ml/kg/min): 2 MET is the amount of oxygen used when walking at 2 kilometres per hour, while 10 MET is roughly equivalent to jogging at 10 kilometres per hour. METs can be measured by exercising the patient on a static bicycle or a treadmill, but an estimate can be gleaned simply from the scale shown in Table 17.2.

Table 17.2 MET score

MET	Equivalent physical activity
1 MET	Watching TV, writing at a desk, eating a meal, washing dishes.
2 MET	Walking from room to room, showering, walking around a supermarket, hanging out the washing, making a bed, playing lawn bowls.
3 MET	Carrying bags of groceries from car, pushing full supermarket trolley, vacuuming floors, and walking up one flight of stairs without becoming short of breath. Playing golf (but not carrying a golf bag).
4 MET	Sweeping yard, raking up leaves, walking up two flights of stairs carrying 7 kg load. Walking 4 km in 1 hour.
5 MET	Walking briskly, climbing four flights of stairs without breathlessness.
35 MET	Olympic athlete running the 400 metres.

If the MET score is less than 4 in a patient having major surgery, then a postoperative adverse cardiac event is likely to occur, either in the recovery room, or later in the ward. This is because there is a large postoperative inflammatory response as well as blood and fluid loss and to perfuse the inflamed tissue the patient must be able to attain, and maintain, a MET score equivalent to 3 to 4 or more. For minor surgery, where the operation is short and there is little tissue damage, then a MET score of 2 to 3 is sufficient.

Electrophysiology and the electrocardiogram (ECG)

The essentials

The heart runs on tiny electrical currents. Unless every cardiac myocyte contracts at exactly the right moment the heart would pump chaotically. To organize and coordinate this activity, the heart uses tiny electrical currents called *action potentials* to kick-start the myocytes.

The sino-atrial (SA) node ticks away like a clock, normally generating about 70 electrical impulses a minute. Each electrical impulse then starts on a journey through the heart as a wave of *depolarization*. The firing rate of the SA nodes is sped up by sympathetic nerves, circulating adrenaline and certain drugs (such as atropine). It is slowed by *parasympathetic nervous system* and certain drugs (such as neostigmine and β-blockers).

Each impulse then plays follow-the-leader through the heart down the same well-beaten path. From the SA node the impulses wash through atrial muscle like a wave, stimulating (*depolarizing*) each myocyte to contract as they pass. As the atrial muscle contracts it pushes blood through the mitral and tricuspid valves into the left and right ventricle respectively. When the wave of depolarization hits the atrioventricular (AV) node it is delayed momentarily to allow time for the ventricles to fill with blood. In less than 120 milliseconds it fizzes, like a lighted fuse, down specialized Purkinje fibres in the bundle of His. Then the depolarizing wave fans out through special conducting tissue along the branches of the right and left bundles to the ventricles to sweep up from the heart's apex jolting each cell into action. All this happens in an orderly sequence, like a cascade of falling dominoes, each activating the one next to it. In this way ventricular contraction squeezes blood, in a twisting anti-clockwise vortex, upwards and out through the aortic and pulmonary valves into the aorta and pulmonary arteries.

It takes about 120 milliseconds to eject the stroke volume from the ventricles during systole, and it takes about another 200 milliseconds for the cardiac myocytes to recover enough to contract again. During diastole the exhausted ventricles relax, receive their oxygen and nutrient supply through the coronary arteries, and fill with blood to be ready to start pumping over again.

At the beginning of diastole, the heart muscles begin to relax, and the backward pressure of blood in the arteries snaps the pulmonary and aortic valves shut. This stops blood refluxing back into the heart. Then the whole cycle starts again.

Monitoring the electrical activity

We routinely monitor the ECG on most patients in the recovery room. The trace is displayed on the monitor's screen (Figure 17.2). Built into the monitors are alarms for cardiac rate, rhythm, and many have facilities for arrhythmia and ST analysis. Although monitors are mostly reliable, you still need to observe your patients carefully.

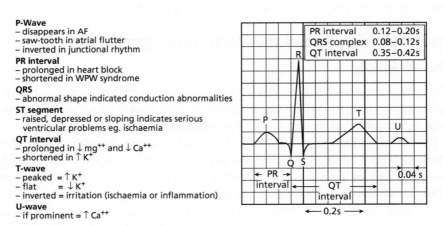

Figure 17.2 The normal ECG complex.

An ECG uses electrodes stuck on the skin to measure the sum of the electrical action potentials on the body surface. Impulses passing towards an electrode record a positive deflection on the trace while those passing away from the electrode cause a negative deflection. Each electrode samples the sequence, direction and magnitude of the impulse as it travels from its origin in the atria to its extinction in the ventricles.

At any instant an ECG trace reveals the overall direction the electrical impulses are going. If the electrical currents are aberrant, or going in the wrong direction, they appear as an abnormal waveform on the ECG trace. Monitors can deceive you. Sometimes false alarms occur or alarms fail to go off when they should. ECG leads can fall off the patient simulating asystole, or electrical interference may simulate ventricular fibrillation. Never silence the monitor alarm without checking the patient's pulse, and blood pressure manually.

> *Do not ignore the monitor, and never ignore the patient.*

Describing ECGs

Learn to recognize and describe ECG traces. Sooner or later you will have to tell someone what is happening over the telephone. This takes practice.

1. If the patient is hypotensive—call for help immediately.
2. What is the heart rate?
   - a bradycardia is less than 60 bpm;
   - a relative tachycardia is greater than 80 bpm;
   - a tachycardia is greater than 100 bpm.
3. Is the rhythm regular? Look at lead II.
4. Is the QRS complex wide or narrow?
5. Is there a P wave in lead II and are they all the same shape?
6. Are there signs of ischaemia? The best lead to detect ischaemia is CM5. Is the ST segment raised above, or depressed below the isoelectric line? Is the ST segment sloping?
7. Is the pulse oximeter showing a decreasing saturation?

Practise explaining these points to each other until you feel confident. If you do not understand something, or what you are doing, or what is wrong with your patient, then consult someone who does.

Pacemakers

Implanted electronic pacemakers are used to maintain cardiac output in patients who are having symptoms caused bradycardias, heart blocks, or recurring or uncontrollable tachyarrhythmias.

Permanent pacemakers

Types of pacemakers

There are two types of implanted pacemakers: anti-tachycardia pacemakers, which terminate arrhythmias, and anti-bradycardia pacemakers that simulate normal pacemaker function. There are also implantable defibrillator/pacemakers. These are for patients with unstable arrhythmias. This device monitors heart rhythms and if it senses dangerous rhythms, it delivers shocks. Many ICDs record the heart's electrical patterns when there is an abnormal heartbeat.

Pacemakers are described by an internationally accepted code. Most patients carry a card describing the make of the pacemaker, when it was inserted, when the battery was last checked and a 5-letter code on specifying what the pacemaker does (Table 17.3).

Table 17.3 Pacemaker code

1st letter chamber paced	2nd letter chamber sensed	3rd letter response to sensed event	4th letter (optional) programmability	5th letter (for implanted devices)
A = atria	A = atria	I = device inhibited	O = not programmable	O = none
V = ventricles	V = ventricles	T = device triggered	P = rate + output	P = anti-tachycardia pacing
D = dual (both atria and ventricles)	D = dual	D = ventricular sensed event with device triggered Atrial sensed even with device inhibited O = off—device unresponsive	M = multiple C = telemetric R = rate responsive	S = shock delivery D = both

For example, DDD = both chambers paced, both chambers sensed. This pacemaker generates an atrial impulse inhibiting the patient's atrium from generating a normal impulse. The pacemaker then senses whether the impulse it generated has arrived at the ventricle. If not, then it generates an impulse to stimulate the ventricle.

Reasons for pacemaker malfunction during surgery include:

- threshold changes where the heart muscle becomes more or less sensitive to the pacemaker's pulse;
- the pacemaker failed to generate an impulse;
- a lead or electrode has become displaced.

VVI pacemakers can be disrupted by tiny electrical currents—even those generated when muscles contract; for instance, fasciculation caused by suxamethonium. Many anaesthetists prefer that VVI mode be switched to VVO mode with a special magnet before they start the anaesthetic.

Temporary pacemakers

Temporary pacemakers are inserted as a stop-gap measure where symptomatic bradycardia, atrioventricular blocks, or sinus arrest cause the cardiac output and blood pressure to fall. The leads are inserted into a large vein, in the same way as a central venous catheter, and fed into the right ventricle to depolarize it. The usual reason for using a temporary pacemaker in a surgical patient is as a precautionary measure, where the patient has a high-grade trifascicular block.

What to check

As soon as the patient with a pacemaker is admitted to the recovery room put on an ECG monitor and do a full 12-lead ECG. If the ECG rhythm strip (lead II), does not show regular pacemaker spikes, the pacemaker may either be faulty, or set in demand mode. Check each pacemaker spike is followed by a widened QRS (similar to an extrasystole).

Sometimes pacemakers are turned off during surgery. Before the patient returns to the ward they should be turned on again using a special magnet, which is placed over the pacemaker. They should also be re-checked by a member of the cardiology team. Pacemakers need normal serum potassium levels to function properly. Check the serum potassium concentrations if arrhythmias occur, or the pacemaker misbehaves.

The electromagnetic fields generated by diathermy or electrosurgery do not upset modern pacemakers, but older models can be damaged by current surges. Cardioversion can damage pacemakers. If possible consult a cardiologist before performing cardioversion on a patient with a pacemaker in place. Do not insert central lines or pulmonary floatation catheters into patients with pacemakers because the catheter may dislodge the pacemaker wire from the right ventricle.

Stents

These are stainless steel tubes inserted into coronary arteries to hold the lumen open and improve the blood flow to the heart. Special precautions are required to prevent them from being covered and blocked by clots. Aspirin and clopidogrel are given initially. Clopidogrel can be stopped after 6 weeks when the stent will be covered by natural tissue but aspirin must be continued indefinitely.

Patients who stop their aspirin preoperatively should be restarted as soon as possible postoperatively. Check the prescription in the notes and if you think this has been over-looked speak to the surgical registrar and ask them to look into it.

Chapter 18

Cardiovascular disease

Introduction

Cardiovascular disease is common. The principal problems, in order of prevalence, are hypertension, cardiac failure, ischaemic heart disease, and valvular heart disease. About 40 per cent of patients over the age of 40 attending a hospital for surgery have some form of cardiovascular disease such as hypertension, vascular disease, or ischaemic heart disease. If these problems are optimized before surgery it reduces the risk of them surfacing in the recovery room.

> *Proper preoperative management*
> *alleviates many problems*
> *in the recovery room.*

Hypertension

Hypertension is due to either an elevated cardiac output, or an increase in peripheral resistance, or both. Increased levels of circulating *catecholamines* cause most hypertension in the recovery room. Adrenaline and noradrenaline are released as the sympathetic nervous system is activated in response to actual or perceived stress. The elevated blood pressure increases cardiac work, which in turn increases the heart's need for oxygen and nutriment.

The left ventricle is mainly perfused during *diastole*. Because tachycardias shorten diastolic time they reduce coronary blood flow and cardiac oxygen supply. If a tachycardia (which reduces coronary perfusion) accompanies hypertension (which increases cardiac oxygen demand), the combination becomes a potential cause of cardiac ischaemia.

> *Tachycardia + hypertension → cardiac ischaemia.*

Acute hypertension

Check the patients' medical records to elicit their preoperative blood pressure. Normal blood pressure ranges from 110/65 to 130/85 mmHg. In the recovery room the patients' blood pressures should ideally remain within 15 per cent of their preoperative blood pressures.

Risks associated with hypertension include:

- arrhythmias;
- myocardial ischaemia, myocardial infarction;

- cardiac failure;
- strokes—subarachnoid, or cerebral haemorrhages;
- bleeding from the operative site.

Causes of acute hypertension include:

- pain;
- hypoxia;
- CO_2 retention;
- full bladder;
- over-transfusion;
- vasopressors;
- obstructed airways;
- shivering;
- hypoglycaemia;
- phaeochromocytoma;
- carcinoid.

Hypertension should be treated if it is associated with:

- a systolic pressure above 180 mmHg or a diastolic over 105 mmHg;
- ventricular premature beats;
- ST changes on the ECG;
- a deteriorating conscious state.

The elderly, or those with pre-existing heart disease, are at risk of cardiac ischaemia and arrhythmias, especially if they also develop a tachycardia. If you see ventricular extrasystoles on the monitor then suspect myocardial ischaemia. Controlling the hypertension usually resolves the extrasystoles.

Chronic hypertension

Chronic hypertension is endemic in the community affecting about half the population over the age of 65 years. In patients with chronic hypertension, haemorrhage or a rapid infusion of intravenous fluids can cause unexpectedly large swings in their blood pressure.

Patients should have taken all their cardiac medication on the day of surgery. Check in their medical record that they have done so. Many patients take a β-blocker (such as atenolol, metoprolol, or bisoprolol). If their β-blockers are withdrawn abruptly then patients may experience rebound hypertension, tachycardia, ventricular arrhythmias, and possibly sudden death.

Malignant hypertension

Fulminating (malignant) hypertension can cause cerebral oedema if the blood pressure rises acutely beyond 220/120 mmHg. Control the blood pressure urgently. Malignant hypertension may cause cardiac ischaemia and cardiac failure with a gallop rhythm, rales in the lung bases, and retrosternal chest pain.

Principles of management of hypertension

Give oxygen, attach a pulse oximeter and an automated blood pressure device.

- Sit the patient up: it sometimes helps.
- Attach an ECG.
- If the patient has new ST segment changes then give sublingual glyceryl trinitrate.
- Eliminate hypoxia and hypoglycaemia as a cause.
- Check that the patient has taken their morning antihypertensive therapy before coming to the operating theatre.
- If patients are in pain then:
  - control it with intravenous analgesia;
  - they may need a regional anaesthetic block.
- Check the intraoperative fluid chart to see if it balances.
- Notify the anaesthetist.

Depending on the cause of the hypertension the anaesthetist may use a vasodilator such as labetalol. To reduce the force of the myocardial contraction and the heart rate a β-blocker may be given. Prepare a syringe pump. Antihypertensive are often given as an infusion. Give each drug infusion though a separate intravenous line and prepare to use intra-arterial continuous blood pressure monitoring.

Hypertension in a healthy patient?
Consider pain or fluid overload.

Antihypertensive drugs

Labetalol

Labetalol is a selective α_1-blocker and a non-selective β-blocker. Bradycardia may become a problem where larger doses are used. It reduces blood pressure by reducing cardiac output and heart rate, and decreasing the peripheral vascular resistance. It has a long half-life of between 3.5 and 6.5 hours depending on the dose given.

Clonidine

Clonidine is a centrally acting α_2-agonist that reduces blood pressure by damping down the activity of the sympathetic nervous system. Clonidine is not a first-line agent. It may cause the blood pressure to rise transiently before it falls and it lasts a long time.

Glyceryl trinitrate

Glyceryl trinitrate (GTN) is a short-acting drug that relaxes vascular smooth muscle and improves myocardial oxygenation. It is suitable for those with ischaemic heart disease, or where you wish to improve pulmonary blood flow. Its effect wears off in 5–8 minutes. *Tachyphylaxis* may become a problem.

Hypertension with myocardial ischaemia

If the patient is showing signs of myocardial ischaemia, with either chest pain or ST changes on the ECG, give sublingual glyceryl trinitrate, and send for the anaesthetist.

If a reflex tachycardia occurs, then the anaesthetist may give a β-blocker such as metoprolol 5–20 mg intravenously over 2 minutes to control the rate. If the patient is hypertensive but does not have a tachycardia, then give a sublingual or an oral spray of glyceryl trinitrate. Since GTN works for about 10 minutes, it will give you time to get help and to set up a glyceryl trinitrate infusion to control the blood pressure. The initial rate for a GTN infusion is 10 micrograms/min, increasing in increments up to 200 micrograms/min. GTN infusions take 3–4 minutes to stabilize blood pressure and the effects wear off in about 8–10 minutes. It may cause a headache.

> *The 12-lead ECG is the centre*
> *of the decision-making pathway*
> *for patients with acute chest pain.*

Hydralazine

Hydralazine is a direct-acting peripheral arteriolar vasodilator. It causes a reflex tachycardia, with increased cardiac contractility, so it may cause cardiac ischaemia. The diastolic blood pressure responds to a greater extent than the systolic pressure.

Hydralazine for moderate hypertension

If the patient is not showing signs of myocardial ischaemia the anaesthetist will probably use hydralazine 5–20 mg slowly intravenously to reduce blood pressure. Hydralazine takes about 15–20 minutes to reach maximum effect, and works for about 3–4 hours. A second dose may be given within 4–5 hours, using about two-thirds of the original loading dose. As hydralazine's effects are unpredictable, dilute it and give in 5 mg increments every 5 minutes. Any reflex tachycardia can be controlled with a small dose of metoprolol 5–10 mg intravenously.

β-blockers

Do not use β-blockers as a first line therapy for hypertension in the recovery room. Both α- and β-receptor stimulation causes hypertension. β-blockers only block β-receptors, leaving unmodified α-stimulation to cause peripheral vasoconstriction. Using β-blockers to reduce the heart's ability to contract, while simultaneously requiring it to pump blood through vasoconstricted vessels, decreases tissue blood flow and may precipitate heart failure.

Phentolamine

Only used occasionally, phentolamine is a short-acting α_1-blocker arteriolar vasodilator. Its effects wear off after 6–10 minutes.

Warning about vasodilators

If vasodilating drugs are used in patients who are unable to increase their cardiac output, they will become profoundly hypotensive.

Antihypertensive medication?
Was it given preoperatively?

Do not use vasodilating drugs in patients with:

♦ aortic or mitral stenosis;

♦ hypertrophic obstructive cardiomyopathies;

♦ cardiac tamponade;

♦ restrictive pericarditis;

♦ head trauma;

♦ hypovolaemia;

♦ epidural or spinal anaesthesia;

♦ closed angle glaucoma.

Hypotension

Hypotension is common in the recovery room. If left untreated it may lead to renal damage, myocardial ischaemia or strokes, and especially so in those who suffer from chronic hypertension.

In the recovery room patients become hypotensive once their mean blood pressure falls below 20 per cent of its preoperative values. A patient with a preoperative mean blood of 100 mmHg is hypotensive if it falls to 80 mmHg. Prepare to correct hypotension once mean blood pressure falls by 15 per cent of its preoperative values, and to treat it when it falls by 20 per cent (see Box 18.1).

When to worry about hypotension

Send for the anaesthetist if your patient:

♦ is restless, anxious or agitated;

♦ has chest discomfort, angina or finds it difficult to get their breath;

♦ complains of nausea, fading vision or their conscious state deteriorates;

♦ oxygen saturation falls below 93%.

Do not worry if the patient's:

♦ mean blood pressure is within 15% of the baseline reading;

♦ **and** they are resting comfortably;

♦ **and** have a good perfusion status;

Box 18.1 **Do not tip hypotensive patients head down**

If a patient becomes hypotensive elevate their legs on pillows but do not tip them head down. Tipping a person head down seriously disrupts oxygen transfer from the lungs to the blood, makes breathing difficult because the diaphragm has to lift the abdominal contents to move. Tipping (Figure 18.1) also slows cerebral blood flow and risks regurgitating stomach contents.

The best way to demonstrate this is for you to put a pulse oximeter on your finger, climb on to a trolley and get someone to tip you 35° head down. Most people's oxygen saturation falls by 2–3 per cent. You will also find it more difficult to breathe and most uncomfortable.

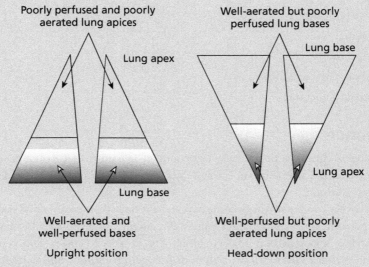

Figure 18.1 Effect of head down tilt.

Why is this so?

The human lungs are designed to operate best when their owner is either upright, or lying flat. They are shaped a bit like tall narrow pyramids. In the upright position the bases of the lungs are better perfused, and better ventilated. Air travels almost in a straight line along axial airways to reach the lower lobes, and blood does not have to be pumped uphill to get there. The bases of the lungs have a much larger surface area available for gas exchange than the apices. When people lie on their back, air passes almost straight to the dependent lungs, which lie in gutter-shaped depressions on either side of their spinal columns.

However, when people are tipped into the head-down position, most of the air is directed to the bases of their lungs, but most of the blood is diverted towards the tip of the pyramid where there is not so much surface area for gas exchange. Consequently there is a mismatch of ventilation (V) to perfusion (Q). In jargon clinicians sometimes call this *V/Q mismatch*.

+ **and** their pulse rate is less than 80 beats/min and greater than 55 beats/min. Elderly people and infants drop their cardiac output if their pulse is less than 55 beats/min.

Management

Immediately

Lift the patients' legs above their *isophlebotic point* using pillows under their knees. Blood runs downhill into their central circulation. The veins in the legs hold about 400 ml of blood: this neither disturbs lung function, nor engorges their brains.

+ Increase the inspired oxygen concentration.
+ Check the ECG trace for asystole, ventricular fibrillation or pulseless ventricular tachycardia. Treat these as a cardiac arrest.

Validate the blood pressure

Check the pulse pressure on the side of the face and in front of the ear. Ensure the non-invasive blood pressure monitor is working properly. Is the blood pressure cuff the correct size? Measure the blood pressure on the other arm. If you are using an arterial line then flush the line, open the three-way tap to air to check the *transducer* is properly zeroed. Check that the waveform is pulsatile and not damped. Check that the oximeter reading is greater than 95 per cent.

Is hypotension expected?

Expect hypotension:

+ Immediately following spinal or epidural anaesthesia.
+ Following cardioactive drugs: vasodilators, β-blockers, or pethidine.
+ In patients who take long-acting vasodilating drugs for hypertension:
  + angiotensin-converting enzyme (ACE) inhibitor drugs with names ending in '-pril'; such as enalapril, and ramipril;
  + or angiotensin receptor blockers (ARB) with names ending in '-sartan'; such as irbesartan or candesartan.

What to do

Raise the patient's legs on pillows and give a rapid infusion of 500 ml to ensure you have adequate vascular volume. Prepare a vasopressor, such as ephedrine, metaraminol or phenylephrine which the anaesthetist will use if the blood pressure does not respond to the volume load.

> *Volume resuscitation is the first priority,*
> *especially after neuraxial blocks.*

Is hypotension unexpected?

Consider:

- tachyarrhythmia: supraventricular tachycardia, atrial fibrillation or ventricular tachycardia;
- bradycardia < 45 beats/min;
- anaphylaxis;
- blood loss;
- impaired venous return, for example, pneumothorax, cardiac tamponade;
- air embolism—has the central line come apart?;
- CO_2 retention (especially after laparoscopy);
- 'trash' emboli (orthopaedic or major trauma surgery);
- amniotic fluid (obstetric surgery);
- water (urological surgery and hysteroscopy);
- myocardial ischaemia;
- transfusion incompatibility;
- septic shock;
- acute adrenal insufficiency;
- rupture of the mitral valve.

Is hypotension unresponsive?

- Get help.
- Check airway, breathing.
- Prepare for chest X-ray, blood gases, 12-lead ECG.
- Prepare to insert central venous lines, or pulmonary artery catheters.
- In the intubated patient, transoesophageal echocardiography can provide useful information about myocardial function, and how adequately the ventricles are filling.

Drugs used to manage hypotension

Vasopressors are drugs that contract the smooth muscle in the walls of arterioles causing them to constrict. These drugs increase the systemic blood pressure in septic shock and during cardiopulmonary resuscitation. Some, but not all, vasopressors are *catecholamines*. Catecholamines include naturally occurring substances such as noradrenaline, adrenaline and dopamine. Non-catecholamine vasoconstricting drugs include ephedrine, metaraminol and phenylephrine.

Adrenaline

Adrenaline is a hormone produced by the adrenal gland. It is the 'hormone of exercise' and a β stimulant. It increases heart rate and cardiac output, and in physiological amounts increases blood flow to skeletal muscle and the heart, while decreasing blood flow to the gut and kidneys.

Noradrenaline

Noradrenaline is the neurotransmitter for the sympathetic nervous system and an α stimulant. It is potent and causes generalized arteriolar constriction everywhere except the brain. It is also produced in the adrenal gland where it is a precursor for adrenaline.

Ephedrine

Ephedrine is a synthetic vasoconstrictor. Its effects are similar to adrenaline although it lasts longer. It is often used to counteract the hypotension caused by vasodilation after the insertion of an epidural or spinal anaesthetic.

Phenylephrine

Phenylephrine is a synthetic vasoconstrictor similar to noradrenaline. It produces profound vasoconstriction and as the blood pressure rises, it triggers a baroreceptor response that causes the heart rate to fall. It has a short half-life and is best administered as an infusion.

Metaraminol

Metaraminol is a synthetic vasopressor with actions similar to phenylephrine. If it is given by infusion then *tachyphylaxis* becomes a problem where more and more drug has to be infused to achieve an effect. A single dose lasts for 20–60 minutes.

Vasopressin

Arginine vasopressin (AVP) is simply another name for naturally occurring *antidiuretic hormone* (ADH). Infused at higher than physiological concentrations it causes profound vasoconstriction in all vascular beds. It acts in an entirely different way to other vasopressors and useful to support the blood pressure in septicaemic shock and increasingly during cardiac arrest in the place of adrenaline.

Acute coronary syndrome

The acute coronary syndrome[1] consists of a collection of ischaemic events with the shared underlying pathology of rupture of a coronary artery plaque, endothelial inflammation, and thrombosis. Clinically the syndrome includes unstable angina,[2] acute ischaemia and evolving myocardial infarction. Emerging from an anaesthetic after major surgery is physiologically stressful. In susceptible patients this may cause *acute coronary syndrome* (ACS) to appear for the first time in recovery room. If staff fail to recognize ACS, the patient will return to the ward at risk of having a myocardial infarct in the next few days.

Physiology

Cardiac ischaemia occurs when the heart's oxygen demands exceed its oxygen supply. When a person is at rest, their heart uses about 8 ml/100 mg/min, however with heavy exercise this may rise to 60 ml/100 mg/min.

Oxygen demands

Oxygen demands depend on how much energy the heart muscle needs to function properly. The harder the cardiac myocytes *work*, the more oxygen they consume. The heart demands a lot more oxygen to sustain a high cardiac output, or a high blood pressure. Unless the oxygen is delivered properly to the heart muscle either the muscle becomes irritable and contracts incoordinately (usually seen as ventricular ectopics on the ECG monitor) or it fails to maintain its output and the patient becomes hypotensive.

Oxygen supply

Oxygen supply depends on the amount of oxygen carried in the blood, and how fast the coronary blood flow can deliver it. The amount of oxygen carried to the tissues by the blood depends on the haemoglobin content of the blood and the oxygen saturation and the coronary blood flow depends on the mean blood pressure, the patency of the vessels, and the viscosity of the blood.

Blood can only flow through cardiac muscle when it is not contracting. Consequently almost all the ventricles' coronary perfusion occurs during diastole.

*Tachycardia decreases
coronary blood flow.*

Cardiac ischaemia in the recovery room

- Postoperative myocardial infarction is the most common cause of death in patients undergoing non-cardiac surgery.
- If patients develop any indication of myocardial ischaemia during the operation or in the recovery room they are at increased risk of arrhythmias, ischaemic episodes, or cardiac failure in the first postoperative week, which probably extends through the following weeks.
- Most postoperative infarcts occur on the second or third postoperative day when the inflammatory response peaks.
- About half of postoperative infarcts are clinically silent with no chest pain; and of those patients who do infarct about half will die.

- Proper preoperative management of *ischaemic heart disease* (IHD) with aspirin, a statin,[3] an ACE inhibitor, and possibly a β-blocker reduces cardiac complications postoperatively.
- Anxiety, fright, or pain is a potent cause of ischaemic chest pain.
- In patients with known ischaemic heart disease prophylactic GTN infusions do not help prevent ischaemia in the recovery room. This is because GTN has a brief action, and a tendency to cause *tachyphylaxis*. For these reasons, it is better to withhold GTN in the recovery room until signs of ischaemia develop.

Who is at risk of ischaemic heart disease (IHD)?

Apply the 40 per cent rule.

40% of patients

with IHD have few or no risk factors;

with IHD don't get classical angina;

with IHD have normal looking ECGs;

with vascular disease have severe IHD;

with diabetes > 10 years have IHD;

smokers > 40 years have IHD;

with eGFR = 50 ml/min/1.73m² have IHD.

In the recovery room be alert for the possibility of myocardial ischaemia in younger people with major risk factors.

Preoperatively:

- men aged > 50, and women aged > 60 years;
- those who have smoked for > 10 years;
- history of dyslipidaemia;
- hypertension;
- diabetes;
- myocardial infarction in a first-degree relative age < 55 years.

Postoperatively:

- major vascular surgery;
- emergency surgery;
- prolonged surgery > 3 hours;
- intraoperative arrhythmias, hypertension or hypotension;
- painful surgery in those aged > 45 years.

PACE

PACE is useful shorthand for *perioperative adverse cardiac events*. It includes such events as cardiac ischaemia, arrhythmias hypotension, shock, cardiac failure, acute pulmonary oedema, cardiogenic shock and death.

For elective surgery the risks of PACE are unacceptably high in those with:

+ a myocardial infarct in the past 6 months, but especially within the past 3 months;
+ a coronary artery stent inserted in the past 3 months, and probably within the last 6 months;
+ unstable angina preoperatively; congestive cardiac failure at the time of surgery.

Such patients should not come to theatre for elective surgery. If they present for emergency surgery you can expect problems to arise in the recovery room.

How to recognize myocardial ischaemia

Diagnosing myocardial ischaemia depends on two features:

+ chest pain;
+ ECG changes.

Chest pain

Patients describe ischaemic chest pain (*angina*) as a heavy crushing pain behind their sternum and often as a tight band around their chest. Cardiac pain may be accompanied by pain radiating down the arm or up into the jaw or neck. In the recovery room these symptoms warn of impending myocardial infarction.

> *Any pain above the umbilicus relieved by rest or GTN,*
> *is angina until proven otherwise.*

More than 40 per cent of postoperative patients with myocardial ischaemia get no warning signs, because they feel no pain. The nerve fibres carrying pain sensation from their hearts are already dead, because their blood supply has ceased. This is especially likely in patients with microvascular disease such as smokers, and diabetics.

As the oxygen supply fails the heart begins to fail. The patient may look grey, sweat, become hypotensive, develop a tachycardia, develop an irregular pulse (ventricular extrasystoles), have poor perfusion status, feel anxious, complain of breathlessness and faintness, or collapse.

Angina does not have to be chest pain. It may present with an aching pain anywhere above the umbilicus. It can radiate to neck, or jaw, or either arm (or both) and even to the top of the head. Occasionally angina is misdiagnosed as pain arising from the gallbladder.

ECG changes

The ECG monitor helps diagnose ischaemia. At first myocardial ischaemia presents with a tachycardia, and a few ventricular ectopic beats. As ischaemia worsens, the ST segment sinks below the isoelectric line. After an infarct the ST segment rises above this point (Figure 18.2).

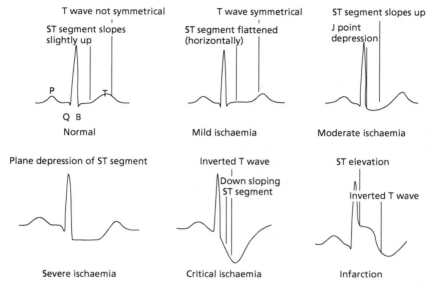

Figure 18.2 ECG stages in ischaemia.

Automated computerized ST analysis in leads II and V5 detects about 80 per cent of myocardial ischaemic episodes. Set the monitor to diagnostic ECG filtering mode. ST analysis may mislead you if the patient is taking digoxin, has a bundle branch block, has a pacemaker, or is a fit young athlete. Isoelectric J-point depression developing for the first time in the recovery room is diagnostic of an ischaemic heart.

How to diagnose acute coronary syndrome

In the recovery room be particularly alert for ischaemia in patients who have:

* previously had coronary artery bypass surgery;
* diabetes;
* chronic kidney disease with an eGFR < 60 ml/min/1.73 m²;
* or a coronary artery stent inserted within the past year.

Signs to look for:

* transient hyperacute tall T-waves;
* flattening of the ST segment;
* down-sloping ST depression is serious;
* new onset left bundle branch block.

Consult the anaesthetist immediately if:

+ The patient has repeated chest pain or discomfort, or if the symptoms last more than 5 minutes.
+ There are persistent ECG changes of ST depression = 0.5 mm, or new T-wave inversion > 2 mm.
+ Transient ST-segment elevation (= 0.5 mm) in more than two contiguous leads on the ECG printout.

Prepare to resuscitate patients if:

+ their systolic blood pressure < 90 mmHg. They have cool peripheries, are sweating, or they develop a mitral regurgitation murmur;
+ their pulse rate > 120 beats/min or worse develops a supraventricular tachycardia;
+ they feel faint and anxious. As though they are 'going to die';
+ they collapse.

ST changes may not occur in a patient with acute coronary syndrome.

Hints

+ Elderly patients, diabetics, long-term smokers, and women may present with atypical symptoms such as neck, jaw, back or epigastric discomfort, sweating, nausea or vomiting.
+ Age is an important factor. The older the patient the more likely they are to have ischaemic heart disease. They do not need to have any of the classic risk factors, although younger patients with acute coronary syndrome generally have one or more risk factors.
+ ST changes on the ECG may not occur in patients with acute coronary syndrome.

What to do if the patient develops cardiac ischaemia

Call for help. At least two trained staff should be attending the patient. Bring the cardiac 'crash cart' to the bedside. Make sure everything is ready in case you need to defibrillate the patient.
   Improve oxygen supply:

+ Give oxygen by mask, and continue it in the ward for the first 2–3 days.
+ Give sublingual glyceryl trinitrate (GTN) 300 micrograms/min.
+ Improve coronary blood flow by treating diastolic hypotension.
+ Patients with ischaemic heart disease who become anaemic are at higher risk, perioperatively their haemoglobin should be maintained above 100 g/L.

Reduce oxygen demands:

+ Treat tachycardia with a β-blocker such as esmolol or metoprolol.
+ Prevent hypertension and tachycardia by treating pain, controlling fluid balance, and treating anxiety.

- Keep blood pressure within 20% of baseline preoperative levels.

- Prevent or correct hypothermia to prevent shivering.

- Start GTN at 10 micrograms/min, and then increase the dose by 10 micrograms/min until the symptoms resolve, or the mean blood pressure falls below 90 mmHg.

What to do next

Give aspirin as soon as possible. Give the patient 300 mg of soluble aspirin tablet dissolved in a glass of water. First discuss this with the surgeon, especially where bleeding may be a disaster such as after neurosurgery, open eye or middle ear surgery.

Persistently raised or lowered ST segments greater than 0.5 mm or new T wave inversion greater than 2 mm suggest severe ischaemia. This means that one or more of the patient's coronary arteries is partly or completely obstructed. The sooner the artery is unblocked, the better the outcome for the patient. Involve a cardiologist immediately. It may be necessary to transfer the patient to a tertiary institution.

Although patients who have just had surgery are not suitable for fibrinolysis they may have *percutaneous intervention* (PCI) such as a coronary stent or balloon angioplasty. Ideally balloon angioplasty needs to be done within 60 minutes of the onset of signs or symptoms, because longer delays result in poorer outcomes. By the time 12 hours have elapsed and where the patient is haemodynamically stable there is little point in performing an angioplasty.

What investigations to order

In the meantime investigations should include 12-lead ECG, full blood examination (FBE), serum electrolytes and creatinine, and blood glucose. Take blood for troponin T levels. These tests must be repeated at least once after 6 hours.

Acute coronary syndrome?
Involve a cardiologist immediately.

How long to monitor patients

Even if a patient develops only transient postoperative myocardial ischaemia in the recovery room, they should be transferred to a special unit to be monitored continuously with an ECG until the stress phase of surgery is over. This phase lasts for several days.

What is heart failure?

Pragmatically, *heart failure* occurs when a person's heart cannot pump enough blood to their tissues. There are only three ways the heart can fail. It can have problems with:

1. rate and rhythm;

2. contractility;

3. excessively high output.

Rate and rhythm problems

Heart rate is too slow:

◆ sinus bradycardia;

◆ heart blocks;

◆ drugs, such as neostigmine, and β-blockers.

Heart rate is too fast:

◆ sinus tachycardia;

◆ uncontrolled atrial flutter or fibrillation;

◆ paroxysmal supraventricular tachycardia;

◆ drugs, such as atropine and adrenaline.

Contractility problems

Cardiac contractility problems occur with:

◆ ischaemic heart disease;

◆ various forms of *cardiomyopathy*.

Pulmonary oedema

Pulmonary oedema sometimes occurs in recovery room. It is caused by fluid reversing into the lung tissue. It can be either cardiogenic or non-cardiogenic.

Cardiogenic pulmonary oedema

In the recovery room acute left ventricular systolic failure presents with *pulmonary oedema*. These patients feel breathless, and are wheezy; if you listen near their mouth you can hear crackles when they breathe. A stethoscope reveals showers of crackles all over their lungs. The patients panic if they are lying flat and struggle to sit up. They usually have a tachycardia. They cannot lie flat (*orthopnoea*) and may be cyanosed or even coughing up frothy pink sputum. Their urine output is low, and they may be sweaty, and cyanosed with cold hands.

These symptoms are easy to recognize, although the early stages may be mistaken for asthma or aspiration. A chest X-ray confirms the diagnosis revealing a snowstorm appearance in both lungs, and pulmonary vascular congestion. Blood gases show signs of tissue hypoxia; typically a metabolic acidosis, and a low PO_2 less than 60 mmHg (7.89 kPa) and a low PCO_2 less than 30 mmHg (3.95 kPa).

Non-cardiogenic pulmonary oedema

Acute pulmonary oedema can also occur without systolic failure. Naloxone not only reverses all the effects of opioids, but also the patient's *endogenous* pain-killing endorphins, and may suddenly catapult the patient into agonizing pain. In younger people the shock may cause such an abrupt rise in pulmonary vascular pressures that intravascular fluid is forced through the alveolar capillary membrane into the airspaces of the lung, causing pulmonary oedema.

Young patients who forcefully inspire against a closed airway can so badly damage their alveolar–capillary membrane that fluids transudate from their blood stream into their alveoli. You sometimes see this after an episode of severe laryngospasm or coughing.

With septicaemia, bacteria release endotoxins, which damages vascular endothelial membranes in all tissues. This event allows fluid to leak out of the capillaries and collect in the interstitium of the lungs causing interstitial pulmonary oedema. This phenomenon is occasionally seen in the recovery room in patients who have had urological surgery, or where abscesses were drained.

How to manage pulmonary oedema

To treat acute pulmonary oedema, first keep your patient alive, then identify the problem, find the cause, and treat it.

First

+ Sit the patient up as much as possible.
+ Give high oxygen concentrations by mask.
+ Inform the anaesthetist.
+ Do a 12-lead ECG to identify ischaemia and arrhythmias.
+ Give furosemide 0.5 mg/kg slowly IV and repeat in 20 minutes if the urine output is < 100 ml/hr.
+ Give morphine 0.1 mg/kg IV slowly to relieve distress, slow their breathing, and lower pulmonary vascular pressures. Use morphine and no other opioid.

Later

The anaesthetist may consider additional measures:

+ Invasive blood pressure monitoring: arterial, central venous, and possible pulmonary artery catheters.
+ GTN infusion to lower vascular pressures.
+ Dobutamine infusion to increase cardiac contractility.
+ Positive pressure ventilation.
+ Intra-aortic balloon pump to assist the circulation.
+ Transfer to intensive care unit.
+ Urgent cardiology consultation.

Monitor

ECG, pulse oximetry, non-invasive blood pressure, urine output, blood gases, serum electrolytes, urea, troponin T levels, and a chest X-ray.

Diastolic heart failure

As each cardiac muscle degenerates and dies, it is replaced by stiff (*incompliant*) collagen tissue and the heart slowly becomes fibrotic. Unable to stretch enough to increase its stroke volume, the only way the heart can increase its output is to beat faster. Usually patients with diastolic failure have preoperative resting pulse rates of 80 beats/min or more.

The commonest reason for chronic diastolic failure is sustained or poorly treated hypertension. The myocytes simply wear out and die from overwork. Once hypertensive patients have established ECG evidence of left ventricular hypertrophy they are destined to get diastolic dysfunction. Unable to increase their stroke volume patients with diastolic dysfunction are susceptible to hypotension if they vasodilate. Vasodilation can be caused by epidural or spinal anaesthesia, and by general anaesthesia. The only way the heart can increase its output to maintain the blood pressure is to increase its rate.

You may encounter other conditions simulating diastolic failure where the stroke volume of the heart is limited by:

- gas embolism, which is occasionally seen after laparoscopy or hysteroscopy;
- acute pulmonary embolism;
- tension pneumothorax;
- pericardial tamponade after thoracic surgery;
- aortic or mitral stenosis.

Features of acute diastolic failure may not be as obvious as those of acute systolic failure, but they include tachycardia, hypotension, nausea, vomiting, and faintness or syncope on sitting up. Peripheral perfusion is poor and urine output is low.

A useful warning is to look at the patient's preoperative heart rate and resting blood pressure. If they have hypertension and a resting heart rate higher than their diastolic blood pressure then suspect chronic diastolic heart failure.

Management

First

- Sit the patient up.
- Give high concentrations of oxygen by mask.
- Inform the anaesthetist.
- Exclude a pneumothorax. See page 263.

Monitor

ECG, pulse oximetry, non-invasive blood pressure, central venous pressures, urine output, blood gases, serum electrolytes, urea, troponin T levels, and a chest X-ray. Continuing management depends on the cause of the failure.

High-output heart failure

High-output cardiac failure occurs, not because there is anything wrong with the heart, but rather that some other disease is making the heart work too hard. If the demands are too great the heart eventually fails. In addition if the patient also has heart disease, then the heart fails sooner, rather than later.

What causes high output failure?

Anaemia

Anaemic patients have less haemoglobin to carry oxygen so their hearts have to pump blood around faster to maintain tissue oxygen supply.

Obesity

With each 10 kg of extra weight the resting cardiac output increases by 1000 ml a minute. A normal person's resting cardiac output is about 5 litres a minute. In contrast, a person who is 40 kg overweight (say weighing 110 kg) has a resting cardiac output of 9 litres a minute. Following a total hip replacement, their cardiac output must increase by an additional 40 per cent. Consequently, on the second and third day following surgery their heart must sustain a resting cardiac output of about 14 litres a minute. This is one reason that obese people are at higher risk of cardiac failure after major surgery.

Thyrotoxicosis

Thyrotoxicosis speeds up tissue metabolism so that their oxygen needs increase hugely.

Paget's disease of the bone

With Paget's disease large blood vessels in the bone allow blood to flow from the arteries into the veins with little resistance. To prevent hypotension the cardiac output has to rise.

Incompetent cardiac valves allow blood to reflux

The ventricles of patients with incompetent heart valves have to cope with a backward reflux of blood in addition to ejecting their stroke volumes. This is analogous to a heart with each beat having to pump two stroke volumes forward into the aorta only to have one stroke volume to reflux back into the ventricle.

Severe intra-abdominal sepsis

Intraperitoneal sepsis may result in up to half the cardiac output being shunted through inflamed peritoneum, thus depriving other organs and tissues of their oxygen supply. This huge afterload reduction causes hypotension, tachycardia and a high cardiac output. Additionally bacterial endotoxins released from the septic source accompanied by circulating shock factors often cause the heart to contract more weakly, resulting in catastrophic septic shock.

Cardiogenic shock

Postoperative cardiogenic shock is usually caused by a massive myocardial infarction, or occurs in a patient with pre-existing severe systolic heart failure. Patients are hypotensive, cyanosed, cold to touch, sweating with almost no urine output. They may have altered conscious state, with dilating pupils. Their blood gases show a severe metabolic acidosis and hypoxia. Perfusion of gut, kidneys, liver and pancreas fails, and skin and muscle circulation almost cease. Once the left ventricular output falls by about 35 per cent the consequent noradrenergically induced vasoconstriction is so intense the patient will not survive.

Cardiogenic shock is managed the same way as severe acute systolic dysfunction. In desperation clinicians sometimes use adrenaline or even noradrenaline infusions to improve cardiac function, but usually to no avail.

Pericardial tamponade

Cardiac *tamponade* occurs when more than 150–300 ml of fluid acutely collects in the pericardial sac. The collecting fluid squashes the heart, preventing it filling enough to eject an adequate stroke volume.

Bleeding into the pericardial sac can occur with chest trauma, a dissecting aneurysm, or after thoracic or upper abdominal surgery (especially hiatus hernia repair, or oesophagectomy). Diagnosing tamponade is not easy; but clinically hypotension, tachycardia, dyspnoea, and especially distended neck veins and facial suffusion give a clue.

On the ECG the QRS complexes look small and low voltages. When patients inspire their systolic pressure may fall by more than 20 mmHg, and their peripheral pulse may even disappear altogether. This *pulsus paradoxus* also occurs with hypovolaemia. Usually patients need to return to theatre to have the fluid drained, but occasionally the surgeon may aspirate the fluid (*pericardiocentesis*) with a wide-bore needle.

Valvular heart disease

Aortic valve sclerosis is common in people older than 65 years, and about 3 per cent of those older than 75 years have severe aortic stenosis. Preadmission clinics usually assess symptomatic valvular heart disease with echocardiography before surgery. This test assesses both the function of the valves and the ventricular ejection fraction. Those with a reduced ejection fraction (EF) of less than 40 per cent are particularly at risk.

People with valvular heart disease such as aortic or mitral stenosis or incompetence have *fixed cardiac outputs* so that they cannot increase their cardiac outputs to meet tissue demand. Mitral valve disease is more common in younger people who have had rheumatic fever, while it accompanies aortic stenosis in older people who have atherosclerosis. To withstand major surgery patients with mitral valve regurgitation need an *ejection fraction* above normal (EF > 45 per cent).

Patients with stenotic valvular heart disease become abruptly hypotensive if their cardiac output falls, or if they vasodilate. Bradycardias may cause hypotension, and tachycardias do not allow enough time between each beat to squeeze blood though the narrow valve openings.

If the patient has aortic or mitral stenosis they may develop pulmonary oedema if given enough fluid to raise their preload; or severe hypotension if they incur peripheral vasodilation with spinal or epidural anaesthetics. People with incompetent valves who have ejection fractions greater than 50 per cent develop a form of high output cardiac failure.

How to manage valvular heart disease

Do not allow your patient to suffer pain, hypoxia, or hypovolaemia; or have any other reason to develop a tachycardia. Patients with valve disease or septal defects are susceptible to bacterial endocarditis. Check that prophylactic antibiotics have either been given in theatre; or give them now. Do not discharge patients to the ward unless they are pain-free, have stable circulations, a good urine output and warm dry hands.

Arrhythmias

Arrhythmias are irregularities in the heartbeat. There are two pathological mechanisms that alter the heart's rate or rhythm: abnormal impulse generation and abnormal impulse propagation.

Arrhythmias are best seen
in lead II on the ECG.

Abnormal impulse generation

Although the cardiac impulse usually originates in the SA node and follows an orderly path through the heart, irritable cells can disrupt the sequence by imposing their own rhythm. Myocardial cells irritated by ischaemia, electrolyte imbalance, or inflammation depolarize spontaneously generating stray *ectopic cardiac beats*.

Abnormal impulse propagation

Arrhythmias can arise at any point on the cardiac impulse's journey from the SA node to its final extinction in the ventricles. Impulses are diverted from their usual path when a group of myocardial cells become hypoxic or die. The abnormal diversion causes the heart to either beat irregularly, or in an uncoordinated way. Impulses blocked or delayed while passing through the AV node cause *heart blocks*. Impulses blocked in one of the major branches of the bundle of His cause right or left bundle branch blocks. Damage to the component branches of the left bundle cause anterior or posterior hemiblocks.

Clinical aspects

Minor arrhythmias are common in patients recovering from anaesthesia. If you notice a slow, fast irregular or absent pulse attach an ECG monitor. It is not always easy to immediately identify the type of arrhythmia on a monitor screen. If the arrhythmia persists do a formal 12-lead ECG to establish its nature.

Patients may complain of one or more of the following: palpitations, chest pain, nausea, faintness, or breathlessness. All these are signs of hypotension or myocardial ischaemia.

Causes of arrhythmias

Patient factors

Factors specific to the patient may cause arrhythmias including pain, hypoxia, myocardial ischaemia, hypercarbia, hypertension, hypotension, electrolyte imbalance particularly potassium, and magnesium; and drugs such as tricyclic antidepressants and digoxin (Figure 18.3).

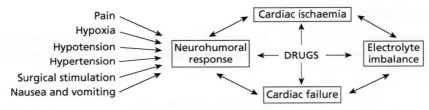

Figure 18.3 The principal causes of arrhythmias in the recovery room.

Surgical factors

Factors caused by the surgery include thoracic operations (especially if the pericardium is damaged), unrelieved pain (particularly from upper abdominal surgery), operations on eyes, ears and upper jaws stimulate the vagus nerve (causing bradycardia), and drugs such as cocaine or adrenaline used to reduce bleeding.

Anaesthetic factors

Anaesthetic drugs can contribute to arrhythmias. These include residual effects of drugs such as fentanyl or neostigmine causing bradycardia, or atropine causing tachycardia. Adrenaline used with local anaesthetics may cause tachyarrhythmias.

*A new wide QRS complex rhythm
needs urgent attention.*

When to worry about arrhythmias

Innocent arrhythmias usually have rates between 60 and 120 beats/min; the ECG shows narrow QRS complexes, the blood pressure remains within 20 per cent of preoperative levels, and the oxygen saturation is greater than 95 per cent.

Notify the anaesthetist if the patient's heart rate is greater than 200 minus the patient's age. Also notify the anaesthetist if the:

♦ pulse rate is < 50 beats/min;

♦ oxygen saturations fall below 92%;

♦ QRS complexes become widened;

♦ regular heart rhythm suddenly becomes irregular;

♦ ST segments rise above or fall below the isoelectric line;

♦ patient feels faint, becomes hypotensive, complains of chest pain, is nauseated, or their conscious state deteriorates;

♦ perfusion status deteriorates.

Arrhythmia with hypotension?
Call for help!

Tachycardia

Tachycardia is defined as a pulse rate exceeding 100 beats per minute, or in children a rate 20 per cent greater than their preoperative baseline rate. Once the pulse rate exceeds 150 beats/min it is either a *supraventricular* (SVT) or *ventricular tachycardia* (VT). An SVT may show P-waves on the ECG trace (although they may be difficult to detect), and ventricular tachycardias do not.

In adults, look for a reason if the pulse rate exceeding 80 beats/min. Tachycardia is a response to an activated sympathetic nervous system, and something must be activating it.

If the heart rate is greater than
80 beats/min then find the cause.

At heart rates above 130 beats/min the ventricles do not have time to fill properly and so their stroke volume progressively declines. Older patients tolerate tachycardia poorly; they readily become hypotensive or develop myocardial ischaemia.

Sinus tachycardia

This is a heart rate of 100–150 beats/min. The P-waves are present; the QRS width is normal (< 120 ms); and the rhythm regular (Figure 18.4).

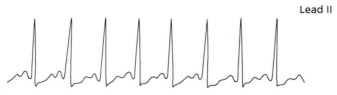

Lead II

Figure 18.4 Sinus tachycardia

Sinus tachycardia is an excellent early warning signs of developing disasters: hypoxia in the early stages, bleeding, hypovolaemia, dilutional anaemia, cardiac failure, early cardiac ischaemia, hypoglycaemia, hypercarbia, malignant hyperthermia and sepsis. Other causes are agitation, developing thyroid storm after a thyroidectomy, pneumothorax, and drugs used to control local bleeding during surgery such as adrenaline or cocaine.

To treat sinus tachycardia you need to treat the cause. Unrelieved sinus tachycardia may progress to supraventricular tachycardia.

Sinus tachycardia warns of
impending problems.

A β-blocker is often used to slow the heart rate if tachycardia is causing signs of myocardial ischaemia. The anaesthetist may start with the short-acting β-blocker, esmolol as an infusion of 50–200 micrograms/kg/min. If this is effective therapy is converted to a long-acting β-blocker, metoprolol or atenolol, once the situation is controlled.

Atrial fibrillation

In *atrial fibrillation* (AF)[2] the P-waves are absent, and the rhythm is irregular, but the QRS width remains normal (Figure 18.5). The usual cause of AF in the recovery room is acute myocardial ischaemia. AF also may occur if the pericardium is disturbed during surgery. Other uncommon causes of AF include acute pulmonary embolism and thyroid storm. If your patient becomes hypotensive then prepare for cardioversion with a synchronized direct-current defibrillator. Seek skilled help.

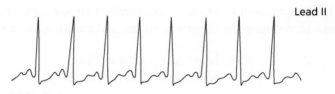

Lead II

Figure 18.5 Atrial fibrillation.

Atrial ectopic beats

Atrial ectopic (AE) beats are common and nearly always benign (Figure 18.6).

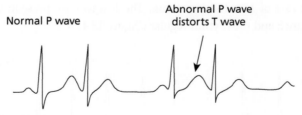

Normal P wave

Abnormal P wave
distorts T wave

Figure 18.6 Atrial ectopic beats.

Multifocal atrial tachycardia

Multifocal atrial tachycardia (MAT) is uncommon. Its irregular rhythm is easy to confuse with AF, but MAT has three or more P-wave morphologies. Look at lead II. It is usually seen in the elderly where it indicates hypoxia or myocardial ischaemia. A bolus of magnesium is often effective at restoring sinus rhythm (Figure 18.7).

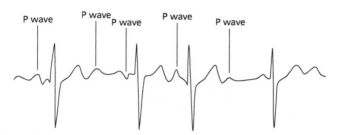

Figure 18.7 Multifocal atrial tachycardia.

Hazardous tachycardias

More serious tachycardias are:

1. Narrow complex tachycardias (QRS complex < 120 ms, that is less than 3 little squares on the ECG paper).
2. Broad complex tachycardias (QRS complex < 120 ms, that is more than 3 little squares on the ECG paper).

Narrow complex tachycardias

Narrow complex tachycardias have a rate exceeding 150 beats/min. Their QRS duration is less than three little squares on standard ECG paper.

Atrioventricular node re-entry tachycardia

With AV nodal re-entry tachycardia the pulse rate may exceed 160 beats/min, but the QRS complex is not widened. It usually starts and stops abruptly (Figure 18.8). The commonest cause is *Wolff–Parkinson–White syndrome* (WPW), a congenital abnormality of the conducting system. The ECG shows PR intervals less than 0.12 seconds, with a slurred upstroke on the R wave. Use DC reversion if the patient is hypotensive.

Do not use adenosine, verapamil, or digoxin to try to slow the rate, because these drugs may, paradoxically, divert the cardiac impulse down the aberrant pathway and cause the heart rate to increase.

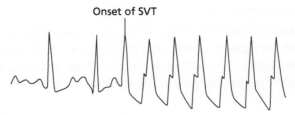

Figure 18.8 Atrioventricular node re-entry tachycardia

Atrial flutter with block

With *atrial flutter* with block can present usually has a fixed number of flutter waves before a QRS complex (Figure 18.9). With atrial flutter with 2:1 block the rate is almost exactly 150 beats/min. Look for saw-toothed flutter waves in lead II. This arrhythmia indicates myocardial ischaemia, or digoxin toxicity. Often, it will respond to a cold wet towel placed on the patient's face. If that fails, prepare to give adenosine 6 mg by rapid IV injection, followed by a saline flush. If necessary another 12 mg dose can be given 3 minutes later. Adenosine often causes bronchospasm in asthmatics.

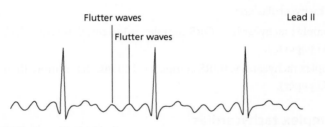

Figure 18.9 Atrial flutter with 3:1 block.

Broad complex tachycardias

Broad complex tachycardias have a rate greater than 150 beats/min, and QRS greater than 120 ms (more than 3 little squares on the ECG paper). They are invariably serious and, apart from torsade de pointes, are almost always due to acute cardiac ischaemia. You will find it difficult to identify the underlying rhythm. Prepare for urgent resuscitation. Give high-flow oxygen by face mask. Call for help. If you cannot feel a pulse then it is a *pulseless arrhythmia*: start the *advanced cardiac life support algorithm*. (See Chapter 19, page 318.)

Ventricular tachycardia

With *ventricular tachycardia* (VT) and the patient is hypotensive then use DC cardioversion; otherwise give amiodarone 150 mg IV over 10 minutes, followed by 300 mg infusion in 1 hour (Figure 18.10). When patients are stable they will be transferred to the intensive care unit.

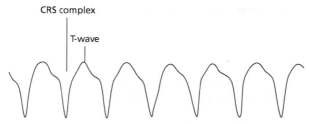

Figure 18.10 Ventricular tachycardia.

Ventricular fibrillation

With *ventricular fibrillation* (VF) there are no clearly identifiable QRS complexes, and the pulses are absent or weak (Figure 18.11). This is a *cardiac arrest*. Start the *advanced cardiac life support algorithm*. Use asynchronized DC cardioversion. When the patient is stable, organize to transfer them to the intensive care unit.

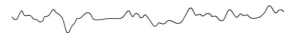

Figure 18.11 Ventricular fibrillation.

Torsades de points

Torsades de points (Figure 18.12) is a vicious polymorphic ventricular tachycardia. The QRS complexes appear to twist about the baseline on the ECG trace. The patient's pre-operative ECG may show a prolonged rate corrected QT interval (*QTc* greater than 400 ms), and possibly U-waves in leads V2 and V3. Most patients have a congenital abnormality of their calcium channels called the long QT syndrome (LQT), but others are taking drugs that prolong the QT interval such as lithium, haloperidol, erythromycin, terbinafine; or cardiac drugs such as amiodarone, sotalol or disopyramide.

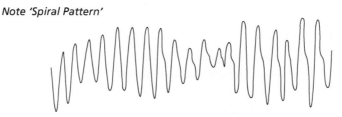

Figure 18.12 Torsades de points.

Hypokalaemia and hypomagnesaemia aggravate the problem. In the recovery room torsades sometimes occurs if a susceptible patient has received isoflurane during the anaesthetic. It is usually treated with magnesium sulfate 2 g IV (4 ml of the 50 per cent solution) infused over 10 minutes. Organize to transfer the patient to ICU for ongoing infusion and observation.

Bradycardia

Bradycardia is defined as a pulse rate less than 60 beats/min. However bradycardia rarely causes problems until the rate is 45 beats/min or less.

> *Bradycardia causing hypotension*
> *is an emergency.*

Sinus bradycardia

With sinus bradycardia the ECG complexes are normal in form, and the rhythm is regular (Figure 18.13). Many athletes have slow pulse rates; other causes include intraoperative fentanyl especially if propofol was used, calcium channel and β-blockers (even timolol eyedrops), residual effects of neostigmine used to reverse muscle relaxation, and after carotid surgery.

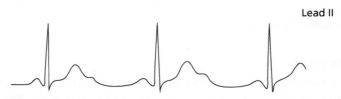

Lead II

Figure 18.13 Sinus bradycardia.

Do not treat bradycardia unless your patient is hypotensive. Then give oxygen, and a small dose of atropine 0.4 mg IV over 1 minute. Serious causes of bradycardia include heart blocks, near-death hypoxia, myocardial ischaemia (especially after anterior infarction), critically raised intracranial pressure hypothermia, high spinal cord injury, and myxoedema.

Trifascicular block

Trifascicular block is misnamed, because the block only involves two fascicles. When two fascicles are blocked simultaneously (such as the right bundle branch and the left anterior hemi fascicle) it is called a bifascicular block. A delay in transmitting the impulse from the sino-atrial node through the atrioventricular node is called an *AV conduction block* (or first-degree heart block). The combination of all three (LAHB + RBBB + AV conduction block) is called a *trifascicular block*. It is caused by ischaemic heart disease, hypertension or other degenerative heart diseases.

First degree heart blocks tend to progress to atrial fibrillation. If you suspect this do a 12 lead ECG and ask your anaesthetist to review the patient.

Complete heart block

Complete heart block (third degree heart block) is a life-threatening arrhythmia (Figure 18.14). The pulse is less than 40 beats/min, and the rhythm irregular. Look for it in lead II. With complete heart block a QRS complex does not necessarily follow each P-wave, because the atria and ventricles are contracting independently from one another.

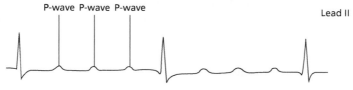

Figure 18.14 Complete heart block.

In the recovery room, the onset of complete heart block strongly suggests acute myocardial ischaemia. Give oxygen. Notify the anaesthetist. The patient may become hypotensive, and feel nauseated. The anaesthetist may try in order: atropine 0.4–1.2 mg IV slowly. If that fails, then an isoprenaline infusion (0.5–20 micrograms/kg/min), or less optimally an adrenaline infusion (2–10 micrograms/kg/min) is used to maintain the pulse rate and blood pressure. This will give you time to organize the insertion of a cardiac pacemaker. Some recovery rooms keep a transcutaneous pacemaker to use as a stop-gap measure.

Other important arrhythmias

Ventricular ectopic beats

Ventricular ectopics (VEs) are also called ventricular premature beats (VPBs) or ventricular extrasystoles (Figure 18.15). These premature contractions arise from an irritable ectopic focus where impulses arrive earlier than expected in the cardiac cycle.

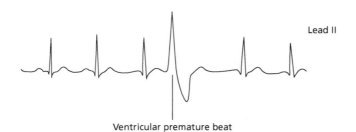

Figure 18.15 Ventricular ectopic beats.

About half the population have occasional ectopic beats, especially if they have recently indulged in caffeine, alcohol, or nicotine. Less than 3 ectopic beats a minute are not a worry. If there are more than 5 ectopic beats, or if the beats have different morphology, then they warn of impending problems. Important causes of VEs include; hypoxia; hypercarbia; myocardial ischaemia; hypertension; pain, anxiety or fear; hypomagnesaemia and hypokalaemia.

Bigeminy

Bigeminy occurs when a normal beat is followed by a ventricular ectopic to be followed by a pause (Figure 18.16). During this compensatory pause the myocytes recover before the next cycle begins.

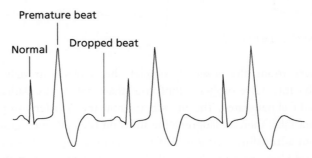

Figure 18.16 Bigeminy.

Bigeminy indicates more serious problems than the occasional VE such as myocardial ischaemia, hypertension, digoxin toxicity; high sympathetic drive; hypokalaemia or hypomagnesaemia. In the recovery room it usually resolves when the cause is corrected, or progresses to ventricular tachycardia. Principles of management are to give oxygen, treat pain, treat hypertension, consider a giving a GTN sublingually or intravenously, and cautiously slow the pulse rate with intravenous metoprolol. A patient with ventricular ectopics, who has myocardial ischaemia or poor peripheral perfusion, is likely to die suddenly.

Anti-arrhythmic drugs

Atrioventricular conduction blockers

Adenosine

Adenosine, an endogenous purine nucleoside, is a potent atrioventricular blocking drug. This drug is used to treat both wide complex and narrow complex supraventricular tachycardias arising in the SA or AV node, but not for atrial flutter. Its therapeutic effect lasts for 20–30 seconds. The dose is titrated starting with 50 micrograms/kg IV, and then give incremental doses of 50 micrograms/kg IV every 2 minutes. The mean dose required to revert AV nodal re-entry arrhythmias ranges from 100 to 250 micrograms/kg. Side effects of dyspnoea, chest pain, hypotension, nausea and flushing and headache are common, but they only last for about 30 seconds. If used in a patient taking dipyridamole it may cause heart block.

Beta-blocking drugs (β-blockers)

β-blockers block the effects of catecholamines, such as, noradrenaline and adrenaline. They slow the heart rate and make the heart contract less powerfully. This effect is useful in hypertension, and angina. Principally they are used to control supraventricular tachycardias. They may cause bronchoconstriction, make asthma worse, and mask the signs of hypoglycaemia, hypovolaemia and hypercarbia. All β-blockers are about equally efficacious. The two most widely available are metoprolol and atenolol. Cardioselective β-blockers have fewer vascular, respiratory and metabolic side-effects, and are less likely to cause bronchoconstriction.

Metoprolol

Metoprolol is a cardioselective β-blocker. The dose is 0.1–0.15 mg/kg IV. Give it over 1 minute. It has a half-life of 3–4 hours, and is metabolized by the liver. It aggravates asthma and cardiac failure, and may cause AV block in patients taking verapamil.

Esmolol

Esmolol is a short-acting, cardioselective β-blocker used to control the heart rate in patients with supraventricular tachycardias. It works in less than 5 minutes, and has an elimination half-life of 9 minutes. It is used as a 10 mg/ml solution, with a loading dose of 500 micrograms/kg over 1 minute. This is followed with a 4-minute maintenance infusion of 50 micrograms/kg/min. The dose is varied to get the desired effect. If the ventricular rate does not fall and the blood pressure remains stable, then repeat the loading dose, and increase the maintenance dose in steps of 50 micrograms/kg/min to a maximum of 200 micrograms/kg/min. Once the heart rate is under control it can be maintained with another agent, such as digoxin, propranolol, or metoprolol. It aggravates asthma and cardiac failure, and will cause AV block in patients taking verapamil.

Drugs prolonging the refractory phase

Once a myocardial cell contracts, it takes a short time to recover before it can contract again. This is called the *refractory phase*. Amiodarone and sotalol are drugs that prolong the refractory phase. They are useful for suppressing abnormal *depolarization* in irritable myocardial cells.

Sotalol

Sotalol is useful for treating atrial fibrillation and flutter, arrhythmias in Wolff–Parkinson–White syndrome, ventricular tachycardia, and ventricular premature beats. Unlike other β-blockers it only slightly depresses the heart's contractility, but may cause sinus bradycardia. The dose is 0.5–1.5 mg/kg IV over 10 minutes. The kidney excretes it, and its effect lasts about 6 hours. Atropine 0.6–2.4 mg IV is used if there is excessive bradycardia causing symptoms, such as hypotension, dyspnoea, or mental state changes. Bradycardia and heart block are more likely if the patient is hypokalaemic.

Amiodarone

Amiodarone is the most effective drug for acute arrhythmias. It is unlikely to reduce cardiac output. Vasodilation causes troublesome hypotension occurs if amiodarone is given too rapidly to patients in heart failure. Make up 300 mg in 50 ml of 5 per cent glucose. (It is not compatible with 0.9 per cent saline.) The oily vehicle causes thrombophlebitis, so infuse it into a central vein.

The initial loading dose is 4–5 mg/kg (about 0.7–0.8 ml/kg) given over 20 minutes. The maintenance dose is 0.3–0.4 mg/kg/hr for the next 24 hours. If the rate control remains poor an extra 1 mg/kg may be given over 1 hour, and repeated if needed. As amiodarone is a non-competitive adrenoceptor antagonist, it potentiates the effects of β-blockers or calcium channel blockers increasing the risk of hypotension and bradyarrhythmias.

Cardiac glycosides

Digoxin

Digoxin usually slows the ventricular rate in atrial fibrillation, but does not revert the heart to sinus rhythm. It is sometimes used in atrial fibrillation to increase myocardial contraction, and slow the rate of impulse transmission through the AV node. The loading dose is up to 10–15 micrograms/kg IV, given over 20 minutes and a further 5 micrograms/kg after 6 hours. The lower dosing range is used in the elderly. Never give digoxin intramuscularly, because it causes massive muscle necrosis.

New onset atrial fibrillation with hypotension?
Use DC reversion.

Calcium channel blockers

Verapamil

Verapamil slows AV node conduction. It is useful to control atrial fibrillation and flutter, but vasodilation may cause the blood pressure to fall. It does not revert the heart to sinus rhythm. It is likely to cause severe bradycardia, heart block, or even asystole if used with β-blockers. The dose is 0.1–0.2 mg/kg IV given over 10 minutes. If an infusion is needed, then give verapamil at a rate of 5 micrograms/kg/min. If the patient is taking a β-blocker do not use verapamil.

For information about the role of magnesium see Box 18.2.

Box 18.2 **Magnesium**

Magnesium is an essential co-factor for the production of *ATP* in biochemical reactions. It is a physiological calcium antagonist. Magnesium deficiency is associated with cardiac arrhythmias, cardiac failure and sudden cardiac death. It can precipitate refractory ventricular fibrillation. Magnesium supplementation may decrease the incidence of post-ischaemic arrhythmias. Suspect magnesium deficiency in patients who have been on diuretics, have had large intestinal fluid losses, or who are hypokalaemic. Since magnesium spreads evenly throughout the extracellular fluid, it needs a large loading dose. The kidneys rapidly excrete magnesium, so to maintain blood levels, the loading dose is followed with a constant intravenous infusion. It works mainly by presynaptic inhibition of neurotransmitter release in peripheral nerves, or by direct inhibition of cardiac muscle, or by vascular smooth muscle dilation. Magnesium also blocks the vagus nerve causing a tachycardia. Apart from its anti-arrhythmic activity it is a bronchodilator, a tocolytic, and has renal vasodilator activity. Calcium is an effective antagonist of magnesium's effects.

References

1. **Acute Coronary Syndrome Guidelines Working Group** (2006) Guidelines for the management of acute coronary syndromes 2006. *Medical Journal of Australia* **184**(8):S1–32.
2. **Wright RS, Anderson JL**, *et al.* (2011) 2011 ACCF/AHA focused update of the Guidelines for the Management of Patients with Unstable Angina/Non-ST-Elevation Myocardial Infarction (updating the 2007 guideline). *Journal of the American College of Cardiology* **59**(19):1920–1959.
3. **Chopra V, Wesorick MD**, *et al.* (2012) Effect of perioperative statins on death, myocardial infarction, atrial fibrillation, and length of stay: a systematic review and meta-analysis. *JAMA Surgery* **147**(2):181–189.

Further Reading

Editorial (2010) Perioperative monitoring of left ventricular function. *British Journal of Anaesthesia* **104**(6):669–672.

Poldermans D, Bax J, *et al.* (2009) Guidelines for pre-operative cardiac risk assessment and perioperative cardiac management in non-cardiac surgery. *European Heart Journal* **30**:2769–2812.

Chapter 19

Cardiopulmonary resuscitation

Introduction

Cardiac arrest is best managed by following the published guidelines and these guidelines have been revised since the previous edition of this book. The A-B-C routine has been changed to C-B-A to give more emphasis to chest compressions and it is hoped that this will mean more bystander participation. Every health care worker must be competent in performing cardiopulmonary resuscitation (CPR) to the level of basic life support (BLS). Competence depends on three things: early detection of cardiac arrest, maintenance of coronary and cerebral oxygenation, and the time to defibrillation. Cardiac arrests will occur. You must be able to commence resuscitation, and be confident about applying defibrillation without a doctor present. Box 19.1 provides a useful guide to terminology in cardiac resuscitation.

Box 19.1 **Terminology in cardiac resuscitation**

- *CPR* = cardiopulmonary resuscitation. This includes external cardiac massage and respiratory support, which may be either bag and mask ventilation, or intubation and ventilation.
- *DCR* = direct current cardioversion with a defibrillator.
- *Pulseless VT* = pulseless ventricular tachycardia.
- *Pulseless electrical activity* (PEA) a hearth rhythm is observed on the ECG that should be producing a pulse but it is not.
- *ROSC* = *resumption of spontaneous circulation* a term used in post cardiac arrest syndrome.
- *Rescue breathing* has replaced the term expired air ventilation (mouth-to-mouth resuscitation), because it includes skilled workers using bag-and-mask techniques.
- *Rescuer* is a term that includes anyone trained in the CPR, whether or not they are a trained health care worker (a nurse or doctor).
- *Two-rescuer* CPR means that while one person is maintain the airway and ensuring adequate tidal air exchange, the other is performing external cardiac massage.
- *VF* = ventricular fibrillation.

Fundamentals

The aim of CPR is to supply enough oxygen to the myocardium and brain to prevent irreversible damage. Success depends on being able to maintain a clear airway, give high concentrations of oxygen, institute efficient cardiac massage, and early defibrillation. The resuscitation technique is based on basic cycles, each of 2 minutes duration.

*A hypoxic heart will not respond
to resuscitation.*

In the recovery room, a number of facts are evident.

- Most cardiac arrests are caused by the profound physiological stresses occurring as the patient emerges from anaesthesia. The effects of these stresses are magnified by underlying ischaemic heart disease.
- Irritable myocardium responds by developing ventricular extrasystoles, this progresses to ventricular tachycardia, and finally ventricular fibrillation.
- Progressive untreated hypoxia ends in an asystolic arrest.
- Pulseless electrical activity is usually caused by unrecognized bleeding.
- Some cardiac arrests in the recovery room have reversible causes. Detect them early.
- Successful cardiac massage depends on pushing fast enough (100 beats per minute) and hard enough. In the elderly this sometimes means fracturing ribs. Ribs heal: brains do not.
- Shock advisory external defibrillators (SAEDs) are useful for inexperienced staff.

*Outcome improves if staff practise
CPR regularly on a mannequin.*

Basic life support

Basic life support (BLS) consists of life-saving techniques, which can be used by trained (but not necessarily medical) responders with only the basic skills to maintain an airway, perform *rescue breathing*, and external cardiac massage (Table 19.1).

In contrast to advanced cardiac life support (ACLS), basic life support does not include using drugs or invasive techniques. Effective basic life support buys time until trained medical responders arrive to provide ACLS. The best outcome is achieved if CPR is started immediately, and if the arrhythmia is VF or pulseless VT.

Advanced cardiac life support

Compression:ventilation ratio

- Press the centre of the chest, at a rate of 100 per minute with minimal interruptions.
- Push hard, push fast. Sing a song to help with the rhythm.
- Universal ratio of 30 compressions to 2 breaths for all two-rescuer CPR for adults.

Table 19.1 The steps in basic life support

D	Danger	**Look for hazards.**
R	Response	Look for signs of life (talk to the patient, shake the patient's shoulder). Send for help.
A	Airway	Tilt the head slightly down, open the mouth and allow material to drain out. Suck out the mouth.
B	Breathing	Look, listen and feel.
C	Compression	If the patient does not show signs of life do not delay by feeling for a pulse. Commence compressions immediately:
		ratio of 30 compressions to 2 breaths; compressions are over the lower half of the sternum; press hard and fast with the heel of your hand, curl your fingers together so that they do not dig into the patient's chest. The rate should be at 100 compressions a minute with 5 cycles (30 compressions and 2 rescue breaths completed over 2 minutes); you will not feel like singing but it will help you get into a regular rhythm. Try 'Happy birthday to you'. Do not stop until you are too tired to go on—minimize any interruptions to CPR.
D	Defibrillate	Attach an automated external defibrillator (AED) as soon as possible and attach the three leads to the patient.

- Universal ratio of 15 compressions to 2 breaths for all two-rescuer CPR for children.
- Attempts to intubate the patient must not interrupt CPR for more than 20 seconds.

Defibrillation

There are three types of defibrillators:

1. *Monophasic defibrillators* sent a direct current in one direction only (Figure 19.1).

2. *Biphasic defibrillators* send the current first one way, and then back again, and deliver the same success rate with lower energy levels, and less myocardial injury. These are better defibrillators.

3. *Automated external defibrillators* (AEDs) are able to detect the type of rhythm and automatically give an appropriate shock.

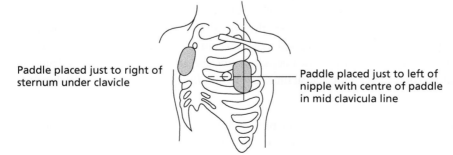

Paddle placed just to right of sternum under clavicle

Paddle placed just to left of nipple with centre of paddle in mid clavicula line

Figure 19.1 Defibrillator paddle positions.

How to defibrillate

Two breaths first and then shock for VF arrests.

- Use shock first for ventricular fibrillation (VF) and pulseless ventricular tachycardia (VT).
- If possible use direct current reversion (DCR) first and then commence CPR.
- All nurses must be trained to use DCR and give it before a doctor arrives.
- Time to defibrillation is the key to survival.
- Use one shock on the first cycle, and thereafter only use one shock.
- When using manual biphasic defibrillators use energy levels of 200 joules.
- When using monophasic defibrillators first give 200 then maximum joules.
- In children use biphasic energy levels of 1–2 joule/kg for defibrillating ventricular fibrillation and pulseless ventricular tachycardia.

Defibrillation will not be successful unless these commonly concurrent problems referred to in Table 19.2 have been diagnosed and treated.

Table 19.2 Detect and correct the 4Hs and 4Ts

Hypoxia	Thrombosis—coronary/pulmonary
Hypovolaemia	Tension pneumothorax
Hypothermia	Tamponade—cardiac
Hyperkalaemia/hypokalaemia	Toxins and drugs

The drugs to use

The effectiveness of drugs in cardiopulmonary resuscitation is less important than chest compression and defibrillation. The best way to give drugs is via a central venous catheter, and failing that a large-bore catheter in a big vein in the arm. After injecting the drugs lift the arm so that the drugs run into the central veins.

Do not inject drugs in leg veins because of the risk of thrombosis. Many drugs used in ACLS, including adrenaline, calcium chloride, sodium bicarbonate, and potassium chloride, are toxic if they get outside the vein and can cause horrendous tissue damage if the patient survives. There is no place for injecting drugs directly into the heart. In desperation a double dose of lidocaine, adrenaline and atropine (but not other drugs) can be instilled down the endotracheal tube. Use the traditional drugs in the following manner.

Adrenaline

Adrenaline is considered to be the best vasopressor to use in cardiac arrest. Give 1 ml of adrenaline 1:1000 every 4 minutes during CPR. If you are injecting it into a peripheral vein make it up to 10 ml in saline first. Long-term prognosis is not improved by higher doses.

Amiodarone

Use amiodarone for pulseless VT and VF. Amiodarone is the only anti-arrhythmic drug that improves short-term outcome. Give amiodarone 300 mg after the third 2-minute cycle. If DCR fails to revert the rhythm then consider giving another 150 mg. Follow this with an infusion of amiodarone 15 mg/kg over the next 24 hours.

Atropine

Atropine has a place in severe bradycardia. Use atropine 1.2 mg intravenously, to a total dose of 3 mg.

Adenosine

If you have a wide-complex tachycardia that is regular and monomorphic, give an initial dose of 6mg. Give this as close to the heart as possible, via a central line or the antecubital fossa. Follow the bolus dose with 10–20 ml of saline. This should result in a transient AV block. If there is no response after 2 minutes give a further 12–18 mg dose.

Calcium

Calcium has no proven place during CPR but it should be used to treat hypocalcaemia, hyperkalaemia or an overdose of calcium channel-blocking drugs. The dose is calcium gluconate 10 ml of 10 per cent solution.

Magnesium

Magnesium has no proven place during CPR. It may be useful in treating *torsade de points*, digoxin toxicity, documented hypokalaemia and documented hypomagnesaemia. It is worth giving when adrenaline and DCR fail to revert pulseless VT or VF. The dose is 5 mmol bolus of magnesium sulfate, which may be repeated once and followed by an infusion of 20 mmol over 4 hours.

Potassium

Use potassium for persistent VF for known or suspected hypokalaemia. Give well-diluted potassium chloride 5 mmol slowly over 5 minutes intravenously (preferably a large vein). Bolus potassium may stop the heart.

Sodium bicarbonate

Use for known or suspected severe acidosis, hyperkalaemia or after 15 minutes of CPR. The trigger for using bicarbonate occurs when blood gases show the pH is less than 7.10. The dose is 1 mmol/kg intravenously very slowly over 3–5 minutes. Do not mix in line with calcium because it will clog the giving set with chalk.

Pulseless electrical activity

Pulseless electrical activity occurs where the heart is generating coordinated electrical activity but there is no discernible cardiac output. Prognosis with this arrhythmia is dismal (as it is with asystole). There is no point in performing DCR. Look for causes for this arrhythmia. In the recovery room particularly look for exsanguinating haemorrhage and tension pneumothorax.

Asystole

Asystole occurs when the heart is not contracting, there is no discernible ECG rhythm—there is a flat line on the monitor. Asystole is often associated with end-stage hypoxia. Unrelieved hypoxia produces a progression of sinus tachycardia to sinus bradycardia to nodal bradycardia to slow wide QRS complexes and finally a flat line on the ECG—asystole.

Asystole has a poor prognosis, few patients are successfully resuscitated, and almost none leave hospital.

Other measures

Fluids

It is lifesaving to give fluids if you suspect the patient is *hypovolaemic*, but otherwise they will not affect the outcome.

Therapeutic hypothermia

Therapeutic *hypothermia* with cooling to 33°C should be induced in patients who are comatose after cardiac arrest.

Post-cardiac arrest syndrome

Patients who survive the insult of cardiac arrest and CPR and who begin spontaneous breathing again still suffer from the after effects of prolonged whole-body ischemia, from post-cardiac arrest brain injury and post-cardiac arrest[1] myocardial dysfunction. There is also a systemic ischaemia/reperfusion response and persistence precipitating pathology. The severity of these disorders vary and the pre-arrest state of the patient's health are all factors in the further management of the patient. A decision will be made by the consultant medical staff involved and a transfer, usually to the intensive care unit will ensue if appropriate.

Reference

1. **Nolan JP** (2010) Post-cardiac arrest syndrome. *International Emergency Nursing* **18**(1):8–18.

Further Reading

Allan R, de Caen ME, *et al.* (2010) Paediatric basic and advanced life support. *Resuscitation* **81**(1):e213–e259.

Hazinski MF, Nadkarni VM, *et al.* (2005) Major Changes in the 2005 AHA Guidelines for CPR and ECC. *American Heart Association* **112**:iv206–iv211.

Chapter 20

Shock

Introduction

Shock is a clinical diagnosis based on a series of events that occur when the circulation is neither sufficient to meet the metabolic demands of the tissues and organs, nor adequate to remove their metabolic wastes.

Clinically established severe shock is easy to recognize. The patient has a low or unrecordable blood pressure, no urine output, and is pale and sweaty, with gasping respiration and a deteriorating conscious state. By the time all these features are present the patient is moribund and unlikely to survive without intensive care. Consequently, it is important to detect and treat shock vigorously long before this potentially irreversible stage.

Recognize the symptoms of impending shock. Get help as soon as you notice your patient's perfusion status is deteriorating. The aim of resuscitation is first to urgently restore tissue oxygen supply, and then find and treat the cause of the shock.

By the time you diagnose shock,
you should already be treating it.

Types of shock

Maintaining satisfactory blood flow to the tissues requires a pump (the heart) and a distribution system (the blood vessels). If either of these components fail, then shock follows. The type of shock depends on which component fails, and in the manner they do so. Shock has many causes, but those most commonly encountered after surgery are acute haemorrhage, acute heart failure, sepsis, and anaphylaxis.

Hypovolaemic shock

Hypovolaemic shock occurs when the blood vessels do not contain sufficient blood to fill the heart. Bleeding is the most common cause, but hypovolaemic shock also occurs where tissue fluid is lost from the circulation with burns, bowel obstruction, or vomiting and diarrhoea.

Normovolaemic shock

Normovolaemic shock occurs when patients' blood pressure falls even though their blood volume is normal.

- *Cardiogenic shock* occurs if the heart fails to pump sufficiently to maintain blood pressure.

- *Septic shock* occurs when bacterial toxins so severely damage the blood vessels that capillaries leak fluid into the tissues, and the smooth muscle in arterioles cannot contract enough to sustain the blood pressure.

- *Anaphylaxis* occurs when an immunological response releases large amounts of inflammatory mediators into the circulation. These biochemicals injure arterioles and capillary membranes allowing intravascular fluid to leak into the tissues.

- *Endocrine shock* occurs if there is insufficient cortisol available for vascular smooth muscle to contract properly to a sympathetic nerve stimulus. Another form of endocrine shock occurs with myxoedema where not enough thyroxine is available for normal tissue metabolism.

Stages of shock

If impending shock is recognized and treated promptly, in most cases its progression through the stages of *compensated* shock, *uncompensated* shock, and *irreversible* shock can be thwarted.

Compensated shock

In the stage of compensated shock the blood flow to the brain and heart are preserved at the expense of the so-called *non-essential organs*: the kidneys, gut, skin and muscles. In this stage of shock the patient usually has a tachycardia, cool skin, and a urine output less than 0.5 ml/kg per hour. Compensated shock generally responds well to treatment, but if not then it progresses to decompensated shock.

> *The blood pressure does not necessarily fall in compensated haemorrhagic shock.*

Decompensated shock

In the stage of decompensated shock the body's compensatory mechanisms begin to fail, and organ perfusion is severely reduced. Oxygen-starved tissues produce lactic acid as they switch from *aerobic* to *anaerobic metabolism* in an attempt to maintain their function. Liver cells are also unable to metabolize lactate.

Hypoxic tissue releases inflammatory mediators. These depress myocardial contractility and damage capillaries allowing intravascular fluid to leak away into the tissues. Damaged or dead tissues release factors that can trigger *disseminated intravascular coagulation* (DIC).

It is only in the later stages of shock that there is profound hypotension. Do not rely on hypotension to diagnose haemorrhagic shock, especially in young people. Their blood pressure may not fall in the stage of compensated shock, and by the time it does fall they may be near death.

It is safer to regard any patient who has cool hands and a tachycardia greater than 100 beats/min as becoming shocked, until some other cause is found to exclude the diagnosis.

Irreversible shock

As shock progresses the tissues are so starved of oxygen that organs fail and die. Irreversible shock is a post-mortem diagnosis.

Signs of shock

Signs of shock include:

- rising pulse rate;
- rapid breathing becoming shallow;
- low urine output;
- anxiety;
- pallor and later sweating;
- confusion.

Bleeding is the most likely cause of shock in the recovery room. Two excellent signs that your patient may be bleeding are that their blood pressure falls by more than 20 mmHg as you cautiously sit them up at 45°, and it takes more than 2 seconds for blood to return when you squeeze a fingernail bed.

Treatment of haemorrhagic shock

Managing shock involves restoring the oxygen supply to the organs, controlling bleeding, and only then finding the cause.

Call for help when you detect deteriorating tissue perfusion. Lay the patient in the position they feel most comfortable, but never head down. If the patient is bleeding they will feel more comfortable lying flat; but if they are developing cardiogenic shock with pulmonary oedema, they may prefer to sit up a little.

Give high flows of oxygen with a rebreathing mask. They should have wide-bore intravenous cannula. If you suspect a patient is bleeding then they need a drip in both arms. To ensure that intravenous infusions run quickly, remove any three-way taps and other plastic paraphernalia because they impede flow.

What happens in the tissues

During the hypoperfusional stage of shock, cells do not receive enough oxygen to allow the mitochondria to make their little packets of chemical energy called adenosine triphosphate (ATP). Cells use ATP to kick start biochemical reactions. As the oxygen supply fails, at first the cells produce a limited emergency supply of ATP using a process called anaerobic metabolism. However, once this limited back-up supply of ATP is exhausted, the cells' membrane pumps fail and fluid leaks through the membranes causing the cells to swell and die. In the meantime anaerobic metabolism releases lactic acid into the blood causing a metabolic acidosis. Metabolic acidosis is a biochemical marker of cellular hypoxia.

Meanwhile the body attempts to compensate for the acidosis. The patient starts to hyperventilate. Hyperventilation removes carbon dioxide from the body, which temporarily restores the blood's pH to more normal levels.

If the crisis is successfully treated, then shock does not progress. If not then, as the body's compensatory mechanisms fail, cells start to disintegrate. The surviving cells stagger along on their emergency energy supply producing more and more lactic acid. Protein-rich fluid leaks from the blood, through damaged capillary walls to collect in the tissues. The remaining blood becomes concentrated and flow in the microcirculation is impeded. The sluggish blood flow further deprives tissues of their oxygen supply, and delays toxic waste removal. Eventually the process becomes irreversible. Brain damage and death follow.

Shock in children

Children who are becoming shocked, present differently to adults. Hypotension in children signals the onset of irreversible shock. This problem is discussed more comprehensively in the chapter on paediatrics (page 205).

Chapter 21

Crisis management

Where to look

Be prepared

Emergencies happen. Be prepared. Before the start of each day check all your trolleys and equipment, including your defibrillator, and make sure all new staff know where everything is kept.

Crisis protocol

A *crisis protocol* is an organized approach to manage the patient whose life is in danger. It is often difficult to diagnose what has happened to the collapsed patient, but the fundamentals of basic life support are the same for all emergencies.

Prepare a set of flow charts (*algorithms*) on 5 × 8 inch filing cards setting out how to diagnose and treat emergencies. These cards are your *crisis protocols*. Put them in a box on the desk where everyone can refer to them. Practise simulated disaster management monthly.

How to practise

In an emergency you must keep your patients alive while you find out what has gone wrong. There are three aspects to resuscitation: first, keeping your patient alive; second, finding out what is wrong; and third is the organization of the resuscitation. Practise resuscitation techniques regularly. Like a ballet, everyone must know their part, and keep out of each other's way.

Successful resuscitation depends on
practise, practise, practise.

As you practise your crisis protocols consider:

- What are the problems?
- What is the worst thing that can happen?
- What is the normal response?
- How do I assess the problem?
- What is the immediate management?
- What is the follow-up?

When patients suddenly deteriorate, for instance, their blood pressure falls, or seizures occur, or they cannot breathe properly, then follow your crisis protocol. Because you will have to act quickly, both diagnosis and treatment must be performed at the same time, even when the cause of the problem is far from clear.

During a crisis make a presumptive diagnosis, consider the differential diagnosis, and plan management. To do this, answer the following questions:

- What is the problem?
- What else could it be?
- What are we going to do about it?

Keep your patient alive

Use the alphabet of resuscitation

Use the A, B, C, D, E, F plan—but first check the patient's conscious state and their carotid pulse. If you cannot feel the carotid pulse or the patient is unconscious then start advanced cardiac life support protocol.

Check the carotid pulse
then
A, B, C, D, E, F

A = Airway

Check the patency of the patient's airway. Gently suck out mucus, blood and other debris with a Yankauer sucker. Use a bag and mask giving 100 per cent oxygen to ventilate your patient.

Oxygen saves lives.

B = Breathing

Check that air is moving in and out of the lungs. If you hold the chin up you can feel this in the palm of your hand. Insert an airway. Check the oxygen saturation. If you are having difficulty in getting oxygen into and out of the patient's lungs then consider upper and lower airway obstruction. Check from outside the airway, to the airway wall, is there a foreign body in the lumen?

C = Circulation

Feel for a carotid pulse. If it is absent start *advanced cardiac life support (ACLS) protocol*. Check blood pressure, pulse rate and rhythm, re-evaluate perfusion status, attach ECG.

What's gone wrong?

D = Drugs

Review drugs for effects or side-effects. If blood, drugs, or plasma expanders are being infused, then consider some form of reaction; turn off the drip. Consider: Wrong drug, Wrong rate, Wrong route.

E = Endocrine

Consider the three Hs:

1. Hypoglycaemia. Check blood glucose with a glucose meter.
2. Hypothyroidism as a cause of delayed emergence.
3. Hypoadrenalism as a cause of refractory hypotension.

F = Fitting?

Consider:

- hypoxia;
- hypoglycaemia;
- hypocalcaemia;
- hyperpyrexia;
- hypocarbia;
- water intoxication;

- epilepsy, eclampsia;
- drugs.

Problem solving

The cause is often obvious such as a cardiac arrhythmia, or laryngospasm, but you will still need to

$$\text{LOOK} \times 5$$
$$\text{LISTEN} \times 4$$
$$\text{FEEL} \times 4$$

Look

1. Wound sites and drains.
2. Appearance: pallor? Cyanosis? Flushing? Sweating? Agitation?
3. Respiration: rates, depth, rhythm.
4. Neck: jugular vein distension? Swelling of tissues? Tracheal deviation?
5. Strip to expose the whole body to ensure you are not missing something.

Blood loss is usually obvious, but it can be hidden beneath the sheets. Blocked chest drains can cause respiratory difficulty. Difficulty in breathing can indicate airway obstruction, inadequate reversal of muscle relaxants, cardiac failure, or allergy. Bleeding into the neck can cause airway obstruction and cause the face to become suffused. Distended neck veins may indicate tension pneumothorax, cardiac tamponade, *TURP syndrome*, or gross fluid overload or pulmonary embolism by clot or air. A tension pneumothorax may push the trachea to the opposite side. Completely uncover the patient to reveal abdominal swelling, and many other problems.

Listen

1. Patient's complaints.
2. Air entry: wheezes with mouth open?
3. Stridor and other breathing noises.
4. Heart sounds: muffled? Murmur gallop rhythm?

If patients say something is wrong, never pass it off as anxiety or attention-seeking. If they cannot breathe properly or are feeling breathless, then something is wrong. Listen to the breath sounds with a stethoscope. Count the rate of respiration for a full minute. Assess adequacy, pattern, and distribution of ventilation. Possible problems include bronchospasm, pulmonary oedema, lobe collapse, pneumothorax, haemothorax, and cardiac tamponade.

Stridor is a sign of impending total airway obstruction. It is a medical emergency—get help immediately. Wheeze suggests: anaphylaxis, aspiration, asthma, acute pulmonary oedema, allergy to drugs or infusions, or embolism. Heart sounds may be muffled if there is a pneumothorax or pericardial effusion—this is a difficult sign to interpret.

Feel

1. Heart and pulse: rate? Intensity? Rhythm?
2. Head: sweaty? Fever?
3. Hands: perfusion? Grip strength, and leg movement on both sides?
4. Head lift to check residual muscle relaxation.

Take both wrists and check that the pulse in each is equivalent. Check the carotid pulse and the femoral pulses. Look for differences in volume and rhythm. A 12-lead ECG may reveal arrhythmias. Cold hands are an excellent sign of noradrenergic discharge, warning of problems such as haemorrhage, hypoxia, hypoglycaemia, and pain. Warm hands and a bounding pulse suggest hypercarbia, thyrotoxicosis. Sweating or fever suggests reaction to blood or drugs, malignant hyperthermia, serotonergic syndrome, thyrotoxic crisis, and neuroleptic malignant syndrome. Loss of grip, strength, or weakness in the legs only on one side of the body suggests stroke, or if on both sides consider the effects of residual muscle relaxants, neostigmine overdose, myasthenia or other neuropathies and myopathies, or massive stroke.

How to monitor resuscitation's progress

Write everything that could possibly be relevant on a special chart, or in the patient's notes. Once you have an established problem list it is much easier to set priorities and follow what is going on.

Organization of a resuscitation

All staff in the recovery room should be adept at managing basic cardiac life support and some should have advanced life support skills. Everyone taking part in resuscitating a patient must know their role, but teaching how to organize resuscitation is often overlooked. At the beginning of each shift each member of the recovery room staff should know what their role would be if an emergency occurs.

Start with the three Cs

1. **Call for help**, summon the anaesthetist or surgeon, emergency trolley and the defibrillator.
2. **Check pulse**, colour, oximeter and ECG.
3. **Check the clock**, and note the time.

Monitor: ECG, blood pressure, pulse rate and rhythm, respiratory rate, oximetry.

Get HELP

H Help—it takes four staff to manage a crisis:

PERSON 1. To manage the airway.

PERSON 2. To monitor the blood pressure, pulse, and perfusion, and perform external cardiac massage if needed.

PERSON 3. To get drugs, equipment, and take blood tests.

PERSON 4. To supervise the resuscitation, liaise with other staff and write the problems and treatment on a white-board where everyone can see it. This person should help the others too.

E Emergency trolley and other equipment as needed.

L Look in the patient's notes for clues: such as allergies, cardiac disease, previous pneumothorax, problems with previous anaesthetics and so on.

P Prepare to take blood for laboratory analysis. Phone the laboratory and warn them of the problem.

Monitoring

Patients who have been involved in multiple trauma or undergone prolonged major surgery with extensive blood loss should be monitored with the following when they arrive in the recovery room:

- ECG;
- nasogastric tube;
- 14 G cannula in their right internal jugular vein to give fluids and measure their central venous pressure;
- 14 G cannula attached to a blood warmer in their right forearm;
- 14 G cannula in their left forearm;
- 20 G cannula in their left radial artery to measure their arterial blood pressure and to collect samples for blood gases estimation;
- urinary catheter attached to 100 ml burette;
- warming mattress or convection heater at 37°C;
- sometimes a pulmonary artery flotation catheter to measure wedge pressures.

Anaphylaxis

A massive release of histamine relaxes vascular smooth muscle, increases capillary permeability and constricts bronchial smooth muscle. Anaphylaxis is life-threatening when cardiovascular collapse, bronchospasm and angio-oedema of the upper airway all occur at once. The anaphylactic response varies. Anaphylaxis is easy to diagnosis if the patient suddenly collapses with wheeze and hypotension immediately after being given an offending antigen. However, it may not be so easily recognized if the signs and symptoms creep up slowly over many minutes or even an hour or more.

Early signs include:

- sensation of warmth or itching, especially in the groin or axilla;
- flushing or mottled rash over the upper part of the body;
- restlessness, acute anxiety, or panic;
- nausea and vomiting;
- feelings of tightness in the chest.

Later:

- erythematous or urticarial rash similar to hives;
- developing oedema of face, eyelids, and neck;
- crampy abdominal pain.

Progressing to:

- hypotension sometimes severe enough to cause coma;
- bronchospasm, cough, dyspnoea, wheeze;
- laryngeal oedema with dyspnoea, stridor, drooling, and hoarse voice;
- tissue hypoxia with cyanosis; arrhythmias and cardiac arrest.

Laryngeal oedema or developing facial oedema is life-threatening. The onset of stridor warns that total airway obstruction is only moments away. If patients are conscious they may panic. At this stage intubation is often difficult, because the normal anatomical landmarks will be obscured. Airway management in the patient needs a skilled anaesthetist. Prepare equipment for intubation, and if that fails, an emergency cricothyroid puncture, or to insert a mini-tracheostomy. In some cases a surgeon may perform a formal open tracheostomy.

Principles

- Suspect any unexpected reaction to a drug as an anaphylactoid reaction.
- Almost every type of drug that can be injected (except ketamine and the benzodiazepines) has been reported to cause anaphylaxis.
- Usually the patient deteriorates rapidly.
- Use adrenaline at the first suspicion of anaphylaxis: it is safe and effective.
- The combination of adrenaline and plasma volume replacement will return cardiac output to acceptable levels. Do not use polygelines, such as Gelofusine® because they occasionally cause allergic responses.
- Although steroids and histamines are used as follow-up therapy, they take many hours to act.
- Pre-existing heart disease increase the risk to the patient of anaphylaxis.
- β-blockers intensify the severity by preventing adrenaline from being fully effective.

Immediate management

1. Call for help.
2. Stop any potentially offending substance.
3. Maintain the ABC—airway, breathing and circulation. Give 100% oxygen. You may need to start advanced cardiac life support.
4. Attach an ECG, pulse oximeter, and automated blood pressure monitor.
5. Get the emergency trolley, and prepare for a rapid infusion of fluids.
6. Lay the patient flat, and raise the limbs. Do not tilt them head down.
7. Insert a large wide-bore drip to infuse large volumes of Plasma-Lyte®, or 0.9% saline. Do not use plasma expanders.
8. Give adrenaline. Patients taking β-blockers need much larger doses than recommended in the following sections. Try metaraminol or a noradrenaline infusion on these patients if they do not respond to adrenaline.

Adults

For adults open an ampoule of adrenaline 1:1000 (1 mg in 1 ml).
   If the patient weighs:

- less than 50 kg then give 0.25 ml of adrenaline;
- between 50 and 100 kg then give 0.5 ml of adrenaline;
- more than 100 kg give 0.75 ml of adrenaline.

Use intramuscular adrenaline initially. If either there is no response to the intramuscular adrenaline, or the blood pressure or pulse is unrecordable then give adrenaline 5 ml of 1:10 000 slowly intravenously over 5 minutes.

Children

For children dilute an ampoule of 1 ml of 1:1000 adrenaline and make it up to 10 ml in saline. The syringe now contains adrenaline 1:10 000. Use this diluted adrenaline and give 0.25 ml per year of age slowly (over 5 measured minutes) into a drip running in a large vein.

Later management

Once your patient's blood pressure is restored:

- Give hydrocortisone 5 mg/kg intravenously 6-hourly. Steroids stabilize mast cells and prevent further mediator release but they take 4 to 6 hours to work.
- Give promethazine 0.5 mg/kg (maximum dose 50 mg) intravenously slowly over 10 measured minutes.
- Treat wheeze with 2 ml of 0.5% salbutamol through a nebulizer and face mask.
- If the wheeze remains unrelieved then give salbutamol 1.5 micrograms/kg intravenously.

- Give H$_2$ antagonists such as ranitidine 1 mg/kg. This will reduce the effect of the circulating histamine.
- Prepare to transfer the patient to ICU for further treatment and observation, recurrence of symptoms can occur. It may be necessary to give an adrenaline infusion for several hours.

Investigations

Have a clear plastic box and label this clearly ANAPHYLAXIS. Have this box readily available and stocked with appropriate tubes for blood samples. Take 10 ml of blood in a plain tube for serum tryptase concentrations. Send another sample 1 hour later. Keep copies of the required paperwork in this box as well. A Medlab form and an anaesthetic allergy referral form will have to be completed by the anaesthetist and photocopied three times. One set of forms should go with the blood, one into the patient's notes and one for the anaesthetist to keep. You might like to make up a chart with the symptoms and signs of anaphylaxis and keep this in your box as well.

Anaphylactoid responses occur when some drug or chemical causes the mast cells to release histamine, either locally or throughout the whole body. The reaction is not usually severe. There is often local erythema and rash but no central effect.

Seizures

A fitting patient?
Exclude hypoxia and hypoglycaemia.

Causes of seizures:

- hypoxia;
- hypoglycaemia;
- an epileptic patient who has not taken their medication;
- water overload, including the TURP syndrome;
- eclampsia;
- malignant hypertension;
- hypocalcaemia, hypomagnesaemia;
- drugs.

Seizures and fits are both terms for the same thing. Drugs that may cause seizures are local anaesthetics, pethidine, rarely propofol and occasionally acute withdrawal of benzodiazepine or antiparkinson drugs. Be cautious about early discharge of a patient if any abnormal muscle movement occurs such as twitching or jerking. If this occurs admit the patient for overnight observation. Pethidine can cause a seizure. Its toxic metabolite 6-norpethidine is excreted only by the kidney. Do not use pethidine in patients with renal failure.

Immediate management

Seizures usually start with the patient losing consciousness and becoming rigid (tonic phase); this is followed shortly by generalized jerking movements (clonic phase), which may persist for some time. Seizures cause cerebral hypoxia and if not quickly treated can cause permanent brain damage.

- Call for help. It takes two competent staff to manage seizures.
- Turn the patient into the recovery position and gently restrain them so they do not fall off their trolley.
- Start the ABC: clear the airway, assist breathing, and give 100% oxygen by mask. Do not try to force anything between their teeth.
- Attach an ECG, pulse oximeter and automated blood pressure machine.
- Do not leave the patient.
- Check that the blood sugar concentration is > 3.5 mmol/L. If they are hypoglycaemic give 50 ml of 50% glucose into a large vein in a free-flowing drip.
- If the patient is even possibly an alcoholic give thiamine 100 mg intravenously to prevent Wernicke's encephalopathy.

Further management

- Thiopental 2–7.5 mg/kg IV is the best option. Usually this immediately terminates the seizure, but you will now have a comatose patient to manage. Continuing seizures are best controlled with a thiopental infusion of 1–5 mg/kg per hour.
- Diazepam 0.15 mg/kg IV (maximum adult dose 20 mg). This is a second-line drug. Midazolam is usually quickly available, give this drug initially but the others are more effective.
- To prevent further seizures give phenytoin 7.5 mg/kg IV into a saline infusion. If the patients are not already taking phenytoin then load them with a further 1000 mg over the next 30 minutes.
- Send bloods for measurement of blood glucose, calcium, magnesium, phosphate, and if relevant, anticonvulsant drug levels.
- If the patient remains comatose, they will need to be intubated, have urinary catheter inserted, and transferred to ICU for further management.

Endocrine emergencies

Consider the three Hs.

1. Hypoglycaemia as a cause of agitation and sweating.
2. Hypothyroidism as a cause of delayed emergence.
3. Hypoadrenalism as a cause of refractory hypotension.

Major disasters

Most hospitals have a detailed Major Disaster Plan designated (Code Brown), with nominated key staff responsible for specific prearranged duties. The operating theatres should already have their own plans in place, with portable packs containing equipment, and drugs prepared for this eventuality.

Apart from the overwhelming number of casualties in a major disaster, most of the problems are logistic, and of these the biggest problem is communication. Your recovery room will work closely with the emergency department (now called a receiving station), the operating theatres, and the intensive care unit.

Do not be surprised if the hospital switchboard is totally overwhelmed and jammed, and the receiving station staff too busy to answer the phones. They will be constantly engaged, and you will not get through. Do not rely on the mobile phone network, because with major disasters, such as 9/11 and the Madrid bombings, the phone networks became so clogged they were unusable.

Allocate the three most experienced senior staff to establish a command centre at the recovery room desk, set up lines of communication, assess priorities, gauge capability and gather information so available resources are used most efficiently. The best way to do this is for each of the commanders to personally visit the ICU, the receiving station and the operating theatres at regular intervals. First-hand reconnaissance by visiting these areas saves a lot of time and makes everything work more efficiently.

Evacuation drills should be practised regularly in order to be effective and expeditious. Effective leadership, communication and coordination of care are critical in efficient emergency evacuation.[1]

Covid-19

In a sophisticated hospital the Covid-19 patients will be operated on in a dedicated operating theatre and two recovery nurses will come into that theatre at the end of the surgery and recover the patient who will then go directly to a dedicated ward and they will not come into your traditional recovery room.

If you are one of the nurses going to that operating theatre take supreme precautions of yourself. Double gloves and gowns and face protection. At the end of the duty, and if possible, strip right off and shower before changing into your street clothes.

Not all, perhaps not even many, hospitals will have these dedicated facilities and some patients will come to your recovery room if they do not require immediate intensive care.

Once you have been told to expect such a patient begin by preparing an area of your recovery room away from your administration desk and as far away as possible from other patients. Some recovery rooms have a special room for infected patients. Use this if you have one. Consider recovering healthy patients in the operating theatre or anaesthetic room. If you have sufficient staff send these patients back to the ward with one of your nurses for 'one on one' care.

The essential aspect of caring for these patients is to limit their ability to spread the virus to staff and other patients. There are other considerations. These patients can deteriorate very quickly and require rapid transfer to the intensive care unit. Have everything prepared for this eventuality. Defibrillator, IV tray with adrenaline and intubation equipment and endotracheal tubes.

Above all, take care of yourself and your colleagues. Wear full protective clothing including masks and eye shields and change your gloves and mask often.

Reference

1. **Hart A**, *et al.* (2018) Have you cored lately? A comprehensive operating room evacuation drill. *American Journal of Disaster Medicine* **13**(4):239–252.

Chapter 22

The kidney

Introduction

Renal failure after major surgery carries 60 per cent mortality, and if systemic sepsis develops then mortality approaches 90 per cent. If the kidneys fail the patient is more likely to develop gastrointestinal bleeding, respiratory infections, cardiac failure, poor wound healing and generalized sepsis. If we can anticipate and recognize developing renal failure, then we have a chance to ameliorate these calamities.

Physiology

Homeostasis

The kidneys help maintain body *homeostasis* by controlling the volume and composition of the extracellular fluid, and by excreting water-soluble wastes. The kidneys regulate the balance of water, sodium, potassium, hydrogen ion and other water-soluble substances in the body. They also produce hormones, erythropoietin, activated vitamin D, renin and *prostaglandins* and excrete water-soluble drugs.

Each kidney is a collection of 1 200 000 nephrons forming a high-pressure blood ultra-filtration system. A *nephron* is a long tube lined with epithelial cells. At the proximal entrance of the nephron is a sieve (*glomerulus*) and the other end of the tube opens into the renal pelvis. Fluid passing through the sieve is called the *filtrate*. As filtrate moves along the nephron useful substances pass back into the bloodstream, while metabolic wastes stay in the nephron to be excreted. Normally the glomerulus will not allow red blood cells, or larger proteins, such as albumin, into the filtrate. If the glomerulus is damaged then albumin or even blood appears in the *urine*.

Glomerular filtration rate

The *glomerular filtration rate* (GFR) is the volume of urine entering the glomerular end of the renal tubule each minute. In a healthy young adult, this is about 125 ml/min or 180 litres per day, but only 2 litres are passed as urine. To reabsorb the remaining 178 litres of filtrate, and to concentrate the urine in the tubules, the kidney needs a good oxygen supply to generate energy for the ion pumps. The kidneys fail to concentrate *urine* if deprived of sufficient blood flow or oxygen supply.

Measuring actual GFR is cumbersome. In the recovery room the best we can do is to measure the urine output. The blood electrolyte results measure the concentrations of a biochemical called *creatinine*.

Creatinine is produced as muscle protein, and is broken down. The amount building up in the blood, the serum *creatinine concentration*, is used as a surrogate marker of renal function. Serum creatinine levels can be misleading in the elderly, obese or those on unusual diets. As a rule, if patients have a raised serum urea level and a normal creatinine then they have kidney disease.

Normal serum creatinine and raised urea?
Then consider chronic kidney disease.

Chronic kidney disease

The two principal markers of the kidneys' health are the volume of urine they form and how effectively they concentrate sodium in the urine. Complications of chronic renal disease increase as the GFR falls. For this reason GFR is the best indicator of the severity of kidney disease.

How the tubules modify urine

Once fluid passes through the sieve of the glomerulus it enters the *renal tubule*. Each tubule has three parts: the *proximal tubule* reabsorbs almost everything that is useful, and excretes most of the unwanted waste; the *loop of Henle* works with the collecting tubule to concentrate the urine; and the *distal convoluted tubule* and *collecting ducts* fine tunes the composition of the filtrate. Most of the waste is urea, a breakdown product from food and cellular metabolism. Importantly, the kidney excretes many drugs.

Kidney blood flow

Each kidney is about the size of your clenched fist. Compared with their size their blood supply is enormous. About 25 per cent of the 5-litre cardiac output passes through them. This blood supply of 1250 ml/min is far more blood than they need for their metabolic requirements. Their high blood flow gives them the ability to rapidly adjust the composition or volume of body fluids to meet the physiological circumstances. They quickly filter out, and excrete the water-soluble noxious wastes in the body. Every hour, the kidneys process about 60 litres of fluid; this is equivalent to the entire volume of the body's water.

Once the mean blood pressure falls below 80 mmHg
the kidneys' health is at risk.

How the kidneys maintain their blood flow

The flow through the glomerular capillaries is *autoregulated*. As blood pressure rises and falls the intrarenal arterioles constrict and dilate to keep the blood flowing at a constant rate. This enables urine to form at an almost constant rate. If the mean arteriolar pressure falls below 80 mmHg autoregulation is lost, and urine output starts to fall.

How the kidneys conserve sodium

Every day the kidneys filter 25 000 mmol of sodium ions, but excrete less than 0.5 per cent of it. The kidneys defend the volume of the *extracellular fluid* (ECF), and if necessary do this at the expense of every other priority. They protect the ECF volume and composition by reabsorbing sodium and other substances and water in varying quantities. Where necessary the kidneys can retain all the sodium in the filtrate, and with it most of the water.

How the kidneys maintain their GFR

To produce urine the kidneys need sufficient perfusion pressure to *force* fluid from the blood through the glomerular membrane to form the *filtrate*. It is a bit like turning a hose on a bed sheet stretched out on a washing line. When the water pressure is low not much water passes through the sheet and most of it runs off. However, if you now turn up the water pressure more will pass through the bed sheet. Likewise with higher pressure more fluid will pass through the glomerulus into the tubules.

Even if the blood flow through the kidney decreases, it can temporarily compensate for this. The kidney maintains the pressure across the glomerular sieve by leaving the inflow (*afferent*) arteriole wide open, while constricting the outflow (*efferent*) arteriole. This causes blood to dam up in the glomerulus. A hormone, angiotensin II, and the noradrenergic nervous system mediate this outflow shutdown.

If the patient has been taking *angiotensin-converting enzyme* (ACE) inhibitors, or *angiotensin receptor blocking* (ARB) drugs then the efferent arteriole cannot constrict effectively. Despite blood flowing freely through the glomerular tuft, there is not enough pressure to form urine.

The kidneys' ability to keep forming urine despite being deprived of their blood supply does not mean that they are well oxygenated, or healthy.

> *Simply because the kidneys are making*
> *urine does not mean they are healthy.*

In a healthy person glomerular filtration stops and urine output ceases once the mean blood pressure falls to 60 mmHg. This pressure corresponds to a driving pressure in the glomerular tuft of about 30 mmHg. In patients with vascular disease (such as diabetics or long-term smokers) glomerular filtration ceases at mean blood pressures higher than 60 mmHg because the kidneys blood vessels are too clogged to maintain enough blood pressure in the glomerular tuft to form urine.

How anaesthesia affects the kidney

Even patients with normal kidneys experience transient renal impairment after anaesthesia. During general anaesthesia, organ perfusion slows because volatile agents depress myocardial contraction, and dilate arterioles everywhere. Blood tends to flow along paths of least resistance; consequently some blood flow is diverted away from the kidneys.

How surgery affects the kidney

The body interprets surgery as a life-threatening physical injury. Evolutionary pressures have finely honed a sequence of survival responses. In anticipation of losing blood or tissue fluid a number of hormones are released: *antidiuretic hormone* (ADH), the *gluco-corticoids*, and *aldosterone*. These hormones prevent the kidney from wasting precious body fluids and help it get rid of excessive potassium released from dead and dying cells. The sympathetic nerves release noradrenaline causing vasoconstriction that slows intrarenal blood flow,

Surgery disrupts renal function and body fluid balance. By far the most common cause of kidney damage is the combination of hypotension and hypovolaemia. Surgery involving an infected field releases showers of Gram-negative bacterial *endotoxins* into the bloodstream. These can damage the glomerular filter, and the capillaries serving the tubules.

If, during aortic surgery, the surgeon clamps the aorta above the renal arteries the kidneys progressively become hypoxic. More than 30 minutes of clamp-time causes substantial ischaemic damage.

Surgery also damages tissues and causes pain, and the more major the surgery, the greater the mass of injured tissue. *Cytokines* released by damaged cells flood into the circulation to damage *basement membranes* everywhere. Unfortunately the kidneys and lungs, with their high blood flows, bear the brunt of this assault.

Hepato-renal syndrome

The hepato-renal syndrome describes the decrease in renal function that a patient with severe liver disease suffers from. Jaundiced patients are at particular risk of kidney damage because of the high levels of bilirubin in their blood. Anaesthesia for these patients is challenging.[1] Drugs and fluid management are difficult during the operation and the recovery period. The combination of hypoxia, low renal blood flows, bacterial endotoxins and bilirubin damage the kidneys. Once established, it is almost invariably progressive and often fatal. In jaundiced patients, check the prescription for fluids ensures adequate hydration. At least one extra litre of crystalloid overnight, and another in the morning should be given. Good pain control also improves renal perfusion. Using either mannitol or furosemide to prompt a *diuresis* does not improve the prognosis.

When urine is not removed from the body and nitrogen-containing waste builds up in the blood stream renal failure follows. The patient passes small amounts of dark coloured urine and often has delirium and muscle jerks. They may not have ascites if the fluid in their abdomen has recently been removed but ascites is usually one of the presenting symptoms.

Hypovolaemia

Unless a hypovolaemic or bleeding patient rapidly receives fluids to restore their vascular volume the kidney blood supply may fall from 1250 ml/min to 250 ml/min or less. The kidneys can survive for 30–60 minutes on as little as one-tenth of their normal blood supply (125 ml/min). Despite deprivation of their blood supply, at first the kidneys are able to maintain a urine output; but they can no longer efficiently concentrate urine. As a priority, the kidneys tend to protect their GFR, rather than supply their tubules with oxygen.

A well-oxygenated healthy kidney responds to hypovolaemia by concentrating the urine, reabsorbing almost all the sodium and most of the water. The urine entering the bladder now has high osmolarity, but a low sodium concentration. If the blood supply fails and the kidney becomes hypoxic, then the ion pumps in the tubules fail (Figure 22.1). Without enough oxygen they are unable to pump sodium back into the blood so it stays in the filtrate and is excreted in the urine. Now the urine has a high sodium content.

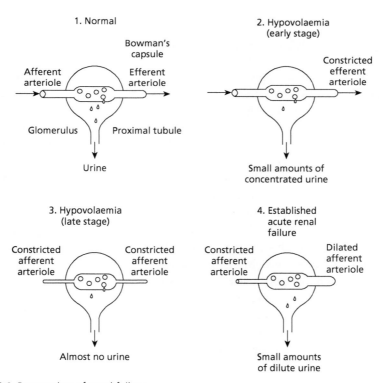

Figure 22.1 Progression of renal failure.

We can measure sodium concentration in the urine with flame photometry. This is a simple procedure for most laboratories. In the recovery room, a urinary sodium concentration greater than 40 mmol/L suggests renal impairment.

Postoperative hypovolaemia can occur because of:

◆ bleeding;

◆ bowel obstruction;

- peritonitis;
- prolonged vomiting.

During surgery the anaesthetist will start to resuscitate the patient but often it is necessary to continue this process in the recovery room.

Bleeding

As a patient bleeds there is an ordered progression of responses (see Box 22.1). These involve the sympathetic nervous system (adrenaline and noradrenaline), and hormones (ADH, angiotensin II, and aldosterone). Initially the urine output is maintained, but as the kidneys become hypoxic they begin to fail to concentrate urine and the sodium content of the urine rises; then urine production falls and finally stops altogether.

Box 22.1 **How kidneys guard their blood supply**

Once the kidneys' blood supply decreases they respond by secreting an enzyme called renin. Renin cleaves a prohormone, *angiotensinogen* into angiotensin-I. Angiotensin-I is converted in the lung by *angiotensin-converting enzyme* (ACE) to angiotensin-II. Angiotensin-II is a potent vasoconstrictor. As it circulates it causes vascular smooth muscle everywhere to spasm including the kidneys' own arterioles. As arterioles shut down, the systemic blood pressure rises. With haemorrhage, the combined effect of angiotensin-II and noradrenaline on the skin's arterioles makes people go white. The shutdown of the blood supply to the gut, skeletal muscle, kidney and skin, diverts valuable blood to the heart, lungs and brain.

The kidney can override this vasoconstriction by producing a prostaglandin. NSAIDs interfere with this process. If the kidneys cannot make the prostaglandin, and the kidneys fate is sealed. Most anaesthetists prefer that patients stop taking their NSAID at least 4 days before major surgery, especially if they are elderly. NSAIDs are a major risk factor for postoperative renal dysfunction.

ACE inhibitors increase the risk of postoperative renal dysfunction because the renin–angiotensin system can no longer compensate if renal perfusion falls. In patients taking ACE inhibitors it is important to maintain *normovolaemia* so that they do not become hypotensive.

As blood is lost the kidneys progressively shut down their circulation. In doing so, they divert up to 1000 ml/min of their 1250 ml/min blood supply to boost the volume of the central circulation. At the same time *aldosterone* primes the pumps in the tubules to retain sodium and water; and the urine output slows and may stop. ADH prevents the kidney from excreting water, while angiotensin II helps raise the systemic blood pressure, and prompts the adrenal glands to release aldosterone to stop sodium loss in the urine.

Bowel surgery

Following abdominal surgery ECF is lost in a number of ways. Fluid transudates into the bowel, or collects as effusions in the peritoneum (this retained fluid is called *third space loss*); or it escapes through drains, or with bleeding. During major abdominal surgery up to 10 ml/kg/hr of water is lost simply by evaporation from the open peritoneum. Dry anaesthetic gases remove water from the lungs. Unless these losses are replaced, the patient will develop *hypovolaemia*, and the kidneys will attempt to compensate by retaining fluid.

Peritonitis

With an inflamed peritoneum large amounts of fluid can accumulate as third space loss in the peritoneum.

Acute tubular necrosis

Unless blood volume and oxygen supply are rapidly restored the kidneys' tubular cells degenerate and die. Damage to the capillaries slows intrarenal blood flow by 40–50 per cent. This process of both endothelial and tubular damage is termed *acute tubular necrosis* (ATN).

At this stage, even if the cardiac output and blood flow is restored, the damaged intrarenal blood vessels prevent blood from circulating properly within the kidney. The patient becomes anuric. Given ideal conditions the dead tubular cells and damaged endothelium will eventually be replaced, and with dialysis, normal renal function usually returns in about 3–6 weeks.

Renal vascular disease, diuretics and nephrotoxins such as gentamicin accelerate the progression of these events.

Who is at risk from renal damage?

The following are at risk of renal damage during, or after, surgery:

- patients over the age of 65 years;
- people with severe arterial disease ('vasculopaths');
- diabetics;
- surgery where the aorta is cross-clamped;
- patients with pre-existing renal disease;
- those undergoing major vascular surgery, especially if they require blood transfusion;
- patients taking NSAIDs;
- patients with systemic sepsis;

- those having bowel surgery;
- pre-eclampsia;
- trauma and crush injury.

How kidneys age

Renal blood flow decreases by about 1 per cent a year after the age of 30 years, and by the age of 90 years has halved. Estimated renal plasma flow falls from about 650 ml/min in 30–40-year-olds to about 290 ml/min in their 80s.

As we age our kidneys' nephrons progressively die, and are replaced by fibrous tissue. Because the elderly have fewer nephrons, a small insult such as a brief fall in blood pressure, may have a large effect.

Any disease affecting nephrons,
affects the GFR.

Drugs and the kidney

How kidney disease affects drugs

With chronic kidney disease the GFR falls, and the incidence of adverse drug reactions rises. Once the GFR falls below 30 ml/min the kidney fails to efficiently excrete water-soluble drugs. Adverse drug reactions may occur because kidney disease prolongs the half-life of some drugs and their metabolites.

Reduce the doses of drugs, and increase the dosing interval in patients with an estimated glomerular filtration rate (eGFR) less than 30 ml/min/1.73m^2.

How drugs affect the kidney

Drugs can damage kidneys by decreasing their perfusion, impairing intrarenal blood distribution, being toxic to tubules, or causing interstitial nephritis.

0.9 per cent saline

In patients with chronic kidney disease, *normal saline* contributes to hyperchloraemia, and probably contributes to postoperative renal dysfunction. If you need to give more than 1 litre of crystalloid fluid then use Plasma-Lyte® or Hartmann's solution.

Avoid large volumes of 0.9 per cent saline
in patients with renal disease.

Diuretics

Loop diuretics increase renal blood flow. Furosemide may shorten the oliguric period, but it has no clinical benefits when used to prevent or treat acute renal failure, and has no effect on mortality and may be harmful. High doses cause ototoxicity and damage a hypoperfused kidney.

Drugs may decrease renal perfusion

Drugs decreasing renal perfusion include diuretics (see Box 22.2), ACE inhibitors (the 'prils', e.g. enalapril), and ARBs (the 'sartans', e.g. irbesartan), and vasodilators. In critically ill patients, especially those with sepsis, these drugs may aggravate hypotension, and impair the kidney's defences that normally preserve glomerular filtration and medullary blood flow.

Box 22.2 **Diuretics**

A *diuretic* is a drug promoting urine output. There are four types of diuretics.

1. *Loop diuretics* e.g. furosemide inhibits chloride (and therefore sodium) reabsorption in the loop of Henle. Furosemide is a powerful drug.

2. *Osmotic diuretics* such as mannitol, which being hypertonic enter the filtrate and drags water along with it.

3. *Potassium-conserving diuretics*; such as spironolactone, an analogue of aldosterone, blocks the uptake of sodium ion.

4. *Thiazide* diuretics such as chlorothiazide and indapamide act at the proximal part of the distal tubule to prevent potassium reabsorption.

Drugs can be toxic to the tubules

Because the kidneys have an enormous blood supply, and the renal tubules concentrate the fluid flowing through them, any toxins present in the tubules are also concentrated. Many drugs are concentrated to toxic levels including gentamicin, high-dose furosemide, and amphotericin.

Drugs can cause interstitial nephritis

Some drugs can cause interstitial (allergic) nephritis. These include β-lactams (penicillins and cephalosporins) and non-steroidal anti-inflammatory drugs.

NSAIDs cause kidney ischaemia

Non-steroidal anti-inflammatory drugs (NSAIDs) disrupt intrarenal blood flow, especially in the elderly. They can disrupt the blood supply to the renal tubules. NSAIDs should be stopped 4 days before surgery, and preferably not used in patients over the age of 65 years, or those with chronic kidney disease.

Morphine

Because morphine is partly metabolized by the kidneys its action may be prolonged in patients with diseased kidneys. Morphine's metabolite morphine-6-glucoronide is a more potent analgesic and respiratory depressant than morphine itself. Although a single loading dose of morphine is well tolerated in patients with kidney disease, increase the intervals between subsequent doses by 30 to 50 per cent.

Pethidine

Avoid pethidine in patients with chronic kidney disease, because its metabolite, 6-pethidinic acid, accumulates and may cause convulsions.

> *Give morphine cautiously and avoid*
> *pethidine in patients with renal impairment.*

Fentanyl

Although fentanyl is metabolized by the liver, and has no active metabolite, the drug's *clearance* is decreased in patients with an eGFR less than 15 ml/min. This prolongs its action. Fentanyl is a useful postoperative drug for pain relief in patients with impaired renal function.

Penicillins and gentamicin

Never combine gentamicin and penicillins in intravenous injections or infusions. Gentamicin splits open-lactam rings of penicillins chemically inactivating both the gentamicin and the penicillin. The problem occurs especially in patients with stage 3 (or worse) chronic kidney disease, who retain higher levels of penicillin for longer than patients with normal renal function.

If patients with renal failure require both gentamicin and penicillin, then separate the doses by several hours.

Benzodiazepines

Because there is increased sensitivity to their effects in patients with kidney disease, reduce the dose of *benzodiazepines*, such as diazepam, oxazepam and midazolam, by 30 to 50 per cent.

Relaxants

Neuromuscular blocking drugs whose effects may be prolonged in patients with kidney disease include pancuronium, doxacurium, pipecuronium, and vecuronium. Atracurium and mivacurium are suitable relaxants drugs for renal patients.

Iodinated contrast media

Iodinated radio-contrast media used in angiography is hypertonic and concentrates in the blood disrupting intrarenal blood flow. To reduce the risk of radiocontrast nephropathy, give 1 litre of 0.45 per cent saline before giving the contrast. Do not try to boost urine output with either mannitol or furosemide because these drugs further desiccate tubular endothelium making the outcome worse.

For calculation of drug doses see Box 22.3.

Box 22.3 **How to calculate drug dose**

The doses of some drugs, such as gentamicin, are modified according to renal function. Check renal function before using any drug that is excreted by the kidney. After you have given a drug to patients with kidney disease, observe them assiduously for untoward effects.

The Cockcroft–Gault equation (1976) is used to estimate creatinine clearance from the plasma creatinine concentration. It is primarily used in the recovery room for determining the correct dose of gentamicin.

$$\text{Creatinine clearance} = \frac{(140 - \text{age in years}) \times \text{lean body weigh in kg.}}{815 \times \text{serum creatinine (mmol/L)}}$$

For women the value is 85 per cent of that estimated by the equation.

Although eGFR has supplanted creatinine clearance, appropriate drug doses in those with kidney disease are still calculated by the Cockcroft–Gault equation.

End-stage renal disease

End-stage kidney disease (ESKD) occurs when the eGFR is greater than 15 ml/min, and dialysis is usually necessary when the eGFR is less than 10 ml/min.

There are two clinical types of ESKD: *oliguric renal failure* with little or no urine produce, and *polyuric renal failure* where urine is formed but cannot be concentrated in the kidney tubules. Both types cause raised serum creatinine and urea concentrations, and are accompanied by the usual retinue of hypertension, anaemia, ischaemic heart disease, calcified heart valves, coagulopathies, chronic steroid dependence, poor wound healing and a susceptibility to infection.

If you have any doubt about the management of patients with ESKD then consult a renal physician. Take care not to overload these patients with intravenous fluids. Most patients have been dialysed before they come for elective surgery, and are relatively hypovolaemic so it is safe for them to receive up to a litre of Hartmann's solution during their operation. If they arrive with their second litre running then, in consultation with the anaesthetist, slow it to an 18-hourly rate.

Patients with chronic renal failure commonly suffer from physical and emotional pain and pain management is difficult in these patients.[2] The margin between an adequate analgesic dose and a toxic dose is small and the patients are physically and psychologically frail.

Veins and arteries are precious

Veins in patients with end-stage renal failure are precious because they may be needed for haemodialysis. Never put drips in around the wrists or in the cubital fossa. Use the smallest possible cannula and a careful sterile technique to insert it (not just wipe with an alcohol swab). Never allow even a hint of thrombophlebitis to occur. If there is any sign of inflammation remove the cannula and re-site it in another place. Replace cannulas within 24 hours. Avoid taking blood gases from their precious radial arteries, use their femoral artery instead.

How to prevent postoperative renal failure

The recovery room has a major role in preventing postoperative renal failure, especially in patients who have risk factors. So:

- Give oxygen.
- Ensure that your patient is not *hypovolaemic*.
- Do not use NSAIDs in patients with an eGFR < 50 ml/min/1.73 m^2.
- Control pain. Pain activates a noradrenergic response, which reduces renal blood flow.
- Do not give nephrotoxic drugs to patients who are hypovolaemic.
- Avoid the so-called 'triple whammy' of furosemide, gentamicin and NSAID.

Classes of acute renal failure

There are three classes of acute renal failure:

1. *Prerenal acute renal failure* is caused by hypovolaemia, which diminishes renal blood flow. This is the most common cause of acute renal failure encountered in the recovery room.
2. *Intrinsic acute renal failure* occurs when there is damage to the renal parenchyma. This is more likely where radiocontrast dyes are used during surgery.
3. *Postrenal acute renal failure* occurs when the urinary tract becomes obstructed, usually with blood clots or stone fragments after urological surgery. However, occasionally the ureter is damaged during pelvic surgery.

What to do if urine output slows or stops

In the recovery room *oliguria* occurs when the urine output falls below 1 ml/kg/hr. *Severe oliguria* occurs when it falls below 0.5 ml/kg/hr, and *anuria* when no urine has been produced for the last 15 minutes.

Consider the likely possible causes for acute renal failure, for example, hypovolaemia (prerenal), toxic drugs (renal) and obstruction (postrenal).

Prerenal causes

Ensure that your patient is not hypovolaemic. Check their perfusion status; cold hands and a tachycardia suggest ischaemic kidneys. A hypovolaemic patient will drop their systolic blood pressure if you sit them up in Fowler's position at 45°.

Cold hands = cold kidneys.

Treat hypovolaemia

- Give oxygen and aim for saturations > 97%.
- Notify the anaesthetist.
- Treat hypovolaemia aggressively because it rapidly causes damage to the kidney.

If they are bleeding then give blood, or:

- Give 500 ml of a colloid first and follow this with Hartmann's solution.
- After each 500 ml of fluid check if they are still hypovolaemic by propping them up at 45°. If their blood pressure falls by > 20 mmHg then prepare to give another 500 ml of Hartmann's solution.

Suppress renovascular constriction

- Give oxygen and aim for saturations > 97%.
- Treat pain, because severe pain reduces renal blood flow. If possible use epidural anaesthesia.
- Be alert for a possible shower of bacteria especially after urological, or gastrointestinal surgery; or where the surgery has involved an infected site such as drainage of an abscess or fluid collection.

Renal causes

Check the patient has not been receiving nephrotoxic drugs leading up to or during their surgery. A common nephrotoxin is radiocontrast dye, especially if the patient is also taking metformin, or the patient is, or has been, hypovolaemic.

To prompt urine output

- Give oxygen and aim for saturations > 97%.
- If the patient's blood volume is normal you can prompt urine output with a small dose of furosemide and mannitol. Start with a combination of furosemide 0.5 mg/kg and mannitol 1 g/kg.
- Use higher doses of furosemide if the patient has pigment associated *nephropathy* following haemolysis, *rhabdomyolysis* or massive crush injuries.

Postrenal causes

- Check the patency of the urinary catheter.
- Is an over-full bladder peeping over the pelvic brim?

In summary and when not to worry

Oliguria is not necessarily a sinister event, and in itself is not a reliable predictor of acute renal failure. This phenomenon of oliguria with well-perfused kidneys is more likely in a patient taking *angiotensin-converting enzyme inhibitors* (ACEIs). If the patient has good perfusion with warm hands, is not in pain, has oxygen saturations greater than 95 per cent and has neither received any nephrotoxic drugs, nor has been assaulted with a shower of bacteria, then the kidneys are probably not at risk.

Providing the patient has not been hypotensive or hypoxic at any time these drugs probably exert a protective effect on the kidney during major surgery. They certainly predispose to perioperative hypotension, especially in patients with cardiac failure. In the case of warm kidneys, urine output will probably improve over the next hour or so. If there has been one or more kidney-damaging events during surgery it is worthwhile provoking an increase in urine output with a small volume load and a low dose of furosemide.

References

1. **Wagener G, Brentjens TE** (2010) Anaesthetic concerns in patients presenting with renal failure. *Anaesthesthesiology* **28**(1):39–54.
2. **Kafkia T, Chamney M**, *et al.* (2011) Pain in chronic renal disease. *Journal of Renal Care* **37**(2):114–122.

Chapter 23

Fluid balance

Introduction

Patients coming to the recovery room from operating theatres may have disturbed circulating and tissue fluid volumes for many reasons: they are fasted, they may have received intravenous fluids or lost fluid during their operation; or have ongoing losses from bleeding or bowel obstruction.

How surgery affects fluid balance

Postoperatively, sensors in brainstem and hypothalamus emerge from anaesthesia to encounter a whole host of neural and *cytokine* messages telling the brainstem and the *vital centres* that the body is injured. These inputs include pain, tissue trauma, hypothermia, hypovolaemia, sepsis, and hypoxia.

If we are injured, evolution has programmed us to hide, without food or water, for several days while recovering. The body uses a barrage of measures to preserve vital body fluids and maintain *homeostasis*. The sympathetic nervous system and several hormones regulate these measures. Hormones that are released include angiotensin, aldosterone, cortisol, and *antidiuretic hormone*. Their net effect is to stop the kidneys excreting precious extracellular fluids, and breaking down skeletal muscle (and some days later, fat) to provide an emergency food source. Some of these responses are potentially harmful, and most are no longer necessary, because we shelter, feed and give fluids to our patients.

The body's fluid compartments

Functionally the body is divided into two compartments: the *intracellular fluid* (ICF) and the *extracellular fluid* (ECF). The two compartments are separated by a cell membrane. Only water can flow across cell membranes, and it does so to keep the ionic concentration (*tonicity*) of the fluid exactly equal on either side of the membrane. The *force* that drives water across the membrane is called *osmotic pressure*. Osmotic pressure is generated by the difference in the number of ions on each side of the cell membrane.

Facts

- The volume of the ECF is about 15 litres, of which 3 litres are *plasma*. The remaining 12 litres are in the interstitial space and bathe the cells in a warm swamp from which they derive their nutrients, and into which they jettison their wastes.

- The volume of the ICF is 30 litres, and about 2 litres of this volume are inside circulating red blood cells.
- Normal blood volume is about 5 litres or 70 ml/kg.
- The capillary endothelium is freely permeable to water, *cations*, and *anions*, but not to larger proteins. Proteins such as albumin are principally confined to plasma.
- The principal cation in the ECF is sodium, but inside the cells it is potassium.

Replacement fluids

Intravenous fluids can be *hypertonic, isotonic,* or *hypotonic*. Most of the intravenous fluids we use in the recovery room are isotonic with plasma. This means they exert the same *osmotic pressure* as plasma. Isotonic fluids include Plasma-Lyte®, 0.9 per cent saline, Hartmann's solution and Ringer's lactate. When these solutions are given as an intravenous fluid into the extracellular fluid, water neither enters nor leaves the cells. These fluids remain entirely in the ECF (Figure 23.1).

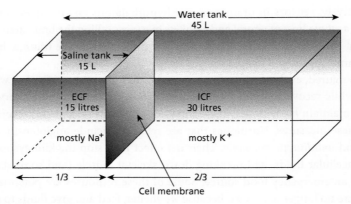

Figure 23.1 Fluid compartments.

Some intravenous fluids are hypotonic. Water from these fluids will flow into cells causing them to swell. Although seldom used, 0.45 per cent normal saline is a hypotonic solution; its osmotic pressure is half that of plasma. Sometimes hypertonic solutions are used to correct serious problems with water balance. Examples of these solutions are 2N saline, 3N saline and 20 per cent mannitol.

Hypotonic solutions

Five per cent glucose in water

5% glucose in water contains 50 g/L of glucose (278 mmol/L) dissolved in sterile water. As soon as it enters a vein it acts as an isotonic solution, exerting exactly the same osmotic pressure as plasma, but within a few minutes the cells take up the glucose, leaving the water behind. The water distributes itself evenly throughout the whole 45 litres of body fluid compartments. Two-thirds of the water enters the ECF, and one-third remains in the ICF.

If you give excess hypotonic fluid its water enters cells causing them to swell and disrupting their function. It may even cause red cells to burst (*haemolysis*) so releasing their haemoglobin into the plasma. Brain cells are confined inside a tight bony box, the skull. If brain cells swell, the *intracranial pressure* (ICP) rises abruptly jeopardizing the blood supply: this can be fatal.

Isotonic solutions

Colloids

Colloids exert enough oncotic pressure to balance the flow of fluid between the intravascular and the interstitial space. Colloids rapidly increase blood volume in hypovolaemic, shocked or bleeding patients, because they stay within the circulation much longer than crystalloids. Colloids include: human albumin, dextrans and starches.

Human albumin 5 per cent

Human albumin 5 per cent (50 g/L) is a purified, sterile, colloid derived from human plasma. It does not need to be cross-matched. Given intravenously it stays in the circulation, but within 18 hours it leaks away to distribute uniformly throughout the ECF. The metabolic half-life of albumin is 20 days, and the turnover in an adult is about 5 g/day. As with all colloids it can cause circulatory overload, particularly in patients with cardiac failure or renal impairment. Occasionally, it can cause hypotension and rigors.

Other synthetic colloids

Hydroxyethyl starch (pentastarch) in sodium chloride is a polysaccharide polymer derived from corn and similar to glycogen used to expand the intravascular volume. It has a plateau effect of 4–6 hours and is excreted by the kidneys more quickly than older solutions of polymers. It has little effect on haemostasis. The advised maximum dose is 15 ml/kg.

Crystalloids

Crystalloids are physiologically balanced salt solutions. They do not cause allergic reactions, they improve renal perfusion more effectively than colloids, and are cheap. However, they have a greater risk of causing pulmonary oedema, and they may aggravate acute respiratory distress syndrome more than colloids.

Normal saline

Normal (0.9 per cent saline) is an isotonic solution containing 154 mmol of sodium chloride in a litre of distilled water. When you give 0.9 per cent saline intravenously it rapidly distributes itself between the circulation and the interstitial fluid, but all of it remains in the ECF, and none of it crosses the cell membrane to enter the cells. Rapid infusions of 0.9 per cent saline can cause a hyperchloraemic acidosis.

Plasma-Lyte®

Plasma-Lyte 148® is a sterile isotonic solution for intravenous fluid therapy. It was introduced as a substitute for 0.9 per cent saline. Rapid infusions of 0.9 per cent saline can cause an acidosis, but Plasma-Lyte® consumes hydrogen ions as the acetate and gluconate are metabolized in the liver to carbon dioxide and water.

Hartmann's solution (Ringer's lactate)

Hartmann's solution is isotonic. When infused into a vein it all stays in the ECF. In addition to sodium ions, Hartmann's solution contains potassium, lactate, chloride and calcium ions. It is useful because it roughly approximates the ionic concentration of plasma, but does not contain any plasma proteins.

How the body controls fluids

The body has two systems for controlling fluid balance. One, the *low pressure baroreceptor system*, responds to the pressure of fluid in the great veins and right atria; in contrast the other entirely separate *osmoreceptor* system responds to changes in *tonicity* in the interstitial fluid.

Grasp this point firmly: there are two separate fluid systems each with its own sensor. Low-pressure baroreceptors respond to stretching the walls of the right atria. As they stretch they release *atrial-natriuretic peptide* (ANP), a hormone that improves renal blood flow. Once they have a good blood supply the kidneys now excrete near-isotonic fluid.

Osmoreceptors in the *hypothalamus* detect changes in concentration of sodium ion in the ECF. This system controls the *tonicity* of the body water. As the tonicity of the ECF rises, the osmoreceptors release *antidiuretic hormone* (ADH). ADH forces the kidney to retain water to dilute the ECF. On the other hand if the concentration of sodium ions in the ECF decreases, the osmoreceptors stop producing ADH and the urine becomes more dilute. This system is a typical example of a physiological negative feedback loop.

What can go wrong

Either of these two systems can become disordered independently of each other. Conceptually, it is easier to regard each of them as separate 'tanks': one containing the 45 litres of *total body water*, and the other 15 litres of *isotonic fluid* in the ECF. The isotonic ECF is predominately a saline solution containing added electrolytes (potassium, chloride, bicarbonate, magnesium and trace elements).

Fluid out = fluid in

Fluid balance is achieved when the rate of fluid going in equals the rate of fluid being lost, and the patient is haemodynamically stable. If you work with this basic formula you will find postoperative fluid balance easier to manage.

$$Fluid\ requirements = continuing\ loss + catch\text{-}up\ fluid + maintenance$$

Disorders of fluid balance

It is best to estimate total body water and ECF volume separately. Replace blood loss with colloid. Replace isotonic fluid losses from the bowel (such as with vomiting or from fistulae) with Plasma-Lyte® or Hartmann's solution. Assess and adjust potassium levels, magnesium and phosphate levels separately. See Box 23.1 for maintenance fluid requirements.

Box 23.1 **Maintenance fluid requirements**

Postoperative fluid therapy is often planned by agreement between the anaesthetist, surgeon and the recovery room nursing staff. The first 8–12 hours of fluid therapy should be organized before the patient is discharged to the ward.

Adult maintenance

Adult maintenance fluids = 40 ml + 1 ml/kg each hour.

A 70 kg man will require 40 + (70 × 1) = 110 ml/hr. This is 2640 ml per day. Add 13.4 mmol of potassium per litre. For a routine adult patient who is expected to drink within a few hours' maintenance fluids would be 1 litre of saline and 2 litres of glucose 5 per cent daily. Give each litre over 8 hours.

Child maintenance

A solution of .18 per cent normal saline and glucose is a commonly used fluid for small children.

For the first 10 kg give 4 ml/kg/hr

Add a further 2 ml/kg/hr for children weighing 10–20 kg

Add a further 1 ml/kg/hr for children over 20 kg

Examples:

5 kg infant would require 5 × 4 = 20 ml/hr or 480 ml/day

15 kg child would require:

for the first 10 kg give 4 ml/kg/hr = 10 × 4 = 40 ml

add 2 ml/kg/hr for the next 5 kg = 5 × 2 = 10 ml

total requirements = 50 ml/hr or 1200 ml/day

28 kg child would require:

for the first 10 kg give 4 ml/kg/hr = 10 × 4 = 40 ml

add 2 ml/kg/hr for next 10 kg = 10 × 2 = 20 ml

then add 1 ml/kg/hr for next 8 kg = 8 × 1 = 8 ml

total requirements = 68 ml/hr or 1632 ml/day

Correct fluid balance problems in the following order:

1. Correct the blood volume to protect and restore the perfusion of the patient's brain, heart and kidneys.
2. Estimate and adjust the ECF volume.
3. Calculate and adjust water balance.
4. Correct other electrolyte disturbances.

Restore the blood volume

In patients who are bleeding or who are saline depleted, the first thing to do is save their kidneys, by quickly restoring the blood volume. Preferably give bleeding patients blood, or failing that a colloid to restore their vascular volume rapidly as possible, and consequently preserve blood flow to their heart, brain, liver, and kidneys.

Next correct the ECF volume

Because isotonic fluids cannot cross cell membranes they are confined to the ECF. Think of the ECF as tank of isotonic fluid (which is 98 per cent saline) that can either can be too full (*saline overload*) or too empty (*saline deficit*).

ECF volume overload

Acute saline overload

In its most dramatic form acute *saline overload* presents with pulmonary oedema. Initially the patient has a tachypnoea (rate greater than 20 breaths/min) and cool hands. Fluid accumulating in the interstitium of their lungs triggers a rise in respiratory rate, and a noradrenergic response. The normal respiratory rate is 12–14 breaths/min. Measure the respiratory rate carefully by putting your hand on the patient's chest to feel it rise and fall.

As the saline overload progresses patients feel breathless, and then start to wheeze. They feel most uncomfortable lying down. At this early stage the chest X-ray shows peribronchial oedema (cuffing) and distended upper lobe veins. Later, the X-rays show a ground glass appearance of interstitial pulmonary oedema.

If you listen at the patient's mouth as they force out a deep breath, you can hear oedematous small airways softly snap, crackle and pop open. As their oxygen saturation falls many patients feel panicky, and grope about the bed. You can now hear showers of crackles at the lung bases that do not go away with deep breaths. The chest X-ray shows the fluffy dense bat's wing appearance of alveolar pulmonary oedema.

How to manage acute pulmonary oedema

Sit the patient up, give high-flow oxygen, and ensure their blood pressure is greater than 100 mmHg. If they are older than 60 years give furosemide 40 mg IV; in patients younger than 60, give furosemide 10–20 mg IV. Wait 20 minutes. If the urine output remains less than 30 ml/hr, check their urinary catheter is not blocked, there is no chance of haemorrhage, and their systolic blood pressure is greater than 100 mmHg. At this point the anaesthetist may double the dose of furosemide to 80 mg IV. If there is still no urine produced seek expert help.

ECF volume deficit

Saline deficit occurs with diarrhoea, protracted vomiting, and diabetic ketoacidosis, but in the recovery room it is most often seen in people who have had surgery to relieve a bowel obstruction, or have suffered severe burns.

The signs of saline deficit are the same as that of haemorrhage: poor peripheral perfusion, a urine output less than 0.5 ml/kg/hr, and tachycardia greater than 100 beats/min. In young people the blood pressure does not fall until the situation is grave. People older than 50 years may become hypotensive, but this is an unreliable sign in a supine patient.

In people of all ages, hypovolaemia is always revealed by a *postural drop* in blood pressure. Take the patient's blood pressure, and then gently sit them up at 45°. If their systolic pressure falls by more than 20 mmHg then their vascular volume is low.

> *Postural drop in blood pressure*
> *is an excellent sign of*
> *low vascular volume.*

Untreated saline deficit progresses to shock and metabolic acidosis. Treat this metabolic acidosis by replacing the fluid loss (deficit) with an isotonic fluid, such as Plasma-Lyte®, Hartmann's solution or 0.9 per cent saline. The patient's electrolyte results help decide whether they need additional potassium, and possibly magnesium too.

Correct total body water

Unlike the saline, water readily crosses cell membranes, so its 'tank' has a volume of 45 litres and includes both the ECF and ICF compartments.

Water overload

The hallmark of water overload is a low concentration of serum sodium ion. In the recovery room it is usually seen after endoscopic urological surgery or hysteroscopy where large amounts of water have been instilled, and then absorbed. Another common cause is the injudicious use of 5 per cent glucose, but it can also occur with severe chronic heart failure, and other more uncommon chronic conditions.

Acute water overload

With acute water overload patients complain of faintness, headache, tingling around the mouth, nausea, breathlessness, and a tight feeling in the chest. They may become progressively restless, confused, disoriented, start retching, develop muscle twitching and then wheeze (a sign of developing acute pulmonary oedema). The blood pressure rises, the pulse may slow, and *haemoglobinuria* causes the urine to turn brown. The ECG may show widening of the QRS complex and T-wave inversion. If not promptly treated the patient becomes cyanotic, hypotensive, and may have a cardiac arrest. All these signs are caused by the osmotic pressure of water entering cells, causing red cells to rupture, cerebral oedema, and disturbing cardiac myocyte function.

Management

Give high concentrations of oxygen by mask. Monitor blood pressure, pulse, respiratory rate, oxygen saturation and ECG. Send blood to laboratory for electrolytes, and haemoglobinaemia, and urine haemoglobin.

Use hypertonic saline as soon as water overload starts to cause symptoms. Give 1000 ml of 3N saline with the aim of increasing the serum sodium ion by 3 to 5 mmol/L over the first 2 hours. The principal risk of using hypertonic saline is saline overload. (Every 1000 ml of 3N saline will convert 2000 ml of the excess water into 2000 ml of isotonic saline; as well as infusing the equivalent of a further 1000 ml of N saline.) To overcome this, use furosemide 20–40 mg IV every 2–4 hours to get rid of the excess ECF volume.

Water deficit

It is uncommon to encounter an isolated water deficit in recovery room. Occasionally you may see water deficit in patients who have been febrile for some time. The hallmark of water deficit is an elevated serum sodium ion concentration ($Na^+ > 142$ mmol/L). It responds readily with 5 per cent glucose. Each 1000 ml of 5 per cent glucose in an adult will decrease their serum sodium ion concentration by 3 mmol/L; conversely each 3 mmol/L rise in serum sodium ion concentrations indicates a deficit of 1000 ml of water.

Correct other electrolytes

Hypokalaemia

Hypokalaemia is a serum potassium concentration of less than 3.5 mmol/L. Hypokalaemia exacerbates residual paralysis from long-acting muscle relaxant drugs. Affected patients are unable to sustain a 5-second head lift. Suspect hypokalaemia if the patient had low serum potassium preoperatively or the ECG shows flattened or inverted T-waves. Hypokalaemia is more likely to cause problems if the oxygen saturation is low, the PCO_2 high, or the patient has had anti-cholinergic drugs. Treat hypokalaemia by adding 26.8 mmol of potassium chloride to 1000 ml of glucose or saline, and give it at a rate of not more than 13.4 mmol (one gram) an hour under ECG control. If extrasystoles occur, slow the infusion rate.

Never inject concentrated potassium chloride directly into the drip—it will kill your patient.

Hyperkalaemia

Hyperkalaemia is a serum potassium concentration exceeding 5.5 mmol/L. Patients at risk include those with renal failure, burns, crush injuries, established muscle paralysis (whatever the cause), incompatible blood transfusions, or where haemolysis has occurred.

The ECG shows high-peaked T-waves especially in the precordial leads, but there should not be any prolongation of the QT interval as happens with other causes of peaked T-waves. As the hyperkalaemia worsens the PR interval becomes prolonged (> 200 ml), progressing to AV conduction defects, the QRS widens, and finally asystole occurs.

Treat arrhythmias with calcium gluconate 1 gram intravenously over two minutes into a fast-running drip into a big vein. If necessary repeat the dose once. If the serum potassium remains greater than 6.5 mmol/L, then treat it with a glucose and insulin infusion. Give one unit of insulin for every 4 grams of glucose. Measure the glucose and potassium levels every half an hour. Watch for signs of hypoglycaemia: sweating, anxiety, tachycardia and confusion. Alternatively you can use the ion exchange resin sodium polystyrene sulfonate (e.g. Resonium A®) 15–30 g as an enema. Persistent hyperkalaemia requires haemodialysis or peritoneal dialysis.

> *Hypokalaemia is easy to correct, but hyperkalaemia*
> *is dangerous and requires intensive care.*

Fluids after surgery

Bowel surgery

For some days after bowel surgery, isotonic fluid transudates into the gut. Because this fluid is lost from the ECF, and is no longer accessible to the circulation, it is called *third space loss*. An atonic bowel can contain 6 litres or more of third space fluid. It may take up to 6 days for the bowel to recover its function, and for the fluid to be returned to the circulation. Following bowel surgery replace four-fifths of the fluid requirements with isotonic fluids such as Plasma-Lyte® or Hartmann's solution. The basic potassium requirement is 1 gram per day. After bowel surgery requirements are usually double this amount. When there has been an anastomosis of bowel tissue surgeons do not want the patients to have too much fluid. Just give enough to support the cardiovascular system and the kidneys, 40 ml of urine output an hour is sufficient. Frequent samples of blood should be sent to the laboratory and an attempt made to keep the patient's electrolytes with the normal range.

Neurosurgery

Many neurosurgeons prefer to keep their patients water depleted with higher than normal serum sodium levels. There is little evidence this reduces cerebral oedema. Indiscriminate fluid restriction causes saline depletion and jeopardizes renal perfusion. Occasionally the surgeon may ask for an infusion of *mannitol* to reduce intracranial pressure.

Urological surgery

Following urological surgery, surgeons are anxious that blood clots do not form in the bladder or ureters where they may cause blockages. To prevent this and for the first few hours surgeons prefer the urine output to be at least 200 ml/hr. Such a high urine output may require a saline load of a litre or more with encouragement of a judicious dose of furosemide 10–40 mg intravenously.

Chronic renal failure

Patients with chronic renal failure are usually dialysed before coming for major surgery and consequently may be relatively volume deplete. In addition to replacing the fluid lost during the surgery, they should not receive more than one litre of Plasma-Lyte® solution while in the operating theatre and the recovery room. Most renal patients have coexisting medical problems, such as diabetes, hypertension, ischaemic heart disease and anaemia. For this reason ask a renal physician to guide postoperative care.

Cardiac failure

If a patient has overt or stable cardiac failure you need to carefully balance the amount of intravenous fluid given against the volume of urine produced. Listen to their chests for developing fine moist sounds or wheeze suggesting saline overload. A respiratory rate rising beyond 14 breaths/min, or the reluctance to lie flat, are early warning signs of problems. A chest X-ray can help you make the diagnosis.

Chapter 24

Metabolism

Homeostasis

At the core of the way we understand how the body controls its internal environment, is the concept of *homeostasis*. This compound word is loosely derived from the Greek meaning: '*to keep things still*'. Most of our work in recovery room is to help the body maintain its homeostasis.

Homeostasis involves a collection of *feedback* mechanisms that keep our internal environment in a steady state despite fluctuations in our external environment. For example, naked individuals can be exposed to temperatures as high as 42°C, and as low as 28°C in dry air and still keep their core temperature constant. Homeostasis is a three-step process. Sensors register the changes, sending a message to a central processor, which coordinates mechanisms to compensate for the change.

For example, as we stand up blood pools in the great veins in our legs, causing our mean blood pressure to fall transiently. Pressure sensors near the heart detect the change in pressure, and send a message to a processor in the midbrain. This signals the heart to increase its output, and the peripheral vessels to constrict. This homeostatic feedback loop (Figure 24.1) prevents us from fainting every time we stand up.

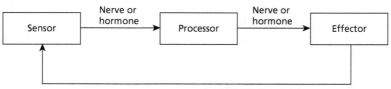

Feedback can either be positive reinforcement or negative inhibition

Figure 24.1 A feedback loop.

What is stress?

A person at rest is almost in equilibrium (homeostatic). In physiological terms, a *stress* is something that moves the body away from its comfortable resting state. Some stresses are minor, such as getting out of a warm bed in the morning, while others are life threatening, such as septicaemia following major bowel surgery. Other stresses include injury, infection, blood loss, dehydration, starvation, hypothermia, poisoning, and fear.

As a rule, the response to stress is proportional to the stress causing it and involves two sets of homeostatic mechanisms. The first is the autonomic nervous system (or *neural*) response, and the other is a hormonal (or *humoral*) response. The neural response works instantly; but the various hormonal responses take time to achieve their effect.

In response to a major stress (Table 24.1) such as surgery, the body blends the neural responses to fit the immediate circumstances, and backs them up with many different hormones to maintain the initial response. Components of the response preserve body fluids, mobilize protein and fat stores to use as energy, prevent infection and heal the wounds.

Table 24.1 Some stresses encountered in the recovery room

Pain	Hypothermia
Fluid imbalance	Starvation
Haemorrhage	Infection
Hypoxia	Hypercarbia
Tissue injury	Anxiety/fear
Vomiting	Nausea

The autonomic nervous system

1. The sympathetic (noradrenergic) nervous system.
2. The parasympathetic (cholinergic) nervous system.

There is an intellectually appealing (but false) notion that these two systems work in opposition to each other. It is true they oppose each other in some aspects; for example, the sympathetic system increases heart rate, while the parasympathetic nervous system slows it down. However, they evolved for two entirely different purposes and for the most part work independently of one another.

The sympathetic nervous system

The *sympathetic nervous system* (SNS) is part of the body's fight and flight response. Its control centre is in the hypothalamus; the nerve fibres leave the spinal cord in the thoracolumbar outflow to *synapse* in the sympathetic chain and then they accompany blood vessels to their target organs.

Fundamentally, an acute stress causes the body to respond either by preparing a person to run away (flight) or stay and face the consequences (fight). Two separate *catecholamines* mediate the two separate responses.

The two catecholamines are:

1. *Noradrenaline* (a neurotransmitter), and
2. *Adrenaline* (a hormone) made by the adrenal medulla.

Following surgery the hypothalamus co-ordinates the effect of the two catecholamines to create an appropriate response that fits the circumstances.

Hormonal back-up

Several hormones back-up the stress response. A steroid, 'cortisol', enables the body to maintain a sustained adrenergic response to prolonged stress. Without cortisol the effects of noradrenaline would soon wear off, and the blood pressure falls. Another steroid, *aldosterone* slows the excretion of sodium ion, for example, in a patient who is bleeding, or has lost some of their extracellular fluid.

Parasympathetic nervous system

The parasympathetic nervous system role is one of housekeeping: a 'rest and digest system'. It attends to the everyday functions of digestion of food, stimulating salivary and other gastrointestinal glands, accelerating peristalsis.

Parasympathetic nerve fibres have their cell bodies in the central nervous system and their neurons run in the cranial nerves (CN III, VII, IX and X). The neurotransmitter of parasympathetic (cholinergic) nervous system is *acetylcholine*.

Simulating the parasympathetic nervous system slows the cardiac rate, constricts bronchi, and constricts the pupils. Drugs simulating the action of acetylcholine cause a bradycardia; they also stimulate bronchial secretions and salivation, and peristalsis. These drugs include neostigmine, physostigmine, and pyridostigmine. Conversely, atropine blocks the effects of acetylcholine on the heart, and causes tachycardia.

Temperature

The *core temperature* is the temperature of blood flowing through the thermoregulatory centre in the anterior hypothalamus.[1] This is not readily accessible so the benchmark is the temperature of blood in the pulmonary artery.

The centre for heat regulation lies in the hypothalamus, which tightly controls the body's core temperature around a *set point* that varies by less than 0.5°C. A normothermic patient has a core temperature between 36.5°C and 37.2°C. Outside this range, cellular metabolism is progressively disrupted.

Heat production and loss

Thermal balance occurs when heat production equals heat loss. In hot environments we use less energy to maintain our body temperature, and in cold environments we use more. In humid atmospheres sweat cannot evaporate to lose heat.

In a *neutral thermal environment* a naked body neither loses nor gains heat. For adults this occurs at 28°C when the *relative humidity* is 60 per cent. In premature babies the neutral thermal environment is 34°C, in neonates 32°C and in babies 30°C.

General anaesthetics abolish the body's ability to raise its metabolic rate, or vasoconstrict, to compensate for heat loss. In contrast, regional anaesthetics block the ability of blood vessels in the skin to vasoconstrict and preserve heat. Patients cool down during surgery because the operating theatre is maintained at 20°C, with a relative humidity of about 50 per cent, which is well below the temperature of their neutral thermal environment.

How much patients cool down during surgery depends on the processes of conduction, convection, radiation and evaporation. For about the first 20 minutes on the operating table the patient's temperature stays stable. Then their core temperature falls rapidly over the following 2 hours, and more slowly after that.

The two main sources of heat loss during anaesthesia are evaporative heat loss from open abdomens, and radiant heat loss from exposed skin.

Hypothermia is common after endoscopic urological procedures where large volumes of fluids are instilled and retrieved. This wash-in, wash-out of fluid is an example of convective heat loss. Giving two units of cold blood at 4°C will cause a fall in temperature of 0.5°C. This is an example of a conductive heat loss.

Cold patients

Waking up cold from an anaesthetic is a miserable experience, and long remembered by many patients; a warmed blanket is most welcome and comforting.

Shivering, particularly in older patients, puts unacceptable demands on the heart and lungs. Do not delay using a convection air heater such as a BairHugger™ or WarmTouch™. Cold patients do not metabolize opioid analgesics efficiently, and are at greater risk of hypoxia, hypoglycaemia, renal impairment, deep vein thrombosis and hypotension.

Air warming devices are not without risk. There have been reports of them contributing to cross-infection, use a new blanket for each patient. It is possible to burn your patient if the blankets are not properly attached to the hose. Simply placing the hose under a sheet or blanket can cause a burn.

Hypothermia

*All patients having surgery
are at risk of hypothermia.*

Occasionally active hypothermia is used to cool patients during cardiac and neurosurgery to protect the patient from brain damage where the blood supply to their brain or heart needs to be temporarily interrupted. Induced hypothermia is also used sometimes to manage patients who have had a cardiac arrest or those with head injuries.

Hypothermia starts to cause clinical problems if the temperature falls below than 36°C, and once it falls below 35.8°C it has significant adverse outcomes.

To delay the onset of hypothermia anaesthetists use warming blankets, and warm infused fluids, humidify inspired air, and try to reduce conductive and convective losses. Warming patients in the recovery room substantially reduces complications and the purchase of warming devices is cost-effective. For risk factors for hypothermia see Box 24.1.

Box 24.1 **What are the risk factors for hypothermia?**

◆ Extremes of ages: thin elderly patients, neonates and infants.

◆ Long surgery (more than 3 hours) especially where the abdomen or thorax has been opened.

◆ Burns victims, especially those having skin grafts.

◆ Cachectic patients.

◆ Patients undergoing emergency surgery for major trauma.

◆ Those who are unable to shiver, such as paraplegics or quadriplegics (or those rendered temporarily so by spinal or epidural anaesthesia).

Neonates become hypothermic quickly. They have poorly developed heat regulatory mechanisms, a relatively high body surface area, no insulation from subcutaneous fat, and they do not shiver. They have a one-off mechanism for restoring their body heat by metabolizing stored brown fat, but once this is gone they are at grave risk of hypothermia.

The effects of hypothermia

Hypothermia slows down the body's metabolism by about 7 per cent per degree Celsius lost. The oxygen dissociation curve shifts to the left, indicating that haemoglobin hangs on to its oxygen more tightly. This means the oxygen pressures in the tissues have to fall further before the oxygen on the haemoglobin is released. Enzymes act sluggishly, or stop working altogether. Blood viscosity increases while the ability of blood to clot progressively fails.

After arriving in the recovery room a patient's core temperature continues to fall, before it begins to rise. This *after-drop* is caused by cold blood returning from the muscle beds and skin as the circulation to these areas is restored.

Hypothermia is a major predictor of serious postoperative problems because it:

◆ promotes bleeding; this is a major problem;

◆ increases the chance of wound breakdown;

◆ increases the risk of pressure injuries;

◆ suppresses the immune system increasing the risk of infection (especially pneumonia);

◆ suppresses the cough reflex increasing the risk of aspiration;

◆ increases blood viscosity, which compromises the circulation to the surgical site. This may jeopardize the viability of skin flaps and patency of vascular grafts;

◆ may cause cardiac arrhythmias, and exacerbate cardiac failure;

◆ delays drug metabolism; especially of opioids, sedatives and muscle relaxants;

◆ delays discharge from hospital after surgery by an average of 2.6 days.

Shivering is not shaking

Shivering is a reflex response to cold. In contrast *shaking* is a complex neuro-metabolic side-effect of general anaesthesia. Both shivering and shaking produce vigorous muscle activity creating lots of heat and using large amounts of oxygen. Oxygen consumption may rise to five- to sevenfold placing huge demands on the cardiorespiratory system to supply it.

Shivering causes the blood vessels in muscle beds to vasodilate abruptly. Once shivering starts you may have to give additional fluid to prevent hypotension. Give warm fluids through an in-line blood warmer.

Epidural and spinal anaesthetics reduce shivering and delay warming. The reason for this is that the nerve fibres relaying information from the skin's temperature sensors to the patient's hypothalamus are anaesthetized. This prevents the hypothalamus from initiating shivering, causing the skin blood vessels to vasoconstrict. Consequently the patient remains vasodilated, radiates heat and only warms slowly.

Once the temperature falls below 34°C patients cease to shiver, and they appear unconscious.

At temperatures below 28°C
the patient may appear dead.

How to detect hypothermia

Place the palm, but not the back, of your hand on the patient's chest. If they feel cold to touch, then measure their core temperature with either an infrared tympanic membrane sensor, or a skin thermistor placed over the temporal artery or an infrared temporal artery scanner. Core temperatures can also be measured by pulmonary artery catheter with a thermistor on its tip, or an oesophageal stethoscope with a thermistor embedded in it.

See Box 24.2 for blood gases in hypothermic patients.

Box 24.2 **Blood gases in hypothermic patients**

Hypothermia increases the solubility of gases in body fluids and slows the thermo-dynamic activity of all chemical reactions in a proportionate way. If you need to measure the pH in a hypothermic patient measure the blood gases as you would for a normal patient at 37°C. This technique is called alpha-stat. There is no need to make corrections for temperature, which is called pH-stat.

Hyperthermia

Fever (pyrexia) refers to core temperatures of 37.8–40°C. *Hyperthermia* refers to a core temperature more than 40°C. At about 42°C brain enzymes are irreversibly damaged and muscle tissue breaks down (*rhabdomyolysis*) releasing myoglobin into the blood stream.

It is rare for a patient to become febrile in the recovery room, but it is always serious when it does happen. For each degree Celsius rise in temperature the body's oxygen consumption increases by about 15 per cent.

A patient's temperature rises if their body produces more heat than it loses. To produce heat the body needs food, energy and oxygen. While at rest the body produces about as much heat as an 80 watt light bulb. This heat keeps the core temperature at about 37°C.

Causes of a rise in heat production

Sepsis, especially following urological surgery or bowel surgery, or the draining of an abscess, or any surgery where Gram-negative bacteria escape into the circulation.

- Thyroid storm.
- Immunological reaction to blood or blood products.
- Shivering or shaking.
- Malignant hyperthermia.
- Drugs causing the serotonin syndrome.

Causes of failure to lose heat:

- Atropine or other anti-cholinergic drugs prevent sweating.
- Core hyperthermia in the grossly obese.

Malignant hyperthermia

Malignant hyperthermia (MH) is a disorder of skeletal muscles. MH affects about 1:15 000 of the general population. It usually runs in families, as an inherited autosomal dominant condition, although there are sporadic isolated cases. The skeletal muscles of affected individuals have abnormal calcium channels in their cell membranes. Certain triggering factors, such as *suxamethonium* and all the volatile anaesthetic agents, allow calcium to flood into muscle cells causing extreme and uncontrolled muscle contraction. This generates enormous amounts of heat, uses lots of oxygen and produces lots of carbon dioxide. Overheated and dying skeletal muscle cells release myoglobin, potassium and creatinine kinase into the bloodstream. The laboratory can detect these markers in the blood.

In the initial stages MH may be difficult to diagnose. Sometimes it presents dramatically as a *metabolic storm* with high fevers, sweating, metabolic acidosis, tachycardia and masseter spasm causing tightly clenched jaws (trismus); but more usually it sneaks up insidiously with a tachycardia and a rising respiratory rate. Slow-onset MH usually presents a few hours later, after the patient has returned to the ward.

Drugs you can use safely in patients at risk of MH include benzodiazepines, droperidol, ketamine, all the opioids and the anti-emetics. Avoid controlling ventricular arrhythmias with calcium blockers such as verapamil and diltiazem, because they cause hyperkalaemia if you use dantrolene.

Thyroid storm

Now rarely seen, a *thyroid storm* occurs where patients with suboptimally controlled thyrotoxicosis present for surgery. It may surface in the recovery room, but more often it occurs 8–16 hours after surgery. It is triggered by preoperative stresses increasing circulating thyroid hormones. These include anxiety, apprehension, iodine withdrawal, pain, hypovolaemia, trauma or infection.

The consequent hypermetabolic state presents with hot flushed skin, tachycardia, atrial fibrillation, hypotension, and high blood pressures. The temperature rises to the range of 38–41°C. Treatment includes β-blockade, potassium iodide, and cortisol.

Acid–base disorders

Our cells are bathed in an isotonic swamp (the extracellular fluid) kept at constant temperature (37°C) and require just the right amount of acidity to flourish. We constantly produce prodigious amounts of hydrogen ions as a product of metabolism. If we did not get rid of the excess hydrogen ions our cells would soon grind to a halt, overwhelmed by acidity.

Our bodies have many mechanisms to control the acidity (or hydrogen ion concentration) of the *body water*. The hydrogen ion concentration is kept at a constant level by the body diluting these ions, excreting them or *buffering* them.[2]

Hydrogen ions

A *hydrogen ion* (H^+) is a single proton (Figure 24.2); it carries a positive electrical charge. Hydrogen ions are present in very tiny amounts in the body, and too much or too little causes havoc to biochemical reactions. Normally homeostatic mechanisms control the hydrogen ion concentration in the extracellular fluid within a range of 38–45 nanomoles per litre.

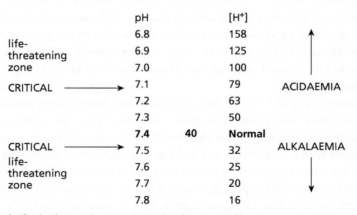

$[H^+]$ = hydrogen ion concentration in nanomol/L

Figure 24.2 Hydrogen ion and pH.

What is an acid?

Acids are substances that *dissociate* in water to donate hydrogen ions to chemical reactions. *Bases* are substances that accept hydrogen ions. Acids and bases are reciprocally related to each other. So, as the concentration of acid rises, the concentration of base falls by exactly the same amount. Every hydrogen ion accepted by a base (OH^-) means that while there is one less hydrogen ion there is one more water molecule (H_2O).

How hydrogen ions affect biochemical reactions

Enzymes are complex proteins whose singular shape is necessary to catalyse biochemical reactions. Too much or too little hydrogen ion in the vicinity of the enzyme distorts an enzyme's shape so that it cannot work properly.

Acid–base disturbances become a life-threatening problem when the pH drops below 7.12 ($[H^+]$ greater than 76 nmol/L) or rises beyond 7.55 ($[H^+]$ less than 28 nmol/L). Outside this range important enzymes progressively fail, and the cardiovascular response to *catecholamines* declines.

How hydrogen ion affects haemoglobin

Excessive hydrogen ion, as occurs in the lactic acidosis of haemorrhagic shock, loosens haemoglobin's bond with oxygen so it is released more readily to the tissues. Conversely, an excess of base tightens haemoglobin's grip on oxygen so that it is not as readily released. In this way mild to moderate acidaemia protects tissues against hypoxia.

Where hydrogen ion comes from

Every day our cell's mitochondria produce staggering amounts of hydrogen ion as glucose is converted into energy. Fortunately more than 99.999999999 per cent of the hydrogen ion (H^+) immediately combines with oxygen (O) to form harmless water (H_2O), which can be either used or excreted at leisure. This still leaves us with 0.000000001 per cent of the hydrogen ion that must be dealt with promptly before it has a chance to upset body metabolism. Even in nanomolar concentrations changes in the amount of hydrogen ion in body fluids disrupts the biochemistry of cells.

Excess hydrogen ion is buffered inside cells by phosphate compounds. Once outside the cell hydrogen ion is counterbalanced by bicarbonate ion (HCO_3^-). In this way hydrogen ion concentration is kept within the normal range. It is only when excessive hydrogen ion is being produced, or it cannot be excreted, that problems arise.

Acidosis and alkalosis

An *acidosis* occurs when too much hydrogen ion accumulates in the tissues. An *acidaemia* occurs when hydrogen ion concentrations in the blood rises beyond 45 nmol/L. Conversely, an alkalosis occurs when there is too much *base* in the tissues. An *alkalaemia* occurs when hydrogen ion concentration in the blood is less than 38 nanomoles per litre.

The body can easily cope with a moderate acidosis, but is almost defenceless against an alkalosis. Fortunately, alkalosis is rare, and usually is caused by some sort of medical intervention. Severe alkalosis can quickly maim or kill.

Acidosis and alkalosis are classified by whatever causes them. An excess or deficiency of carbon dioxide results in a respiratory acidosis, or alkalosis respectively; while an excess or deficiency of bicarbonate ion results in a metabolic acidosis or alkalosis (Box 24.3). The lungs control carbon dioxide levels, while the kidneys control the absolute levels of bicarbonate.

Box 24.3 **Four steps to interpret blood gases**

Step 1. What is the hydrogen ion concentration [H⁺]?

- If [H+] > 45 nmol/L (pH < 7.35) the patient has an acidaemia.
- If [H+] < 35 nmol/L (pH > 7.45) the patient has an alkalaemia.

Step 2. What is the arterial PaO₂?

- If PaO2 < 60 mmHg (7.9 kPa) then the patient is hypoxaemic.
- If PaO2 < 35 mmHg (4.6 kPa) then the patient is dying.

Step 3. What is the arterial PaCO₂?

- If PaCO2 > 45 mmHg (5.5 kPa) then the patient is hypoventilating.
- If PaCO2 < 35 mmHg (4.6 kPa) then the patient is hyperventilating.

Step 4. What is the actual bicarbonate?

- If it is nearly normal and the pH is abnormal then there is an acute respiratory component.
- If it is abnormal and the pH is abnormal then there is a metabolic component.

Tell the laboratory the inspired oxygen concentration or FiO₂

When you send blood gases to the laboratory make a note on the request slip about the fractional *inspired oxygen concentration* (FiO₂). In a person with healthy lungs the FiO₂ and the PaO₂ rise in parallel. However, if there is something wrong with the lungs, for instance pneumonia or asthma, then this parallel rise does not happen.

The balance between acids and bases

Since too much or too little hydrogen ion concentration or activity in the body disrupts cell metabolism, the balance has to be just right for the enzymes and protein pumps in cells to function properly.

In the body several chemical reactions are involved in acid–base balance, but the principal extracellular reaction involves a balance between carbon dioxide, water on one side of the equation and hydrogen ion and bicarbonate ion on the other.

$$H_2O + CO_2 \rightleftharpoons HCO_3^- + H^+$$

Each component is in *dynamic equilibrium* with the others. They balance each other in much the same way that a weighing scale does.

If you add CO_2 to the one side of the balance the pointer will swing towards a low pH (and higher hydrogen ion concentration). You can restore the balance to normal by either removing the CO_2, or adding HCO_3^- to the left side to counterbalance it. Similarly adding HCO_3^- to the left-hand pan will swing the pointer to a higher pH (and lower hydrogen ion concentration). You can restore the balance by either adding CO_2 to the right-hand pan, or removing HCO_3^- from the left hand pan.

Respiratory causes of acid–base disorders

Carbon dioxide (CO_2) is produced in mitochondria as a waste product of oxidative metabolism. The pressure exerted by CO_2 in arterial blood is about 40 mmHg (5.3 kPa) and in venous blood about 46 mmHg (6.1 kPa). If a patient fails to breathe deeply enough to *blow off* carbon dioxide as fast as the tissues produce it then the excess CO_2 dissolves in body water releasing hydrogen ion (a strong acid) and bicarbonate ion (a weak base) to cause a *respiratory acidaemia*. Conversely, if patients blow off carbon dioxide faster than they produce it, the hydrogen ion levels fall in the blood and the patient will have a *respiratory alkalaemia*.

It is commonly believed that hydrogen ion is 'blown off' as carbon dioxide, but this is a mistake because there is no hydrogen ion (H^+) in carbon dioxide (CO_2). Instead, the mitochondrial enzymes shuffle the highly reactive hydrogen ion around to eventually link it to oxygen to make water (H_2O).

How hypoventilation causes respiratory acidosis

Hypoventilation is caused by:

* a side-effect of the opioids:
* residual effects of muscle relaxants;
* sedation caused by benzodiazepines such as midazolam or diazepam.

While at rest we produce about 200 ml of CO_2 every minute. Our total body stores of carbon dioxide are about one hundred times this amount (20 litres). If the patient has been *hyperventilated* during their anaesthetic, their body stores of CO_2 become depleted, and bicarbonate ions accumulate in the blood. This is revealed by a reluctance to breathe up in the recovery room, and blood gases will show a respiratory alkalosis. However, the CO_2 soon builds up to normal levels. During this time give high concentrations of oxygen to compensate for the patient's diminished *minute volume*.

An uncommon cause of an acute respiratory alkalosis, with low arterial $PaCO_2$ levels, (*hypocarbia*) is interstitial pulmonary oedema. Fluid accumulating in the lung's interstitial space triggers a reflex to make the patient hyperventilate to blow-off CO_2. The causes of interstitial pulmonary oedema include fluid overload, acute or chronic cardiac failure, septicaemia, fat or gas emboli, gastric aspiration or early acute respiratory distress syndrome.

Metabolic causes of acid–base disorders

A metabolic acidosis occurs if the liver fails to metabolize lactic acid, or the kidney fails to excrete acids.

The causes include:

- hypoxia, where the tissues produce lactic acid faster than it can be metabolized;
- unstable diabetics, where keto-acids accumulate;
- septicaemia, where bacterial endotoxins have damaged the liver so that it cannot deal with organic acids as fast as normal;
- renal failure, where the kidney can't excrete the acids.

Metabolic alkalosis is uncommon. Usually it is the result of severe potassium depletion, or injudicious use of sodium bicarbonate. Massive blood transfusion may cause a metabolic alkalosis, because the liver metabolizes sodium citrate (used as an anti-coagulant in the stored blood) to sodium bicarbonate. Metabolic alkalosis becomes a clinical problem once the pH exceeds 7.55.

Is the acid–base disorder an acute or chronic problem?

Disturbances that occur within minutes or hours are known as *acute disturbances*. Others creep up slowly over days or weeks, and are known as *chronic disturbances*. Patients with acute disturbances have an abnormal hydrogen ion concentration (pH) in their arterial blood. In patients with chronic disturbances, the kidneys or lungs have adjusted the balance of CO_2 and HCO_3^- to ensure the patient's pH is normal.

What to monitor in acid–base disorders

- Blood pressure, pulse rate, temperature.
- ECG.
- Respiratory rate, tidal volume and minute volume.
- Urine output.

Prepare to take:

- Arterial blood gases: pH, hydrogen ion concentration, PaO_2, $PaCO_2$, and bicarbonate.
- Blood samples for sodium, potassium, chloride, urea, creatinine, bicarbonate, anion gap, lactate, and glucose.

How to manage an acid–base disorder

Get help from someone who understands this complex problem. Never use sodium bicarbonate to treat respiratory acidosis, not only is it inappropriate, but it will make the problem worse.

Dangers with bicarbonate

Sodium bicarbonate corrects a metabolic acidosis, but it is difficult to use and best reserved for patients near death. In general bicarbonate is only used for patients with an arterial pH < 7.12 who are not responding to therapy, as is the case of a diabetic with ketoacidosis who is not responding to insulin; or when the patient is not responding to catecholamines during cardiac arrest.

Problems with bicarbonate

* In patients who have a metabolic acidosis bicarbonate slows their respiratory rate, causing excessive carbon dioxide to build up in body fluids.
* It alters the shape of haemoglobin molecules so that they do not release oxygen to the tissues as readily.
* It takes some days for the kidneys to excrete the excess in the urine.

Diabetes

The incidence of diabetes is increasing in most countries. There are two principal forms of diabetes: type 1 and type 2 diabetes. These are two quite different diseases, with different causes, different natural histories, and requiring different management.

* *Type 1 diabetes*, formerly known as insulin-dependent diabetes mellitus (IDDM), is caused by insufficient insulin secretion; and occurs in about 10 per cent of diabetics.
* *Type 2 diabetes*, formerly known non-insulin-dependent diabetes mellitus (NIDDM), is caused by tissue resistance to the effects of insulin; and occurs in about 90 per cent of diabetics.

What is diabetes?

The World Health Organization (WHO) defines diabetes mellitus as 'a chronic disorder of carbohydrate, protein and fat metabolism caused by an absolute or relative insulin deficiency, fasting hyperglycaemia, glycosuria, and a striking tendency for atherosclerosis, microangiopathy, nephropathy and neuropathy'.

How surgery destabilizes diabetes

Surgical mortality rates are five times higher in diabetics than in non-diabetics. Surgery damages tissues. The injured tissues release biochemicals into the circulation irritating the already sick endothelial cells and the additional osmotic effect of hyperglycaemia is too much to bear. The sick endothelial cells retreat to form scattered heaps on the walls of blood vessels. Clots form in places they should not, small arterioles become blocked, and atheromatous plaques rupture leaving raw surfaces for platelets to adhere to and form clots. These processes are most noticeable in the small vessels in the eyes.

All these events give diabetics a much higher risk of suffering cardiac ischaemia, stroke (both haemorrhagic and embolic), venous thrombosis, renal dysfunction and disruption of blood flow to the surgical site.

Properly functioning insulin promotes wound healing, white cell function, phagocytosis of bacteria, clotting, and prevents fat breakdown that causes ketone production (Box 24.4). Postoperatively diabetics are at a higher risk of dying from primary infection, anastomotic breakdown, pneumonia, pulmonary emboli, and adverse cardiac and cerebrovascular events. All these problems can be traced back to insufficient insulin, excessive blood glucose concentrations, and tissue glycation.

Box 24.4 Insulin

Insulin has two principal functions. First, it packs any glucose, fat and amino acids that are excess to immediate needs into storage as glycogen, triglyceride and cellular protein respectively. Second, and more importantly insulin prevents glycogen and protein stores being raided unnecessarily to provide energy. Without insulin, the liver frenetically mobilizes glycogen and cellular protein stores back to glucose. As glucose is released into the circulation blood glucose levels rise sharply.

The triglyceride in fat cells (lipocytes) is not converted back to glucose, but released as fatty acids, ketones and glycerol. All the tissues (except for brain) can use these compounds as a fast food energy source, but like fast food it may become indigestible in large quantities and then ketones appear in the blood.

The problem with type 1 diabetes is too much glucose production, rather than too little uptake by the cells. In contrast, the problem in type 2 diabetes is that the cells can neither use nor store the glucose delivered to them.

In both types of diabetes excess glucose slowly sticks to connective tissue and cell membranes. This process is called glycation, which essentially means the tissues are turning to caramel. The endothelial linings of small blood vessels take the brunt of glycation. The eventual result is atherosclerosis everywhere, but most importantly in the eyes, heart, brain and kidneys.

Diabetes in the recovery room

Postoperatively there are two big risks for diabetics: hyperglycaemia and hypoglycaemia. The normal range of blood glucose concentrations is 3.5 to 5.5 mmol/L. In the recovery room the blood glucose concentration of normal people, especially if they are in pain, may exceed 14 mmol/L. It is well known that untreated hypoglycaemia rapidly causes brain damage. However, it is less well known that if the blood sugar in a diabetic exceeds 12 mmol/L in the recovery room the risks of postoperative infection, strokes, myocardial infarction, ischaemia and deep vein thrombosis rise more than sevenfold.

To prevent postoperative complications keep, the blood glucose levels within the normal range.

Type 1 diabetes

Before coming to theatre for major surgery type 1 diabetics should be stabilized on a continuous infusion of insulin and glucose. They need a baseline infusion of 150 grams of glucose over 24 hours. To this baseline infusion is added a continuous infusion of regular insulin equivalent to their normal total daily requirements. For example, if a patient normally takes 20 units of protamine zinc insulin in the morning, 12 units of regular insulin at lunch time, and 40 units of protamine zinc insulin at night, the total 24-hourly dose of insulin would be 20 + 12 + 40 = 72 units or 3 units per hour. This means the patient should come to theatre with an infusion of 50 grams of glucose running over 8 hours, and a regular insulin infusion of 3 units an hour. A sliding scale is not appropriate (Table 24.2).

Table 24.2 Insulins

Class	Example	Onset (hr)	Duration (hr)
Rapid-acting	Lispro	0.25	4–5
Short-acting	Neutral	0.5	6–8
Intermediate-acting	Isophane	1–2.5	16–24
Long-acting	Ultralente	2–4	24–36

Why sliding scales are harmful

The *sliding scale* technique of controlling blood glucose levels relies on tailoring the dose of insulin or glucose to the amount of glucose in either plasma or urine. This technique should be avoided, it chases the problem and allows dangerous swings in blood glucose. Following surgery it only takes a few minutes of high blood glucose levels to harm a diabetic patient's endothelium. By the time you discover the hyperglycaemia, the damage may already be done. A proper plan prevents hyper- or hypoglycaemia.

Check the blood glucose frequently when you have a diabetic patient in the recovery room.

Why nerves are damaged

If a patient has had diabetes for more than 5 years, especially if the diabetes is not well controlled, they are prone to developing peripheral and autonomic neuropathy. Patients with malfunctioning autonomic nerves respond unpredictably to fluid loads. They become hypotensive if you sit them up, and they may not feel chest pain (*angina*) if myocardial ischaemia occurs.

Type 2 diabetes

Type 2 diabetes is controlled with oral hypoglycaemic drugs. Most type 2 diabetics use metformin, but sometimes they need an alternative drug, or a supplement with one of the sulfonylureas: gliclazide, glimepiride, or glibenclamide; or one of the glitazones such as pioglitazone. Some patients may also be taking a supplementary drug, sitagliptin. All these drugs are usually omitted on the day of surgery.

Problems with metformin

- Metformin decreases glucose absorption from the gut, increases glucose entry into cells and lowers the appetite. Lactic acid is produced by hypoxic tissue. Metformin prevents the liver metabolizing lactic acid efficiently. For this reason it is stopped 36 hours before surgery where tourniquets or vascular clamps are used (e.g. leg surgery), big operations where lots of tissue is damage (e.g. total hip replacements) or where large blood transfusions are necessary (e.g. abdominal aneurism repairs).
- Metformin induced lactic acidosis may present in the recovery room. The first sign will be a rapidly rising respiratory rate.

If a type 2 diabetic becomes acidotic, then suspect metformin as the cause.

- Metformin-induced lactic acidosis is lethal in 50 per cent of cases and needs urgent and expert management.
- Metformin may cause acute renal failure if the patient receives X-ray radio-contrast media for angiography or intravenous pyelograms. To prevent this metformin is ceased 48 hours before the procedure and for 5 days after it.
- In patients taking metformin it is better to avoid large volumes of Hartmann's solution because it contains lactate.

Diabetic patients in recovery room

When managing diabetic in the recovery room aim to:
- keep the blood glucose concentrations within a range of 6–10 mmol/L;
- prevent, detect and treat hyperglycaemia and hypoglycaemia;
- prevent large swings in blood glucose concentrations;
- give enough insulin to prevent ketosis;
- detect and treat lactic acidosis;
- prevent and treat hypokalaemia, hypomagnesaemia and hypophosphataemia.

Why hypoglycaemia is harmful

Hypoglycaemia occurs when blood glucose concentration is less than 3.5 mmol/L. Healthy people experience symptoms of an adrenergic alarm response once their blood glucose falls below 2.5 mmol/L. These include tachycardia, feeling alarmed and light-headed, pallor, palpitations, sweating and double vision. As it progresses patients can become confused, agitated or aggressive, with slurred or confused speech. They soon convulse and lapse into coma. If blood glucose concentrations fall below 2 mmol/L then hypoglycaemia causes irreversible brain damage and death.

Risk factors for hypoglycaemia include: type 1 diabetics, alcoholics, neonates, those with septicaemia, and severe liver disease. In the recovery room the warning signs of hypoglycaemia may be camouflaged by β-blockers, residual anaesthesia or opioids. For this reason measure the blood glucose levels of all those at risk as soon as they are admitted to the recovery room, then every half hour thereafter, and just before discharge to the ward.

Every recovery room
needs a glucose meter.

How to manage hypoglycaemia

If the blood glucose is 3 mmol/L or less then give 30 grams of glucose intravenously into a large vein. You should see an improvement in the patient's conscious state within 2 to 3 minutes. Repeat the dose after 5 minutes. Start a 6-hourly litre of 5 per cent glucose. Check the blood glucose levels at 20-minute intervals until they stabilize at about 5 mmol/L. You may need to change the rate of the glucose drip.

Hints

- Dextrose is the American name for glucose.
- Use 300 ml of 10% glucose or 600 ml of 5% glucose.
- One litre of 5% glucose contains 50 grams of glucose.
- One litre of 10% glucose contains 100 grams of glucose.
- Keep a litre of 10% glucose with your emergency drugs.
- Glucose is cheaper and safer than glucagon.

Why hyperglycaemia is harmful

Hyperglycaemia occurs when the blood glucose concentration rises above 10 mmol/L. Normally blood glucose concentrations lie within the range of 3.5–5.5 mmol/L. With the physiological stresses of surgery, even in normal patients the glucose concentration may rise to 18 mmol/L or more. Generally the higher the stress levels (pain, hypovolaemia, or hypoxia) the higher the blood glucose concentrations.

*Hyperglycaemia is a sign
of a stressed patient.*

In diabetics, within 20 minutes of their blood glucose concentration exceeding 12 mmol/L their vascular endothelium is damaged. Non-diabetics whose endothelium is healthy are not as easily affected.

Hyperglycaemia in a diabetic immediately after surgery is a disaster. The combination of high blood glucose, catecholamines, and *cytokines* released from injured tissue, wreak havoc on already diseased endothelial cells. Within 20 minutes they are so damaged there is an immediate risk of myocardial ischaemia or stroke.

*Keep the blood glucose
of diabetics < 12 mmol/L.*

Hyperglycaemia in the immediate postoperative period carries over into the ward to cause a 15-fold increase in risk of vascular disasters such as stroke, myocardial infarction, deep vein thrombosis, and renal impairment in the first postoperative week. These effects are additional to the increased risks diabetics already have of infection, osmotic diuresis and poor wound healing.

How to manage hyperglycaemia

Measure the blood glucose concentration when the patient is admitted into the recovery room and check their urine for ketones. If their blood glucose is above 12 mmol/L then give one unit of regular insulin for every 10 kg of lean body mass. Notify the patient's physician so that control can be continued in the ward.

Hints

+ Insulin requirements usually rise in the recovery room.
+ One unit of regular insulin (in a stable adult diabetic) lowers the blood glucose concentration by about 1.5 mmol/L, but after surgery one unit of insulin only decreases the blood glucose levels by about 1 mmol/L.
+ Maintain the glucose infusion at a constant rate of 50 grams 8-hourly and vary the insulin dose. Not the other way around.
+ 10 grams of intravenous glucose raises the blood glucose in an adult by about 1.5–2 mmol/L.
+ Ketosis is a sign of insulin lack, and not excessive glucose. If your patient is ketotic then check the blood sugar levels and give additional insulin. Initially one unit for one mmol/L of glucose above 12.
+ Monitor potassium levels because insulin causes potassium to enter cells, resulting in hypokalaemia.
+ To convert mmol/L of glucose to mg/100 ml multiply the mmol/L by 18.

- Although insulin is adsorbed by glass and plastic, there is no need to initially prime the apparatus with glucose and insulin.
- Never use sliding scales to control insulin doses.

What is hyperosmolar plasma?

Poorly controlled diabetics become much worse after surgery. This places them at risk of a hyperosmolar crisis. A hyperosmolar crisis occurs when the blood glucose rises beyond 25 mmol. The concentrated glucose in the extracellular fluid osmotically sucks water out of cells. Middle-aged and elderly diabetics are at the highest risk. Initially the brain and kidney suffer most.

Ketosis may or may not be present. The urine output rises, and as the brain cells shrivel the patient becomes confused, sleepy and may convulse. You can check the stability of the patient's diabetes over the previous 2–3 months by measuring their glycolysated haemoglobin levels (HbA1c). 5–7 per cent is 35–53 mmol/mol, 8 per cent is 64 mmol/mol, and 9 per cent is 75 mmol/mol.

Postoperatively all diabetic patients who have been starved for procedures must have their ketones checked as soon as possible and 4 hourly thereafter. For further reading on the management of post-surgical diabetic patients please refer to https://www.drtamaraeichel.com.au.

Obesity

Many obese patients present for surgery either directly as a result of their obesity, *bariatric procedures*, or incidentally for other operations. Bariatric patients are more likely to have major joint replacement and back surgery. Procedures such as high gastric reduction, ileojejunal bypass, and laparoscopic stomach banding are also performed to treat life-threatening obesity.

Problems arising in the recovery room increase progressively and steeply once a patient's BMI > 40.

Body mass index

Body mass index (BMI) is one way of classifying obesity. It is not ideal because it does not assess muscle mass. A super-fit body builder may well be classified as obese on the BMI scale (Table 24.3).

$$BMI = \frac{\text{weight in kg}}{\text{height in metres}^2}$$

Most very obese people have life-threatening comorbid chronic diseases, such as hypertension, heart disease, diabetes, and *dyslipidaemias*.

Table 24.3 Body mass index

Status	BMI (kg/m2)
Starving	< 17
Underweight	17–19
Normal	19–25
Overweight	25–30
Obese	30–35
Very obese	35–40
Morbidly obese	40–50
Super-morbidly obese	> 50

How to manage obese patients

Obese patients weighing more than 150 kg need special reinforced beds, trolleys and lifting apparatus. Special pillows are available on the market. If you do not have these pillows you will need a great number of towels which can be rolled to support the vulnerable parts of the obese body against the trolley sides for example. Have these available before the patient comes to the recovery room.[3,4]

Hover mattresses, e.g. HoverMatt®, are useful for transferring the patients.

Book an ICU bed for those patients with BMI greater than 50 or those with pre-existing cardiac or respiratory disease, CO_2 retention, or where the surgery is expected to last for more than 3 hours.

Following open abdominal and even laparoscopic procedures consider admitting morbidly obese patients (BMI > 40) overnight for continuing observation. Obese patients seem to tolerate laparoscopy quite well.

Respiratory problems

Preoperative respiratory function tests do not always predict postoperative problems.[5] Obstructive sleep apnoea (OSA) and obesity hypoventilation syndrome (OHS) are common problems. Two weeks of continuous positive airway pressure (CPAP) can correct the abnormal respiratory drive in these patients. Longer periods improve other aspects of their abnormal physiology and reduce their risk of postoperative problems. This is only possible for planned procedures. Those coming for emergency surgery are very high risk patients.

With their low *functional residual capacity*, obese patients are vulnerable to postoperative hypoxia. Plan to send them to HDU or intensive care once they leave recovery room where they can be given give supplemental oxygen, particularly at night.

Morbidly obese patients have kilos of fat lying across their chests and bellies. If they lie on their back their fat sits on their chest like a sandbag, which makes breathing difficult.

This becomes a problem especially after major abdominal or thoracic surgery. Once obese patients are fully awake, prop them up at about 45° on their trolley. This move takes the weight off their chest and diaphragm and lets them deep breathe and cough more effectively. Sitting them up also reduces the risk of aspiration.

Obese patients have precarious airways that easily obstruct. Access to their pharynx is made difficult by a fat face, big breasts, short necks, limited cervical spine movement, high anterior larynx, and restricted mouth opening. This is especially true for obese men who often have a pad of very solid fat at the back of their necks making neck extension difficult. If the obese patient comes to recovery room with a laryngeal mask take special care with this airway and if possible turn the patient to the side as well as sitting them up. Laryngeal masks can cause problems in obese people. If they regurgitate the laryngeal mask can divert stomach contents down the trachea.

Encourage obese patients to breathe deeply, and cough. These manoeuvres blast open small airways increasing the functional residual capacity and improving oxygenation. Never tip obese patients head down. As their intra-abdominal fat pushes their diaphragm up it squashes the bases of their lungs. They will almost immediately become hypoxaemic, and usually panic. In a head-down position they are also more likely to regurgitate and aspirate stomach contents.

Sleep apnoea

Snoring, with or without overt *sleep apnoea*, occurs in most morbidly obese people. During sleep they get a bradycardia when they stop breathing and a tachycardia when they start again. In the recovery room these patients need constant attention to maintain an unobstructed airway. If they start to snore then protect the patency of their airway. A nasopharyngeal airway is often useful to bypass their floppy soft palate. Many obese patients use a CPAP mask at home, and in some cases they will bring them to recovery room. This equipment can be effectively applied once the patient is fully awake and sitting up.

Deep vein thrombosis

The perioperative risk of venothromboembolism (VTE) in obese patients is more than twice that of normal patients. This particularly applies to those with *android obesity* ('beer bellies'). Start their leg exercises in the recovery room. Ensure they have received low molecular-weight heparin prophylaxis, and have their compression stockings properly fitted. Use sequential compression devices if these are available.

Predisposing factors include polycythaemia, prolonged immobilization leading to venous stasis, increased intra-abdominal pressure retarding venous flow from the legs, cardiac failure, and decreased fibrinolytic activity with increased concentrations of fibrinogen. VTE is the commonest complication of obesity surgery with an incidence of about 5 per cent.

Gastro-oesophageal reflux

Obese people often have as much as 75 per cent more fluid in their stomach than a normal patient. Even if they report no heartburn or reflux most obese patients have hiatus hernias, and this puts them at risk of regurgitation and pulmonary aspiration. The risk of aspiration is augmented by raised intra-abdominal pressure exerted by the mass of fat in their abdominal wall and cavity. A prudent approach would be to neutralize their stomach acids with oral pantoprazole (or ranitidine) 2 hours before surgery, and 0.3 M sodium citrate 30 ml orally just before induction. Aspiration of gastric contents into the lungs remains a danger well into the postoperative period after the patient returns to the wards.

Cardiac and circulatory problems

You will need especially large blood pressure cuffs. Normal-sized cuffs either will not fit, or if they do they overestimate the blood pressure. Obese patients have a lower relative blood volume (50 ml/kg) than a normal person (60 ml/kg). Because their large capacitance veins are squashed by fat, and are less able to distend to hold additional fluids, they are at risk of pulmonary oedema if given injudicious intravenous fluids.

When very fat people lie flat, the huge mass of fat in their abdominal cavity tissue falls back to tamponade their inferior vena cava. With the impeded venous return to the heart, their cardiac output plummets. Some super-morbidly obese patients cannot lie flat, and panic if they attempt to do so. They may even have a cardiac arrest. Have assistance at hand to help the patient sit up again if they begin to panic.

Nerve damage

Obese patients have a higher risk of intraoperative neural compression injury and pressure sores, so check pressure areas and movement and feeling in limbs. If the patient has been in the lithotomy position where there is risk of stretching the sciatic nerve then check that they can bend their knees and flap their feet up and down.

Transport

Transport morbidly obese patients on their beds. Limit the number of transfers between beds, trolleys and tables to the minimum. Use a HoverMatt® if you have it available. Occasionally you may need to use special hydraulic lifting devices to manoeuvre super-morbidly obese patients around. Remember that many nurses have injured their backs while lifting patients. Do not attempt to move them on to hospital trolleys because it is possible the patient may accidentally slip on to the floor.

Drugs and doses

Calculate the drug dose in obese patients on their estimated *lean body weight* (LBW), not on their actual weight. Their lean body weight is approximately their height in centimetres minus their weight in kilograms. Be especially careful with drugs with low therapeutic indices, because their toxic dose is a hair's breadth from the therapeutic dose; these drugs include digoxin, lithium, dipyridamole, and the aminoglycosides.

In some cases fatty changes in liver may not be reflected in routine liver function tests. Drugs such as opioids and others metabolized by the liver may be cleared slowly, requiring longer dosing intervals and smaller incremental doses.

In the recovery room it is best to give drugs intravenously. If it is necessary to give intramuscular drugs, use special long needles otherwise 'intramuscular injections' may never reach the muscle, and just stay in poorly perfused fat.[6]

Benzodiazepines

Benzodiazepines do cause problems in the obese by exacerbating the effects of the *sleep apnoea syndromes*.

Opioids

Using opioids is particularly hazardous in morbidly obese patients. There is a danger when sedated obese patients, with reduced respiratory drive, are propped up in bed. When they fall asleep and their head flops forward to obstruct their airway they quickly and silently die (*Ondine's curse*).

Sleep apnoea is a cause
of unexpected postoperative death.

References

1. **Hooper VD, Chard R**, *et al.* (2010) ASPAN's evidence-based clinical practice guideline. *Journal of PeriAnesthesia Nursing* **26**(6):346–365.
2. **Grogono AW** (2011) *Stewart's strong ion difference.* <http://www.acid-base.com/strongion.php>
3. **Schumann R** (2011) Anaesthesia for bariatric surgery. *Best Practice & Research Clinical Anaesthesiology* **25**(1):83–93.
4. **Kirkham L, Thomas M** (2011) Anaesthesia in obese patients. *British Journal of Medicine* **72**(9):515–520.
5. **Simha V**, *et al.* (2019) Perioperative Glucose Control in Patients with Diabetes Undergoing Elective Surgery. *JAMA* **321**(4):399–400.
6. **Hamblin PS** (2019) SGLT Inhibitors Increase the Risk of Diabetic Ketoacidosis Developing in the Community and During Hospital Admission. *J Clin Endocrinol Metab* **104**(8):3077–3087.

Further Reading

Corrie KR, Chilliston S, *et al.* (2011) The effect of obesity and anesthetic maintenance regimen on postoperative pulmonary complications. *Anaesthesia and Analgesia* **113**(1):4–6.

Mace HS, Paech MJ, *et al.* (2011) Obesity and obstetric anaesthesia. *Anaesthesia and Intensive Care* **39**(4):559–570.

Chapter 25

Chronic disorders

Introduction

Diseases covered in this chapter are not found elsewhere in this book. They were chosen because they are either common, like alcoholism, important, because errors in management can cause harm, for example, hepato-renal syndrome, or the disease represents useful principles applicable to many other diseases.

ASA classification is shown in Box 25.1.

Box 25.1 **The ASA classification**

Unfit patients frequently come to surgery. Their illness may be a result of their lifestyle of smoking, drinking or over-eating, or an acquired or inherited disease. In the 1940s the American Society of Anesthesiologists published a scale known as the ASA class to grade the fitness of patients presenting for anaesthesia. The classification has proved remarkably robust and remains one of the better predictors of surgical and anaesthetic outcome.

ASA I Fit for their age.

ASA II Mild systemic disease not interfering with daily activities.

ASA III Severe disease interfering with daily activities.

ASA IV Severe disease that is a constant threat to life

ASA V Moribund. Submitted for surgery in desperation.

ASA V1 Organ donor.

E. The letter E is added if the operation is an emergency; e.g. ASA IV E

Adapted with permission from Owens, W.D., Felts, J.A., Spitznagel, E.L. Jr. ASA physical status classification: a study of consistency of ratings. *Anesthesiology*, 49: 239–243. Copyright © 1978, Wolters Kluwer Health. DOI: 10.1097/00000542-197810000-00003

AIDS/HIV

Those at high risk of HIV/AIDS include homosexual and bisexual men and their partners, older haemophiliacs, intravenous drug users and children of affected mothers. Heterosexually transmitted HIV is common in many countries. In some poorer countries it occurs tragically, because of inadequately sterilized medical or dental equipment and where syringes and needles are reused.

HIV (*human immunodeficiency virus*) is the quiescent phase of the disease. Most of these patients are taking immunosuppressive drugs and are at risk of acquiring nosocomial infections. Use standard precautions to protect the patient and yourself. The biggest risk to staff is through needlestick injuries.

AIDS (*acquired immune deficiency syndrome*) is the active phase of the disease where the patient is infected with one or more of a bizarre variety of organisms. These patients are usually frail, often with severe lung infections and recent weight loss. Patients with end-stage AIDS seldom come to surgery and are rarely encountered in the recovery room. Read more about HIV and AIDs in Chapter 28 on infection control.

Alcoholics

Alcoholism occurs when a person's drinking is either damaging their health, or causing disruption to their lives, or the lives of their families and associates. It is a hidden disease and far more prevalent than suspected. In Australia and the UK and many other parts of the world it is a big problem affecting about 15 per cent of the adult population. It is a major cause of perioperative morbidity, and the elderly are not exempt. Alcoholism hides behind diseases such as hypertension, dilated cardiac myopathy, atrial fibrillation, dementia, postoperative delirium and liver disease.

People who drink more than four standard alcoholic drinks a day tend to be tolerant to many sedative drugs. As they emerge from anaesthesia they may be restless, and move about in a semi-purposeful manner before they awake properly. They may try to sit up, and open their eyes before spitting out their airway. During this time they appear dazed, will not respond when you speak to them, and occasionally become violent. Do not remove their airway; let them take it out themselves.

Alcoholics are susceptible to spontaneous hypoglycaemia, especially when physiologically stressed after surgery. If they remain mentally obtunded, or become sweaty or restless then check that their blood glucose level is greater than 4 mmol/L. If not, give 20 ml of 50 per cent glucose slowly through a freely running drip into a large vein.

Thin alcoholics can become hypothermic during surgery. Do not discharge them until their temperature is greater than 36°C.

Drug addicts

Marijuana

Marijuana smokers can emerge from anaesthesia in a very restless and combative way. Use clonidine 150 micrograms in 10 ml of normal saline and give 2 ml boluses, as required, to calm them. Check their blood pressure between doses. They also sometimes cough excessively after general anaesthesia. This settles quickly with a vaporizer of salbutamol 5 mg in 5 ml of saline.

Heroin

Following general anaesthetics heroin addicts are susceptible to respiratory depression in the recovery room. Their respiratory centres remain partially insensitive to rising carbon dioxide levels for 3 or more months after their last 'hit'.

If you give naloxone to a using heroin addict it may trigger acute *opioid withdrawal syndrome*. This presents with abdominal cramps, sweating, itch, and lacrimation and simulates all sorts of postsurgical disasters. Addicts too, are entitled to good postoperative analgesia. Titrate opioid analgesics intravenously to achieve an effect. Some recovering addicts are apprehensive that perioperative opioids will reignite their addiction. They are not wrong to think this, it can happen. If possible substitute opioids with NSAIDs or local blocks.

Cocaine and amphetamine

Cocaine, amphetamine (speed, ecstasy) and methamphetamine users can become alarmingly hypotensive after surgery. Continual use of these drugs depletes neuronal stores of noradrenaline. Consequently with the stress of surgery there may not be enough noradrenaline stored in the nerve endings to maintain the blood pressure. The blood pressure of cocaine and amphetamine users responds readily to normal doses of direct-acting vasopressors such as adrenaline, but they may need additional hydrocortisone supplements to sustain the response. If they are regular users of cocaine they may not respond to indirect-acting vasopressors, drugs such as ephedrine or metaraminol.

Many intravenous drug users have hepatitis C (or occasionally hepatitis B). Take precautions and wear gloves when you are recovering them. Chronic liver dysfunction prolongs the sedative effects of anaesthetic drugs, which may require patients to stay longer than usual in the recovery room. They also have an increased risk of bleeding, and a higher susceptibility to infection.

Epilepsy

Epilepsy is caused by uncoordinated, spontaneous and uncontrolled neuronal discharge somewhere within the brain. The type of seizure depends on where the abnormality occurs. To prevent perioperative seizures epileptics should take their usual medication on the day of surgery.

There are two types of seizures: a one-off *isolated seizure* associated with fevers, head trauma, hypoxia, hypoglycaemia; and *recurrent epileptic seizures*. An isolated seizure may occur in men after transurethral resection of the prostate if water from the irrigation fluid enters their circulation.

Epileptics sometimes have a fit in the recovery room, and the seizure can take many forms. Frank seizures are obvious, but a subtle seizure in a semicomatose or paralysed patient may only be revealed by twitching around the mouth. Seizures cause brain damage and must be controlled quickly. Seizures respond well to benzodiazepines such as diazepam. All seizures respond well to thiopental. If this is available in your recovery room offer it to your anaesthetist. He or she may use it to stabilize the seizures while assessing the situation and starting other measures such as a phenytoin infusion.

Facial twitching in a comatose
patient may indicate an epileptic seizure.

Drugs that may trigger seizures are propofol, sevoflurane, methohexital, pethidine, and anti-cholinergics. Pethidine, with its neurotoxic metabolite nor-pethidine, is a major offender, particularly if the patient has renal impairment.

Liver disease

The liver is the largest organ in the body. It is a factory for many biochemicals including coagulation factors and it is the headquarters for carbohydrate, fat and protein production and breakdown. Its enzyme systems metabolize many drugs, and toxins. The liver only needs about 20 per cent of its metabolic capacity to fulfil its day-to-day functions. The remaining, or spare metabolic capacity, is reserved to break down lactic acid produced during exercise. Postoperatively the liver mobilizes essential glucose from protein and glycogen stores.

In patients with liver disease spontaneous hypoglycaemia can occur without warning. Check their blood glucose levels when they are admitted to the recovery room.

The liver's oxygen supply comes from the hepatic artery. During general anaesthetics the hepatic artery blood flow may halve and reduce the liver's oxygenation. A diseased liver tolerates this poorly. After general anaesthetics it is not surprising that those with liver disease are slower to metabolize drugs and this prolongs their recovery.

The liver metabolizes many anaesthetic drugs. When tourniquets or vascular clamps are released large amounts of lactic acid from hypoxic tissues flood into the circulation. A healthy liver is able to metabolize lactic acid quickly, but not if the patient is acidotic, hypoxic, hypoglycaemic or cold, or they have been taking metformin for diabetes.

Metformin-induced lactic acidosis

Metformin, used to treat type 2 diabetes, blocks the liver's ability to metabolize lactic acid. Usually metformin is withdrawn 36 hours before surgery where it is anticipated that tourniquets or vascular clamps will be used, or large amounts of tissue damage are expected.

An acute lactic acidosis can present in the recovery room. If it occurs it is potentially fatal and more than half the patients die. Lactic acidosis is more likely if the liver is already affected by cirrhosis, jaundice, gallbladder disease, Gram-negative sepsis, or where volatile anaesthetic agents have reduced liver arterial blood flow during long operations.

Patients with a developing lactic acidosis have a rising respiratory rate, they feel breathless, and want to sit up to get their breath. They develop a tachycardia, skin flushing and may start to sweat.

Send blood for blood gas analysis, lactate levels, electrolytes and urea, blood glucose concentration, and full blood examination. Lactic acidosis becomes severe once lactic acid levels rise higher than 3 mmol/L.

The patient will need to go to ICU. Management of metformin-induced lactic acidosis includes correcting hypovolaemia, and oxygen therapy. Using bicarbonate to correct the acidosis is hazardous.

Managing patients with liver disease

Principles include:

+ Keep patients well oxygenated, and if necessary maintain tissue perfusion with an inotrope.
+ If opioids are given, watch for respiratory depression. This may cause acidaemia and hypoxia, which are not well tolerated by a sick liver.
+ Keep patients with liver disease warm.
+ Suspect clotting factor deficiency when a patient with liver disease has prolonged bleeding from venous or arterial puncture sites, or the surgical site.

Hepato-renal syndrome

To avoid renal failure in jaundiced patients (hepato-renal syndrome) the aims of management are to:

+ keep their urine output above 1 ml/kg/hr;
+ insert a urinary catheter to monitor the urine output;
+ ensure hydration is adequate. Give at least 2 litres of crystalloid at 6-hourly intervals;
+ treat systemic infection with appropriate antibiotics.

Neither mannitol nor furosemide improve the prognosis and may be harmful.

Multiple myeloma

Multiple myeloma is a relentlessly progressive bone marrow plasma cell tumour. Patients often have fragile vertebra and ribs, so move and position them gently. The excessive protein they excrete can damage their kidneys, so keep their blood volume normal, and do not allow them to become hypotensive or dehydrated. Their plasma is often syrupy and protein-laden, placing them at risk of deep vein thrombosis. Prophylaxis against deep vein thrombosis depends principally on adequate fluid replacement, doing stir-up exercises to prevent venous stasis, and giving a low molecular-weight heparin, such as enoxaparin. Graded compression stockings are helpful.

Musculoskeletal disease

Patients with a wide variety of musculoskeletal disease and myopathies are susceptible to malignant hyperthermia. This may present in the recovery room so monitor their temperature, and watch for the signs of sweating, rising respiratory rate (reflecting hypercarbia) and tachycardia.

Patients with muscular dystrophy are weak. They require smaller amounts of all anaesthetic agents than normal patients and are especially vulnerable to the residual effects of muscle relaxants. Make sure they can sustain a 5-second head lift from the pillow, and that they can deep breathe and cough before the anaesthetist leaves the recovery room. Where possible, use regional blockade for pain relief. If you need to use opioids then give increments of about one-fifth of the estimated dose and watch for slowing respiratory rate and depth before repeating.

Normal doses of muscle relaxants may overwhelm patients with low muscle mass. Watch for signs of inadequate reversal; this is especially likely to occur as the neostigmine wears off about 45 minutes after it was given. Use sugammadex if you have it or give a second dose of neostigmine. Start with a half dose of neostigmine and atropine or glycopyrronium bromide and monitor the effects with a 5-second head lift.

Patients with connective tissue disorders often have thin atrophic skin and pressure sores are common especially if they have been lying on the operating table for some time. It is so easy to tear their fragile skin if you drag them across a bed sheet, or tear off adhesive dressings carelessly.

Myasthenia gravis

Myasthenia gravis (MG) is a chronic autoimmune disease characterized by episodes of muscle weakness. It is caused by an autoimmune attack on acetylcholine receptors, so that nerve impulses cannot reach the muscles. It mainly affects muscles innervated by the cranial nerves. It is treated with anticholinergic drugs such as pyridostigmine.

Occasionally patients with rapidly progressing MG undergo a thymectomy in order to relieve the symptoms of the disease. Usually these patients need ventilatory support for a few days after surgery and are transferred directly from the operating theatre to ICU.

Many patients with MG are intermittently treated, over the years, with huge doses of prednisolone. They may need hydrocortisone supplement if their blood pressure falls while they are in the recovery room.

Avoid benzodiazepines, such as midazolam or diazepam, in patients with MG. These drugs make patients extremely weak, and at risk of aspiration. Opioids are safe, but reduce the dose in line with their reduced muscle mass. Other drugs likely to exacerbate MG symptoms are gentamicin, β-blockers, and calcium channel blockers. If a patient with MG drops their blood pressure, then consider giving 100 mg of hydrocortisone.

The weakness in patients with MG is treated with one of the anti-cholinesterase drugs. These drugs include pyridostigmine, neostigmine or physostigmine. If a patient becomes weak while in the recovery room, it is difficult to know whether they are having a *cholinergic crisis* caused by too much anti-cholinesterase, or a *myasthenic crisis* where the patient has not received enough anti-cholinesterase. The two conditions can be separated if the anaesthetist gives the rapid-acting anti-cholinesterase, edrophonium 10 mg IV slowly over 5 minutes. If the patient gets stronger then it is a myasthenic crisis, if they get weaker then it is a cholinergic crisis. In the latter case the anaesthetist may need to support the patient's breathing with a *bag and mask* for a few minutes until the drug has worn off.

Eaton–Lambert syndrome

Eaton–Lambert syndrome is an immune mediated disease, with similar features to myasthenia gravis that occurs in some patients with small-cell carcinoma of the lung. It occurs if *acetylcholine* is not released from nerve terminals and the muscle weakness does not respond to anti-cholinesterases.

Multiple sclerosis

Multiple sclerosis (MS) is a slow progressive episodic disease caused by patchy demyelination of nerve fibres in the brain and spinal cord.

The main problems in the recovery room with patients with MS are laryngeal incompetence predisposing to aspiration, and autonomic instability causing erratic fluctuations in blood pressure and pulse rates.

Fever triggers severe relapses; even a rise in temperature as small as 0.5°C causes their condition to worsen dramatically. Warn ward staff to monitor postoperative temperatures carefully, and treat fever aggressively.

Although general and neuraxial anaesthesia are safe in patients with MS, spinal and epidural anaesthesia are usually avoided. MS often worsens temporarily after surgery, and these neuraxial blocks will be inevitably blamed even though there is no evidence to support this assumption.

Myotonic dystrophy

Myotonic dystrophies are a group of inherited genetic disorders that cause selective muscle weakness. They tend to progress as the years pass. The most common is myotonic dystrophy (*Steinhart's disease*)which can occur at any age and predominately affects distal muscles. Patients with muscular dystrophy are susceptible to malignant hyperthermia. Monitor their temperature and report it to the anaesthetists immediately if their temperature rises beyond 37.4°C. Patients suffering from myotonic dystrophy are highly sensitive to muscle relaxants and may develop signs of residual paralysis in the recovery room. They also have great difficulty in coughing effectively.

Paget's disease

Paget's disease is a chronic disease that causes the bones in elderly adults to become honeycombed. Localized areas of bone become hyperactive, and are replaced with highly vascular porous bony tissue. Since most patients have no symptoms, the diagnosis is easily missed on preoperative assessment. These people typically have a prominent forehead, and a prominent tibial ridge. They shunt large volumes of blood from their arteries straight to their veins, bypassing tissues. They need a high cardiac output simply to maintain their blood pressure. Patients with Paget's disease become hypoxaemic easily, so continue supplemental oxygen in the ward. Be prepared for overwhelming blood loss following orthopaedic surgery.

Parkinson's disease

Parkinson's disease is a slowly progressive degenerative CNS disorder usually affecting older men. It has three main features: slow movement, muscular rigidity, and resting tremor. Because they cannot move quickly to readjust their posture, people with Parkinson's disease are particularly prone to falls, and often come to surgery to repair the damage. In the recovery room these patients are at risk of aspiration and are unable to mount an effective cough. Those with advanced disease are usually frail. Urinary retention can also cause a problem.

Severe Parkinson's disease is often treated with the dopaminergic drugs, levodopa and carbidopa. They may develop arrhythmias or hypertension in recovery room, because their adrenergic nerve endings are chocked full of noradrenaline, waiting to be released when triggered even by a trivial stimulus. Their blood pressures can surge without warning. Monitor them with an ECG and be prepared to give a β-blocker, such as metoprolol, to control tachyarrhythmias.

Take care not to give drugs with antidopaminergic activity, such as metoclopramide, droperidol or prochlorperazine, to control nausea. These drugs will render the patient rigid and unable to move (*acute Parkinsonian crisis*). This is treated with intravenous benzatropine. Ondansetron is safe for them. Patients are also prone to unexpected drops in blood pressure, attacks of breathlessness and anxiety. Rotigotine is a dopaminergic patch which is useful.[1] Opiates, especially fentanyl increase their rigidity. A case of severe rigidity on emergence from anaesthesia has been treated with crushed co-careldopa and amantadine through a nasogastric tube.[2]

Peptic ulceration

Peptic ulcer disease (PUD) is often exacerbated by surgery. It can also occur acutely in accident victims. Over the perioperative period patients with peptic ulcers or reflux oesophagitis should be covered with a proton pump inhibitor such as pantoprazole. Ranitidine, a 5-HT3 antagonist, is often used because it can be given intravenously, but it is not as effective as the protein pump inhibitors.

In the recovery room keep patients with PUD on their sides until they are fully conscious and able to care for their own airway.

Phaeochromocytoma

Phaeochromocytomas are tumours that secrete catecholamines. The main problems following their resection are hypovolaemia and hypotension in the recovery room. They sometimes need surprising amounts of colloid or blood to maintain their blood pressure. If the tumour has been active for more than a few months the patient may also have a cardiomyopathy. In this case the blood pressure and cardiac output may need to be supported with inotropes.

Uncommonly a patient may come to surgery with an unsuspected phaeochromo-cytoma. Induction of anaesthesia is an unintended and sometimes alarming provocation. Patients abruptly develop the traditional signs of hypertension, pallor, and palpitations.

Their systolic blood pressure may exceed 300 mmHg. The operation is usually postponed and the patient sent to the recovery room for further management. See 'Principles of management of hypertension', page 285.

Porphyria

Porphyrias are a family of inherited diseases of errors in the synthesis of haeme, the porphyrin unit of haemoglobin. It is more common in Nordic people who have carried it with them as they migrated to other parts of the world. The biochemical precursors of haeme are toxic, and cause a plethora of confusing symptoms: acute abdominal pain, vomiting, neuropathies, epilepsy, psychiatric disturbance, and even coma. Surgical stress, and anaesthetic drugs, especially barbiturates, such as thiopental, may trigger all three types of hepatic porphyria.

Psychiatric disease

Brains get sick too. At some time in their lives more than 20 per cent of the population suffer from some form of mental illness (including dementia) and 4 per cent are severely disabled by it. Many patients are taking psychotropic medication that interacts with anaesthetic drugs and analgesics.

Anxiety is part of a spectrum of emotions that blends into fear, agitation, panic and terror. Do not dismiss these emotions lightly. They are associated with neurohormonal responses that trigger hypertension, myocardial ischaemia, and arrhythmias. Acutely anxious patients profit from an anxiolytic premedication such as midazolam 15 mg orally 30 minutes before coming to theatre.

Patients with chronic anxiety disorders are often taking psychotropic medication and there is a high comorbidity with other psychiatric conditions especially alcohol, cigarette and drug abuse, which they use to self-medicate to numb their anxiety.

Phobias are disproportionately severe responses to a potentially threatening stimulus. Needle phobias and mask phobias are common, and can cause panic ending in a *vasovagal reaction* where the patient develops bradycardia and faints. There is no point in trying to overcome phobias with logical reasoning; it never succeeds. In the recovery room do not challenge a patient's mask phobia; they will often accept nasal prongs for oxygen therapy. Better still cut the top third, including the metal shaper, off a plastic face mask and use this. Most mask-phobic patients will accept a mask as long as they cannot see it.

Similarly, needle phobias are overcome if the patient cannot see the needle. Obscure the patients view so that they cannot see what you are about to do and ask the patient if they will now accept a sharp slap to the puncture site to disguise the prick of the needle to follow.

Management

In the recovery room most anxious patients respond to gentle words of reassurance and a compassionate touch.

Agitation is not a defined medical term, but describes a state of acute high anxiety. Patients do not hallucinate, and are oriented in time and place; however they may behave in an irrational manner.

> *Always remember that agitation is a*
> *cardinal sign of developing hypoxia.*

Other causes of agitation include awareness under anaesthesia, youth, preoperative anxiety, mutilating operations; or occasionally acute withdrawal from heroin, benzodiazepine or alcohol.

Depression

Depression is an overwhelming and pervasive feeling of despair, sadness and pessimism with an inability to get enjoyment out of life. We are not talking about a mood here, certainly not sadness or grief: we are talking about an illness.

> The only reason I got out of bed this morning was that I hadn't died during the night. There is no pleasure to be found in anything. I have lost music and birdsong, sunsets and my daughter's blue eyes... and I grieve terribly for the loss.

It is hard to imagine a more profound cry of despair.

The brain in a depressed person functions slowly, and repercussions are reflected throughout the body. Depression adversely affects many physiological processes causing autonomic dysfunction, insulin resistance, increased platelet aggregation, and decreased cellular immunity. Depressed patients metabolize drugs slowly, especially opioids and benzodiazepines; they heal poorly, their immunological systems malfunction and they are six times more susceptible to infection and wound breakdown, and have a three-fold higher incidence of ischaemic heart disease and venothromboembolism. Depressed patients are four times more likely to die in the postoperative period than a patient without mental disease. Most surgeons do not do elective operations on depressed people until they are treated; and depression is treatable.

Electroconvulsive therapy

Electroconvulsive therapy (ECT) is used on profoundly depressed people who are not responding to drug treatment. ECT is astoundingly effective and a few sessions can turn a patient who is in a semi-vegetative state into a functioning individual. ECT is a very safe procedure, but requires a trained anaesthetist to administer the anaesthetic and a psychiatrist to apply the electrodes and give the shock. ECT treatment is often administered in the recovery room. There is sometimes a marked parasympathetic response, with bradycardia and salivation before the patient recovers consciousness.

Once the fitting has stopped turn them on to their left side, and give them oxygen. Check their vital signs. If patients continue to salivate and their heart rate is less than 50 beats/min then you may need to give further atropine.

Patients with pacemakers can safely have ECT with ECG monitoring. Have an appropriate magnet nearby to convert the pacemaker to a fixed mode if the patient gets a bradycardia.

Schizophrenia

Schizophrenics have *psychotic thought disorders* affecting the way they feel and behave. Untreated, the patient's mind and personality slowly disintegrates. Withdrawn schizophrenics are so wrapped up with their delusions and hallucinations that they cannot communicate with anybody else. Anti-psychotic drugs allow patients to lead fairly normal lives. Acutely disturbed schizophrenics are highly delusional, and may become physically combative to protect themselves from perceived dangers. They may not verbalize their fears, but their faces betray their feelings. They must take their medication on the day of surgery. Almost all their anti-psychotic medication interacts adversely with pethidine and tramadol, however morphine and fentanyl are safe. Ketamine, propofol and fentanyl seem to decrease emergence confusion in schizophrenic patients.

Do not discharge schizophrenic patients from the recovery room if they appear unsettled, or agitated. A small dose of haloperidol can help to allay their distress.

Bipolar disorder

Bipolar disorder was once called manic depression. Patients swing between episodes of major depression, curled up in a miserable ball on a bed, and flights of frenetic activity where the patient's exuberance precludes sleep, and normal prudent judgement is lost. Awaking one morning the patient might buy a sports car, or not sleep for several days on end. Bipolar patients must take their lithium as usual on the day of surgery. Ensure that their lithium levels were checked before surgery.

Avoid pethidine, and tramadol in these patients (Table 25.1), their reaction is similar to those with schizophrenia. Do not give patients on lithium either haloperidol or droperidol, because the combination can cause a fatal encephalopathy.

Table 25.1 Possible problems with anti-psychotic drugs

Drug	Possible problems
Tricyclic antidepressants, e.g. amitriptyline, doxepin, olanzapine	Exaggerated response to catecholamines. Avoid ketamine, tramadol and pethidine
Serotonin reuptake inhibitors, e.g. paroxetine, sertraline, olanzapine	Serotonin syndrome with tramadol and pethidine. Mild antiplatelet activity
Monoamine oxidase inhibitors, e.g. tranylcypromine, isocarboxazid	Possible fatal response with pethidine and tramadol
Lithium	Avoid droperidol, metoclopramide and tramadol
Phenothiazines, e.g. promethazine, prochlorperazine, chlorpromazine	Excessive sedation with pethidine. Possible hypotension with metoclopramide, tramadol
Quetiapine, risperidone, valproate, ziprasidone	Avoid pethidine and tramadol

Antipsychotics and the ECG

Many of the anti-psychotic drugs cause a prolonged QT interval on the ECG. A prolonged QT interval will warn you of lithium toxicity. Lithium interacts with a number of neurotransmitters and receptors decreasing noradrenaline release and increasing serotonin synthesis.

Psychiatric patients on medication often have abnormally functioning calcium channels in their cardiac cell membranes, and may flip into a serious form of ventricular tachycardia called torsades de points if given trigger drugs such as pethidine, tramadol or the butyrophenones (droperidol or haloperidol). If a patient who is routinely taking antipsychotics is given one of the trigger drugs, then monitor them with an ECG while they are in the recovery room, and organize for them to have a full 12-lead ECG when they return to the ward.

Quadriplegics and hemiplegics

Patients who are partially or completely paralysed have unused peripheral nerves innervating muscles, and underused autonomic fibres serving blood vessels. These nerve endings are packed with noradrenaline and other neurotransmitters.

In the recovery room pain or hypoxia can cause the nerves to abruptly dump all these transmitters into the circulation (*autonomic hyperreflexia*) to cause fulminating hypertension and cardiac arrhythmias. Once the hypertension is treated the arrhythmias usually resolve spontaneously.

Be aware that people with complete spinal cord injuries do not sweat below the level of the injury and many quadriplegics cannot even sweat above the injury. With the loss of the ability to sweat or vasoconstrict within affected dermatomes the patient becomes poikilothermic and needs careful control of their environmental conditions.

Rheumatoid arthritis

Rheumatoid arthritis is characterized by inflammation of peripheral joints with progressive destruction of articular and periarticular connective tissue. It affects about 1 per cent in the general population. Women are affected three times more often than men.

Assume all elderly patients with rheumatoid arthritis have ischemic heart disease. Patients with rheumatoid arthritis are more susceptible to opioid-induced respiratory depression than normal people. They are also more prone to respiratory obstruction, and particularly sleep apnoea. They have stiff necks and brittle bones, so be careful when turning them or transferring them from the trolley to the bed. Their cervical spines are frequently unstable, so extend their necks gently, or you may damage their spinal cords and render them quadriplegic. They sometimes have temporomandibular joint destruction, so be careful, when inserting or removing airways, and do not over-extend their lower jaw.

Their atrophic skin tears easily when you remove adhesive dressings. Similarly their veins are fragile; so make sure drip cannulas cannot move up and down in the veins. Do not put needles in the backs of their hands. Patients with severe rheumatoid arthritis are often thin and hypothermia may become a problem: keep them warm.

Many sufferers are moderately anaemic and some have pulmonary fibrosis. Consequently they tend to have a higher resting respiratory rate than normal, and find it difficult to cough or deep breathe effectively. They may be taking steroids and may need hydrocortisone supplement.

Sickle cell syndromes

Sickle cell syndromes are a serious problem. Patients occasionally die in the perioperative period unless they are carefully managed.

Sickle cell syndromes included a cluster of inherited autosomal recessive diseases causing chronic haemolytic anaemia. It occurs almost exclusively in black people and those people from the malaria belt of Africa, Central America and around the Mediterranean Sea. Those who inherit one gene (*heterozygotes*) get sickle cell trait (HbAS), and those who inherit a gene from both parents (*homozygotes*) get sickle cell disease (HbSS). The full-blown sickle cell disease (HbSS) occurs in about 0.4 per cent of black people who are usually anaemic, have multiple bone painful infarcts and are severely affected. In contrast about 6 per cent have heterozygous sickle cell trait and are not anaemic, have no painful episodes, or thrombotic complications and may be unaware they have a problem. All patients from affected parts of the world must have a Sickledex® screening test before surgery, and if necessary a confirmatory haemoglobin electrophoresis.

Problems occur, either with the trait or the disease, if patients become *hypoxaemic* (that is where their arterial oxygen tensions fall below 60–70 mmHg (8–9.3 kPa)). If an affected patient's oxygen saturation falls below 93 per cent or if the patient becomes febrile, hypothermic, or acidotic their haemoglobin molecules deform into spiky tactoids. These tactoids deform the red cell into their distinctive sickle shape, and eventually destroy them.

Less obviously, hypoxaemia can occur in just one limb if a tourniquet is applied, or the blood pressure is repeatedly measured with a non-invasive blood pressure monitor. The sickle-shaped red cells clog the microcirculation causing multiple organ and tissue infarcts. Then as red cells rupture they release haemoglobin into the circulation. This *haemolytic crisis* can precipitate renal failure, particularly if the patient is also septic.

Patients may present for routine surgery or because of complications of their disease, for instance to graft leg ulcers or debride dead bone from their limbs.

Those patients with the full sickle cell disease (HbSS) presenting for elective surgery usually require a series of preoperative exchange transfusions to raise their haemoglobin levels above 100 g/L and treatment with hydroxyurea to reduce the number of abnormal circulating red cells.

In the recovery room never let patients with sickle cell syndromes become hypoxaemic, acidotic or cold. Keep their inspired oxygen high and keep them warm. Continuously monitor their perfusion status. Do not allow them to develop signs of poor peripheral perfusion. Replace blood loss early. Test their urine for haemoglobin before discharge.

To guarantee red cell oxygenation patients with sickle cell syndromes should return to the ward; and remain on oxygen for at least 4 hours. Manoeuvres such as the routine use of anti-coagulants, or anti-platelet agents, giving high concentrations of oxygen or alkalizing their blood with sodium bicarbonate, or magnesium glutamate do not improve the outcome.

Pain is a huge problem for patients with sickle cell disease. Many suffer from pain in their fingers and toes most of the time due to emboli in the small blood vessels. They may be on chronic pain treatment and require large doses of opioids post operatively.

Smokers

Elderly smokers usually have ischaemic heart, cerebrovascular and peripheral vascular disease. Smokers often cough uncontrollably especially after bronchoscopy. Persistent cough can often be controlled by lidocaine 1.5 mg/kg made up to 5 ml in saline and given by a nebulizer.

On the other hand some older smokers make no effort to cough. They seem oblivious to the sputum rattling in their airways, or are unable to muster the lung reserves necessary to cough it up. Unless the sputum is cleared it will dry into thick plugs, block the airways and go on to cause segmental lung collapse or pneumonia. Give them humidified oxygen. Encourage them to take deep breaths and cough. They should have oxygen by mask for several hours after their surgery and sit up if that is not going to interfere with their wound care.

Strokes

Cerebrovascular disease is common; it has the same risk factors as ischaemic heart disease: smokers, aged over 60 years, hypertension, diabetes, dyslipidaemia, obesity, and sedentary lifestyle. There are two forms of stroke: embolic and haemorrhagic. Embolic stroke is more common, and occasionally occurs during surgery especially after carotid endarterectomy. In the worst cases, the patient develops localizing signs, such as weakness down one side, or may not even regain consciousness.

Major surgery within 3 months of a stroke or transient ischaemic attack increases the risk of a further stroke or cardiac ischaemia in the early postoperative period. Elective surgery is usually deferred until the danger period has passed, if not then monitor these patients carefully for signs of cardiac ischaemia.

Patients who are disabled by previous strokes may have difficulty coughing, problems in adjusting their position, telling staff they are in pain or that their bladders are full. Make a small signboard, so that patients can point to simple pictures representing pain, nausea, full bladder and so forth. You can also use this board for patients who do not speak English. A relative or close friend who really know the patient well can help you to interpret their needs. Ask them to join you in the recovery room as soon as the patient is stable.

Thyroid disease

Hyperthyroidism

Hyperthyroidism occurs when the thyroid gland produces excessive hormones called tri-iodothyronine and thyroxine (T3 and T4). Although not as common as hypothyroidism overt hyperthyroidism is usually easy to recognize, but subtle undiagnosed hyperthyroidism may cause problems in the recovery room. Many symptoms of hyperthyroidism are similar to adrenergic excess. Monitor patients with an ECG. The patients are thin, heat intolerant, and almost invariably have a resting tachycardia. Watch for atrial fibrillation, this is not uncommon in hyperthyroid patients. With the postoperative stress of emerging from their anaesthetic, they may develop rapid AF or even ventricular tachycardias.

> *Think of thyroid disease if the patient is taking amiodarone.*

In the frail and elderly the diagnosis of hyperthyroidism is sometimes missed. It may present as a wasted, elderly woman with an agitated dementia (*thyrotoxic madness*) and atrial fibrillation or a resting tachycardia.

Hypothyroidism

Hypothyroidism occurs when the thyroid gland produces insufficient thyroid hormones. Subtle hypothyroidism occurs in 10 per cent of elderly women, and frequently the diagnosis is overlooked for years. Typically the patient feels 'tired and run down', but the diagnostic hint is their dislike of the cold. Occasionally unsuspected hypothyroid patients undergo anaesthesia.

If the diagnosis of hypothyroidism is missed at preoperative assessment patients will come from theatre cooler than expected, be slower to wake up, and become unduly sleepy with sedative drugs or opioids. Think of hypothyroidism if an older woman is 'difficult to wake up'.

Myxoedema

Myxoedema is a severe form of hypothyroidism. It is easily overlooked during the pre-anaesthetic work up since the patient is a slow thinker and consequently classed as 'a poor historian'. They are usually obese elderly women, but may not have the classic dry, coarse hair, podgy features and a large tongue described in textbooks. Typically they come to recovery room cold, comatose, with a bradycardia, hypotensive and are 'slow to emerge'.

In patients with myxoedema all drugs are metabolized slowly. Muscle relaxants are difficult to reverse and the patients may have to go to ICU for further management. These patients are particularly sensitive to opioids and normal doses may cause profound respiratory depression.

References

1. **Mariscal A, Medrano IH,** *et al.* (2011) Perioperative management of Parkinson's disease. *Neurologica* 27:46–50.
2. **Stagg P, Grice T** (2011) Nasogastric medication for perioperative Parkinson's rigidity. *Anaesthesia and Intensive Care* **39**:1128–1130.

Chapter 26

The bleeding patient

Introduction

We have divided this chapter into three sections: the physiology of blood; the bleeding patient in recovery room; and the science and technology of blood transfusion. This is a long and quite complicated chapter. Read it slowly, one section at a time.

Part one—the physiology of blood

Blood is composed of red cells (erythrocytes), white cells (granulocytes and lympho-cytes), and platelets suspended in honey-coloured plasma. Plasma contains clotting factors, proteins for transporting various substances, and electrolytes. As a clot forms into a jelly-like blob, the clotting factors are removed from the plasma, leaving behind serum.

Anaemia

Red blood cells contain haemoglobin molecules, which carry oxygen. *Haemoglobin* (Hb) is a tangled ball of protein chains with a ferrous *ion* in a cleft. The ferrous ion slides out of its cleft to bind oxygen as the blood passes through the lungs turning crimson in the process, and slides back releasing it into the tissues' capillaries turning a bluish hue. When fully saturated with oxygen, haemoglobin inside red cells carries 650 times more oxygen than is dissolved in plasma.

Anaemia occurs when the total *mass* of haemoglobin is less than normal for the patient's age and sex. The normal concentration of Hb in blood is about 140 g/L (14 g/dL). For practical purposes patients become anaemic once the Hb level falls to less than 110 g/L, although this does not automatically require treatment.

Physiology of oxygen supply

Our core responsibility in the recovery room is to ensure sufficient oxygen is delivered to patients' brains and hearts to prevent hypoxic damage.

While resting, an adult uses 250 ml/min of oxygen for basal metabolic needs. During exercise, or with shivering, fever or emotional stress, the amount of oxygen the body uses increases many fold. Damage quickly occurs if the heart or brain is even temporarily deprived of its oxygen supply.

How oxygen gets to the tissues

The volume of oxygen delivered to the cells depends on the amount of haemoglobin present in blood, and how fast the circulation carries the red cells to the tissues.

Oxygen content of blood

The oxygen content of haemoglobin (Hb) depends on the:

- number of grams of haemoglobin in each litre of blood;
- percentage oxygen saturation of haemoglobin;
- number of millilitres of oxygen carried by each gram of haemoglobin.

The laboratory measures haemoglobin concentration, and we can measure oxygen saturation with a pulse oximeter. The carrying capacity of haemoglobin remains fairly constant at about 1.34 ml of oxygen for every gram of haemoglobin.

Oxygen content of blood	=	Hb concentration	×	Hb saturation	×	Hb capacity for oxygen
	=	150 g/1000 ml	×	98/100	×	1.34 ml O_2/g of Hb
	=	200 ml of oxygen carried by each litre of blood				

How fast the heart can deliver blood to the tissues depends on the cardiac output. In a resting adult the cardiac output is about 5000 ml/min. In healthy young adults this can increase five-fold with exercise or to cope with other physiological stresses, however many elderly people, or those with heart disease have a limited capacity to increase their cardiac output.

Calculating the oxygen supply to the tissues

Oxygen supply to the tissues = volume of oxygen carried by blood
× how fast it is delivered

Oxygen supply to the tissues = oxygen content of blood × cardiac output
= 200 ml / L × 5 L / min = 1000 ml / min

Of the 1000 ml of oxygen delivered to the tissues each minute, an adult at rest uses only 250 ml. The remaining 750 ml of oxygen remains bound to haemoglobin. In the extreme circumstances of shock, extreme exercise or hypoxia, an extra 250 ml of oxygen can be extracted from the haemoglobin. This means that the usable amount of oxygen in fully oxygenated blood is only about 500 ml/min. So if your patient's oxygen delivery falls to a *critical point* of about 500 ml/min they will be near death.

Patients can only cope with one disturbance of either anaemia, or low oxygen saturation or a low cardiac output. If two of these factors combine then the tissues will become hypoxic; and the combination of all three factors is often lethal. For example, bleeding patients can cope quite well with the developing anaemia provided they are not hypoxic, but if they also have low oxygen saturations and cardiac failure they are likely to die.

Physiology of coagulation

When a blood vessel is damaged little strands of collagen fibrils from the wound poke out into the blood stream and flap about like water-weeds. When passing platelets collide with the collagen they instantly discharge their granules, and shrivel into burr-shaped grappling hooks that catch on to and *adhere* to the collagen fibrils. The platelets also *aggregate* together in clumps. Passing fibrinogen strings get entangled in the hooks and are converted to fibrin.

Circulating coagulation factors use calcium ions to convert prothrombin in the plasma into an enzyme called *thrombin*. Thrombin turns inactive fibrinogen into strings of *fibrin* that quickly mesh and ensnare more passing platelets, red and white cells. In this way the process snowballs to form a gelatinous tangled clot (Figure 26.1).

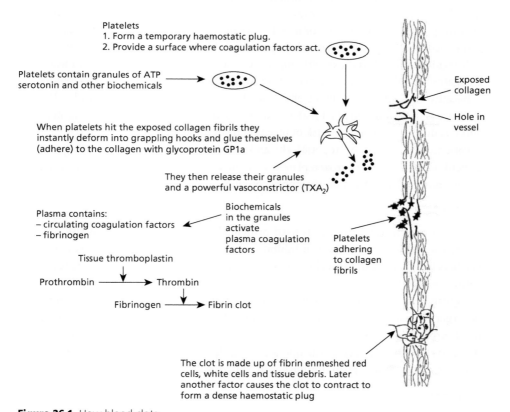

Platelets
1. Form a temporary haemostatic plug.
2. Provide a surface where coagulation factors act.

Platelets contain granules of ATP serotonin and other biochemicals

Exposed collagen

Hole in vessel

When platelets hit the exposed collagen fibrils they instantly deform into grappling hooks and glue themselves (adhere) to the collagen with glycoprotein GP1a

They then release their granules and a powerful vasoconstrictor (TXA$_2$)

Plasma contains:
– circulating coagulation factors
– fibrinogen

Biochemicals in the granules activate plasma coagulation factors

Platelets adhering to collagen fibrils

Tissue thromboplastin

Prothrombin ⟶ Thrombin

Fibrinogen ⟶ Fibrin clot

The clot is made up of fibrin enmeshed red cells, white cells and tissue debris. Later another factor causes the clot to contract to form a dense haemostatic plug

Figure 26.1 How blood clots.

Once a gelatinous clot has formed, the mesh shrinks into a tight dry fibrin plug that blocks the hole in the vessels. It takes about 6 minutes for the vessel to stop bleeding, but some hours for the clot to mature into a tight plug.

Normally, blood neither clots unless it needs to, nor in places where it should not. *Prostacyclin*, one of the prostaglandins, stops the process snowballing out of control. It is secreted by vascular endothelium, preventing platelets from sticking to undamaged vessel walls so that unwanted clots do not form there.

Drugs interfering with clotting

Drugs that react with serotonin, prostaglandins, prostacyclin, vitamin K, or any other biochemicals involved with clotting will upset the coagulation process. Many patients are taking drugs that impede blood's ability to clot. If patients continue to bleed after surgery then check their clinical notes to see if they have been taking any of these drugs.

Dabigatran

Dabigatran[1] is an oral thrombin inhibitor. It binds directly with thrombin and there is no delay of onset of effect. It is prescribed for patients with atrial fibrillation and to prevent deep vein thrombosis in vulnerable patients. It is also sometimes given after major orthopaedic surgery. The main risk to patients is bleeding. There is an increased risk in older patients as well as those with impaired renal function. The anticoagulant features of dabigatran are also enhanced when it is used concomitantly with aspirin or clopidogrel.

Because of dabigatran's direct effect on thrombin the INR is not reliable. The best measure is thrombin time (TT). aPTT can be used but it is less sensitive to higher doses and it is difficult to assess the risk of bleeding from these test results.

Patients who bleed postoperatively and are known to have taken dabigatran are difficult to manage. Fresh frozen platelets are the first option. Other treatments including tranexamic acid and dried prothrombin complex can be tried as well.[2]

Aspirin

Low-dose aspirin (60–150 mg) is used principally in patients who are at risk of stroke or myocardial infarction. Aspirin inhibits prostaglandin synthesis, which is needed for platelets to aggregate to form clots. It permanently disables the affected platelets for their entire 10-day life span.

Aspirin is usually stopped a few days before major surgery (but continued on the day of surgery in patients with cardiac stents). This allows blood to clot effectively enough for most surgery. Bleeding with neuro- or urological surgery is so serious that most surgeons stop aspirin 7–10 days before the operation. Platelet transfusion given 12 hours after the last dose of low-dose aspirin diminishes its anticoagulant effects.

Clopidogrel

Clopidogrel is an anticoagulant used in patients who have had coronary stents implanted. It is not as effective as warfarin and it cannot be reversed. Clopidogrel permanently prevents platelets aggregating, and thus lasts for the whole of the platelet's 10-day life span.

Clopidogrel is usually withdrawn 7–10 days before surgery. However, if it is withdrawn in patients who have recently had a cardiac stent inserted and the epithelium has not yet covered the lumen there is a risk of the stent clotting and causing myocardial infarction.

Clopidogrel and aspirin

When used together, the synergistic combination of clopidogrel and aspirin is a highly effective anticoagulant. Both agents block platelet aggregation for the whole of their 10-day lifespan. Even if the last dose of the combination was given more than 5 days ago consider them as a potent cause of bleeding. Platelet transfusion will generally correct bleeding if it is given 8–12 hours after the last dose of the combination.

Dipyridamole

Dipyridamole inhibits platelet function. It is occasionally used in patients with mechanical heart valves, or a secondary prevention of embolic strokes. It is readily reversed by platelet transfusion. Its vasodilating properties can cause hypotension.

Other drugs

Other drugs affecting blood clotting (Figure 26.2) include all the NSAIDs, and all the SSRIs. Their individual effects are equivalent to low-dose aspirin, but when used together the effects are amplified. If postoperative haemorrhage occurs in these patients treat it with aprotinin or aminocaproic acid.

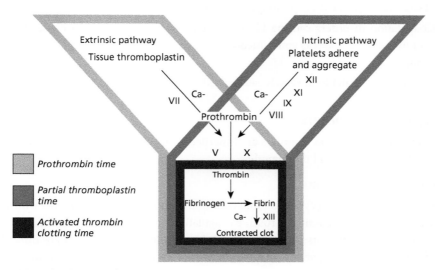

Figure 26.2 Clotting cascade.

Drugs affecting clotting factors

Warfarin

Warfarin is the most widely used anticoagulant. Usually warfarin is stopped 5 days before surgery. Warfarin's effect is monitored with an INR. The INR needs to be less than 1.5 for most surgery. The effects of warfarin can be reversed over 18 hours with vitamin K, or immediately with fresh frozen plasma.

Heparin

Unfractionated heparin (UH) is often used during vascular surgery to prevent clots forming. Its clinical half-life is 50 minutes, but this is prolonged if the patient is hypothermic. The anaesthetist usually reverses the effects of heparin with protamine before the patient leaves the operating theatre.

If patients continue to bleed the anaesthetist may give an additional dose of protamine. Protamine 1 mg IV will reverse the effects of approximately 100 units of heparin. Give protamine slowly (over 10 minutes), otherwise it may cause hypotension and pulmonary artery vasoconstriction. Paradoxically, excessive protamine depresses platelet function and so aggravates bleeding.

Low molecular-weight heparins (LMWHs) are used perioperatively in patients who are at risk of developing deep vein thromboses. The two most commonly used are enoxaparin and dalteparin. Remember these LMWHs are given subcutaneously and not intramuscularly.

Bleeding disorders

Disorders causing bleeding fall into the groups.
1. Those causing immediate prolonged bleeding during surgery.
2. Coagulation disorders causing bleeding after surgery. Haemophilia causes bleeding later in the ward, whereas von Willebrand's disease may cause bleeding in the recovery room.
3. Disorders of small blood vessels cause bleeding during surgery.

Coagulation disorders

Most chronic coagulation disorders are inherited genetic diseases. Usually they are well known to the patients and their families.

von Willebrand's disease

von Willebrand's disease (vWD) is more common than haemophilia. Patients with vWD have a normal platelet count and routine coagulation profiles are usually normal.

There are many variants of this genetic disease. Mild forms of vWD are difficult to diagnose, consequently patients may be unaware they have inherited it. However, they may have bled after tooth extraction, or had menorrhagia and know of 'bleeders' in their family.

Fortunately, patients with vWD who are surgically stressed have other changes in their blood that make them clot readily Bleeding is not usually a problem but watch them carefully, they can bleed postoperatively in the recovery room.

Pressing on the bleeding site with a sterile pad will usually control superficial bleeding. If this fails then a haematologist or anaesthetist will prescribe specially derived factor VIII, which contains von Willebrand's factor if this is available. Another drug used to treat patients with vWD who bleed is *desmopressin*. This drug should be kept refrigerated, it is often given before surgery. Desmopressin is related to antidiuretic hormone and it can interfere with urine output so this should be monitored carefully. It can make the patient turn impressively pale and cause nausea.

Haemophilia

The *haemophilias* are a group of inherited bleeding disorders caused by clotting factor deficiencies (Table 26.1), usually involving factors VIII and IX. Most haemophiliacs have been treated with factor VIII concentrates before coming to surgery. Virus inactivated cryoprecipitate or fresh frozen plasma can be used as a substitute. Haemophiliacs usually do not bleed immediately after surgery, but may do so in the ward some hours later. Bleeding from superficial wounds, although staunched by pressure, resumes when the pressure is released. Do not give intramuscular injections. Some older haemophiliacs have HIV or hepatitis C, because they received blood transfusions before effective screening for these diseases were in place.

Table 26.1 Special transfusions

Disease	Haemostatic defect	What to use
Haemophilia A	Absent/low factor VIII	Desmopressin
Haemophilia B	Absent/low factor IX	Factor IX concentrate
von Willebrand's	Defect in vWF	Desmopressin

Disseminated intravascular coagulation

Disseminated intravascular coagulation (DIC), sometimes called consumption coagulopathy, causes uncontrollable bleeding. It may occur in patients who have suffered acutely life-threatening disasters where a lot of tissue is damaged; such as multiple trauma, severe systemic sepsis, and obstetric emergencies.

Spontaneous clots form everywhere. The clots plaque out like cobwebs along the inside of blood vessels, snaring red blood cells and damaging them. The mangled red cells seen under a microscope appear as *microangiopathic haemolytic anaemia*.

Meanwhile the fibrinolytic system tries to dissolve all the cobweb clots. As they dissolve the clots release fibrin degradation products (FDP) and fibrin split product (FSP) into the plasma. Elevated levels of FSP and FDP with a falling platelet count are signposts to the diagnosis. Eventually, the patient runs out of clotting factors and platelets, and starts to bleed uncontrollably. A warning sign of developing DIC occurs when old venipuncture sites start to bleed. These patients should return to the operating theatre urgently. DIC is a life-threatening problem that needs expert advice from a haematologist. The only way to manage DIC is to identify and treat the underlying cause; for example, using antibiotics to treat sepsis, or evacuate the uterus of retained necrotic tissue.

Platelet disorders

The normal platelet count is 150,000–300,000/ml. Platelets are put out of action by drugs, such as aspirin, clopidogrel, NSAIDs, SSRIs, calcium channel blockers and dipyridamole. The platelet count is normal, but the platelets do not function normally. This condition is sometimes called *thrombasthenia*.

A lack of platelets, *thrombocytopenia*, rarely causes spontaneous bleeding, although it may do so after surgery. Patients tend to have lots of superficial bruises on their arms and legs.

There are many causes of thrombocytopenia including:

◆ idiopathic thrombocytopenic purpura (ITP);

◆ alcoholic with liver disease;

◆ patients with bone marrow suppression.

Patients with ITP may come to theatre for splenectomy with the aim of preventing the spleen from removing platelets from the circulation. As soon as the spleen is removed, the patient is transfused with platelets. This transfusion may be continued in the recovery room.

Diseases of blood vessels

Many diseases weaken blood vessels so that they bleed more easily or fail to retract properly to prevent bleeding. Common diseases include scurvy, amyloidosis, vasculitis, and connective tissue disease such as rheumatoid arthritis. Patients on long-term prednisolone therapy often have bruises on their arms and legs, and thin skin that tears easily. Take care not to tear their skin while moving them or removing dressings.

Part two—bleeding in the recovery room

A patient bleeding on the operating table or in the recovery room is at risk of harm from myocardial infarction or stroke. Blood transfusion is life-saving therapy. If a patient is bleeding and you anticipate that you will need more than 2 units of blood then give ample warning to your hospital's blood bank and haematologist. Delegate one member of the staff to organize the blood transfusion and liaise with the blood bank technicians and the haematologist as well as the surgeon and the anaesthetist.

Assess the bleeding

Slow bleeding—microvascular ooze

Microvascular ooze occurs slowly enough for the body to compensate. The cardinal sign is a decreasing haemoglobin and packed cell volume. Microvascular ooze is caused by either metabolic disturbance or more usually hypothermia. Some drugs lingering in the body aggravate ooze.

+ Check if the patient is taking any anticoagulant drugs.
+ Treat hypothermia.

Hypothermia is the cause
of most microvascular ooze.

+ Now check the coagulation profile.
+ If that ooze continues use fresh frozen plasma.
+ Then give 4 units of platelets.
+ The ultimate, but rarely used, therapy is a direct blood transfusion from a compatible donor directly into the patient.

Rapid blood loss

Rapid blood loss causes hypovolaemia. Treat ongoing rapid blood loss with blood transfusion. Such *pre-emptive transfusion* in an actively bleeding patient reduces the incidence of problems later.

Rapid blood loss after an operation usually arises from problems with surgical haemostasis: either a vessel has started to bleed, or a surgical tie has slipped off a blood vessel. Monitor wounds and suction bottles frequently for excessive loss. If the loss is more than 100ml in 30 minutes call the surgeon. If the bleeding is coming from the wound wear sterile gloves and press firmly on the area.

Revealed haemorrhage is easy to recognize; it is either coming out of the wound or is in the drain bottles. On the other hand, *concealed bleeding* into the peritoneum, thorax, or big muscle beds is less obvious. Concealed bleeding following a total hip replacement can exceed 1500 ml before local swelling becomes obvious; with a fractured pelvis or bleeding into the abdomen many litres of blood collects before the abdomen distends. Once a patient becomes hypovolaemic his life is in danger.

What to do immediately

+ Call for help.
+ Lay the patient flat.
+ Give oxygen by mask of at least 6 L/min.
+ Lift the patient's legs onto a pillow (Figure 26.3). This runs about 400 ml of blood into their central circulation. Never tip them head down; not only is it distressing for the patient but it alters the distribution of blood flow within the lungs, and pushes abdominal contents up against the diaphragm reducing the patient's *functional residual capacity*. This severely impairs oxygen uptake.

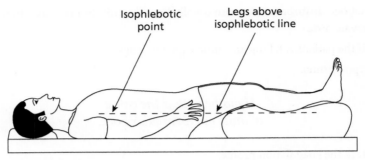

Figure 26.3 Place legs on pillow.

- Start basic monitoring: ECG, pulse, blood pressure, attach a pulse oximeter and measure their core temperature.
- Check that you have a large cannula and a freely flowing infusion of normal saline running. Consider inserting another cannula.
- Check the intraoperative blood loss, and replacement. Are they balanced? From this you will get an idea of how much blood you will need to give.
- If your hospital has a Massive Transfusion Protocol consider activating this.
- Give blood. If available use the patient's own blood type, or else use low titre O-negative blood. While you are waiting for blood transfuse the patient with either crystalloid or colloid fluid. Change this to saline to flush the line before beginning the blood transfusion.
- Warm all fluids with an in-line blood warmer such as the Level 1®. Aim to maintain: systolic blood pressure > 100 mmHg; pulse rate < 100 bpm; Hb > 80 g/L or the haematocrit > 25%.

If you are giving more than 2 units of blood then use a microfilter to prevent post-transfusion lung injury. Give each unit in less than 60 minutes. Do not allow it to warm in its bag because it will deteriorate rapidly at room temperature.

Blood is a living substance. It deteriorates
quickly at room temperatures.

How much blood to give

Give colloid or blood until the patient's jugular venous pressure (JVP) rises, or they no longer feel faint when they sit up. At this point the patient will probably still have poor perfusion status with cold hands and a low urine output, but their pulse rate should be slowing, and their mean blood pressure rising. It may take up to an hour before perfusion to their hands and feet improves. You will need to top-up their blood volume as their vasculature dilates.

Giving blood?
Give oxygen too!

How to manage ongoing bleeding

◆ Use a central line to assess continued bleeding and to guide your fluid therapy.

◆ Aim to keep the CVP in the range of +5 to +8 cm H_2O.

◆ If you are not certain whether the patient's blood volume is roughly normal then rapidly infuse 5 ml/kg boluses of blood, or colloid. If the CVP rises for a minute or two and then falls again keep repeating the boluses until the CVP remains above 5 cm H_2O.

◆ Listen to the lung bases. Crackles, followed by a wheeze, indicate the patient's blood volume is becoming overloaded.

◆ You will know when you are gaining on the blood loss if the pulse progressively slows over the following 5 to 10 minutes, and the urine output increases beyond 1 ml/kg/hr.

How to use coagulation profiles

◆ Coagulation studies help you work out why the blood does not clot, and what to do next.

◆ Send blood for INR, aPTT, haemoglobin, platelet and fibrinogen levels.

◆ If the INR is >1.8 then clotting factors are less than 30% of their normal levels. This is the minimum acceptable level; below this level microvascular bleeding (ooze) is almost certain to occur.

◆ Other useful predictors of microvascular bleeding are platelets < $50,000 \times 10^3$/L, fibrinogen < 1 g/L, and an aPTT > 1.5 its normal time.

Do not give platelets, fresh frozen plasma, or clotting factors in anticipation of bleeding. The coagulation system is remarkably robust and will form clots with as little as $10,000 \times 10^3$/L platelets. The vascular endothelium quickly promotes clotting providing the patient is warm, and has a well oxygenated liver.

Part three—blood transfusion

The spread of HIV, hepatitis C and other diseases transmitted by blood transfusion has altered the way we use blood, during and after surgery. Anaesthetists are more reluctant to give blood, and patients are more reluctant to receive it. Advances in understanding the physiology of tissue oxygenation makes it possible to reduce the amount of blood transfused, and in many cases avoid it completely. Intraoperative salvage and reinfusion of blood enables many major operations to be done without blood transfusion.

Transfusion is life-saving therapy, and when properly screened is safe. If you need blood to save a life, do not withhold it because of fear of transfusion-transmitted disease. Blood transfusion is ultimately needed to prevent your patient having a myocardial infarction, a stroke, or developing cardiac failure.

Transfused blood is a tissue transplant

Transfused blood is an expensive and limited resource. It is a living tissue transplant, and like all transplants the donor blood must be immunologically compatible with the recipient blood otherwise transfusion reactions occur. Serious transfusion reactions are always dangerous and sometimes lethal.

A patient with Group O blood
must always receive Group O blood.

Blood groups

There are four principal blood groups: O, A, B and AB. Each of these blood groups can be further divided into two main rhesus subgroups: Rh positive and Rh negative (Table 26.2). The recipient's serum may have antibodies against many other antigens in donated blood. These antigens reside on the donor's red cell membranes. There are many antigens with names like Lewis, Duffy, and Kell.

Table 26.2 Blood groups

Blood group	Red cell antigen	Serum antibodies	Prevalence in population (%)
O	None	Anti-A	45
		Anti-B	
A	A	Anti-B	43
B	B	Anti-A	10
AB	A and B	None	7

Typing and cross-matching

To prevent transfusion reactions donor blood is first typed and then cross-matched against the recipient's blood before infusion (Figure 26.4).

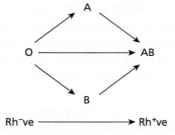

Figure 26.4 Blood or platelet groups theoretically safe to give.

Blood typing

Patients must receive compatible blood. Before issuing blood your hospital's blood bank will type the patient's blood into its respective blood group and rhesus group (Box 26.1). The technician will hold a sample aside, in case more blood is needed later. The typing process takes about 10 minutes.

Box 26.1 **Typing blood**

The patient's blood is typed to see which of the four major blood groups it belongs. This is done by adding the patient's serum to four little white dishes containing a solution of special reference red cells of blood groups A, B and AB and O. If the patient's serum causes the red cells to clump together then it contains antibodies to the antigens stuck on the surfaces of the reference red cells. For instance, if the patient's group is O then the patient's serum will clump the red cells of groups A, B, and AB, but not O. In contrast, if the patient's group is AB, then it will not clump any of the cells.

Blood cross-match

After grouping the patient's blood the hospital laboratory then tests it against the donor's blood to make sure that they are compatible. Blood cross-match ensures that the many other antigens that may be either in the donor's or recipient's blood are not going to trigger an antigen–antibody reaction in the patient. A full cross-match takes about 45 minutes, sometimes longer.

In an emergency you can use typed blood without going through the whole cross-match. Typed blood is less than 1 per cent likely to cause a transfusion reaction.

A HemoCue® is a useful guide for blood transfusion requirements.

Principles of blood transfusion

Do not delay blood transfusion if the patient is showing signs of hypoxia including confusion, ST changes on their ECG, a tachycardia greater than 100 beats/min, their blood gases reveal an acidosis, or they have a poor perfusion status.

Patients who cannot tolerate a low haemoglobin include those with:

◆ coronary artery disease;
◆ myocardial ischaemia;
◆ congestive cardiac failure;
◆ a history of transient ischaemic attacks or suspected cerebral ischaemia;
◆ symptomatic valvular heart disease such as severe aortic stenosis;
◆ a history of previous ischaemic stroke.

Patients who have acute or chronic problems with bleeding or anaemia including those with:

◆ disseminated intravascular coagulation;

◆ inherited bleeding disorders such as haemophilia or von Willebrand's disease;

◆ thrombocytopenia;

◆ bone marrow failure.

For information about warming blood see Box 26.2.

Box 26.2 **Warming blood**

If you anticipate giving more than 100 ml/min, or more than two units of blood in an hour, then use an in-line blood warmer to warm the blood to 37°C. Warm blood for those at risk of hypothermia: the young, the elderly, and the infirm; and those patients who have cold agglutinins. If you give cold blood at 4°C, each unit will decrease the patient's core temperature by about 0.25°C. Cold blood is painful to infuse through peripheral veins. It may cause red cells to clump, impeding flow through the microcirculation, and it is a major cause of bleeding. Do not transfuse cold blood rapidly through a central venous line; it is likely to cause arrhythmias and the cardiac output to fall.

It is extremely dangerous to warm the pack of blood in warm or hot water, because this will cook the blood, haemolyse the red cells and destroy the clotting factors. Never put blood in a microwave oven, because microwaves do not heat uniformly. They concentrate intense heat in separated small areas, boiling the red cells. In-line blood warmers are essential for massive transfusions. Warming blood from 4°C to 37°C decreases its viscosity 2.5-fold, and dilates the patient's veins allowing transfusions to run faster.

Blood transfusions run slowly through standard blood warmers. To overcome this difficulty there are a number of newer systems such as the Level-1™ which delivers 500 ml/min, while the Rapid infusion System™ delivers 1500 ml/min. Water bath blood warmers are less commonly used now. Dry heat blood warmers such as the Atom™ do not require dedicated disposables and accept any standard giving set.

Every blood warmer should indicate the temperature, have a thermostat control and warning alarms. The temperature must never exceed 41°C. Blood warmers can be dangerous if they malfunction so they need maintenance checks every 12 months.

Therapeutic goals

The therapeutic goals are to maintain the patient's blood pressure within 20 per cent of their preoperative levels, keep the pulse rate between 60 to 80 beats/min, and maintain a urine output of more than 50 ml/hr.

While waiting for the blood, Plasma-Lyte® or Hartmann's solution is appropriate. Infusion of large amounts of crystalloids can cause problems. They seep into the tissues causing peripheral oedema, and may migrate into the lungs later to cause pulmonary oedema. Over the coming days the kidneys need to excrete this excessive fluid. Limit the infusion of synthetic colloids.[2] High doses of colloids are associated with renal failure.

How to estimate the amount of blood loss

How to replace blood if you do not know the volume lost

Most of the time it is difficult to know how much blood or fluid has been lost. In this case use other criteria such as clinical signs, haemoglobin concentration, and give blood once the transfusion threshold has been crossed.

How to replace blood if you know the volume lost

Some hints for managing patients who are bleeding slowly:

- Check the haemoglobin or haematocrit frequently.
- Start giving blood once the haemoglobin falls to the transfusion threshold; predetermined by the surgeon.
- Treat hypovolaemia separately from anaemia.
- Replace blood volume first.
- Prepare to give blood if the patient pulse rate rises above 100 bpm.
- If a patient is developing an acidosis then use blood straight away.
- Notify the blood bank early about the situation. Aim to maintain:
  - the systolic blood pressure > 100 mmHg;
  - pulse rate < 100 bpm;
  - Hb > 80 g/L or the haematocrit > 25%.
- If giving more than 2 units of blood then use a microfilter to prevent post-transfusion lung injury.
- Give each unit in less than 60 minutes. Do not allow blood to warm in its bag because it will deteriorate rapidly at room temperature.

Massive blood transfusion

Most hospitals have guidelines. These should be printed out and displayed in your recovery room (Figure 26.5). In an emergency you can use typed but uncross-matched blood of the same blood group as the patient's. There is less than 1 per cent chance of a severe reaction. Most operating rooms keep 4 units of low antibody titre Rh-negative blood to use in emergencies. Where possible do not give Rh-positive blood to a Rh-negative patient, however you may give Rh-negative blood to a Rh-positive patient.

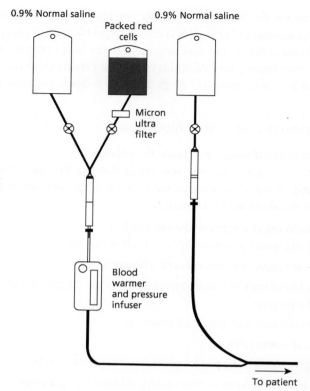

Figure 26.5 Set up for a massive blood transfusion.

How much O-negative blood to use

Once the patient has received more than 4 units of group O-negative blood you will need to continue with O-negative blood. If, at this stage, you revert to the patient's own group the O-negative blood you have used may contain antibodies to the cross-matched blood you get from the blood bank.

When the laboratory has the time to carefully cross-match a fresh blood sample from the patient you can revert to the patient's own blood group.

You can make an improvised pressure bag (Figure 26.6). Carefully cut open one end of the tough outer plastic container in which many bags of intravenous fluid are delivered.

Reinforce the container with non-stretchable cloth surgical adhesive (such as zinc oxide tape or Sleek®) so that it can withstand pressure. Then attach a blood pressure cuff inflation bulb to an empty litre bag. Slip the litre bag inside the reinforced outer bag to act as inflatable bladder. Insert a bag of blood or other fluid with its giving set attached. As you inflate the bladder the bag of fluid is compressed against the reinforced outer container.

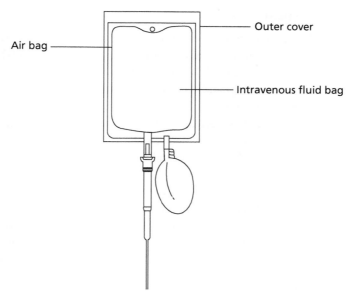

Air bag

Outer cover

Intravenous fluid bag

Figure 26.6 Improvised pressure bag.

How to know if the coagulopathy is severe

After about 10 units of blood 40 per cent of patients develop a severe coagulopathy (INR or aPTT double normal) with thrombocytopenia (platelets less than $50 \times 10^9/L$). However, you cannot predict the severity of the coagulopathy from the number of units of blood you have transfused. Haemostasis is affected by many factors, particularly: hypothermia, liver blood flow, acid–base status, the mass damaged tissue, and tissue oxygenation.

Practicalities

Blood should either be running into your patient or stored in the special blood fridge at 2–6°C. Blood deteriorates rapidly as it warms. Do not leave it lying around on bench tops. Most blood packs have a temperature-sensitive label to indicate if this has happened. Never store blood in an ordinary household refrigerator. Frozen red cells are dead red cells. If they are transfused into a patient they will rupture, releasing their haemoglobin to clog the kidney. Warm blood with an in-line blood warmer (see Box 26.2, page 416). Cold blood infused faster than 100 ml/min may cause cardiac arrest. Use a blood warmer if you are giving more than two units in one hour, or in patients who have cold agglutinins. Blood must not be warmed above 41°C.

To prevent the lungs becoming clogged with microemboli filter blood through special 20–40 μ microfilters to remove cellular debris from the blood bag. They reduce the risk of adult respiratory distress syndrome, non-haemolytic febrile reactions and thrombocytopenia. Packed cells flow through micro-filters much faster if they are diluted with 0.9 per cent saline.

How to identify patients

Giving the wrong blood to the wrong patient is the commonest cause of serious or fatal adverse reactions to blood transfusion. Such clerical errors are totally avoidable.

Every hospital should have a Blood Transfusion Committee. It is their responsibility to formulate a policy to document and trace a unit of blood on every step of its journey beginning with its collection from the vein of the donor, to its infusion into the vein of the recipient. To reduce the risk of clerical error many hospitals use portable barcodes to ensure the right blood gets to the right patient. Because of the problems with vCJD legislation, many countries require that all blood and blood components must be traceable to the recipient for 15 years.

Two trained staff must independently check each unit before it can be transfused. Meticulously check each unit of blood before giving it: check the labels on the blood pack, the transfusion slip accompanying it, the patient's identification bracelet, and the patient's record. EVERY detail must match exactly. The blood's identification number, the blood group, and its expiry date must exactly match the details on the transfusion slip.

Tips about technique

- Do not directly mark intravenous bags with solvent marking pens because the ink penetrates the plastic and contaminates the solution.
- Do not vent plastic containers with needles.
- Wear gloves and eye protection when putting up blood.
- Be careful not to put your fingers on the needle in such a way that it may carry contaminants into the bag (Figure 26.7).

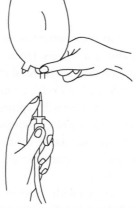

A common mistake when setting up a drip. Note the forefinger contaminating the sterile needle as it is being inserted into the bag of intravenous fluid.

Figure 26.7 An error.

- Before putting up blood, invert the bag a few times to mix the components.

- Apart from 0.9% saline do not add anything whatsoever to blood or components. This includes drugs.

- Crystalloids (Hartmann's solution or Ringer's lactate) and polygeline colloid solution (Haemaccel® or Gelofusine®) contain calcium ions, which reverse the citrate anticoagulant, and the blood will clot in the lines. Glucose 5% solutions cause red cells to aggregate and will eventually cause haemolysis.

Blood and its components

Whole blood

Packs of whole blood usually contain about 400 to 500 ml. Fresh whole blood is the best blood but not easily available in larger hospitals where there is a blood bank.

*If bleeding will not stop, then ask
for fresh 4-day old blood.*

Packed cells

Red cell concentrates (packed cells) come in bags of about 300 ml. They contain no effective clotting factors or platelets. The sticky viscous packed cell concentrate does not pass easily through micro-filters. To make them run through a filter more quickly you can dilute them in 0.9 per cent saline. Do not use Ringer's lactate or Hartmann's solution, since calcium ions in these solutions cause blood to clot in the intravenous line.

One pack of blood in a 70 kg adult raises the haemoglobin by approximately 1 g/L (or 100 mg/100 ml). Red cells should be infused rapidly. Most patients easily tolerate a unit in 60 minutes, and no infusion should take longer than 3 hours.

Storage lesion

Blood can be stored in a special refrigerator at 2–7°C for up to 35 days. During storage potassium continuously leaks out of the red cells into the plasma, and may cause arrhythmias if infused too quickly down a central line. After rewarming the red blood cells quickly take up the potassium.

After a few days in the refrigerator blood starts to suffer *storage lesion*; platelets disintegrate, and clotting factors degrade. Stored red cells pick up oxygen readily enough, but they will not release it to the tissues. It may take up to 18 hours for the surviving red cells to start functioning properly.

Boutique blood

Special types of blood are available for specific patients. Cytomegalovirus (CMV) seronegative blood is used for cytomegalovirus seronegative patients who are on immunosuppressive chemotherapy, have lymphoma or leukaemia, or are pregnant. Gamma radiation kills white cells (T-lymphocytes). Use irradiated blood for immunosuppressed patients.

Prestorage leucocyte-depleted blood is used for those who have had previous febrile non-haemolytic transfusion reactions. If these latter patients are taking ACE inhibitor medication they may be unexpectedly hypotensive.[3]

Platelets

Surgical bleeding is most unlikely to be a problem if the platelet count is greater than $50,000 \times 10^6$/L. In some cases of chronic thrombocytopenia surgery can be performed with counts as low as $10,000 \times 10^6$/L.

Platelets come in packs of 70 to 100 ml and are stored at room temperature. They are issued in O, A, and B groups only. If Rh-positive platelets are used in Rh-negative women then give them anti-D immunoglobulin. Give each unit of platelets through a fresh standard blood-giving set. Each unit should be infused in no longer than 30 minutes, but may be given rapidly over 5 minutes if necessary. One unit of platelets usually raises the platelet count by about $10,000 \times 10^3$/mm^3.

Store platelets at 22°C (room temperature), and not in the refrigerator. Treat them gently. Their role in life is to burst, which they readily do at the slightest provocation. Do not suck them into a syringe through a needle, or slap the packs around on the bench.

When to use platelets

Indications for platelet transfusion in recovery room are:

♦ Continued bleeding after surgery when the platelet count is $< 50,000 \times 10^3$/mm^3.

♦ Continued diffuse microvascular bleeding (ooze) when the platelet count is $< 50,000 \times 10^3$/mm^3.

♦ Dysfunctional platelets where the patient has been taking drugs such as dabigatran, clopidogrel, aspirin, NSAIDs, calcium channel blockers, SSRIs, β-blockers.

A few units of platelets will be very effective once the patient is warm and oxygenated and red cells are being transfused.

Five per cent albumin

Five per cent human albumin (50 g/L) is a purified, sterile, colloid derived from human plasma. It does not need to be cross-matched. It can be useful as a plasma expander in resuscitation while you wait for blood to arrive. Rarely, it may cause hypotension. Although never reported there is a theoretical risk of transmitting Creutzfeldt–Jakob disease (CJD), but not HIV or hepatitis viruses.

Fresh frozen plasma

Fresh frozen plasma (FFP) contains all the clotting factors (especially factor VIII). Normally the body contains the equivalent of about 12 units of FFP. Even in extreme cases, 12 units should restore coagulation factors to normal levels.

Reserve Group O plasma
for Group O recipients.

FFP is stored at −25°C. It is delivered in 150–300 ml bags of beige coloured ice. Usually the blood bank defrosts them for you. Use the ABO group compatible with the recipient's red cells. Fresh frozen plasma can be infused rapidly.

When to use fresh frozen plasma

- To restore labile coagulation factors in massive transfusions once the INR or aPTT > 1.5, or when factors V and VIII are < 25% of normal.
- To immediately reverse the effects of warfarin.
- To treat DIC where there is active bleeding.
- With surgical bleeding in patients with severe liver disease.

Do not use fresh frozen plasma simply to expand plasma volume, or when the patient is hypothermic. Empirically, you can use fresh frozen plasma after every 2–3 units of packed cells. If specific therapy is available, such as cryoprecipitate, factor VIII, or other specific factor concentrates, then use these in place of fresh frozen plasma.

Do not defrost fresh frozen plasma in a microwave oven, or in hot water, because you will denature the enzymes. Use FFP within 6 hours of thawing.

> *The biggest risk of blood transfusion*
> *is iatrogenic pulmonary oedema.*

Cryoprecipitate

Cryoprecipitate is prepared from a single donation, frozen at minus 30°C and takes 30 minutes to thaw. Cryoprecipitate contains fibrinogen, factor VIII (to see drugs decreasing transfusion requirements see Box 26.3), factor XIII and von Willebrand's factor.

Box 26.3 **Drugs decreasing transfusion requirements**

Desmopressin, a synthetic analogue of vasopressin, causes intense vasoconstriction—the patient goes 'white as a ghost'. It releases factor VIII from endothelium and pro-coagulant components of factor VIII. It is useful when patients with von Willebrand's disease bleed following surgery, and where bleeding is caused by platelet abnormalities associated with uraemia. It is sometimes used where large blood losses are expected, for example in major spinal surgery.

Antifibrinolytics

Tranexamic acid and epsilon-aminocaproic acid stabilize existing clots, and prevent primary fibrinolysis. They are given to patients having hip and knee surgery to reduce the blood loss. Aprotinin inhibits fibrinolysis and also kallikrein-induced activation of the clotting cascade. It diminishes postoperative blood loss. Antifibrinolytics occasionally promote pathological thrombosis.

When to use cryoprecipitate

Microvascular ooze is likely if fibrinogen is greater than 50 g/L. Consider using cryopre-cipitate when the fibrinogen values are trending towards 0.75 g/L. Start with 1–1.5 donor units per 10 kg body weight. Cryoprecipitate is not treated to remove viruses. Do not use it to treat haemophilia or von Willebrand's disease, if alternative therapies are available. Use the correct ABO group.

Recombinant factor VIIa

Factor VII is one of the enzymes in the clotting pathway. In severe haemorrhage the body may not be able to make factor VII fast enough. Recombinant factor VIIa (rhFVIIa) was originally developed for treating haemophiliacs. It is increasingly being used to treat uncontrollable haemorrhage.

Problems with blood transfusions

Risk of transmitting disease

The risk of transmitting disease from allogeneic (donor) blood is very low indeed. The risk of transmitting HIV is far less than 1 in 5 million, and the risk of hepatitis B or C is approaching this level too.

To put these risks into perspective, the risk in any single year of an urban dweller being killed in a car accident is 1:10,000. For people who live in rural areas, the chance of being killed by a bolt of lightning is about 1:20,000 in a given year. It is worth noting that, in a teaching hospital, the risk of giving too much blood to a patient and causing pulmonary oedema is about 1 per cent.

Blood transfusion reactions

Microbial contamination

Sepsis is the leading cause of transfusion mortality. Bacteria can get into the blood as contamination from skin organisms when the blood is collected from the donor. If the bag of blood is frothy, or chocolate brown or is distended, it is probably infected. Do not open it! Return it to the blood bank.

Because platelets are stored at room temperature they are more likely than blood stored in a refrigerator to be a culture medium for bacteria.

Variant Creutzfeldt–Jakob disease

Variant Creutzfeldt–Jakob disease (vCJD) is a human *prion* disease, which is an abnormal host-encoded glycoprotein that accumulates in the brain. Another form of the disease is bovine-spongiform encephalopathy BSE, or 'mad cow disease' which can be passed on by blood transfusion. Because of this concern most blood banks will not accept blood donors who have lived in the UK for a period prior to 1992. There is no known reliable test for this disease but processes are being developed to remove prions from blood component.

Acute haemolytic transfusion reaction

The most tragic transfusion reactions occur when ABO-incompatible blood is accidentally given to a patient. These accidents are usually caused by clerical lapses—giving the wrong blood to the wrong patient. Almost everyone has naturally occurring antibodies (including anti-A and anti-B) in their blood. If challenged these *autoantibodies* activate a special plasma protein called complement that rapidly ruptures circulating red cells to cause shock and renal failure. This can be fatal, even if only a small volume of incompatible blood was transfused.

ABO-Rh typing alone results in a 99.8 per cent chance of a compatible transfusion. This means that in an extreme emergency you are fairly safe giving typed but uncross-matched blood.

Signs

Signs of blood transfusion reaction are those of haemolysis and an acute immune reaction. Mild reactions present with: fever, tachycardia, sweating, and urticaria. Severe reactions occur with additional: back and chest pain, hypotension, oliguria, haemoglobinuria and progress to disseminated intravascular coagulation, renal failure, and sometimes death.

Febrile non-haemolytic transfusion reaction

A *febrile non-haemolytic transfusion reaction* (FNHTR) is defined as a rise in body temperature of 1°C or more during a transfusion. It usually occurs towards the end of the transfusion. It is the most common adverse effect of transfusion occurring in about 1 per cent of transfusions. Bioreactive substances, such as interleukins or complement fractions that accumulate when blood is stored, usually cause FNTHR. These reactions are seldom dangerous and are treated by simply stopping the transfusion. If the patient has had a previous febrile reaction use leucocyte-depleted blood for subsequent transfusions.

Allergic reactions

Transient hives (*urticaria*) and itching occur in about 1 per cent of transfusions and indicate a minor allergic reaction to the donor's plasma proteins. Treat it by stopping the transfusion. However if the patient also starts to wheeze, or becomes hypotensive, then you are dealing with much more serious anaphylaxis.

Anaphylaxis

Anaphylactic reactions occur rarely; in about 1:50,000 transfusions. Coughing is usually the first sign, followed shortly by wheeze, urticaria, hypotension, and abdominal cramps. See page 332.

Transfusion-related lung injury

Transfusion-related lung injury (TRALI) is an immune-mediated life-threatening syndrome with symptoms and signs similar to acute respiratory distress syndrome (ARDS). Transfusions of FFP are the main culprit. In most cases, there is an antibody in the donor's plasma that reacts with the recipient's white cells. TRALI presents with respiratory distress, hypoxia and fever, which progresses over several hours to a chest x-ray revealing a bilateral white-out with diffuse alveolar and interstitial infiltrates. More than 80 per cent of patients with TRALI recover with appropriate management in ICU.

How to manage transfusion reactions

If, shortly after starting a blood transfusion, your patient starts to cough or develops an itchy rash all over their body that looks like hives, then they are having a blood transfusion reaction.

Turn off the transfusion. Summon help. Notify the anaesthetist. Monitor vital signs, and perfusion status. Give high-flow oxygen by face mask. Change the drip sets and continue the infusion with 0.9% saline. Re-identify the patient and blood pack. Inform the blood bank and return the unused blood and pack. Take the giving set that has the blood in it and seal both ends so that the laboratory can sample blood in the IV line. Recheck the data label on the unit of blood with the blood cross-match form and the patient's wrist name band. Notify the hospital's blood bank. Take three samples of blood from the arm opposite the infusion. Put a sample of blood in each of three tubes: a white capped (*serum*) tube, in a blue capped (*citrated*) tube and a pink capped (*EDTA*) tube. Fill out a pathology request slip labelling it: 'Transfusion reaction investigations'. Send the three specimens of blood, the sealed IV line and any previously empty bags to the haematology laboratory in a large sealed plastic bag.

If the patient starts to wheeze then treat them for anaphylaxis. If the patient's urine turns dusky brown, this could be haematuria; treat this with mannitol 1.5 g/kg IV to promote a diuresis. Mannitol works within minutes and lasts for 2–3 hours.

If the patient develops only a slight fever (< 1°C rise) then the reaction is probably a febrile non-haemolytic reaction. If they develop rigors, chills, shivering, or they become restless or short of breath, or their temperature rises higher than 38.5°C then the reaction is more severe. Patients with very severe life-threatening reactions go on to develop one or more of these symptoms. Loin or back pain, hypotension, tachycardia, blood oozing from drip sights or wounds, or hypotension and collapse. These reactions indicate one of the following: a haemolytic reaction, bacterial contamination, anaphylaxis, or developing hours later, a transfusion-related lung injury. To survive the patient will need skilled specialist care from the anaesthetist, haematologist and other medical and nursing staff.

References

1. **van Ryn J, Stangier J,** *et al.* (2010) Effect of dabigatron on coagulation assays. *Thrombosis and Haemostasis* **103**(6):1116–1127.
2. **Finfer SR, Boyce NW,** *et al.* (2004) The SAFE Study. *Medical Journal Australia* **181**(5):237–238.
3. **Muller L, Lefrant JY** (2010) Transfusion alternatives in transfusion medicine. *Medical Education Global Solutions* **11**(3):10–21.

Further Reading

The Australian Red Cross has an excellent manual, *Transfusion Medicine*, freely available over the internet, which covers all aspects of blood transfusion.

In New Zealand the NZ Blood Service publishes the *Transfusion Medicine Handbook*.

In the UK the Blood Transfusion & Tissue Transplantation Services publish the *Handbook of Transfusion Medicine*, 4th edn, 2007.

There are many additional guidebooks and information online available. Here are a few:

Callum JL, Lin Y, *et al.* (2011) *Bloody Easy 3: Blood Transfusions, Blood Alternatives and Transfusion Reactions: A Guide to Transfusion Medicine*, 3rd edn. Canada: Ontario Regional Blood Coordinating Network.

Canadian Blood Services (2011) *Clinical Guide to Transfusion*, online edition: <http://www.transfusionmedicine.ca/resources/clinical-guide-transfusion>.

Harmening DM (2012) *Modern Blood Banking & Transfusion Practices*, 6th edn. Philadelphia, PA: F.A. Davis Company.

Klein HG, Anstee DJ (2006) *Mollison's Blood Transfusion in Clinical Medicine*, 11th edn. Malden, MA: Oxford: Blackwell Publishing. E-book available (12th edition published in 2014).

McClelland DBL (ed) (2007) *Handbook of Transfusion Medicine*, 4th edn. London: The Stationery Office.

McCullough J (2012) *Transfusion Medicine*, 3rd edn. Oxford: Blackwell Publishing.

Mintz PD (ed) (2010) *Transfusion Therapy: Clinical Principles and Practice*, 3rd edn. Bethesda, MD: AABB Press.

Roback JD (ed) (2011) *AABB Technical Manual*, 17th edn. Bethesda, MD: American Association of Blood Banks.

Chapter 27

Surgical issues

Drains and catheters

Surgical tubes (catheters) and drains are inserted with the intention of preventing unwanted fluid accumulating in surgical wounds, hollow organs or body cavities. Unwanted fluids such as blood, pus, intestinal fluids or lymph can collect in spaces entered into (e.g. the abdomen) or created by surgery. This can improve patient comfort, prevent swelling and hopefully avoid infection. In the chest drains can be used to remove air from around the lung to allow the lungs to expand. In some situations drains can be lifesaving, for example, chest drains in tension pneumothorax or a nasogastric tube in acute gastric distension. Having a urinary catheter following surgery has the dual benefit of facilitating comfort and allowing urinary output to be accurately documented.

Drains are usually made from biologically inert silicon rubber (Silastic®) and cause little tissue damage (Figure 27.1).

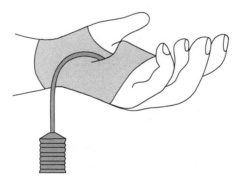

Figure 27.1 Mini-concertina drain.

Drains can be open to the air or closed to prevent contamination. Passive drains rely on body pressures and gravity for expulsion. Suction applied to drains facilitates their action and many companies produce simple closed suction drainage systems where a vacuum can be applied. Open drains include corrugated sheets of rubber or plastic, simple tubes or sheets of small tubes allowing for capillary action. The fluid collects externally in gauze, or a stoma bag. Being exposed to the external environment increases the risk of infection with these drains. Closed drains allow fluids to escape into sealed containers—these include chest and abdominal drains. There is less risk of infection with closed drains or contamination of medical staff with their contents.

Nasogastric tubes

If the stomach cannot empty satisfactorily because of intestinal obstruction or paresis (ileus) following handling at surgery then it can become distended leading to nausea and vomiting. Of great concern is the risk of aspiration in an obtunded patient with resulting chemical and infectious pneumonia. Handling bowel at surgery typically reduces gastro-intestinal mobility for a few days. During this time fluid transudates and collects in the gastrointestinal tract. Nasogastric tubes (Figure 27.2) drain the fluid accumulating in the stomach and proximal small bowel. While they are typically used in the setting of intes-tinal obstruction they are used routinely only infrequently in abdominal surgery, most likely when the stomach or oesophagus is operated on directly.

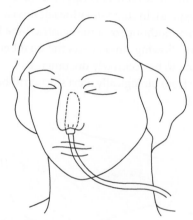

Figure 27.2 Fastening the nasogastric tube.

Nasogastric tubes are left to drain freely. For their siphoning action to work properly, keep the bag below the level of the bed. Sometimes the surgeon will request 4-hourly aspiration. Aspirate these tubes very gently. The fluid should almost flow freely into your syringe with little or no suction. Never apply vigorous suction to the tube because you will damage the stomach's delicate mucosa and create haemorrhage. Do not kink off the nasogastric tube 'to prevent air flowing back into the stomach'—it won't. (Consider the consequences of applying the same amount of suction to the mucosa in your mouth.)

Urinary catheters

Urinary catheters are another form of drain. They are used to relieve or prevent urinary retention and bladder distension, or to monitor urine output. Most are inserted through the urethra, but where this is impractical the patient may need a suprapubic catheter. Urinary catheters are usually made of a form of silicon plastic, or occasionally latex rubber. Men need 38 cm long catheters, and women need 22 cm long catheters. Adult diameters range from 10 Fr to 24 Fr, but 14 Fr is the most useful size. There are many different types used for specialized purposes, including whistle-tipped, Gibbon, Tiemann, Malecot, and Nelaton catheters.

To lower the risk of introducing infection, use an aseptic technique to insert catheters. Use ample lubricant. If you select the appropriate size they should simply glide in. Do not inflate the balloon until you see urine flowing from the catheter. Never use force when inserting a catheter. If you have difficulty then the patient may need a suprapubic catheter. Do not use a catheter introducer unless you have been trained in its use. When you first place the catheter, make a note of the residual urine volume in the patient's record.

Laparoscopy

Laparoscopic surgery is now the preferred technique for many intra-abdominal and pelvic procedures with numerous innovative developments.

The advantages of laparoscopy are smaller wounds with less tissue damage, less handling of the bowel with quicker recovery, and a magnified view is available to the theatre team which aids the surgeon and enhances interest and teaching. The result for the patient is less postoperative pain, less physiological disturbance, and shorter hospital stays. For the theatre team, there is much better understanding and appreciation of the procedure.

Problems with laparoscopic surgery include accidental damage to intra-abdominal structures, and the risks of introducing carbon dioxide under pressure. Under pressure gas can escape into the tissues causing subcutaneous emphysema, or even enter blood vessels, causing gas embolism. Carbon dioxide is routinely used as it is rapidly absorbed compared to nitrogen.

Absorption of carbon dioxide can cause hypercarbia and acidosis resulting in cardiac tachyarrhythmias. Patients may come to recovery room flushed, with a tachycardia and a wide pulse pressure.

In the recovery room the patient may still be breathing-off the excess carbon dioxide and consequently feel short of breath. This resolves within a few minutes. The insufflated carbon dioxide has to be excreted eventually through the lungs.

Following abdominal laparoscopy the gas, fluid and distension may irritate the diaphragm causing referred pain to the shoulder tip. Typically patients feel as though someone has wrenched their shoulders. The pain resolves with conventional analgesia usually over 24 hours.

Abdominal surgery

General principles

Postoperative hypoxaemia is common after abdominal surgery. This is partly a result of pain stopping the patient from taking deep breaths and coughing effectively. The best pain relief is provided by epidural analgesia, although this is not without hazard. Some surgeons inject local anaesthetic into the abdominal wound. Once your patient has adequate pain relief you can safely encourage deep breathing and coughing. You may need to support their wound while they do so.

The closer the incision is to the diaphragm,
the more painful it will be.

For 3 to 5 days after major gastrointestinal surgery, such as a Whipple's procedure, large amounts of fluid *transudate* into atonic bowel. This fluid is now not available to the general circulation. Unless the fluid is replaced the patient will become hypovolaemic. The hidden fluid in the bowel is called *third space loss*. A central venous catheter is often useful to guide fluid therapy. To avoid urinary retention and guide fluid therapy many patients need a catheter after major surgery.

The sick laparotomy

A *laparotomy* is a procedure to open the abdomen so that the surgeon can explore the cavity with the intention of finding or confirming an underlying problem and providing a surgical solution.

Emergency laparotomies for intra-abdominal catastrophes are a greater risk than elective laparotomies. Patients are often hypovolaemic and additionally may have systemic sepsis, hypothermia, hypotension, myocardial depression, renal impairment and malfunctioning lungs. Following the procedure patients are usually transferred directly from the operating theatre to the intensive care unit. Recovery room nurses often accompany the anaesthetist on the journey to the intensive care unit.

Moving such a patient from the operating table is fraught with hazard. There are lines, and wires and tubes and drains everywhere begging to be pulled out. Many hands make light work. Do it gently. As soon as the patient is on their bed stop everything and check their vital signs. The simple act of moving sick patients often destabilizes their blood pressure.

During transfer to the ICU make sure you have an emergency box containing everything you might need on the way. Carry a spare oxygen cylinder.

One difficulty is keeping the multitude of lines, cables, tubes and drains from tangling. Do not disconnect or try to sort the lines. Just move them in bulk. Do make sure they are clearly labelled, both where they leave the pumps, and where the other end of the line enters the patient. A useful technique is to use white sticky paper labels and fold them in half around each line then sort them out and unravel them later. One common error is to spend 10 minutes sorting out the lines, during which time the patient is virtually ignored.

It is well worthwhile, at some convenient time, to spend an hour or so planning and practising how to transfer these sick patients; where to put the pumps, how to carry the infusions, what to do with the monitors and where to hang the drains and so on.

Splenectomy

Splenectomy is an operation to remove the spleen. Splenectomy is used to treat some types of thrombocytopenia; but occasionally, being delicate and friable, the spleen is damaged during incidental surgery. It starts to bleed and has to be removed. A simple elective splenectomy causes few problems in the recovery room. Apart from pain control, concealed bleeding is the principal immediate risk. Watch for deteriorating skin perfusion, and tachycardia. Do not depend on hypotension to warn you of haemorrhage. Following splenectomy the platelet count increases dramatically, and 2 to 3 days later may reach $750,000 \times 10^3/mm^3$. This predisposes the patient to forming clots in their great veins.

Colon and rectal surgery

Colon and rectal surgery is usually for cancer and involves opening the abdomen and operating deep inside the pelvis. It is painful so many patients return to the recovery room with epidural analgesia. Test the upper level with ice.

If they have a colostomy or ileostomy, note the volume and nature of the drainage. If there is profuse loss of small bowel content from the stoma, it may intensify the patient's metabolic derangement in the recovery room.

Abdominoperineal resection

During abdominoperineal resection the lower sigmoid, rectum and anus are removed. The ends of the proximal colon are exteriorized to form a permanent colostomy. Check the colour of the colostomy to make sure it is pink. If it looks blue, or congested tell the surgeon. Abdominoperineal resection is a formidable procedure, with considerable tissue damage and blood loss. Patients frequently become hypothermic.

The final phase of the operation, the excision of the rectum, is done with the legs in the lithotomy position. When the legs are lowered blood re-enters the capacitance veins from the central circulation revealing hypovolaemia. Usually the anaesthetist will give the patient a colloid load just before the legs are taken down. Carefully watch the patient for signs of developing hypovolaemia for the first 20 minutes after they return to the recovery room.

Whipple's operation

Whipple's operation is major surgery to resect a carcinoma of the head of the pancreas. It is sometimes called a *pancreaticoduodenectomy*, which involves the removal of the gallbladder, common bile duct, part of the duodenum, and the head of the pancreas.

For 3 to 5 days after major bowel surgery large amounts of fluid transudates into atonic bowel as a hidden third space loss. Unless this fluid is replaced as it is lost the patient will become hypovolaemic. A central venous line is useful to guide fluid replacement.

Cholecystectomy

Cholecystectomy is the surgical removal of the gall bladder when it is inflamed or obstructed, if gallstones have caused pancreatitis, or where cancer is suspected.

Laparoscopic resection is the commonest way of removing the gallbladder. However, about 5 per cent of patients, usually those who have had previous abdominal surgery or a very severe chronically inflamed gall bladder require a laparotomy. Following this laparotomy the most common complication is right lower lobe atelectasis. In the recovery room encourage deep breathing and coughing to prevent this complication. Coughing is painful and your patient needs excellent analgesia. Morphine can precipitate biliary pain in patients who have had a cholecystectomy. Use fentanyl instead.

Internal bleeding can occur, especially if a tie slips off the cystic artery or there is an unnoticed minor laceration of the liver. Back in the ward concealed haemorrhage remains undetected until the patient becomes severely shocked. In the recovery room be suspicious if the patient develops a tachycardia, or their peripheral perfusion deteriorates. Confirm your suspicion by testing for a postural drop in systolic blood pressure.

Abdominal lipectomy

Abdominal lipectomy sometimes called an *apronectomy* or 'tummy tuck', is a traumatic operation. The long incision traverses the lower abdomen, large masses of fat are removed, and the incision is closed under tension. Sometimes blood loss exceeds a litre. The patients are obese, and have similar problems to all obese patients. Watch out for these. Pain is often the first sign of a developing haematoma. Check that there is no swelling or wound ooze before giving analgesia. Sit the patient up by raising both the foot and the head of the bed into the 'banana position' (Figure 27.3) to take the tension off the stitches. Take care when giving pain relief not to sedate the patient. They must remain alert and focus on deep breathing to fully expand their lungs.

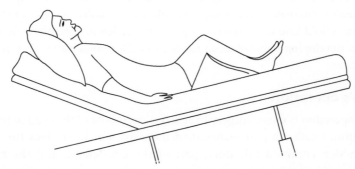

Figure 27.3 Banana position for recovering after abdominal lipectomy (cot sides would normally be in place).

Perineal surgery

Operations on the perineum, such as haemorrhoidectomy, are painful. Often this is usefully controlled with a caudal block, but these blocks can wear off abruptly. Warn the patient to ask for analgesia when they first start to feel pain.

Thoracic surgery

General principles

Many patients having thoracic surgery are elderly, and debilitated with malnutrition; some have cancer, others severe lung disease. They need skilled staff to monitor them closely during their stay in the recovery room.

The patient's posture and position affects the ventilation and perfusion of their lungs. If the patient is on a ventilator, the uppermost areas of the lung are better aerated. If the patient is breathing spontaneously then the dependent areas of the lung are better aerated. In both situations the dependent areas of the lungs get more perfusion. To achieve the best outcome you need to position your patient so that aeration matches with perfusion of their lungs. A spontaneously breathing patient in the recovery room has better gas exchange if they are nursed semi-sitting at 45° in Fowler's position.

After thoracic surgery there are four principal acute threats: concealed bleeding, pneumothorax, pneumomediastinum, cardiac tamponade and arrhythmias. A chest x-ray will help with the diagnosis. Pneumothorax presents with dyspnoea, sometimes with pleuritic pain, and a deviated trachea. Tension pneumothorax progresses rapidly to abrupt cardiovascular collapse. With cardiac tamponade the patient first develops a tachycardia, followed by a falling blood pressure, and their JVP rises.

Pneumomediastinum occurs when air leaks into the mediastinum. The air can track into the neck. So feel for crackles (*crepitus*) under the skin in the sternal notch. If you feel crepitus notify the surgeon because the patient may need to return to the operating theatre to patch the leak.

If the pericardium is damaged during surgery the patient may develop cardiac arrhythmias, particularly atrial fibrillation, while in the recovery room. Unrecognized hypomagnesaemia can contribute to this.

Check that the drain tubes are patent and swinging correctly. Never tie drain tubes to beds, the linen or anything else: if patients roll over they may pull them out. To avoid damaging delicate lung never apply high-pressure suction to the drains or 'milk' the tubing with an old-fashioned roller pump clamp. Never clamp thoracic drains, particularly if they are bubbling or the patient is being ventilated. Air that is unable to escape will quickly build up to cause a tension pneumothorax. Do not lift drain bottles on to the bed. Keep the drain bottles below the patient otherwise fluid in the bottle may drain back into the patient (Figure 27.4).

Occasionally air leaks occur, and the patient becomes acutely breathless. Notify the surgeon and prepare to return the patient to theatre to control the leak.

If the surgeon opens both the peritoneal and the thoracic cavity or divides the diaphragm, then the patient usually remains intubated, and will be extubated later in ICU. Otherwise patients come to recovery room extubated. As soon as possible sit them up. This improves their oxygenation and ability to breathe and cough effectively. They should return to the ward on continuous humidified supplemental oxygen overnight.

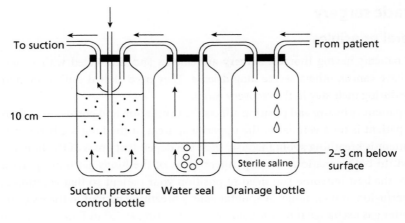

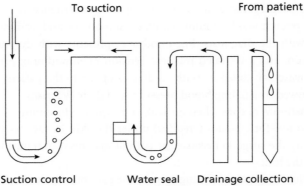

Figure 27.4 Set-up for continuous three-bottle low-pressure drainage of the thoracic cavity. Note how the principle of the three-bottle drainage is incorporated into a plastic drainage system moulded to form three chambers.

Bronchoscopy

Bronchoscopy is used to inspect the airways and to help diagnose lung disease, also, to take a biopsy, or remove a foreign body, and occasionally to insert airway stents. Occasionally it is used to treat certain lung conditions. Fibreoptic bronchoscopy is usually done under local anaesthetic as an outpatient procedure, whereas rigid bronchoscopy requires a general anaesthetic because an instrument resembling a 40 cm pipe is passed into the trachea.

If the patient returns to the recovery room still unconscious after a bronchial biopsy then nurse them on their side with the biopsy side down so that if they bleed, the blood will not enter the unaffected lung on the opposite side. As soon as they are awake sit them up, and support them on two or three pillows.

Following rigid bronchoscopy patients often cough uncontrollably. The anaesthetist will probably have sprayed the throat and larynx with lidocaine before the patient comes to the recovery room; but despite this they may cough violently, become hypoxic and distressed. Lidocaine 1 mg/kg made up to 5 ml in saline and given by a nebulizer is useful. Take care that nothing the patient coughs up touches any part of you. Wear a gown, gloves and goggles.

Mediastinoscopy

The *mediastinum* is the space that separates the lungs and lies between the sternum and the spinal column. It contains the heart, oesophagus, trachea, large blood vessels, the thymus, and lymph nodes. During mediastinoscopy a lighted instrument called the *mediastinoscope* is inserted through a small incision in the neck. This enables the surgeon to directly view the structures in the upper thorax. Mediastinoscopy enables examination of the lymph nodes in a patient with lung cancer, and if necessary a biopsy of suspect areas is used to stage their disease.

Patients come to recovery room with a small wound and no drains. However, their thoracic cavity may conceal much mischief, such as massive occult bleeding from a damaged great vein or pneumothorax from a breached lung. Watch for signs of airway obstruction, deviation of the trachea and developing dyspnoea. A chest x-ray will reveal widening of the mediastinum or air outside the lungs. Air can track into the neck, so feel for crackles (*crepitus*) under the skin in the sternal notch or neck. If you feel crepitus notify the surgeon and prepare to insert a chest drain. The patient may need to return to the operating theatre.

Oesophagectomy

Oesophagectomy involves the surgical removal of part of the oesophagus for cancer, or high-grade dysplasia of the lower oesophageal mucosa (*Barrett's oesophagitis*). This procedure is usually performed with laparoscopic and thoracoscopic instruments, reducing the extent and severity of the surgery. If the chest and abdomen are opened this becomes a major, long and often bloody exercise. A length of bowel with its blood supply replaces the excised oesophagus. The principal risk is disruption of the anastomoses followed by frequently fatal mediastinal infection.

Most patients remain intubated after surgery, and are then transferred to ICU for a short period of ventilation. Their stay in recovery room is usually brief. Those who do stay in the recovery room need intensive and experienced nursing. Plan to allocate two nurses to care for them. Watch the ECG carefully. About 60 per cent of patients develop postoperative cardiac arrhythmias (particularly atrial fibrillation) and 20 per cent get major respiratory complications.

If patients are extubated in the recovery room, wait until their temperature is greater than 35.8°C. Check that you can hear normal breath sounds over the right side of the chest, and the underwater seals on the chest drain tubes are swinging or bubbling correctly. Check that the nasogastric (NG) tube is stitched through the frenulum of the nose so it cannot be accidentally pulled out. The NG tube prevents accumulating fluid distending the relocated bowel and tearing the stitches out. Make sure the NG tube is draining freely. Aspirate it gently.

Thymectomy

Thymectomy is excision of the thymus gland that lies in the upper mediastinum. This is usually done in an attempt to relieve the symptoms and modify the progress of myasthenia gravis. Thymectomy is typically done through a sternal split. Postoperatively there is a slight risk of pneumomediastinum.

Myasthenics commonly take the anticholinergic drug (pyridostigmine) to counteract the muscle weakness. Pyridostigmine is often omitted for a few hours before surgery and recommenced in the recovery room. Some patients need postoperative ventilation until they are able to breathe and cough adequately, especially those who have had respiratory failure in the past, or who are taking more than 750 mg of pyridostigmine a day. Do not extubate them until they can sustain a 5-second head lift. They must return to their maintenance anti-cholinesterase drugs as soon as possible. If necessary give these drugs down a nasogastric tube.

Sometimes neostigmine is used as an alternative to pyridostigmine. For every 30 mg of pyridostigmine they are taking preoperatively, use intravenous neostigmine 1 mg postoperatively. You will need to give atropine with the neostigmine to prevent bradycardia, salivation, abdominal cramps and bronchorrhoea. Start with intravenous neostigmine 2.5 mg and atropine 1.2 mg given over 2 minutes. Continue giving neostigmine in 1 mg boluses every 3 minutes until you reach the equivalent dose of pyridostigmine. For instance, if the patient is taking 120 mg pyridostigmine, the maximum dose of neostigmine is 4 mg. You may need to repeat the neostigmine in 2 to 4 hours' time depending on their ability to lift their head off the pillow.

Vascular surgery

General principles

Vascular surgery is used to repair major blood vessels, damaged or obstructed by trauma or disease. Vascular surgery is physiologically stressful. Major vessels are clamped diverting blood flow through unaccustomed routes. Blood loss may be large, renal and gut blood flow is often abruptly compromised, the operations are long, and the patient usually has associated illnesses, such as ischaemic heart disease, cerebrovascular disease, and frequently diabetes.

Intensive monitoring

Many patients are intensively monitored with an arterial line, triple lumen central venous catheter, 5-lead ECG, and possibly a pulmonary artery catheter in their right subclavian or left internal jugular vein, and a urinary catheter.

These patients need close observation in the recovery room. They are at high risk of coronary ischaemia, and more than half do not get the warning chest pain.

Major aortic surgery

Abdominal aortic aneurysm repair is the commonest major abdominal vascular procedure. An aneurysm occurs when a blood vessel swells, stretching its walls and ballooning abnormally outward. The normal diameter of the aorta is about 2.5 cm. If the lumen swells to more than 6 cm the aorta is likely to acutely rupture and the patient will probably bleed to death.

At the end of major vascular surgery patients may appear haemodynamically stable. Watch them carefully, however. As soon as they are moved on to their bed for transport, they can drop their blood pressure and central venous pressure, revealing that they are hypovolaemic.

If they are not transferred directly to ICU or HDU postoperatively, they may remain in the recovery room for a lengthy time. Keep them warm, fully oxygenated and pain free.

Potential problems

* Hypothermia. Patients will fare better if they are electively ventilated until their temperature rises beyond 36°C.
* Myocardial ischaemia is common. Monitor closely for ST changes using a 5-lead ECG (leads II and V5).
* Cardiac support. The patient may well be receiving ionotropes or vasodilators delivered through syringe pumps.
* Renal hypoperfusion. Up to 25 per cent of patients develop renal impairment after aortic surgery. Closely monitor urine output. If urine output is < 30 ml/hr, then try a fluid challenge of 5 ml/kg of saline.
* Pain. Analgesia is best achieved with a T6–T11 epidural infusion preferably with diamorphine, which is more effective than fentanyl. Those who do not have an epidural will need patient-controlled analgesia.
* Ongoing bleeding. Hypothermia is the usual cause. Check the preoperative transfusion threshold and give blood if it has been exceeded. Check the activated clotting time; it should not exceed 140 seconds. Use platelets first and fresh frozen plasma only if needed.
* Spinal cord ischaemia causing paraplegia is a rare and devastating complication.

Carotid surgery

Carotid endarterectomy is a surgical procedure to open the lumen of the internal carotid artery and remove plaque so that blood flow can be restored to the brain. It is usually performed when carotid stenosis is greater than 70 per cent or the patient is experiencing neurological symptoms.

The danger is not over once the surgery is completed. The two most likely complications are stroke and myocardial infarction. Complications can appear within minutes, so keep patients under close observation in the recovery room for at least 3–4 hours postoperatively rather than transferring them to ICU.

Postoperatively about 5 per cent of patients develop a blood clot on the raw lining of the artery, usually within 2 hours of surgery. This causes signs of a stroke. If the artery is unblocked within 30 minutes the stroke will, most likely, resolve.

Patients should be able to lift each leg off the bed, and strongly grip two of your offered fingers with each hand. Ask patients to show you their teeth, and watch for asymmetry in their grin.

Watch for bleeding causing swelling in the neck; it may progress to cause respiratory obstruction. Check the drain tubes are allowing blood to escape. Notify the anaesthetist and surgeon if the patient develops noisy breathing, or stridor.

Because of trauma to the baroreceptors up to 65 per cent of patients become hypertensive and up to 35 per cent become hypotensive. Hypertension forewarns of deterioration in cerebral function or stroke, and also cardiac ischaemia. Notify the anaesthetist if the systolic blood pressure exceeds 160 mmHg. Use short-acting glyceryl trinitrate to control blood pressure, and avoid longer-acting agents such as hydralazine.

Cerebral hyperperfusion syndrome may cause a migraine like headache. As the blood supply is restored the weakened cerebral vessel walls stretch; they may even burst, causing stroke.

Watch for signs of cerebral hypoperfusion, such as nausea, and deteriorating conscious state. Stroke tends to cause unilateral signs. In contrast whereas cerebral hypoperfusion causes more global dysfunction with agitation, clouding of consciousness, seizures, and unless relieved, stroke.

Breast surgery

Mastectomy

Mastectomy involves the surgical removal of an entire breast, usually to treat breast cancer.

There are four types of mastectomy: subcutaneous mastectomy; total or simple mastectomy; modified radical mastectomy; and radical mastectomy.

While most breast cancers can now be treated with conservation of the breast, total mastectomy is still a common procedure. If axillary lymph nodes are involved an axillary dissection will be required. A sentinel lymph node biopsy is often performed to try and accurately determine if any axillary lymph nodes harbour metastatic disease. Radical mastectomy where the underlying chest muscles are removed is really a historic procedure.

After mastectomy (Figure 27.5) nurse patients on their back with their heads turned to one side in case they vomit. If they are obese sit them up as soon as they are fully conscious. Tight breast-binding dressings achieve little. The pressure they exert is insufficient to stop bleeding or prevent haematoma, and they severely impede the patient's ability to deep breathe and cough effectively.

On the side of the operation elevate the patient's arm on two pillows. Extension of surgery into the axilla may impede venous return causing the arm to become congested and blue. If this happens notify the surgeon. To avoid putting tension on her stitches, help her to change position if she is uncomfortable.

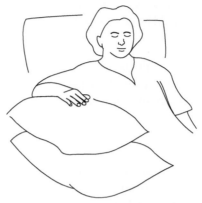

Figure 27.5 The mastectomy position.

Breast reduction surgery

Breast reduction surgery is done for women to reduce the bulk of massive breasts. Sometimes kilograms of breast tissue are removed, and 1500 ml or more blood can be lost. Pain can be a problem.

Gynaecology

General principles

Gynaecological surgery is pelvic surgery conducted on women's reproductive organs. It may involve opening the abdominal cavity, but many operations can be done through the vagina.

Higher risk of deep vein thrombosis

Gynaecological surgery often subtly disturbs venous blood flow back from the legs. These women are at a higher risk of deep vein thrombosis. Most deep vein thromboses start in the recovery room, so encourage leg movements. Make sure they are written up for suitable thromboprophylaxis.

Patients who have had their legs in lithotomy position for more than 30 minutes frequently become hypotensive when their legs are laid flat again. When their legs are elevated about 400–600 ml of blood runs down into their central veins. As their legs are let down, the blood re-enters their legs, their central venous returns falls, and they become abruptly hypotensive. Nurse these patients with their legs elevated on pillows for the first hour, and give them 5 ml/kg of intravenous fluid during that time.

Nausea and vomiting

Because surgery on the uterus and ovaries stimulates the vagus nerve, nausea and vomiting are common. Antiemetics should be given prophylactically.

Vaginal surgery

Vaginal surgery is performed with the legs in lithotomy. Over-abduction of the legs causes postoperative hip or knee pain. If the patient has hip or knee pain, then record this fact in the notes and notify the surgeon. Check their pads for continued vaginal bleeding.

Hysteroscopy

Hysteroscopy involves a visual inspection of the lining of the uterus with a fibreoptic hysteroscope. To allow a view, irrigation fluid is instilled into the uterus opening up the cavity. Some of this fluid may be absorbed. Irrigation fluid causes the same problems as the *TURP syndrome*. Unlike men, premenopausal women and children risk fatal cerebral oedema if their serum sodium falls abruptly below 130 mmol/L, whereas men and postmenopausal women do not run this risk until their serum sodium falls below 125 mmol/L. In the recovery room cerebral oedema first shows up as a headache which is made worse when patients move their head around.

Tubal surgery

Cauterization of the Fallopian tubes is painful. Some surgeons drip 0.5 per cent bupivacaine into the cut end of the tubes, which provides excellent pain relief for the first hour. Nausea and vomiting can be troublesome. If the pain is spasmodic it may respond to hyoscine butylbromide more than morphine.

Surgery on the limbs

Hand surgery is often done under regional blockade. The usual local anaesthetic used for brachial plexus blocks is lidocaine because it has a 2–3 hour action. If the anaesthetist has used bupivacaine then reassure the patient that feeling will return eventually though it may take a day or more. Since the arm is both numb and paralysed, warn the patient not to try to move their hand because it can fly about uncontrollably. Patients have hit themselves in the face while attempting to investigate their new place; some have even broken their noses. Following hand surgery the arm is usually splinted, with at least a plaster back-slab. Elevate the arm in a box-sling (also known as gallow's sling) to reduce swelling (Figure 27.6). Monitor the perfusion of the fingers.

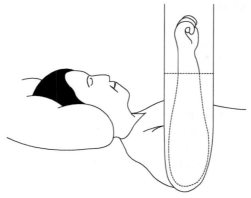

Figure 27.6 Gallow's sling.

Amputations

Amputation of a lower limb is occasionally performed for trauma, but more often for arterial insufficiency. In the latter case the patients are usually old, sick and frail with a combination of ischaemic heart disease, malnutrition, diabetes, and the accumulated ravages of decades of smoking. Apart from the diabetics, who are protected by numbness from peripheral neuropathy, most patients have considerable pain, and have received high doses of opioids over the preceding days or weeks. This means they need proportionally higher doses of opioids that you would otherwise expect.

Amputation is best done under spinal anaesthetic or epidural anaesthesia, as this reduces the risk of postoperative *phantom limb pain*. Having protracted, excruciating pain in a limb that no longer exists affects about 65 per cent of amputees, and the pain is refractory to most therapy. This pain is a form of chronic pain. To help alleviate this problem patients require outstanding analgesia postoperatively.

Send patients back to the ward with an Esmark's bandage taped to the top of their bed, so that should a ligature come off a major artery a tourniquet can be applied immediately before they bleed to death.

Orthopaedic surgery

General principles

Operations on bones are painful. Do not be alarmed if young patients especially, need more than the usual amount of opioids to control their pain. It is best to start analgesia before they reach the recovery room, and use a multimodal technique. Orthopaedic surgery performed under either spinal or epidural technique will effectively control pain while the patient is in recovery rom. Make sure there is an adequate prescription for the ward. For patients who have had spinal anaesthesia still need to begin treatment with other analgesics, both opioids and NSAIDs.

Carefully check for nerve damage if the patient has been operated on in the 'deck chair' position.

Tourniquets

Operations done under tourniquet, such as knee replacements, may bleed vigorously, up to a litre or more, while the patient is in the recovery room. Monitor the drain bottles for blood loss. Check the patient's records for a cause such as aspirin, NSAIDs, SSRIs or even herbal remedies. Also check that blood is available should a transfusion become necessary.

Type 2 diabetics who take metformin are at risk of severe lactic acidosis unless this drug has been ceased at least 36 hours before surgery. Metformin prevents the liver metabolizing the huge flood of lactic acid which suddenly enters the central circulation when the tourniquet is released. If the patient starts to hyperventilate or their pulse rate rises, then notify the anaesthetist immediately.

Arthroscopy

Arthroscopy is painful. It is usually done as a day case procedure. Local anaesthetic injected into the joint capsule helps control pain. This treatment is controversial and can cause damage to the articular surfaces. When the patient is young and healthy he can be given NSAIDs. If the patient complains of pain in the recovery room it may indicate bleeding into the operation site. Notify the surgeon.

Hip surgery

Patients having hip replacement surgery tend to lose blood, and they continue to bleed into the surgical site for some time after they have left theatre.

Several litres of blood can be lost during hip replacements and after fractures of the femoral neck. Blood spilled on the floor and drapes make it difficult to estimate the loss, and the patient may come to recovery room either hypovolaemic or fluid overloaded. Often patients continue to bleed in the recovery room. The loss may be concealed inside the wound, and unless detected the patient may be discharged to the ward still bleeding. Up to 1500 ml of blood can be lost into a thigh before it starts to swell noticeably.

Hypoxia is a constant threat to
elderly orthopaedic patients.

It is usually the elderly, with all their concurrent medical problems, who have hip surgery. Elderly patients with fractured necks of femurs are almost always hypoxic before they get to theatre; and the hypoxaemia becomes worse postoperatively. Following hip surgery patients often become hypoxaemic in the recovery room, especially if they have had a general anaesthetic. Periodic hypoxaemia can recur for up to 5 days after surgery.

'Grandma was never the same after she broke her hip.' Hypoxaemia usually occurs at night during sleep, and remains mostly unrecognized. It contributes to postoperative confusion and the residual cognitive damage may be permanent. This tragedy is avoidable. Mandatory supplemental oxygen, especially for the first few nights, reduces the risk substantially.

Contributing factors to the risk of hypoxia are opioid infusions, fat emboli; and although not often considered malnutrition contributes to muscle wasting so that these elderly patients cannot cough or deep breathe effectively.

Abduction pillow

After hip replacement surgery, a Charnley (*abduction*) pillow is used to keep the legs apart, strapped in the abduction position. Before you put on the pillow check the circulation to the feet. Put the wide end between the ankles. Apply the straps in such a way that you can easily slip your fingers between the strap and the skin. Be careful not to compress the peroneal nerve with the straps.

Routine orthopaedic observations

+ Check the drain tubes every 15 minutes. Make sure they are patent. Record the volume of drainage, and its colour and nature: serous, clotted blood, or bloodstained fluid.
+ Check the neurovascular status every 15 minutes. This includes: volume of peripheral pulses, limb colour and temperature, rate of capillary refilling; as well as occurrence of numbness, tingling, swelling and if possible movement.
+ Keep the limb in the correct position set by the surgeon.
+ Check for evidence of fat emboli.

Plaster checks

If a patient has a plaster applied check the exposed limb distal to the plaster to see that circulation is not impaired.

Observe and record:

+ Warmth, colour and capillary refilling.
+ Movement of fingers or toes.
+ Sensation and presence of pain, numbness or tingling.
+ Pulses.
+ State of plaster; whether it is showing signs of bloodstains or seepage.

Hints about plasters

+ Elevate the arm or leg on a pillow to help prevent swelling.
+ You cannot rely on numbness or tingling to warn of nerve compression if the patient has had a regional anaesthetic.

- Capillary refill is the most useful sign. Gently squeeze a finger or toenail bed. Blood should flush back pink within 2 seconds.
- Pain in a plastered limb is an ominous sign of ischaemia. Tell the surgeon immediately.
- Occasionally, muscles cramp or spasm inside the plaster. This usually responds to a small dose of diazepam 2 mg given intravenously.
- Outline any oozy stains on the plaster with an indelible pen. Put the date and time on the boundaries.
- Always ask the surgeon to review the plaster before the patient returns to the ward.

Surgery of the head and neck

General principles

Following head and neck surgery, the principal worry is the patency of the patient's airway. Bleeding behind the deep fascia in the neck can obstruct lymph and venous drainage from the surgical site without much obvious swelling on the outside, however the swelling inside may rapidly obstruct the airway. Check the drain tubes are draining. The first sign of airway obstruction will be noisy breathing. Notify the anaesthetist immediately.

The vagus nerve is often disturbed during surgery, and this predisposes to nausea and vomiting. Surgery around the bifurcation of the carotid artery can disturb baroreceptors, so that blood pressure may be unstable for some hours after the operation.

Blepharoplasty or meloplasty

After facelifts or eyelid surgery sit the patient up. The eyes are sometimes bandaged. If the patient complains of pain it may mean a haematoma is developing beneath the dressings. Sterile iced water-soaked pads help reduce the swelling. Do not disturb these patients, or encourage coughing. Let them recover quietly. Before discharging patients back to the ward check for double vision, a sign of a developing haematoma.

Faciomaxillary procedures

Major jaw surgery may take 4–6 hours. These patients are often young, the surgery is painful and they require deep anaesthesia. It may take some time to for them to wake up. They sometimes come to the recovery room still intubated. The anaesthetist cannot extubate the patient until they are sufficiently awake to look after their own airway. After mandibular surgery the teeth may be fixed together with elastic bands.

Nasal surgery

Following nasal surgery the nose is usually packed with stuffed glove fingers, gauze, silk, or yellow BIP paste. Partially conscious patients find it difficult to breathe through their mouths, and are distressed at having their airway blocked, they may become restless and thrash about. The anaesthetist should remain with patients until they are fully conscious.

Sit them up as soon as possible. This helps reduce venous bleeding into the soft tissues around the eyes, and postoperative facial swelling.

Opioids are best given intra-operatively and NSAIDs postoperatively. Pain is not usually a problem as the surgeon injects local anaesthetic. Opioids, if they are used, may suppress ventilation. They can also cause the patient to get a very itchy nose, which he may attempt to rub vigorously. A small dose of promethazine 6.25 mg IM usually resolves the problem. Naloxone will remove the itch, but plunge the patient into pain.

Sometimes a piece of tissue or blood clot will fall on to the vocal cords causing laryngospasm, coughing or a hoarse voice. If you suspect this has happened the anaesthetist may check the larynx and pharynx with a laryngoscope.

A large blood clot can easily be hidden in the nasal pharynx where it cannot be seen. This *coroner's clot* can be aspirated without warning into the trachea, to totally block the airway (Figure 27.7). After surgery on the upper airway gently use a dental sucker to explore the nasopharynx.

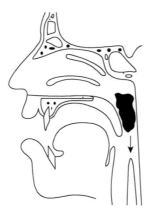

Figure 27.7 The coroner's clot.

An excessively dry throat may make patients restless. Once they are fully conscious, give them a piece of wet gauze to suck or little sips of water.

Sometimes small bits of plaster get into the eyes and irritate them. If this happens, notify the surgeon, and record the fact in the history. Irrigate the eyes with sterile 0.9 per cent saline. Check the eyes are not red before discharging the patient to the ward. Cold wet swabs to their eyes are comforting, and help prevent peri-orbital bruising.

Tonsillectomy

Following tonsillectomy bleeding into the pharynx is a grave danger. Nurse these patients on their side without a pillow until they are conscious (Figure 27.8). With patients weighing less than 50 kg put a pillow under their hips and tilt them slightly head down so that the blood can drain from their mouth.

Tonsillectomies are painful, but there are problems if the patient is deeply sedated after this operation. Check with the surgeon or anaesthetist before giving additional opioids. Patients with sleep apnoea are at particular risk of obstructed airways, and silently become apnoeic. Always have a working sucker tucked under their pillow. Use soft plastic catheters, which will not dislodge stitches, or damage friable surgical site, rather than the standard metal sucker.

A bleeding tonsil is a major recovery room emergency. Ensure every patient has freely flowing intravenous infusion sited, just in case it is needed. If it is accidentally pulled out replace it immediately. If you are continually aspirating blood from the pharynx notify the surgeon. Remember that babies and infants are seriously compromised with as little as 10 per cent blood loss. This may only be two well-soaked small swabs in infants.

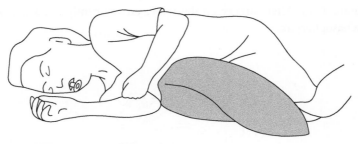

Figure 27.8 Tonsillectomy position.

Cleft palate

After repairing a cleft palate the surgeon may put a loose looping suture through the tongue. To clear the airway, gently pull the loop forward. Leave the suture in place for 36 hours until the facial swelling subsides. Pain can be a problem, so give analgesia early. Keep the face clean and watch for oozing from the nose or mouth. Notify the surgeon if it continues. It may be necessary to splint the arms of children so they cannot suck their fingers. Monitor their oxygenation with an oximeter. Never turn your back on children, because respiratory obstruction may occur quickly, silently and without warning. You will find it easier to monitor the child's heart rate by feeling the apex beat, rather than the carotid or radial pulse.

Dental surgery

Many of the problems with the care of postoperative dental patients are those of tonsillectomy. Hypoxaemia and airway problems remain a risk. Nurse the patient on their side. Check that those with valvular heart disease have received antibiotic prophylaxis against endocarditis. In young and healthy dental patients diclofenac or ibuprofen gives good postoperative pain relief.

Intellectually disabled patients

It is almost impossible to do dental procedures in intellectually handicapped patients under local anaesthetic. These patients need general anaesthesia for even minor procedures. Many will have Down's syndrome; of these 40 per cent have valvular heart disease and need antibiotic prophylaxis against endocarditis. People with Down's syndrome have a lower intelligence than normal, and are easily confused by unfamiliar routines. They may become frightened when away from people they know and trust. Adult patients can be very strong indeed, and some become combative when frightened or in pain. Sometimes they have 'security blankets'—a favourite object—these can come to theatre and recovery room with the patient.[1]

Intellectually disabled patients require one nurse dedicated to the patient. You may need strong attendants. Midazolam quickly controls agitation, but the effective dose is highly variable. Some are easily sedated with a small dose, while others are quite resistant. Patients with Down's syndrome are particularly sensitive to opioids, and require about half the dose of a normal person. Their biggest risk is airway obstruction. They have short stiff necks and large tongues, and are particularly susceptible to laryngeal stridor. Some patients have unstable atlanto-occipital joints. Be especially gentle when extending their bull-necks, because you may dislocate their cervical spine and render them quadriplegic.

Thyroid and parathyroid surgery

After thyroid or parathyroid surgery, sit the patients up as soon as they regain consciousness. Check and re-secure their dressings. These patients are frequently nauseated because the surgeon has retracted on, or near, the vagus nerve in the neck. Check which anti-emetic they have received during their anaesthetic, and choose another from a different group. Suitable alternatives are prochlorperazine 12.5 mg IM, or metoclopramide 15 mg IV, or ondansetron 4–8 mg IV. If they have received preoperative instruction, properly applied acupressure is surprisingly effective in these patients.

Concealed bleeding, usually from the superior thyroid artery, beneath the deep fascia in the neck, blocks lymphatic and deep venous drainage, and can quickly cause airway obstruction. The problem is not tracheal compression, but rather obstruction of veins, and especially lymph drainage, which rapidly causes submucosal oedema. If you look in the mouth you will find the mucosa of the pharynx ballooning into the lumen. If the patient develops noisy breathing or stridor then notify the anaesthetist immediately (see Box 27.1).

The internal swelling generally makes re-intubation either hazardous or impossible. In this case sit the patient up. Give high concentrations of oxygen. Wherever possible the patient should return to the operating theatre for the surgeon to control the bleeding. If not, you must act alone. Take out the skin clips or sutures and the wound will fall open. Using sterile instruments take out the deep sutures running transversely across the deep fascia at the bottom of the wound. Blood will gush out, and the tissues will fall

Box 27.1 **Management of stridor after thyroid operation**

Step 1. Put the patient on high inspired oxygen, and sit him up.

Step 2. Take out the skin clips or sutures. The wound will fall open (Figure 27.9).

Step 3. Using sterile instruments take out the sutures running transversely in a straight line in the bottom of the wound. The tissues will fall open, and allow the blood to drain out. No harm can be done by this procedure, and it may save the patient's life.

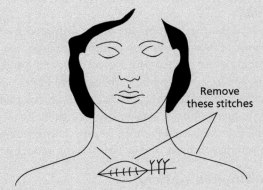

Remove these stitches

Figure 27.9 The stitches to remove should stridor occur.

away exposing the trachea. If necessary you can push a percutaneous tracheostomy tube beneath the first tracheal ring to gain an airway.

Send the patient back to the ward with a sterile pack containing all the instruments needed to take out the stitches. The pack should be fastened to the head of the bed so that the instruments are available immediately should the stitches need to be removed in a hurry.

Radical neck dissection

Radical neck dissection is a traumatic operation for cancer of the oropharynx or salivary glands. It involves en-bloc resection of all the lymph nodes and vessels from the mandible to clavicle along the course of the jugular vein. Airway obstruction is a major risk, and most patients will return to recovery room with an elective tracheostomy, and a number of drains inserted to allow blood to escape. Watch for swelling in the operative field indicating bleeding below the deep fascia. The risk of swelling in the neck is similar to that of a thyroidectomy.

Operations on the left side of the neck may damage the thoracic duct, in which case milky *lymph* may appear in the drain bottles.

Pneumothorax can follow major neck surgery. Suspect it if the patient develops stabbing chest pain or difficulty in breathing. The larynx may be pushed away from its midline position toward the affected side. Percuss the chest. A pneumothorax has the same deep hollow quality you will hear if you percuss a pillow.

Urological surgery

Because common urological operations have long names they are usually abbreviated:

+ Transurethral resection of the prostate = TURP.
+ Transurethral bladder tumour resection = TURBT.
+ Percutaneous nephrolithotomy = PCNL.

General principles

Patients undergoing urological surgery are usually elderly people with multiple intercurrent diseases. They are prone to developing complications in the first 2 hours after surgery. Keep them a little longer, and do not discharge them until you are sure they are stable. If they have had spinal anaesthesia they should stay under close observation for 1 hour from the time of insertion of the block. Hypotension can occur at any time during this period.

Sepsis

A urinary tract can host a variety of bacteria. During TURPs, or when the surgeon relieves a chronic obstruction, a shower of bacteria may enter the bloodstream. The cell membranes of Gram-negative bacteria contain incredibly potent *endotoxins*. This endotoxic shower manifests as a short episode of hypotension, sometimes with severe chills, and flushing. If the temperature rises then it indicates septicaemia. Gentamicin 2 mg/kg is the usual prophylaxis against this event. A single dose of gentamicin will do no harm, but another dose should not be given until the patient's creatinine clearance is calculated; otherwise there is a risk of kidney damage and irreversible deafness. Furosemide greatly accentuates gentamicin's toxicity.

Transurethral resection of the prostate

Those who have had a spinal anaesthetic for TURPs are especially vulnerable to complications. They have been flooded with irrigation fluid, sometimes 20 litres or more, some of which they may have absorbed and they have had their legs raised in lithotomy position for a long time.

Hypothermia is a big problem. Patients can get very cold. The elderly do not tolerate this well. Prevention is better than cure. Warm all irrigating and intravenous fluids. Use convection warming blankets on the patient in the recovery room. Do not discharge the patient back to the ward until his temperature is greater than 36.5°C.

When the patient's legs are taken down from the lithotomy position, up to 800 ml of blood can rush back into the leg veins and the blood pressure may suddenly fall. To prevent this elevate the legs on pillows while the patient is in the recovery room. Give intravenous colloid continuously until the patient is stable.

TURPs are not particularly painful. If the patient complains of pain then suspect clot retention or even a ruptured bladder.

TURP syndrome

TURP syndrome is a serious problem. It occurs when irrigation fluid enters the circulation causing a combination of acute hyponatraemia and acute fluid overload. The most usual irrigating solution contains 1.5 per cent glycine in water. If the patient has had more than 15 litres of irrigation fluid, or has been on the table for longer than 45 minutes then expect problems. On the patient's arrival in the recovery room send blood to check the haemoglobin levels and serum sodium concentration. Elderly patients and children are especially at risk.

Acute hyponatraemia causes the conscious state to deteriorate. The patient initially describes tingling or numbness around the mouth, and then may find it difficult to form thoughts and talk coherently. Headache, vomiting, confusion soon follow. Finally the patient may have convulsions and lose consciousness. Symptoms appear when the serum sodium (Na^+) drops below 130 mmol/L, becomes severe when Na^+ concentration is less than 125 mmol/L and is often fatal when less than 120 mmol/L.

Acute volume overload presents first with a rising respiratory rate, decreasing oxygen saturations, then cough, then wheeze; and finally overt pulmonary oedema. At this stage the patient is unable to lie flat and is coughing up frothy pink fluid.

Once the central nervous system is affected, consider using hypertonic 3 per cent saline. Using this requires judgement and experience, and is better done in an intensive care unit.

Glycine toxicity

Glycine toxicity occurs if sufficient glycine enters the circulation. This may cause transient blindness with or without cardiac failure. Other signs are a sequential progression of nausea, vomiting, slowing respiratory rate, confusions, and convulsions.

Burns

Managing patients with burns is a challenge. After surgery they are physiologically unstable and may respond unpredictably so assign your most experienced staff to look after them.

Burns oedema and limb ischaemia

The patient becomes oedematous about 18 hours after major burns. As oedema develops, circumferential burns on a limb act like a non-flexible tourniquet. Regularly check peripheral capillary return, if a limb becomes congested, or white, an *escharotomy* is urgently needed. This involves cutting the tight band of dead tissue strangling the limb. It is a relatively painless procedure, and does not require an anaesthetic, but it may bleed vigorously so be prepared to give a rapid transfusion.

Airway burns

Patients with facial burns always have airway burns too, and probably smoke damage to bronchi and lung tissue. As the airway becomes progressively oedematous and swollen, wheezing, or noisy breathing warns of impending airway obstruction. Watch for agitation, or restlessness heralding hypoxia.

If the lips and tongue swell to close the airway you may need to gently insert a soft nasopharyngeal airway as a temporary measure. Lubricate it well with 2 per cent lidocaine gel. Even in a conscious patient these airways are well tolerated. Avoid rigid plastic tubes as these can damage tissues, rupture nasal cartilages, and introduce infection into the paranasal sinuses.

Burnt face = burnt airway.

Monitoring

It can be difficult to find somewhere to put the ECG dots, or blood pressure cuffs. If the arms are burnt then use a large blood pressure cuff on the thigh to measure blood pressure. The ECG dots can go anywhere on the limbs, and they can even be put on the head if necessary. Just place them so they form the corners of an equilateral triangle around the heart.

Pain

With full thickness burnt skin the nerve endings are destroyed so the burn is painless. Debridement of burns, especially the hands or feet, is very painful. Donor sites are more painful than the grafted area. If the debrided areas are extensive local blocks are impractical.

Patients with acute burns are often in a lot of pain. Their pain is made worse because they are frightened. Take time to comfort and reassure them. As you remove their anxiety much of their pain will dissipate. One remembers the compassionate nurse who stroked a burnt man's forehead—his pain disappeared and he fell asleep.

If high doses of opioids are ineffective, or only give short periods of pain relief, and the blood pressure is stable, clonidine increments (30 micrograms boluses) can be alternated with morphine. Pain relief can also be supplemented with small doses of ketamine. Use a loading dose of ketamine 0.1 mg/kg followed by an infusion of 1–4 mg/kg/hr. Use the larger dose in a young person, and lower in the elderly. To reduce the chance of hallucinations, keep the environment quiet, and do not disturb the patient.

Hypothermia

Hypothermia is an especially grave problem for burned patients. In the operating theatre the ambient temperature is low and the evaporative losses are high. Burnt patients are invariably hypothermic on their return to the recovery room. To minimize further heat loss, increase the ambient air temperature to above 30°C. Cover the patient with a warm air blanket, space blanket and warm towels. Warm all intravenous or dialysate fluids. Heat and humidify the inspired air if possible. Monitor the patient's core temperature with a temporal artery infra-red scanner, oesophageal probe, or tympanic membrane sensor.

Fluid balance

Monitor central venous pressure and urinary output. It is well known that patients with burns lose a lot of fluid, but over-enthusiastic resuscitation risks pulmonary oedema. Conversely, renal failure and shock occur if fluid replacement is not adequate. Maintain the central venous pressure 9–12 cm of water above the level of the right atrium. Avoid diuretics, the hourly urine output is a useful guide to volume replacement in the early stages of burns resuscitation.

If a burnt patient becomes sweaty and hypotensive consider either septicaemia or hypovolaemia.

Bleeding

Grafted and donor sites can bleed extensively. Watch the bandages carefully for signs of further blood or fluid loss. Monitor the patient for signs of impending hypovolaemia: tachycardia, a urine output less than 30 ml/hr and poor peripheral circulation.

Reference

1. **Arif-Rahu M, Grap MJ** (2010) Facial expression and pain in the critically ill non-communicative patient: State of science review. *Intensive and Critical Care Nursing*, **26**(6):343–352.

Chapter 28

Infection control

Three ways to prevent infection

1. Wash your hands
2. Wash your hands
3. Wash your hands

Rates of hospital acquired infection in the UK are falling. This decrease is mainly attributed to the successful control of ribotype 027.[1]

Transmission of infectious diseases between patients and staff, and between one patient and another is preventable. There are two main issues: keeping yourself safe from infections the patients may be carrying, and keeping the patients safe from infections carried by other patients or health care workers. If staff do not adhere to strict protocols they place everyone at risk.

How infections occur

There is a clearly recognizable chain of events that lead to infection. Each link in the chain is necessary, and the more links we remove the less likely it is that cross-infection can occur.

The chain comprises:

- a source;
- a mode of transmission;
- a breach in body defences;
- leading to infection.

The chain of infection

1. There must be an infectious agent: virus, bacteria, fungi, protozoa or prion.
2. An infectious agent needs a source or reservoir where it can thrive and replicate; or at least settle. Patients are a good reservoir, especially as they are a source of pus, blood, faeces, or flakes of skin (called *squames*). Some organisms remain for long periods on equipment, linen, benches and stethoscopes simply waiting to hitch-hike to a suitable host. Hepatitis B can survive for 7 days, and hepatitis C for 13 days or more at room

temperature on dried blood. HIV is fragile and survives outside the host for only a few minutes.

3. If a patient is infected, then there has to be some way the micro-organism can leave their body. The vehicle may be droplets from a sneeze or cough, or secretions, blood, skin squames, urine, or faeces.

4. The micro-organism then has to travel to the next person. This can occur through direct contact, or indirect contact (e.g. hitch-hiking on a stethoscope, blood pressure cuffs or your hands). It can be airborne spread; transmitted through a vector (such as a malarial mosquito, or house fly), ingested in contaminated food, or it can be inoculated through a breach in the skin (needle stick injury) or absorbed through a mucous membrane (influenza).

5. People vary in their susceptibility to infection. While some are already immune, others are immunologically compromised in the presence of disease. Many elderly patients are suffering from severe degrees of unrecognized malnutrition, which leaves them open to infection.

Important organisms

Some infections are more hazardous to staff, such as HIV or hepatitis B or C, whereas others are more dangerous to sick patients such as meticillin-resistant *Staphylococcus aureus* (MRSA) or vancomycin-resistant *Enterococcus* (VRE). Staff and patients may unwittingly and without ill effect be colonized with MRSA or VRE.

HIV/AIDS

The human immunodeficiency virus (HIV) is a blood-borne retrovirus first described in 1981. It had probably been around for many years before this. In industrialized nations, about 1:350 people carry it, but the prevalence rises to more than 40 per cent in some parts of Africa. After a short illness with symptoms similar to infectious mononucleosis (glandular fever), people with HIV have no further symptoms for many years, and often do not know they have the disease. Eventually, as the immune system breaks down the patient is infected with uncommon infections such as herpes zoster, or cryptosporidiosis; or they develop a lymphoma. In this later symptomatic stage the disease is called acquired immunodeficiency syndrome (AIDS).

HIV is diagnosed with serological testing. *Seroconversion*, where anti-HIV antibodies appear in the victim's blood, occurs about 3 months after the initial infection.

HIV is transmitted by blood, and other body fluids from infected people. The virus can be transmitted horizontally through sexual intercourse, blood donations, and donated organs, or sharing infected needles as well as through needlestick injuries (see Box 28.1). It can also be transmitted vertically from mother to child.

Box 28.1 **Needlestick injuries**

HIV has been transmitted to health professionals, but worldwide this is fortunately rare. The main risk to staff is through needlestick injury. Fortunately seroconversion is uncommon, and is estimated to occur on about 1:300 needlesticks.

About 75 per cent of needlestick injuries are potentially preventable.[2] Recapping needles is the commonest cause of needlestick injury. A feeling of being hurried, tired or ill also puts you at risk. A needle should either be in the patient, or in the sharps' container. Never put a used syringe and needle down. Never remove a used needle from its syringe; drop the whole unit into a sharps container. Do not allow your sharps containers to become so full that people need to stuff objects into it.

For injuries with needles, sharp instruments, bites or deep scratches encourage bleeding, but do not suck and do NOT squeeze the wound. Wash well with soap and water. HIV is very water soluble. Immediately report the injury to your hospital health service unit for management. Most hospitals have forms for you to fill in and a protocol for both you and your patient to follow for blood testing.

Early treatment with antivirals can prevent infection becoming established in people exposed to HIV and hepatitis B virus and can eradicate evidence of viruses in more than 90 per cent of people with acute hepatitis C virus infection.

To be effective a combination of the anti-HIV drugs indinavir, lamivudine and zidovudine is best administered within 72 hours of exposure, and continued for 4 weeks.

What is the long-term risk?

The estimated mean risk for a full-time nurse working for 30 years in the operating theatre suite of contracting HIV is 0.049 per cent, and for hepatitis C is 0.45 per cent. This means that for every 1000 recovery nurses working for 30 years about 5 may contract HIV from a contaminated percutaneous injury (PCI). Statistically you are six times as likely to be killed in a car accident in any given year.

Hepatitis B

Hepatitis B (HBV) is a DNA virus spread via blood products, sexual intercourse, intravenous drug users, health care workers and substandard sterilization of surgical instruments in developing countries. Seroconversion after a needlestick injury is about 3 per cent. The incubation period is 60–120 days. It progresses to chronic liver disease in 2–10 per cent of people. The surface antigen Hbs-AG is present from 1–6 months after exposure. A genetically engineered vaccine is 95 per cent effective and should be offered to all staff working in the recovery room. Passive immunization (anti HBV antibody) can be given to non-immune contacts after high-risk exposure.

Hepatitis C

Hepatitis C (HCV) is an RNA virus spread by blood transfusion, drug addicts sharing needles, tattoo needles, skin piercings, and barber shop razors. It is not spread by sneezing, coughing, oro-faecal routes or through intact skin.

One serious and major source of infection is substandard sterilization of surgical and dental instruments in developing countries (where more than 1 per cent of the population are affected), but in 40 per cent of cases the cause remains unknown.

Seroconversion after a needlestick injury is about 30 per cent. About 15 per cent of those infected progress to chronic infection. About 20 years after the initial infection for every 100 people infected: 15 get cirrhosis, 10 die of liver failure, and 10 develop hepatocellular carcinoma. Treating the acute infection with double combination therapy with interferon and ribavirin now gives a 50 per cent cure rate.

There are no tests available to differentiate acute, chronic or resolved infection; however a persistently elevated ALT level suggests chronic disease. There is no vaccine for hepatitis C.

Other hepatitis viruses

Hepatitis D (HDV) co-habits with HBV. Hepatitis E (HEV) is similar to HBA, and may be encountered in patients from the Indian subcontinent. Hepatitis GB causes usually asymptomatic post-transfusion hepatitis, but HGB-C may cause acute liver failure.

Tuberculosis

Pulmonary tuberculosis (PTB) is making a comeback in the community. Some strains are now resistant to all antibiotics—*multiple drug resistant tuberculosis* (MDRTB). *Tuberculosis* (TB) is an airborne bacterium (*Mycobacterium tuberculosis*) transmitted as an aerosol by coughing or sneezing, and common in most developing countries. It most commonly occurs in the lungs but it may occur in other sites of the body (e.g. kidney, lymph nodes, liver, abdomen, brain, and bone). Adults with non-pulmonary tuberculosis are regarded as non-infectious, and outside the operating theatre are safe to treat as normal patients, but treat as infectious aerosol-generating procedures such as wound irrigation, and abscess incision.

Patients with MDRTB require special precautions outside the capabilities of most hospitals.

Recovering tuberculous patients

Use disposable anaesthetic circuits and bacterial filters. Immediately after use, put all contaminated articles in designated infectious waste containers. Wear gown, disposable gloves, and N95 mask and cover your head. This is particularly important for the staff who may encounter sputum, bronchial secretions or aerosol droplets from coughs or sneezes.

Ideally, only those with a BCG inoculation will look after the patient with TB. The patient must be recovered in the operating theatre, and not in the recovery room. Do not accompany the patient back to their isolation unit. Leave all your potentially contaminated clothing in the operating room, and shower yourself and wash your hair.

Notify your Occupational Health Authorities of the names of all staff who were exposed to the patient, or handled infectious material in any way.

MRSA

Meticillin-resistant *Staphylococcus aureus* (MRSA) bacteria are resistant to meticillin, flucloxacillin and other beta-lactam antibiotics. MRSA are commonly found in hospitals, but found far less commonly in the wider community. MRSA seem no more virulent than antibiotic-sensitive organisms, but because of their resistance they are more difficult to treat. They are spread around the hospital on people's hands, and for this reason these infections are largely preventable. Some health care workers become *reservoirs*, because they carry MRSA as part of the resident skin flora.

Risk factors for developing the disease are prolonged hospital stay, severe underlying disease, and malnutrition. These bacteria enter the body through open wounds, drain tubes, skin lesions and pressure sores (also see Box 28.2).

When perfectly healthy people come into a hospital ward their skin becomes transiently colonized within hours. This is the reason that orthopaedic surgeons prefer patients for major joint surgery to be admitted on the day of their operation, go straight to the operating theatre, and not pass through the ward first.

Box 28.2 **N95 mask**

The National Institute of Occupational Safety and Health (NIOSH), which is part of the Centers for Disease Control and Prevention in the United States, sets standards for respirators and masks. Air must pass through respirators, but can leak around the sides of masks. However the terms are used casually to mean the same thing. The number (95, 99, 100) refers to the efficiency the devices filter particles. An N95 respirator filters out 95 per cent of the particles that attempt to flow through the device. Similarly an N99 respirator filters out 99 per cent of the particles and an N100 respirator filters out 100 per cent of the particles that attempt to flow through it. N means not resistant to oil. Many viruses are small, from 0.04–0.8 μm in diameter. Particles of this size readily pass through an N95 filter, however airborne micro-organisms are carried on water droplets generated when someone sneezes or coughs. These 5 μm droplets are far too large to pass through an N95 respirator.

VRE

Vancomycin-resistant enterococci (VRE) are causing troublesome wound infections in some surgical units. VRE is resistant to all antibiotics apart from rifampicin. This disease is transmitted from a colonized individual's faeces to a surgical patient by hitch-hiking on the hands of a member of staff. This cross-contamination is easily prevented if staff wash their hands after coming into contact with potentially contaminated material, including bed sheets.

Barriers to transmission

Innate defences

Humans have evolved elaborate and efficient defences against invading microorganisms. Every day each of us shrugs off an assault by micro-organisms with no ill-effect. However, if our defences are compromised by malnutrition, or disease, or our natural defence barriers are breached by surgical incisions, intravenous infusions, drains or catheters then we run the risk of being overwhelmed (see Box 28.3).

Cross-infection in hospitals occurs where pathogenic micro-organisms migrate from one infected patient to another. Hospitals tend to breed particularly virulent *nosocomial* bacteria, which invade readily and are resistant to antibiotics.

Box 28.3 **Protect your own skin**

If you are using good-quality handwashing lotions then skin cracks should not be a problem, but if they do occur skin cracks may get infected. Cover small wounds with occlusive membrane dressings such as Tegaderm® or Op-Site® spray to provide a good barrier. Gloves will easily slip on and off over the plastic dressing. Use them on knuckle-scrapes too instead of Bandaid®-type dressings which tend to come off under gloves. Change the membrane at the end of the shift or your skin will become macerated. Also change it if it starts to lift off.

You can contaminate your hands
by merely taking the patient's pulse.

Skin

Your most important piece of protective equipment is your skin. Intact skin is a superb barrier to infection. Look after it even when you are not on duty. Most bacteria and other micro-organisms do not survive long in its acid environment, and the resident flora such as micrococci, *Staph. epidermidis* and diphtheroids crowd out newcomers.

Bacterial colonization is measured by counting *colony-forming units* (CFU). Different areas have different bacteria counts. The scalp has an average of 1,000,000 CFU cm^2 whereas hands range between 40,000 and 4,000,000 CFU cm^2.

Bacteria on the hands can be divided into two groups: resident and transient. Resident flora live in deeper layers of the skin, and they are usually benign. Transient bacteria colonize the superficial layers. They are usually picked up by staff during direct contact with patients or contaminated objects. Resident bacteria are not removed by normal hand washing, but transients are. Unfortunately some staff pick up pathogenic bacteria, such as MRSA, which then become part of their resident flora population. MRSA like warm wet places: the nose, groin and axilla. Some patients are taking broad-spectrum antibiotics. These can selectively kill parts of the resident population, which makes way for antibiotic-resistant bacteria to set up home. Once the skin is disrupted by surgery, these antibiotic-resistant bacteria can invade to cause serious wound infections.

Respiratory tract

Most inhaled micro-organisms are entrapped in mucus secreted by the mucous membranes lining the respiratory tract. The mucous membranes are guarded by a variety of white cells, macrophages, complement, and by special immunoglobulins called IgA. Bacteria rarely penetrate these defences, but some airborne viruses may; the recurring epidemics of influenza are an example.

Gut

Our gut houses more bacterium and micro-organisms than there are cells in our body. Most are harmless commensals, some help by producing vitamin K, and excluding unwelcome bacteria, but others are pathogenic. If ordinary commensal bowel flora contaminates the peritoneum, say after colon surgery, the resulting peritonitis and septicaemia is frequently fatal.

Urinary tract

The one-way flow of urine usually flushes unwelcome bacteria out of the urinary tract, but indwelling catheters can provide nooks and crannies where pathogenic bacteria can survive and grow.

How to prevent transmission

Bacteria are everywhere. In non-medical offices high bacterial counts can be found on light switches, telephones, computer mice, and other work surfaces, while the communal coffee cups revealed a 40 per cent contamination with faecal bacteria. If an ordinary office is such a cesspool, then consider the organisms lurking in the nooks and crannies of your recovery room.

Hand hygiene

Hand hygiene is the essential core for *Standard Precautions*. It is the most ignored, but most effective way of reducing cross-infection. It is tempting to take short cuts in personal hygiene when working in a busy recovery room, but lapses not only cause increased infection rates among patients, but increase your risk of infection too.

In 2002 the Centers for Disease Control and Prevention in the United States produced a detailed 48-page document, *Guidelines for Hand Hygiene in Health Care Settings*. Everyone should read this clearly written and excellent report.

Essentially, its recommendations were:

- When your hands are visibly dirty wash them with antimicrobial soap and water, and then decontaminate them with an alcohol-based hand rub.
- If your hands are not visibly dirty decontaminate them with an alcohol-based rub.
- Alcohol-based hand rubs must be available at every patient site.
- If your hands come into contact with any bodily fluids or potentially contaminated sites such as dressings or mucous membranes, then wash your hands with antimicrobial soap to decontaminate them.

Decontaminate your hands—the 5 Moments of Hand Hygiene:

- before you touch patients or their surroundings
- before any procedure or body fluids exposure
- after touching patients or after body fluids exposure
- after any procedure
- after touching patients' surroundings

> *Alcohol-based hand rub kills almost every germ.*
> *Soap and water merely cleans them.*

Additional tips

- Post the maker's directions above the alcohol-based rub's dispenser.
- Do not top-up dispensers. Replace the bottles with new ones when they are empty.
- The best-alcohol rubs contain n-propanol because they denature proteins (n-propanol is not widely available in the US).
- Although dermatitis caused by alcohol rubs is rare, this is no place for false economy. Use good-quality rubs that are acceptable to the staff. Avoid those rubs containing perfumes because they are more likely to cause allergies and skin reactions.
- Avoid bar soaps, because they are warm wet places where bacteria can grow.
- Take off hand jewellery, and bracelets.
- Wash your hands with soap for at least 30 seconds (put a clock above the sink to time it).
- For sterile procedures you may need a surgical forearm scrub. This takes 2–5 minutes.
- Scrub your nails.
- Pat your hands dry with paper towels. Do not rub them dry because you will damage the skin.
- Use a dry towel to turn off the tap.
- Do not install hot air-blowers because they contaminate the whole room.

♦ Alcohol-based rubs are flammable. Bulk-store them safely, because they have *flash points* when they spontaneously ignite between 21–24°C.

In 2009 WHO published a similar document of 270 pages, *WHO Guidelines on Hand Hygiene in Health Care*.[4] This is due to be reviewed but essentially the message is the same. Wash your hands.

Fingernails

Keep fingernails short and clean. Do not wear artificial nails because they shelter a zoo of potentially pathogenic micro-organisms, even after hands have been washed. Freshly applied nail polish does not seem to be a problem, but there is a potential for chipped nail polish to harbour organisms.

Jewellery

Wedding rings and hand jewellery are better off than on, because they interfere with hand hygiene, collect *microbes*, damage gloves, and tear patient's skin. Some hospitals allow staff to wear a flat wedding band.

Overshoes

There is little evidence overshoes reduce theatre contamination from microorganisms carried on the footwear. Overshoes help prevent staff footwear being contaminated with blood or body fluids; and this is especially so where there is a risk of blood-borne viruses. Get your own footwear. Make sure it is impervious to blood, body fluids, and falling needles, and can be decontaminated if necessary. For high-risk situations, thick-soled Wellington boots are best.

Aprons or gowns

Wear an appropriate plastic apron or gown (Table 28.1) whenever you are dealing with fluids, or there is a chance of being contaminated with blood, secretions or other body fluids, or dealing with infectious patients. Many staff prefer to wear gowns rather than aprons as they provide better coverage.

Table 28.1 Plastic aprons' colour code

Colour	Function
Red	In contact with blood, or bowel secretions
Blue	Directly dealing with patients, changing beds etc.
Yellow	Dealing with patients in isolation
White	For doing clean procedures, e.g. wound dressings

Gloves

Where appropriate, use latex gloves because they give better protection than non-latex gloves.

Choose the type of glove worn appropriate to the task, as follows:

Sterile gloves are worn to protect the patient. They must be worn for invasive and aseptic procedures requiring a sterile field, involving normally sterile areas of the body.

Non-sterile gloves are worn to protect staff members. They are worn for non-sterile procedures where there is a perceived risk of contaminating your hands through contact with blood or body fluids, secretions (excluding sweat), contaminated patient care items, non-intact skin or mucous membranes.

General purpose non-sterile utility gloves are worn for housekeeping chores including *cleaning*. These rubber gloves are worn to protect the wearer's hands from cleaning agents and prolonged immersion in water.

*Each time you change your gloves,
decontaminate your hands.*

Masks, goggles, spectacles and visors

Wear protective eye guards whenever there is a risk of body fluids splashing into eyes or mouth for example when managing or removing a patients' airway.

Hats

Theatre caps prevent hair and skin squames from escaping, and to stop your hair being contaminated by splashes of body fluids. Although there is no need for non-scrubbed staff to wear caps, it is a good thing to keep your hair covered while in the theatre block.

Standard precautions

Universal Precautions against transmission of infection were introduced more than 25 years ago when HIV/AIDS was first recognized as a hazard to hospital staff. Universal Precautions are now called Standard Precautions. *Standard Precautions* requires all health care workers to assume that all body substances from all patients be treated as potential sources of infection regardless of diagnoses or perceived risk.

*All staff are to assume
all patients are always infectious.*

Safe working practice demands standardized procedures to protect staff, other patients, and visitors from cross-infection.

Standard precautions include policies on hand hygiene, gowns, gloves, face protection, safe use and disposal of sharps, safe handling of specimens, safe handling of linen, safe disposal of clinical waste, and decontamination of spills and accidents (Table 28.2). If you have cuts or abrasions then cover them with waterproof dressings.

Staff with breaches in their skin such as dermatitis, psoriasis, eczema, skin wounds or other skin disorders must not come into contact with potentially contaminated material.

All body fluids are potentially infectious.

Wear clean latex gloves whenever you are touching potentially infective substances, and change them between tasks.

Table 28.2 A standard precautions checklist

Question	
Do staff wear gloves appropriately?	Yes/No
Do staff decontaminate their hands at the correct moments?	Yes/No
Are the following available?	
◆ Aprons/Gowns	Yes/No
◆ Face-protection goggles, and visors	Yes/No
◆ Gloves (including non-rubber latex ones)	Yes/No
◆ Masks	Yes/No
Are single use items ever reused?	Yes/No
Is linen dealt with appropriately?	Yes/No
Are stethoscopes, and blood pressure cuffs cleaned regularly?	Yes/No
Are sharps handled safely?	Yes/No
Is there a formal policy for handling biological spills?	Yes/No
Is there a formal policy for needlestick injuries?	Yes/No

For information on hazardous health care workers see Box 28.4.

Box 28.4 **Hazardous health care workers**

In 2001 the Department of Health (UK) set up a committee to assess the potential for health care workers to be a hazard to patients. Accordingly they proposed that new health care workers be tested for blood-borne viruses (BBV): HIV, hepatitis B, hepatitis C, and tuberculosis, and those who are positive be excluded from doing exposure-prone procedures (EPP). This did not exclude such workers from working in the NHS,[3] but restricted them to working in clinical areas where they posed no hazard to patients. These tests are not compulsory, but health care workers new to the NHS who decline to be tested are not cleared to perform EPP.

Spills

Quarantine all spillages of blood and body fluids, and deal with them immediately. Make the area safe. Soak up the spill with paper towels and wash the area with neutral detergent. For blood spills on hard surfaces throw sodium hypochlorite solution on the area, leave it soak for 10 minutes, and then rinse the area with neutral detergent and water and allow it to dry. Discard contaminated articles: paper towels, gloves and apron into the yellow clinical waste container. Do not use hot water because it coagulates proteins, which then sticks to surfaces offering shelter for microorganisms.

Waste

All clinical waste contaminated with body fluids or tissue must be discarded in yellow waste bags and sealed securely. Never transfer clinical waste from one container to another.

Use transparent plastic bags for household waste only. Some hospitals use black plastic bags for this purpose, however these can conceal inappropriately jettisoned waste.

Linen

All linen is infectious, but the risk of transmission is low. Use standard precautions. Contaminated linen goes into special bags. If the linen is wet, put it in double bags, so that contaminated fluids cannot seep through to the outside.

Additional precautions

Fortunately in the operating theatre and recovery room the risk of transmission from one patient to another is small, and if it does occur then, it is almost always because of a lapse by a member of staff.

Standard Precautions are a basic risk minimization strategy. Use *Additional Precautions* when Standard Precautions are not enough to prevent transmission of infection. *Additional Precautions* are used for highly transmissible pathogens including airborne transmission or droplet of highly contagious agents such as influenza, chickenpox, tuberculosis, and pertussis; and direct or indirect contact with dry skin or contaminated objects colonized by MRSA or VRE.

> *Microbes don't fly.*
> *They hitchhike.*

Additional precautions include using personal protective equipment such as a particulate filter respirator for tuberculosis, or assigning already immune staff to attend a patient, for example, those who had chickenpox (varicella) in the past.

All blood and body fluids, tissue, secretions, and products, are potentially infective regardless of the perceived risk of the source (Table 28.3).

Screening and isolating patients only work if people tending the patient are not carrying the bug.

Table 28.3 Sources of contamination

Potentially infectious body fluids	
Major	**Minor**
Blood	Urine
Faeces	Nasal secretions
Wound ooze	Gastric secretions
Pus	Peritoneal dialysis fluid
Sputum	Ascitic fluid
Saliva	Pleural and pericardial fluid
Potentially infectious body sites	
Major	**Minor**
Wounds	Nasal passages
Skin lesions	Mouth
Drainage sites	Intravascular access sites
	Peri-anal area
	Armpits

Eleven sensible precautions

1. Most hospitals have an Infection Control Unit as part of the administration structure. Its duty is to set standards, write protocols and enforce them with regular quality assessment procedures.

2. Staff in the recovery area should wear theatre gear. Do not wear your street clothes or shoes. Visitors should wear a gown, not necessarily for infection control, but to reinforce the idea that they are in a restricted area.

3. Ensure your recovery room has the minimal possible flat surfaces such as shelves. Do not allow the room to become a storage area.

4. Have a regular cleaning schedule.

5. If a member of staff has an infectious illness such as a 'cold' then they must stay at home. It is easy to transfer airborne viruses to already compromised patients with disastrous consequences. Postoperatively a patient who has picked up a cold from a sniffling member of staff is highly likely to get pneumonia.

6. Ensure every site has facilities for washing hands.

7. Nebulizers can be a source of infection because they spray a fine aerosol into the air which may disperse infective particles.

8. Neutral detergent is adequate to make surfaces biologically safe.

9. Insist on immediate repairs to cut linoleum or broken woodwork, chipped surfaces. These places harbour pathogens.

10. Never clean, wash or place instruments in handbasins.
11. Ensure curtains/blinds are cleaned and changed regularly.

Cleaning

Cleaning involves washing with water, *detergents* and scrubbing or using ultrasound to dislodge foreign material such as dust, blood, secretions, excretions and micro-organisms from objects and people. Cleaning simply removes, but does not inactivate, micro-organisms. Cleaning keeps things looking good, and is one of the most cost-effective procedures a hospital can do. Organic residue shelters micro-organisms and prevents sterilizing agents or disinfectants from coming into contact with the surfaces of the item being sterilized. Protein in particular inactivates some chemical disinfectants.

If an item cannot be cleaned, then it cannot be disinfected or sterilized.

Disinfection

Disinfection is a process for removing all organisms except bacterial spores from an object.

Points to note

♦ Automated thermal washer-disinfectors are effective, but make sure you select the appropriate cycle.

♦ Make sure you use a properly certified instrument-grade disinfectant. Usually these are used alone or in an automated chemical washer-disinfector.

♦ Disinfection is not a sterilizing process.

♦ Disinfection is not simply a convenient substitute for sterilization. Do not use thermal disinfection for instruments that need to be sterile. However, thermal disinfection is more effective than chemical disinfection (Table 28.4).

Table 28.4 Which disinfectant to use

Disinfectant	Indication
Alcohol	
70% alcohol impregnated wipes	Wiping down dressing trolleys, stethoscopes.
Hypochlorite solutions	
Sodium hypochlorite solution 1 in 20 dilution (500 ppm available chlorine)	Decontamination of environmental surfaces (e.g. after a blood spill).
OPA (orthophthaladehyde)	High-level disinfection for heat-sensitive equipment that is unsuitable for autoclaving, e.g. transoesophageal echo transducer probes, thermistors.
Peracetic acid	High-level disinfection of heat-sensitive equipment that is unsuitable for autoclaving, e.g. endoscopes in a washer/disinfector machine

How to use disinfectants

◆ Use sachets of antiseptics and disinfectants once only, and then throw them away.

◆ Before using any disinfectant or antiseptic check that the solution is clear and there is no particulate matter visible.

◆ If you open a flask of a water-based solution, such as aqueous chlorhexidine, then it must be discarded within 24 hours.

Antiseptics and their use

Antiseptic agents (Table 28.5) are substances that are rubbed on the hands or applied to surfaces to reduce the population of micro-organisms.

Table 28.5 Antiseptic agents

Antiseptic name	Indication
Aqueous chlorhexidine solutions	
Chlorhexidine 2% (green)	Handwashing before an aseptic procedure
Chlorhexidine 4%	Surgical handwashing in OR
Aqueous chlorhexidine 0.1% (blue)	Urinary catheter insertion, perineal wash-downs
Chlorhexidine and cetrimide (yellow)	Perineal wash-downs. Lacerations
Alcoholic chlorhexidine solutions	
Chlorhexidine 0.5% in 70% alcohol (pink)	Skin preparation where an alcohol swab is inappropriate (e.g. blood cultures, IV insertion)
Chlorhexidine 1% in 70% alcohol (pink)	Decontaminating hands that are not visibly soiled
Alcohol	
Microshield™ (61% ethanol & emollients white)	Decontaminating hands that are not visibly soiled
Alcohol swab—saturated with 70% isopropyl	Preparing small areas of skin
Povidone iodine solutions	
Povidone iodine scrub (0.75% povidone iodine)	Handwashing (in specialist areas)
Povidone iodine solution (10% povidone iodine)	Skin preparation for surgery

Sterilization

Sterilization is a process that eliminates or destroys all forms of microbes including, virus, bacterial spores and fungi.

Principal techniques for sterilizing equipment include:

◆ moist heat using steam under pressure;

◆ dry heat;

◆ ethylene oxide;

◆ automated sealed low-temperature peracetic acid, hydrogen peroxide plasma and other chemical sterilant systems;

* ionizing radiation.

All of these give a minimum sterility assurance level (SAL), but the process must be validated to make sure it has worked properly.

Do not use, or trust ultraviolet light units, incubators, microwave ovens, domestic ovens and pressure cookers, because they do not guarantee sterilization.

Keep permanent records so that, if necessary, you can trace the source of an infection to at least a batch level, and preferably to an individual patient.

References

1. **Health Protection Agency Centre for Infections** (2009) *Healthcare-Associated Infections in England 2008–2009 Report*. London: Health Protection Agency.
2. **Raghavendran S, Bagry HS**, *et al*. (2006) Needlestick injuries. *Anaesthesia* **61**:867–72.
3. **NHS Estates** (2004) *The NHS Healthcare Cleaning Manual* (2004). London: Department of Health.
4. **World Health Organization** (2009) *WHO Guidelines on Hand Hygiene in Health Care*. Geneva: WHO.

Chapter 29

Working with people

Perioperative care

Knowledge and practical skill is the background to everything we do to help the patients have a successful recovery. We all aim to do everything possible to avoid problems, and one way to avoid problems is to have a careful production line approach to routine surgical procedures. As well as an orderly sequential process of preoperative assessment and optimization, operative care, recovery room and the surgical ward rehabilitation we need to develop our ability to identify problems rapidly and respond in a communicative way with our colleagues to make sure the patient gets the best care and nothing is omitted or overlooked.

Staffing

Standards for the staffing levels of recovery room vary from country to country, and according to the workloads, the type of surgery and the fitness and age of the patients. Many countries have set standards and guidelines on these matters. Each recovery room must establish its own staffing protocols, and insist that they are given the resources to adhere to them.

*Staff must be proficient
in cardiac life support.*

Every member of staff working in recovery room must be proficient in *basic life support*, and ideally recovery room nurses should receive training in *advanced cardiac life support* (see page 318).

If patients are physiologically unstable or potentially may become so, two nurses should be present when they first arrive in recovery room. However, if the patients are stable, the surgery is minor and the anaesthetic uncomplicated then such intense supervision is not warranted.

Communication and trust between staff

Trust and team work along with communication will help prevent emergencies getting out of hand.[1] Breakdown in communication between staff leads to a loss of awareness of the patient's condition. Take care not to be distracted from your focus which must be on the patient at all times. If an emergency occurs identify a leader immediately. It should be someone who is present and already knows the patient (it could be you).

Communication and trust between the staff and the patient

The patient will trust that you know your job and they will understand that you will look after them while they are at one of the most vulnerable times of their life.[2] You should receive a careful handover from the scrub nurse and the anaesthetist. If they do not come out with the patient and hand over to you, ask that they do come. This link in the chain of communication and patient care is a very important one. It is not only the words spoken but the concern and care that these people from the operating theatre convey. An atmosphere of goodwill and a sense of trust both to the patient who is barely awake as well as to the nurse who now knows this person by name and can count on them to come back swiftly to help if there is a problem.[3]

As soon as your preliminary observations have been done study the preadmission assessment, the clinical pathways, the informed consent and the operating theatre 'time out'. *Informed consent* includes discussion of both the perceived benefits and the possible harms of the procedure and the operating theatre 'timeout' will have a record of concerns expressed by the surgeon and the anaesthetist just prior to beginning the operation.

Clinical pathways started in the preadmission clinic guiding the patient's care through a standardized sequence of best practice protocols should also be in the patient's notes. The patient's postoperative care is planned from the time they first consult the surgeon to the time their rehabilitation is complete and their welfare is handed back to their own doctor and local health facility. The aim is to ensure that the patient's hospital stay is free from unexpected adverse events, and they recover from their surgery and are able to resume their normal lives as quickly as possible.

Time Out is a check list designed by the World Health Organization to minimize risk just before surgery begins.[4]

Communication is vital
for good patient care.

Cultural and religious issues

Recovery staff need to be sensitive to customs of patients from diverse cultural, ethnic and religious backgrounds. Practising cultural sensitivity is essential in recovery room nursing. The patients' traditional methods or religious beliefs need to be taken into account.

Sometimes patients' beliefs seem to be not in their best interests. For instance Jehovah's Witnesses have sincere and deeply held beliefs that do not allow them to accept blood or blood product under any circumstance. To staff faced with a patient bleeding to death in front of them this is a challenging and painful dilemma. Jehovah's Witnesses believe that personal commitment to their faith is more important than their family or their own life.

They may refuse surgical or medical intervention for themselves or their children. In some countries the law will not allow treatment to be withheld from minors under a certain age. If you foresee conflict or have doubts about the situation involve your hospital's legal and ethical consultants immediately.

Family involvement is of ultimate importance in some cultures and patients may feel more comfortable if they have had three or four opinions before they decide on treatment. Some cultures require all messages to be transmitted through the oldest male member of the family; others preclude men caring for women in the recovery room or women caring for men.

It is easy to accidentally offend some patients by the way you say things, or with non-verbal communication. Direct or prolonged eye contact in some cultures (such as North American Indian, and some Australian aborigines) is considered aggressively disrespectful, whereas in some other cultures (South American and European) to avoid eye contact is a sign of a lack of interest. Vietnamese, Thais and some South Pacific people are deeply offended if you touch their head without their permission. Always ask before taking the paper theatre hat off the patient. New Zealand Maori patients do not like pillows that would normally be under their heads being used under other parts of their bodies. It is appropriate to have different coloured pillow cases for these situations. A warm smile, gentleness, genuine concern and a respectful soft voice, will ease the path through this cultural minefield.

Some cultures and religions have certain articles of clothing or jewellery they wish to wear, or have nearby. As far as possible accommodate their wishes.

Interpreters

If a patient is not fluent in English or impaired in some other way you may need an interpreter in the recovery room. As far as possible use family members. Pain is best assessed by these people who have known the patient before surgery and are familiar with their normal behaviour.

Study the preadmission
assessment.

Recovery stages

The patient's stay in recovery room is just the first step in a process that may take months or years to complete. Recovery from anaesthesia and surgery is divided into three stages: Stage 1, Stage 2, Stage 3 recovery.

Stage 1 recovery includes physiologically unstable patients, and those patients who potentially could become unstable and are consequently at risk of harm. These are patients whose *vital signs* deviate significantly from their preoperative baseline values. They may still be:

- comatose;
- receiving ventilatory support;

- intubated, or require a laryngeal mask to preserve their airway;
- receiving vasoactive drugs;
- hypothermic;
- bleeding;
- or have a major metabolic disturbance.

Ask the question is: 'Is it likely that the patient may encounter an incident that would cause harm?' If the answer is 'yes', then they are in Stage 1 recovery, if the answer is 'no', then they can step down to Stage 2 recovery.

Ideally two nurses will attend patients in Stage 1 recovery until they are stable. One of these nurses must be proficient at advanced cardiac life support. An anaesthetist should remain within the operating suite while there are any unstable patients in the recovery room.

Supervision

Stage 1 recovery requires at least one nurse with advanced cardiac life skills training be present in the recovery room for nurse with basic training.

Double care = two nurses to one patient

Patients require *double care* if one or more of the following:

- physiologically unstable;
- critically ill;
- being ventilated;
- agitated or combative.

Dedicated care = one patient to one nurse

If the patient is one or more of the following:

- unstable with vital signs outside their preoperative baseline;
- intubated with either an endotracheal tube or laryngeal mask (including ventilated patients);
- receiving vasoactive drugs;
- is receiving a transfusion or blood or blood products;
- under the age of 8 years whether conscious or not.

Shared care = two patients to one nurse

If:

- one patient is conscious and stable, and the other is unconscious and stable;
- both patients are conscious and stable.

Potentially unstable patients

Whether a patient will become physiologically unstable in the future is not easily quantified, but specialist recovery room nurses will readily recognize factors that put the patient at risk.

As a guide potentially unstable patients have one or more of a combination of the following:

+ cardiovascular instability;
+ respiratory insufficiency;
+ metabolic problems (such as diabetes, acid-base disturbance, or hypothermia);
+ or where the patient bled during the surgery (raising the possibility of functional anaemia).

Any one of these components alone is unlikely to cause worrying physiological instability. However, should one or more other components intervene there is the potential for a cascading chain reaction that may result in the patient suffering cerebral, cardiac or tissue hypoxia.

Extended Stage 1 recovery includes patients discharged to ICU or coronary care unit, or other high-care units where the specialist nursing staff caring for the patients have equivalent training and abilities of specialist recovery room nurses.

Stage 2 recovery

Stage 2 recovery includes stable patients who are conscious and competent (although they may still have residual effects of a local anaesthetic or neuraxial block). The patients should have stable vital signs comparable to their preoperative baseline for at least 30 minutes before they are discharged to the ward.

Patients may be attended by non-specialist nursing staff who are proficient at basic life support.

In the ward (extended Stage 2 recovery)

Here the patient will be cared for by staff who have equivalent skills and training of a non-specialist recovery room nurse.

During Stage 2 recovery at least one specialist nurse should be immediately available, but the care of patients can be left with non-specialist qualified nurses.

Supervisory care = one nurse to three patients If the patients are:

+ over the age of 8 years;
+ under the age of 8 years but with a parent present.

Special supervisory care = one nurse to two patients

If the patients are one or more of the following:

+ under the age of 8 years;
+ receiving intravenous fluids;
+ at potential risk for some untoward event to occur such as bleeding;
+ require plaster checks.

Standard care = one nurse to five patients

Standard care is the level of care normally available on a surgical ward. This should never be less than one nurse for every five patients.

Stage 3 recovery

Stage 3 recovery applies to patients who have yet to recover fully from the effects of their surgery or anaesthetic no matter how long this takes.

After day case procedures *Stage 3 recovery* applies to patients who are discharged into the care of a competent and informed adult who can intervene in the case of untoward events. This carer may have no skills in cardiac life support techniques, or any medical knowledge, but must be capable of recognizing problems and know what to do about them. The carer must have clear written instructions of what to do about pain, nausea and vomiting, continued ooze from the wound site, or attacks of faintness. In case problems arise the carer needs a phone number to call, and a plan in place to bring the patient back to the hospital (or day care centre) if necessary. In other words do not send a patient to a remote location without a telephone and transport to bring them back should it become necessary.

Stage 3 recovery also applies to those who have been discharged from hospital, but remain at risk from complications of their surgery or anaesthetic, no matter how remote. Hospital staff tend to assume that once a patient leaves the hospital, even after days or weeks in the ward, they have recovered and all will be well. As any family doctor will tell you this is not necessarily so because of the occasional wound breakdown, deep vein thrombosis, or pulmonary embolism occurring after the patient has gone home. Recent surveys have shown a surprising number of elderly people die in the first 6 weeks after discharge from major surgery, some without ever coming to the attention of the hospital. Furthermore the psychological repercussions of serious illness, such as depression, can haunt patients for months to years. For this reason *Stage 3 recovery* involves a holistic view of the patient, and their family, as part of a continuum of health care and welfare, and not merely simply their stay in the recovery room.

Who must be present in the recovery room

Every member of staff working in recovery room must be proficient in basic life support, but additionally specialist recovery room staff must be proficient with advanced cardiac life support including defibrillation. As a basic requirement someone proficient in advanced cardiac life support must always be present in the recovery room while any patient is in Stage 1 recovery.

Should the recovery nurse do preoperative visits?

It would seem ideal for recovery room nurses to see their prospective patients before surgery. In many operating suites the preoperative ward is close to the recovery room and this visit is possible. The patients then know what to expect during their stay in the recovery room, and will be reassured by a familiar face when they emerge from anaesthesia. The nurse, knowing the patient's condition, can make a nursing plan before the patient arrives.

Administration

The recovery room is usually supervised by either the Nursing Director of the Operating Theatre Suite or the Director of the Department of Anaesthesia. A trained and certified nurse should manage the area. Clerical staff are needed to answer phones, take messages, keep track of supplies, handle medical records and so on.

Planning is usually delegated to an Operating Theatre committee composed of nurses, medical staff, and administrators. Some tips to make this committee run smoothly are that it should:

◆ be small with no more than six members;

◆ hold regular meetings;

◆ have defined written responsibilities;

◆ have an agenda circulated some days before each meeting.

One of the principal roles of the committee is to establish guidelines and protocols.

Protocols and guidelines

Protocols are designed to be followed precisely, whereas *guidelines* allow latitude for common sense. *Policies* lay out a course of action for the future (also see Box 29.1). Protocols ensure everyone does the same thing in the same way. Most clinical and administrative problems occur again and again, and every hospital has its own way of dealing with these issues. It is not easy or appropriate to transplant routines from one hospital to another, so develop your own policies and protocols. Protocols, policies and guidelines make auditing performance easier.

Box 29.1 **Policies, protocols and guidelines**

Policies set down the general principles of what you are to do under defined circumstances. For instance hospital policy does not allow you to disclose medical information about your patient to other persons, without the patient giving written and signed permission.

Protocols set down the details of procedures to follow under specific circumstances. These procedures are not optional; they are rules to be obeyed. The rules are usually laid out in a step-wise manner.

Guidelines are suggestions of what to do under certain circumstances. They do not carry the weight of compulsion, but are there to guide you. Guidelines require that you use common sense. However, common sense is not always a common commodity. Ultimately common sense relies on *education*, which enables you to understand why you are doing something; *experience* in that you have seen and done it before and can quickly recognize it again; and *training* so that you can respond rapidly and uniformly to the circumstances.

You will need protocols for:

- checking equipment and drugs;
- transferring patients from one area to another;
- handover of patients from one area to another: from theatre to recovery room staff, and from recovery room staff to ward staff;
- documentation;
- emergency procedures;
- discharge criteria;
- and responsibilities of the various categories of staff.

Routines and protocols help prevent mishaps and errors. Written guidelines help staff manage the more complex postoperative problems such as epidural catheters, or airway problems after thyroidectomy.

Guidelines and protocols need to be concise. There is much helpful information on the Internet. Type out clear notes and keep them in a ring binder in the recovery room where everyone has access to them. You will know if they are being consulted because they will soon look well-thumbed and dog-eared.

To formulate a protocol you need:

- up-to-date and accurate information on the topic;
- practical ideas on how to modify or control risk;
- clear ideas on how to implement the protocol;
- to regularly review and revise the protocol.

Good protocols set out in the simplest and clearest language:

- the purpose of the protocol;
- the medical/nursing/administrative reasons for the protocol;
- how to do it—equipment and resources required;
- special rules—who can do what, and where;
- precautions and contraindications;
- where to get help if things go wrong;
- definitions—explaining the meaning of the technical words;
- where to get more information;
- a future date when the protocol will be reviewed.

Problems with protocols:

- the information may not be current or accurate;
- protocols might not be applicable to a particular individual;
- they may not allow for flexibility in clinical practice.

Reference books

A small library with a set of reference books is useful. Make sure it includes *The Complete Recovery Room Book* by Anne Craig and Anthea Hatfield. Do not lock these books away after hours. You never know when you may need to consult them. Do not allow staff to take books home. Reference books on practical pharmacology and nursing procedures help cope with situations that might not be covered by your protocols or guidelines.

Message book

A message book is useful to pass messages on to staff on following shifts. Use it to keep track of equipment you have loaned to other parts of the hospital, to follow up good ideas, and even staff requests for roster changes.

Maintenance books

Maintenance books ensure the weekly check of equipment, such as the defibrillator, has been done properly.

Weekly meetings

Weekly meetings should be part of your quality assurance programme.

Audits

Audits are part of the quality control process. They help you find potential problems, and may reveal information to improve patient care. They also provide a benchmark so that you can compare your performance with that of other equivalent recovery rooms in your area. Once you have corrected a problem, repeat your audit to make sure it really was solved. This check is called *closing the audit*. Audits can be a tedious chore, but they really do make a difference.

Risk management

Personal risk

You are in harm's way working in the recovery room. Needlestick injury is an obvious one, and there are many other physical risks which you must guard against, and clearly record if they happen. During emergencies take care to follow all normal safety routines such as sharps disposal. Wear gloves and change them often. Stay out of the way of X-rays, as you double your distance from the source of the beam you reduce your exposure by a factor of 4 (this is the inverse square law). If you need to stay close to the patient wear a lead apron and thyroid shield.

Take precautions to protect yourself as well as your work mates against mental harm. You must talk to the appropriate person if you are suffering from emotional stress or becoming too tired to work effectively.

Managing difficult behaviour

Patients or relatives can exhibit challenging behaviour such as anger in the recovery room. It is important to acknowledge feelings and attempt to de-escalate the situation. Careful documentation is imperative. Be aware of the codes to call for security back-up and perform practice scenarios regularly to ensure all staff are familiar with the codes and protocols for managing difficult behaviour.

Clinical governance

One in ten patients suffers an adverse event while in hospital. Preventing or controlling these adverse events is the role of risk management. Risk management is merely one large cog in the much larger wheel of clinical governance.

Clinical governance is a *system* designed to integrate education, clinical audit, best practice, risk management, research, and effective communication. It is necessary to identify and document each one of these factors to detect when things go wrong, analyse what went wrong, fix the problem, and try to make sure that it does not happen again. All this sounds simple, reasonable and logical, but it is difficult to implement on a large scale. Difficulties arise when a single component of a complex system is modified. This throws the rest of the system into disarray. So it is tempting to simply patch each problem as it arises, and leave an outdated or hazardous *system* intact. Think about the implications of closing the recovery room for a week to install a better suction system: lists cancelled, staff not working, urgent cases transferred elsewhere, political ramifications, dust, dirt and much more. It is easier to put a patch on the problem by installing inferior portable suckers.

Adverse events

The recovery room is a high-risk area where there is ample opportunity to accidentally harm otherwise well people. Risks arise whenever you do something that might have an uncertain outcome. Where risks are present adverse events are eventually inevitable.

Adverse events are those that cause unintended harm to patients through any action, either directly or indirectly, by a member of hospital staff. These unintended complications or injuries either prolong the hospital stay, or require additional measures to manage them. Complications of surgery, such as wound infection or deep vein thrombosis, are adverse events. There are two things to look at when analysing adverse events: was it predictable, and could it have been better managed? Each component can be rated on a scale from low to high. For instance the risk of a patient vomiting could be predicted as high, but even though it was predicted the subsequent management of the vomiting may have been suboptimal.

Not all adverse events are preventable, but those that are preventable are called *errors*. Just because an adverse event occurs does not mean anyone has been negligent or that it was avoidable. All medical care entails risk and bad things happen despite the most scrupulous, rigorous and conscientious care.

Near misses occur when something goes wrong, but the event is detected and averted before anyone is harmed. For instance someone notices that the wrong drug is about to be given to the patient before it occurs.

Incidents occur when an event has occurred that harms or could harm someone within the hospital precincts. (This includes staff, patients and visitors.)

Sentinel events are serious clear-cut events that occur because of errors made by health care workers, for instance amputating the wrong leg, or giving blood of the wrong group to a patient causing a haemolytic transfusion reaction, or intravenous gas embolism by detaching a central venous line. Sentinel events occur when protocols are not followed. These events need thorough investigation using the techniques of *root cause analysis*.

Types of risk

Risk management falls into two categories: proactive and reactive risk management.

Preventative (*proactive*) risk management involves identifying risks before they occur, and then putting in place strategies to prevent them happening. Preventative strategies include such things as preoperatively identifying patients who are likely to vomit in the recovery room, so that they can be given prophylactic anti-emetics during their anaesthetic, or washing your hands to prevent cross-infection.

Responsive (*reactive*) risk management involves dealing with adverse events once they have occurred. Examples include policies and protocols to deal with death in the recovery room, aspiration of stomach contents, or needle-stick injuries to staff. (To see some reasons why things go wrong, see Box 29.2.)

Box 29.2 **Reasons why things go wrong**

1. *Slips* result in an unintended action and are usually caused by human error.
2. *Lapses* are caused by rule-based mistakes. That is by applying a bad rule or failing to apply a good rule.
3. *Knowledge-based mistakes* occur because you don't know what you are doing.
4. *Violations* occur when rules are deliberately broken.
5. *Mishaps* are unpredictable events, statistically certain to occur.
6. *System errors* occur when the managerial frameworks are flimsy.
7. *Communication errors* occur when people don't pass the message on.

Why errors happen

We all make mistakes: humans do. But in some jobs mistakes can harm, injure or kill. Working in recovery room is one of these jobs. No one ever makes mistakes intentionally. Good people do not come to work in the morning saying: 'I'm going to purposely harm someone today'.

*Errors are preventable
adverse events.*

Mishaps are not preventable

Mishaps are not preventable, but they are inevitable. Sooner or later you will encounter a patient who has an anaphylactic reaction despite having no known drug allergies, or a patient who becomes violent on emerging from an anaesthetic. Where patients or staff are harmed the outcome is called a *serious adverse event*.

Errors are preventable

Slips, lapses, poor training, violations or protocols, system errors and communication errors are all preventable. Errors occur at all levels of care, not only with high-risk procedures. Good governance prevents errors.

Human error causes slips

Slips are caused by human error. Many slips occur because of absent-mindedness or lack of concentration. Slips are preventable, but they rarely occur simply because of one single factor. Slips tend to occur in familiar and routine settings where staff are preoccupied or distracted.

Brains on autopilot

Our brains can only cope with so much information without going into meltdown. Slips occur if our attention is constrained by something else going on around us, or some worry on our mind. Have you ever done something like putting salt in your tea, or a grapefruit skin in the dishwasher? These slips are not as stupid as they might first appear. One rarely thinks about automatic tasks. Your brain was simply on autopilot.

These virtues of economy, of delegating attention to autopilot while doing routine tasks, free up our mind to think of other things. It's part of our make-up. You rarely play close attention to what you are doing while having a shower before going out for the evening; your mind is off elsewhere.

If the same error occurs more than once, then look for a system error. Do not blame the individual.

If you are on autopilot while tending patients in the recovery room then slips are likely. Two most common slips in the recovery room are giving the wrong dose of a drug, or allowing an intravenous infusion to run in too quickly. One way to avoid the autopilot phenomenon is to vary your tasks during each shift as much as possible: recover a patient, go to the ward with the next, and teach, and so on.

Causes of errors

Human errors

Knowledge-based errors occur where training is inadequate, experience is lacking, or facts are unknown or unavailable. A common preventable error is to prescribe two or more drugs without realizing that they may interact with each other, such as giving metoclopramide to someone on a dopamine infusion. The facts are well known, but unless the knowledge is remembered, and then applied—an error occurs. Computer systems for dispensing drugs reduce the risk of such lapses.

Fatigue is a common cause of error. A member of staff who is sleep deprived or has been working too long without a break cannot think quickly and will inevitably sooner or later make a mistake.

Working in unfamiliar environments or settings, or having to cope with time pressures, or with complex clinical problems also creates situations where errors are more likely to occur.

Lapses occur when protocols
are not followed.

Adverse events increase logarithmically as patient to nurse staff ratios increase. Things are missed, short cuts taken: hurried staff make mistakes.

Lapses occur where protocols and rules, for one reason or another, are not followed. This is rarely due to laziness, or incompetence. The protocols and guidelines used in recovery rooms are part of an integrated and extremely complex *system*. Protocols and guidelines cannot possibly cover every situation, and when they do not, then staff are tempted to improvise or take short cuts. No one error, no one technical failure causes disaster. It usually takes a diabolical combination of factors aligning each other through tiny windows of opportunity for a lapse to cause a problem. This phenomenon is sometimes called the '*Swiss Cheese Effect*'. Think about a stack of slices of Swiss cheese; the holes in the cheese may not align, but as circumstances change and holes overlap then gaps in the system are revealed.

Disasters are always predictable—
in hindsight!

Most errors are systematic

Honest analysis of an adverse event will probably reveal up to 20 or more factors contributing to the disaster. Many of the factors are systematic such as inappropriate rostering, insufficient staff or supervision, lack of knowledge, high workloads, time pressures, inadequate equipment, tired or distracted, or out-of-sorts staff, and almost inevitably poor communication

Good recovery rooms are not necessarily the ones where errors never seem to occur, because errors happen every day. If there seem to be no errors, then the slips and lapses are probably being concealed. Good recovery room managers recognize error-prone situations, detect adverse events when they occur, and have contingencies in place to correct them.

Proper training and ongoing education
help prevent errors.

Lack of communication causes disasters

A common system error occurs where there are unclear lines of authority for doctors, nurses, and other health care workers. Unless there are clearly defined lines of responsibility and authority about patients' care, the recovery room can become a high-risk zone where the surgeon and the anaesthetist give conflicting instructions, or worse still think the other is taking the responsibility. This is a scenario for a disaster. Under these circumstances it is easy for the recovery room nurse to end up in a void, and enticed to act independently without knowing the full surgical or anaesthetic implications of the case. This puts the nurse in an untenable position. As a general rule the anaesthetist is the head physician responsible for the patients' medical care in the recovery room. If an adverse event occurs notify the anaesthetist immediately.

Poor communication is a root cause of many problems. This is one reason to employ specialist perioperative nurses. They know their patients. They know the system. The patient's specialist perioperative nurse has information, much of which is not in the patient's notes.

Audits and quality of care

Audits collect and record data about outcomes. Good practice demands this is done regularly, and systematically. Good governance gives us the resources to do so. Audits are designed to improve practice and the care of patients. For this reason the data must be recorded honestly. Apart from helping identify adverse events the data may well be used in confidential enquiries. It is not about how good we are, but about how bad we are. If we can stop bad things happening then what remains is better than it was. Each little improvement is a step towards better care for our patients.

Quality assessment

Quality assessment answers the question, 'Is what we are doing in the recovery room working properly?'. This involves identifying risky situations, evaluating them, assessing the available resources, determining a course of action, and planning for contingencies.

Quality assurance

Quality assurance answers the questions, 'Are we achieving what we set out to achieve? And if not; then why not? And what are we going to do about it?'.

Risk management

Risk management relies on identifying risky situations, and then putting in place measures to counteract them. These measures include creating policies, protocols and guidelines; while other measure includes appropriate education, proper training, repeated practice and regular review of outcomes.

The secret of risk management is to create successive layers of defence involving checking, and rechecking and checking yet again. Other examples of multiple layers of defence include coloured labels for syringes, two staff independently checking drug doses, patients having labels on both wrists and ankles, different coloured containers for different levels of waste, or fail-safe alarms on monitors.

Quality assurance involves continuous monitoring,
and regular review.

Risk management and the law

Some hospital policies are mandated by statute law. For instance a patient who dies in recovery room becomes a coroner's case. Some are subject to common law and precedent, such as what constitutes patients' consent to decisions about their care, and how their consent must be obtained.

Nurses are not immune from their
legal responsibilities.

How to protect yourself from legal problems

You must keep your knowledge and skills up-to-date. This includes your knowing the laws and statutory regulations affecting the way you practise.

+ Ignorance of the law is not a legal defence.
+ Preferably join both a professional nursing association, and a union.
+ Maintain adequate indemnity insurance. This is especially important if your employer does not cover aspects of your practice.
+ Keep your patients' records conscientiously. Write everything down. If an event is not in writing, then it effectively it did not occur. You will have difficulty, perhaps in 5 years' time, proving events in a courtroom.
+ Do not use abbreviations in the patient's medical record unless they conform to your hospital's guidelines.
+ Write only what you see, do and hear in the patient's record. Clearly separate opinion from fact. Do not pass judgment. 'The patient was rude and stupid' is not acceptable. 'I feel the patient was impolite and ignorant of the facts', is barely acceptable. 'The patient appeared upset, and I believe does not understand what I told him', is an acceptable observation.
+ Never criticize colleagues or the hospital in front of patients, and never in the medical record.
+ If you disagree with hospital management, or disagree with your colleagues then, as soon as possible, write everything down, and date it. Keep your notes as a personal record.
+ Follow your hospital's policies and procedures. If you feel they are inadequate then work through appropriate channels to address your concerns.

- Foster relationships. Be considerate, polite, respectful and truthful.
- Treat your colleagues fairly. Do not allow your views on their lifestyle, religion or culture to prejudice your professional relationship with them.
- Talk to your colleagues because communication breakdown is the most frequent and serious cause of errors.
- Take legal threats against you seriously. Seek help immediately.

Risk management is
everybody's responsibility.

How to get feedback

Risk management involves managers listening to patients, and staff, and carefully considering what they have to say: their criticisms, suggestions, solutions and ideas.

Good managers listen with the ears of their heart, but analyse with the logic of a computer.

Good managers are realistic, and non-critical, and able to temper enthusiasm with experience. They need to cultivate an easy non-threatening relationship with their staff and patients. They avoid micromanaging staff under their control by allowing competent people to get on with their job, and give them the resources to do so.

Good communication is the key. Managers need tact and empathy to tell their staff what is expected of them, and correct them when they are wrong. Managers need to establish formal structures, for reporting adverse events and, just as importantly, near-misses (slips and lapses).

Compliment in public.
Criticise in private.

Ensuring compliance and accountability

Once policies and protocols are in place it is essential to check compliance to find out if staff are following them, and if not, then why not. If there is a system problem it may be that the protocols are impracticable.

Sometimes staff feel that a change in direction is unwarranted. To counteract this requires a change in the culture of the unit. For fear of criticism, ostracism, or ridicule staff may be reluctant to report adverse events, or near misses. Possibly there is a culture of covering up mistakes, or taking shortcuts.

Direction and strategy

It is management's role to set direction, and establish strategies. *Direction* is a statement of intent; it defines exactly and precisely where we want to go in the long term. *Strategies* are the plans we make to get there.

To put strategies in place you will need to clearly determine your objective, have sufficient data to make sensible decisions, identify possible obstacles, have the necessary resources (knowledge, human resources, and finance), and develop a timetable to implement your plan. At each step you will need to re-evaluate your progress.

An organization may change direction when existing strategies are hazardous, or no longer work; or because new superior techniques come along. A change in direction occurred with the move away from general anaesthesia for Caesarean section to spinal anaesthesia. The strategies put in place to achieve this included setting up a climate for change by educating patients and staff.

Our goal might be to reduce the level of pain patients have when they are discharged from the recovery room. The strategies include a wide variety of analgesic techniques. For most problems there is no one simple answer; instead you will need many different strategies to achieve a satisfactory outcome. For example, consider all the different ways to control pain in the recovery room. No one strategy suits every patient.

Elegant solutions evolve
from collaborative problem-solving.

Changing the culture

As anyone who has tried to get doctors to wash their hands before and after touching a patient will know, changing culture requires many qualities including patience, empathy, tact, discretion, reason, coercion, and humour.

To change hospital or unit culture, means to change the way people think. If we can change the way people think then they will change the way they act.

Ethics and morality

Even in recovery room we sometimes we have to make extremely difficult decisions: what to do about a Jehovah's Witness who has just had a Caesarean section and is now bleeding to death. We know that a couple of units of fresh frozen plasma will save this young mother's life; how to cope with death in the recovery room; how to deal with dangerously incompetent colleagues. These are difficult and serious questions. The study of ethics and morality helps guide us in dealing with such quandaries.

Morality

It is the privilege of our profession to care for people. Our patients trust us with this care; they have faith in us to honour their welfare. The privilege of this trust, this honour, sometimes gets lost in the busy-ness of our day. Often the office politics, problems and personalities of the moment are more prominent in our thoughts. But they are not more important. Without continually reinforcing feelings for morality and ethics, it becomes tempting to take shortcuts in our work, or to become disrespectful to others, or be inconsiderate or even unkind to our patients.

Ethics

Ethics is about the proper and moral conduct of our profession. To be ethical we need to be competent, have integrity, and conform to professional etiquette.

It is our patients' welfare that, and above all else, is our first consideration. Over the years, academics, philosophers, lawyers, theologians, politicians and others have argued and debated and tried to lay down principles of what this means. But it is simple. It means: 'treat others as you would have them treat you or those you love'. It is as basic as that.

The most important person in the room is the patient;
any room, at any time and any patient!

Although this is a simple notion it is not always possible to achieve if our morals and beliefs get in the way. Take abortion for instance. Some regard this practice as heinously repugnant, while others see it as a woman's basic right. We must treat patients with all the care and concern we can summon; to nurture their physical, mental, psychological, spiritual and emotional welfare, and put this care above our feelings.

There are four principles to help us find the way to do this:

1. *Autonomy* is the right of individuals to make decisions on their own behalf.
2. *Beneficence* is the duty, where possible, to do good.
3. *Non-maleficence* is the duty to do no harm.
4. *Justice* is a broad concept that includes ideas of equity and fairness.

Treat every patient as you would your sister,
parent or child, and demand that others do too.

Don't blame the individual

When adverse events do occur, it is almost instinctive to find the person who caused the problem and load the responsibility on them—to blame them. Blaming one person for an adverse event is a delicious emotion. Naming, shaming and blaming is easy, satisfying, and extremely unjust. When we do load blame on someone else, then bad things follow. Blame nails responsibility on one individual. Everything becomes their fault. This lets the rest of us off the hook. Blame ignores the circumstances leading up to the event, and unless we dispassionately analyse these circumstances, nothing will be done about it.

Blame is never appropriate.

Competent administrators understand this. It then becomes their job to do a rigorous *root cause analysis* to find out why the adverse event occurred in the first place, and then resolve to put good systems in place to ensure that it does not happen again. Unfortunately the term root cause suggests there is simply one single cause behind an adverse event. This is almost never the case.

Don't shoot the messenger

There have been many tragedies over the years because the administrative framework, procedures, equipment, or facilities have been inadequate. Competent hospital administrators are aware of this too, but if they do not have the facts they cannot deal with the problem.

Sometimes things are not as they should be. If you have sound reason to think your ability to manage your patients safely is compromised by inadequate staffing levels, equipment or other resources then draw the matter to the attention of the management. Keep written records with dates, times and names about your concerns, and what steps have been taken to try and resolve them.

Respect the skills and work of your colleagues, but if you have well-founded fears about the performance or conduct of either yourself or other staff members then you are obliged to bring them to the attention of the management in a respectful, and private way. Most hospitals have contingency plans to deal with such matters. They have done so in the past, and they will do so in the future.

Whistleblowers

It would be comforting to believe that administrators, senior staff and government authorities always respond appropriately to reports of inadequacy or incompetence, but there have been terrible disasters either because staff at the coal face have been afraid to speak up, or because they have been ignored, and regrettably at times even persecuted and forced to leave their work.

This situation is especially difficult for nurses who often do see and understand problems but do not feel brave enough to say anything. Their fear is justified, but also difficult to make a plan for. Possibly the best approach is a group one with a number of nurses who have a concern voicing them together.

Bullying, harassment and stress in the workplace

Bullying and harassment has increasingly become highlighted as a major problem in surgical teams. It is important to show respect and kindness towards colleagues especially towards more junior colleagues such as trainee nurses and registrars. We must create a culture where staff feel safe at work. There must be sympathy for staff struggling with stress and appropriate help readily available. Stress in the workplace has been associated with depression, burnout, compassion fatigue and poor work performance.

It is important to speak up if you witness bullying or intimidating behaviour and document it. Bullying has been associated with distress, anxiety, absenteeism, training withdrawal and suicide.[5]

References

1. **Giswold SE, Fasting S** (2011) How do we know that we are doing a good job? *Best Practice and Research Clinical Anaesthesiology* **25**(2):109–122.
2. **Smith AF, Mishra K** (2010) Interaction between anaesthetists, patients and the anaesthetic team. *British Journal of Anaesthesia* **105**(1):60–68.

3. **Smedley P** (2010) Staffing in PACU. *British Journal of Anaesthetics and Recovery Nursing* **11**:3–8.

4. **WHO** surgical safety checklist and implementation manual. <http://www.who.int/patientsafety/safesurgery/ss_checklist/en/index.html>

5. **Royal Australasian College of Surgeons**. Operating with respect. <https://youtu.be/zUsLoPKzY7g>

Further Reading

BMJ Quality and Safety journal. <http://qualitysafety.bmj.com>

Chapter 30

Working with facts

Introduction

In this chapter we will examine some very basic ideas in the science of statistics, and then see how to use them to help our patients (at least not harm them) by applying these techniques in evidence-based practice.

Statistics

We cannot cover the full scope of statistics in a few paragraphs, but instead let us browse through some common concepts you might encounter in journals and books.

Statistics is the study of the methods of collecting and analysing data. We collect data by taking *samples* from *populations* of individuals. Statistical analysis measures what is happening in a few people and then *extrapolates* the results to make predictions about what is happening in the population as a whole. To increase our *power* to get to the truth, and to reduce *bias*, which may confound us, our samples are usually collected randomly from a defined group (called a *set*) of the population.

Let us do a study on the effects of morphine on blood pressure. Seems simple? But selecting good samples and collecting valid data is difficult. To prevent *errors* we need to research and define exactly what we want to do. For example, if you measure blood pressures simultaneously in your right and left arm the readings may differ by up to 20 mmHg. So our study needs to take these factors into account.

For the most part statistics is a study of *probability*. If you think about it, probability is the only way to deal with uncertainty. We are uncertain whether it will rain today. Looking at the low grey clouds we might predict that it probably will.

Statistical analysis can never prove something to be true, it can only estimate how likely (or unlikely) it is to be false.

There are two main branches of statistics: *descriptive* and *inferential statistics*. *Descriptive statistics* describe how to summarize, organize and simplify data so that we can manage it more easily. For example: how to find the *mean* (average) of a number of measurements, or the *mode* (the most common value), or the *median value* (the middle of the range of series of values).

Inferential statistics allow us to determine the chance that a real difference exists between observations in one group, and another. Examples of inferential statistical techniques include *correlation* and *confidence levels*. We use correlation every day; for instance, cyanosis correlates with hypoxia and stridor correlates with respiratory obstruction. We use confidence levels to measure how confident we are that something hasn't happened simply by chance. When we look at the laboratory reports of electrolyte results we find that the normal range of serum sodium is 135–145 mmol/L. Studies using inferential statistical methods show that we can be confident that 95 per cent of normal people have serum sodium levels within that range (called a *confidence interval*), but 5 per cent of the sodium levels of perfectly normal people lie outside that range. The *normal* serum sodium concentrations are between 135–145 mmol/L. We can predict this with 95 per cent *confidence* or with *confidence levels* of positive 2.5 per cent and negative 2.5 per cent.

Sensitivity and specificity

The terms *sensitivity* and *specificity* are widely used to make logical decisions about the diagnosis and management of patients. For example, some, but not all, bacteria make chemicals called nitrites. If we test urine with a dipstick and find that it contains nitrites and lots of white cells then it is almost certain that the patient has a urinary tract infection. The presence of nitrites and white cells gives this test 100 per cent *sensitivity* for a urinary tract infection. The bad news is that about 50 per cent of patients with urinary tract infections do not have both nitrites and white cells in their urine. Thus, the *specificity* of this dipstick test is only 50 per cent. If we rely only on nitrites and white cells to find urinary tract infections then there is a 50 per cent *false negative result*. Similarly *false positive* results can occur with many tests; in which case the test says something is wrong, when in reality nothing is wrong and everything is normal.

Number needed to treat (or harm)

In the past decade statisticians have introduced a number of new techniques. The *number needed to treat* (NNT) is one of the more useful. In adults the NNT with paracetamol 1000 mg for moderate postoperative pain is 3.8. This means you would have to give almost four adults 1000 mg of paracetamol for one of them to get effective pain relief. Similarly, some drugs and treatments can be harmful (such as anti-cancer drugs) in which case we measure the *number needed to harm* (NNH).

Evidence-based practice

In our day-to-day practice it is easy to be led astray and either give unnecessary treatment or withhold effective treatment when it is needed. How do we know what is best for our patients? In the past doctors and nurses have relied on the opinions of experts to guide them on what to do. Too often that is all they were: merely opinions. Treatments were based on belief and experience, usually without solid evidence to support them. Sometimes these opinions were simply wrong, and occasionally tragically lethal. One of the saddest events occurred when doctors and nurses recommended that mothers place their sleeping babies on their stomachs instead of their backs. It seemed a good idea at the time, but tens of thousands of babies died from cot death before researchers showed how dangerous this practice was.

Every day recovery room nurses use harmful or ineffective treatments, such as tipping hypotensive patients head down (harmful), or using metoclopramide to treat opioid-induced vomiting (ineffective).

It is easy to be misled into believing some intervention works when it does not, especially when we base our ideas on incompletely understood physiological or pharmacological principles. Just because we have always done something in a particular way does not mean it is either beneficial or that it does no harm: nor does it mean that there may not be better options.

The only way out of this conundrum of doing good and preventing harm is, as far as possible, to do things that are proven to work. This is the basis of *evidence-based practice (EBP)*. EBP is the process of making decisions about patient care based on the best available research evidence, and then integrating decisions with clinical expertise and the patient's wishes.

How the facts are discovered

Evidence comes from carefully conducted clinical trials. The most valid trials are properly conducted randomized controlled trials (RCTs).

Over the past decade tens of thousands of RCTs have been done, especially involving drugs. More recently anaesthetists and nurses have taken an objective look at the quality of recovery. Using a postoperative quality recovery scale they can demonstrate that although patients' recovery improves over time it is possible to assess and predict outcomes before surgery for individual patients and procedures.[1]

How evidence is collected

There are more than two million papers and articles published in English-language medical and nursing journals each year. How can we possibly find ones that directly benefit our patients?

It takes skill and time to find and analyse available data critically. Has the study been properly conducted? Are the statistics appropriate? Is the sample large enough? How can we use the evidence? Answering these questions is not easy; so most of us have to rely on reputable journals and reviews, and special searches by organizations devoted to gathering and analysing evidence, and formulating guidelines.[2] These organizations include the Cochrane Collaboration based in the UK, McMaster University (Canada), the National Institute for Nursing Research in the US, and the National Health and Medical Research Council (Australia). There is also EmBase, an internet site covering important biomedical literature, and Elsevier, which has information from a large number of academic journals.

How evidence is analysed

It is easy to be influenced by our hopes, beliefs and prejudices, and even easier to be led astray by bias (Table 30.1). *Bias* occurs when the information we have about something does not give an accurate picture of what is really going on. Bias is a systematic deviation from the truth. Occasionally rogue researchers intentionally introduce bias for profit, glory, honour or status, but most bias simply occurs because of haste, ignorance and ineptitude.

Table 30.1 Analysing evidence

Level of evidence	Where does the evidence come from?
1. Evidence with a high degree of reliability.	Studies that use well-tested methods to make comparisons in a fair way and where the results leave very little room for uncertainty. Trial design: usually Level 1 studies are systematic reviews or large, high-quality randomized controlled studies.
2. Evidence with reliability but open to debate.	Studies that use well-tested methods to make. comparisons in a fair way but where the results leave room for uncertainty (for example, due to the size of the study, losses to follow-up or the method used for selecting groups for comparison). Trial design: usually Level 2 studies are systematic reviews without consistent findings, small randomized controlled trials, randomized controlled trials in which large numbers of participants are lost to follow-up, or cohort studies.
3. Some evidence without a high degree of reliability.	Studies where the results are doubtful because the study design does not guarantee that fair comparisons can be made. Trial design: usually Level 3 studies are systematic reviews of case–control studies or individual case–control studies.
4. Some evidence but based on studies without comparable groups.	Studies where there is a high probability that results are due to chance (for example, because there is no comparison group or because the groups compared were different at the outset of the study). Trial design: usually cohort or case–control studies where the groups were not really comparable, or case–series studies.

A *meta-analysis* is the mathematical synthesis of the results of two or more separate trials addressing the same hypothesis in exactly the same (*homogenic*) way. This data is then statistically analysed, and the results compared. This process is called a systematic review.

A *systematic review* is a summary of the scientific evidence gathered from two or more randomized trials. The evidence it provides is stronger than the results from a single randomized trial. Preferably systematic reviews answer just one question, and present it in a manner we can easily understand. Systematic reviews need to fulfil specific requirements: they must be comprehensive, minimize bias, and use statistically valid information.

It is easier to understand a good meta-analysis than it is to plough through piles of original primary research papers. The downside of meta-analysis is that it is easier to be misled by faulty (or even fraudulent) methods. A weak point with meta-analysis *is* heterogenicity. *Homogenicity* means that each trial is done under exactly the same conditions, collects data in the same way and uses the same statistical techniques. *Heterogenicity* occurs when they are not. Homogenicity compares apples with apples. Heterogenicity compares apples with pink-footed gerbils; or the renal function of dehydrated greyhounds with human patients.

Not all evidence is equally valid. Some evidence is obtained from randomized controlled trials, while other evidence is based on solid observation. For these reasons evidence is classed on its strength, as set out in Table 30.1.

There are several dozen classifications of levels of evidence. Some are more complex than others. The sensible one tabled here is used by the New Zealand Guidelines Group. The Oxford Centre for Evidence-based Medicine uses a similar system for evaluating the levels of evidence (LOE) with categories labelled A, B, C and D, while the USA uses a more complex one with six levels of evidence.

How to ask the right questions

If you ask the following questions, then they demand an evidence-based answer:

+ What are the options for treatment?
+ What are the possible outcomes of those options?
+ How likely is each of these outcomes to occur?

Are there any drawbacks to evidence-based practice?

For most of our nursing and medical practice there is little, and often, no hard evidence to support the way we do things. Unfortunately many clinical trials are performed so poorly that their data is worthless or misleading.

Hormone replacement therapy (HRT) was for years advocated to prevent heart disease and stroke in postmenopausal women. The evidence for its benefit came from a single trial that was not *powered* to look for these outcomes anyway. Millions of women were prescribed HRT. It took a huge US government survey—the Women's Health Initiative—to prove that HRT contributed to heart disease and stroke.

On the other hand some professionals argue that:

+ the principles of evidence-based care discount clinical experience;
+ qualitative trials also provide valid information;
+ usually there are no trials or guidelines for the problems of a particular patient. It suppresses clinical freedoms;

- it opens the door for insurance companies to refuse to reimburse for procedures that have not been proven (yet) to be effective;
- it is unethical to have a placebo trial in diseases where effective therapy is available.

Much of our practice is common sense. It is obvious folly not to have cot sides on trolleys, or to leave comatose patients unattended. However, other practices we take for granted are not so clear. Strangely, there is little direct data in the literature to prove that giving a general anaesthetic to a patient with an active respiratory tract infection predisposes to pneumonia, but every anaesthetist knows from experience that this is true. See 'Randomized controlled trials', Box 30.1.

Box 30.1 **Randomized controlled trials**

Randomized controlled trials[3] compare patients receiving one treatment for a particular disease with another group of patients who are receiving either a placebo (*sugar pill*), or a different treatment. Both groups contain patients selected at *random*, and the trials are done under tightly controlled conditions. Some trials are *double-blinded* in that neither the patients nor the people running the trial know which group is getting which treatment. Blinding increases the *power* of a trial.

Randomized controlled trials are designed to eliminate bias. When selecting samples to study, the data will be biased if, on the average, your samples do not accurately reflect what is going on in the population you are studying.

Suppose you wish to study the frequency of age groups in the general population. You could stand on a busy city railway station at 8.30 a.m., select people at random and ask their ages. But your sample would be biased. Young children are at school, and the retirees are probably still in bed. Your survey would be biased towards office workers who probably do not own cars.

Randomized trials need to be properly powered to extract the data you are seeking. If you were doing a study on weight loss, but chose to measure people's weight in 100 kg increments, then a weight loss of few kilos would be missed. Your study is insufficiently powered to give meaningful results. However, if your survey is designed to find the proportion of the population who weigh 100 kg or more, then the power of your study is sufficient.

References

1. **Royse CF, Newman S**, *et al.* (2010) The Post-operative Quality Recovery Scale. *Anesthesiology* 113(4):892–905.
2. **Rothman B, Sandberg WS**, *et al.* (2011) Using information technology to improve quality in the OR. *Anesthesiology Clinics* 29(1):29–55.
3. Guide to Biostatistics. <http://www.medpagetoday.com/>

Further Reading

Giswold SE, Fasting S (2011) How do we know that we are doing a good job? *Best Practice and Research Clinical Anaesthesiology* **25**(2):109–122.

NHMRC (2012) *A Guide to the Development and Evaluation of Clinical Practice Guidelines.* Canberra: NHRMC.

Trolley set-ups

Emergency trolleys are best prepared in advance and stored for easy access. Those that are rarely required, like malignant hyperthermia and bronchoscopy, can be shared with the operating theatre. Photograph the layout and tie the photograph, encased in plastic, to the trolley. This makes it easy to check the set-up each day. Discourage people from borrowing from these trolleys. Keep the trolleys as near as possible to the fridge and the defibrillator. If you are a remote hospital without piped oxygen you will need to keep a full cylinder and regulator close too.

Trolleys include:

- IV access;
- reintubation and difficult intubation trolley;[1]
- cardiac arrest;
- paediatric—this can be a tray on the bottom shelf of the main trolley which can be lifted up when required;
- anaphylaxis;
- thoracic aspiration and chest drain insertion;
- malignant hyperthermia;
- bronchoscopy;
- local anaesthetic trolley.

General emergency trolley

If you have a small recovery room you may wish to combine your main trolley.

A typical set-up for a general emergency trolley would include:

- an intravenous tray with all sizes of cannulas, spirit wipes and gauze;
- tubes for taking blood studies and a key to their coding;
- tubes for blood gas studies;
- boxes of non-sterile gloves, all sizes;
- two laryngoscope handles with batteries;
- extra batteries;
- laryngoscope blades (all sizes);
- stylettes and guide wires (malleable metal or plastic);

- water-soluble lubricant;
- oropharyngeal airways, all sizes;
- nasopharyngeal airways, all sizes;
- laryngeal masks (including an intubating laryngeal mask);
- cricothyroidotomy kit;
- retrograde intubation kit;
- self-inflating manual resuscitation bag, such as Ambu® or Laerdal®;
- face masks to fit this bag;
- oxygen tubing to connect the bag to the oxygen source;
- bronchoscopes with their light source: small, medium and large;
- cuffed endotracheal tubes, all sizes;
- catheter mounts and tight connections;
- 20 ml syringe for inflating tracheal cuffs;
- Magill forceps;
- wooden mouth-gags.

Drugs should be kept on the trolley or in the fridge, as appropriate. Leave a list of the drugs kept in the fridge on the trolley.

The following drugs are suitable for the trolley, you will probably add others:

- ketamine;
- propofol;
- suxamethonium, put out two ampoules each day and keep the main supply in the fridge;
- clonidine
- midazolam;
- atropine 0.6 mg;
- lidocaine 1% and 2%;
- glucose 50%;
- adrenaline 1:1000 and 1:10,000;
- hydrocortisone 100 mg;
- intravenous fluids and drip tubing.

Massive blood transfusion

Keep a Red Box with instruction sheet, investigation and cross match paperwork, and colour coded tubes for blood ready as far as possible. An example of a Red Box instruction sheet is shown in Box A1.1, but you can make your own. Remember the chemicals in the blood tubes have a definitive life and will need refreshing from time to time.

Box A1.1 **THE REDBOX CONTENTS**

PHONE NUMBERS
Blood Bank...
Haematology Lab...

OTHER USEFUL PEOPLE TO CONSULT
....
....
....

BLOOD BOTTLES
PURPLE top..2 ml ....CBC
GOLD top................................10 ml ....U and E's LFT and Calcium
BLUE top..................................3 ml ....PT/APTT and Fibrinogen
PINK top..................................6 ml ....Cross match
Forms are typed and all filled in as much as possible.
Handwriting on bottles is required by the laboratory.
The box will also contain Y connections and large giving sets specific for massive transfusions.

AND OTHER CONSIDERATIONS
Calcium... If ionized Ca is < 1 give 10 ml CaCl slowly
Warfarin reversal...................................... Vit K 10–20 mg slowly
Heparin reversal.. Protamine 1 mg/100 units of heparin slowly
(60% of enoxaparin and other fractionated heparins will be reversed.)
Desmopressin............................. for patients in renal failure 0.3 micrograms/kg 20 mg
in a 70 kg patient
Aspirin reversal... Tranexamic acid 30 mg/kg
Platelets < 75.. give one extra pack
Fibrinogen less than 1gm/L.................... consider 3 × Cryoprecipitate
APPT greater than 1.5 control................. FFP 10–15 ml/kg (1000 ml/70 kg)
rVIIa.. Consider after 10 RBCs
and if pH is > 7.2
if platelets > 50
fibrinogen <1 g/L
the dose is 90 micrograms/kg to nearest vial.

Local anaesthetic trolley

A local anaesthetic trolley should be ready at all times for the urgent insertion of a spinal or epidural. This should include:

- gown and sterile gloves, all sizes;
- four sterile drapes;
- sterile gauze;
- sponge holders;
- preparation solution such as cetrimide;
- local anaesthetic drugs;
- commercial packs for spinal and epidural procedures;
- spare needles and other individually packed sterile items if available;
- needles and syringes of various sizes;
- lidocaine 1% for skin analgesia.

Difficult intubation trolley

Before preparing your difficult intubation trolley consult the internet. There are several very comprehensive sites. Begin with <http://www.das.uk.com>.

Thoracic drain trolley

This trolley should hold the following:

- one medium stainless steel tray, or similar commercial packed tray;
- one small kidney dish;
- two small gallipots;
- one scalpel handle size 3;
- one toothed dissecting forcep;
- two pairs of artery forceps;
- one suture scissors;
- one needle holder;
- one 1/0 atraumatic silk suture;
- one scalpel blade size 10;
- sterile packs of cotton wool swabs;
- sterile packs of gauze;
- three sterile drapes.
  Add to this:
- lidocaine 1%;
- disposable syringes and needles;

- povidone skin preparation;
- drain tubes of various sizes including children's sizes;
- trochars, Argyle® or similar.

Malignant hyperthermia trolley

This trolley should be kept right beside the fridge and a supply of Ringer's lactate and normal saline should be set aside in the fridge for use in this crisis, if it should occur. Also in the fridge, dedicated to this emergency, keep:

- nasogastric tubes;
- dantrolene sodium, at least 20 ampoules (shelf life is 3 years);
- regular insulin.

On the trolley keep the following:

- urinary catheter and insertion tray;
- a urinometer;
- fresh breathing circuit;
- temperature probe and recorder;
- cooling blanket (or note where this is stored);
- rectal tube;
- intravenous, central venous and pulmonary artery catheters;
- tubes for blood gas and haematological studies;
- equipment for administering high-flow oxygen;
- sterile distilled water, at least 2 litres;
- a sterile bowl for mixing dantrolene and this water;
- mannitol;
- furosemide;
- sodium bicarbonate 8.4 mg in 100 ml;
- glucose 50%;
- procainamide hydrochloride.

Requirements for resuscitation of the newborn

These include:

- a high-sloping trolley;
- a radiant heater;
- oxygen, a flow meter, limited to a flow of 4 L/min, and tubing;
- a suction which is set at 40 cm water pressure;
- suction catheters, sizes 5–10 F;

- a bulb syringe;
- a meconium aspirator;
- sterile gloves, all sizes;
- a stethoscope;
- a laryngoscope with straight blades;
- extra bulbs and batteries;
- airways, sizes 000, 00 and 0;
- small masks;
- endotracheal tubes, sizes 2.5 to 3.5. Check that the tube has an end on it which will fit into the mask mount if you need to intubate;
- laryngeal mask, size one;
- a neonatal Ambu® or Laedal® resuscitation bag;
- pulse oximeter with appropriate sensor for a baby;
- ECG;
- umbilical catheter, 3–5 F;
- sterile umbilical vessel catheterization tray;
- needles and syringes, all sizes;
- three-way taps;
- IV giving set with a burette;
- 0.9% saline, 4% glucose, 1/5 N saline;
- albumen 5%;
- glucose 10%;
- adrenaline 1:10,000;
- naloxone 0.4 mg/ml;
- sodium bicarbonate 840 mg in 10 ml ampoules;
- sterile water and saline 10 ml ampoules;
- adhesive tape;
- scissors.

Reference

1. **Baker PA, Flanagan KB,** *et al.* (2011) Equipment to manage a difficult airway during anaesthesia. *Anaesthesia and Intensive Care* **39**(1):16–34.

Appendix 2

Infusions

Some drugs need to be administered at a constant rate for a number of hours or longer. This is best achieved by an infusion. A solution is prepared with a known concentration of drug. This is delivered at a rate calculated to keep the blood concentration of the drug at a fairly constant level. A loading dose is needed for most drugs. The advantages of an infusion are that the effect of the drug is smoother, a lower overall dose is required and the need for repeated injections is eliminated.

There are two ways to administer an infusion:

1. *Syringe drivers* give small volumes of concentrated drug through a catheter placed in one of the large central veins such as the superior vena cava. The drugs are usually so concentrated that they will injure smaller peripheral veins and may cause severe tissue damage if extravasation occurs.

*Never infuse concentrated drugs
through peripheral veins.*

2. *Infusion pumps* give larger volumes of fluid. Generally the drugs are less concentrated and often it is possible to safely infuse them into smaller peripheral veins.

Prepare written protocols

Prepare written protocols for each drug used. In them, set down the dose of the drug and the required pump or syringe drive settings. Include details of the expected effects, complications and management of these complications. Staff should be familiar with all the effects and expected problems before the infusion starts. Establish clear written instructions about limits of the parameters of blood pressure, pulse rate, respiratory rate and other variables.

Each drug needs its own dedicated separate intravenous line. It is unwise to use one catheter for infusing a number of drugs. Do not 'piggy-back' lines by using multi-entry ports or plug infusions into intravenous lines carrying other intravenous infusions. For safety potent drugs should be infused through a multi-lumen central venous catheter, with each lumen carrying only one drug.

To prevent errors, always have two trained staff independently check the drug concentration and the rate of infusion. The staff must understand how to use the equipment.

In the doses recommended in Table A2.1, the concentration of drug has been chosen so that the pump settings in millilitres per hour represent some simple numerical function of the drug dose in units per hour. For example if morphine is to be given then a setting of 4 ml/hr will give a dose of 4 mg/hr.

Attach an intravenous additive label to bags, flasks, or syringes containing drugs (Figure A2.1).

Patient's name_____Unit record number_____

Ward_____ Date_____Time prepared_____

Prepared by_____ Checked by_____

DRUG AND DOSE ADDED_____

_____

_____

_____

Concentration _____ Duration of infusion _____ Time to finish _____

Figure A2.1 Example of a drug label.

Use a central venous catheter

Many of these drugs are highly concentrated and cause severe thrombophlebitis and tissue necrosis if infused into peripheral veins. They should only be infused through a central venous line.

Multi-lumen catheters

Multi-lumen catheters are more expensive and are associated with more catheter complications. Each potent drug needs its own dedicated separate intravenous port. See Box A2.1.

Box A2.1 **Important notice**

Most of the drugs in Table A2.1 are highly concentrated and will cause severe thrombophlebitis and tissue necrosis if infused into peripheral veins. So infuse them into central veins only through a central venous catheter.

When infusing vasoactive or cardiac drugs always monitor cardiac rate and rhythm with an ECG and continuous record blood pressure, preferably an intra-arterial blood cannula.

Patients receiving infusions need constant monitoring and careful nursing care. Patients must never be left unattended. Everyone needs to be familiar with the pharmacology of the drugs, their actions, and side effects. Written protocols are needed and patient cardiovascular and other parameters need to be carefully specified.

Box A2.1 **(Continued)**

Table A2.1 Typical drugs including dilution and dose

Drug	Dilution	Dose
Adrenaline Epinephrine in USA 1 ml of 1/1000 = 1 mg 10 ml of 1/10,000 = 1 mg	Adrenaline 3 mg Make up to 5 ml in 5% glucose	1 ml/hr = 10 micrograms/min 1–30 micrograms/min Increase dose by 1 microgram/min until desired effect
Amiodarone	Amiodarone 300 mg in 50 ml of 5% glucose. (Not stable in saline.)	Loading dose: 25 micrograms/kg/min for 4 hrs May be given at 5 mg/kg over 20 min if urgent Maintenance: 5–15 g/kg/min
Dobutamine	Dobutamine 250 mg Make up to 41.5 ml in 5% glucose	1 ml/hr = 100 micrograms/min 2.5–15 micrograms/kg/min
Dopexamine	Dopexamine 10 mg Make up to 41.5 ml in 5% glucose	1 ml/hr = 4 micrograms/min
Furosemide	Furosemide 100 mg Make up to 50 ml in normal (0.9%) saline	1 ml/hr = 2 mg/hr Loading dose: 0.5 mg/kg Maintenance dose: 0.1–1 mg/kg/hr Protect from light.
Glyceryl trinitrate, GTN	Glyceryl trinitrate 100 mg Make up to 41.5 ml in 5% glucose	1 ml/hr = 40 micrograms/min Maintenance dose: 1–5 micrograms/kg/min Increase dose by 2–40 micrograms/min
Heparin 1 mg = 100 units	Heparin 25,000 units Make up to 25 ml in 5% glucose	1 ml/hr = 1000 units/hr Low dose: 75 units/kg stat then 10–15 units/kg/hr Full heparinization: 200 units/kg stat then 15–30 units/kg/hr
Insulin	Insulin 50 units Make up to 50 ml in 5% glucose	1 ml/hr = 1 unit/hr
Isoprenaline	Isoprenaline 3 mg Make up to 50 ml in 5% glucose	1 ml/hr = 1 micrograms/min 1–20 micro/min Increase dose by 1 micrograms/min until desired effect
Lidocaine	Lidocaine 1000 mg Make up to 41.5 ml in 5% glucose	1 ml/hr = 0.4 mg/min Run at: 8 ml/hr for 1 hr 6 ml/hr for 2nd hr 4 ml/hr for next 24 hrs

(Continued)

Box A2.1 **(Continued)**

Drug	Dilution	Dose
Morphine	Morphine 50 mg Make up to 50 ml in 5% glucose	1 ml/hr = 1 mg/hr Loading dose: 0.1–0.5 mg/kg Normal requirements 0.02–0.1 mg/kg/hr
Noradrenaline Norepinephrine in USA	Noradrenaline 3 mg Make up to 50 ml in 5% glucose	1 ml/hr = 1 micrograms/min 1–30 micrograms/min Increase dose by 1 micrograms/min until desired effect
Nitroglycerin	see Glyceryl trinitrate	
Verapamil	Verapamil 50 mg Make up to 50 ml in 5% glucose	1 ml/hr = 1 mg/hr Loading dose:1 mg/min up to 10 mg (10 ml of 10% calcium gluconate may be needed to control hypotension) or 0.1–0.1 mg/kg IV over 10 minutes

Be careful of dead space

Be careful of dead space in lines and catheters. *Dead space* is the volume fluid you need to inject into the line before it reaches the patient's bloodstream. If you do not fill the catheter with the drug (prime the line) it will take some time to fill the dead space and reach the patient. Furthermore if you flush the line you may wash unwanted drug into the patient.

Check your doses with someone else

Always independently check your dose regime with another member of trained staff who understands the infusion pumps and how to use them.

What to monitor

If you are infusing vasoactive drugs, then monitor the patient with an ECG, and continuously record intra-arterial blood pressure.

Useful data

Resources

Acid-base
http://www.acid-base.com

Acupuncture
http://www.acupuncture.com

American Heart Association
http://www.americanheart.org/aha.html

American Pain Foundation
https://uspainfoundation.org

American Society of Pain Management Nursing
http://www.aspmn.org

American Society of Peri-anesthesia Nurses
http://www.aspan.org

Association of Peri-operative Registered Nurses
http://www.aorn.org

Australian and New Zealand College of Anaesthetists
http://www.anzca.edu.au

Australian College of Critical Care Nurses
http://www.acccn.com.au

Australian College of Nursing
http://www.acn.edu.au

Australian College of Operating Room Nurses
http://www.acorn.org.au

Australian Institute of Health and Welfare
http://www.aihw.gov.au

Australian Lung Foundation

http://www.lungnet.org.au

Australian Pain Society

https://www.apsoc.org.au/

Australian Resuscitation Council

http://www.resus.org.au

British Anaesthetic and Recovery Nurses' Association

http://www.barna.co.uk

British Medical Journal

http://www.bmj.com

Cancer Council of Australia

http://www.cancer.org.au

Capnography

http://www.capnography.com

Centers for Disease Control and Prevention

http://www.cdc.gov

Cochrane Collaboration

http://www.cochrane.org

College of Emergency Nurses Australasia

http://www.cena.org.au

Epidural manual (Royal Marsden)

http://www.blackwellroyalmarsdenmanual.com/sample/mars29.htm

Johns Hopkins Center for Tuberculosis Research

http://tbcenter.jhu.edu/

Journal of Perianesthesia Nursing

http://www.jopan.org

Malignant Hyperthermia Association of the United States

http://www.mhaus.org

National Association of Theatre Nurses

https://www.afpp.org.uk/

National Heart Foundation of Australia

http://www.heartfoundation.org.au

North American Nursing Diagnosis Association

http://www.nanda.org

Operating Room Association of Canada

http://www.ornac.ca

Perioperative Nurses' College of New Zealand

https://www.nzno.org.nz/groups/colleges_sections/colleges/perioperative_nurses_college

Postoperative Pain

http://www.postoppain.org

Royal Australasian College of Surgeons

http://www.surgeons.org

Royal Children's Hospital

http://www.rch.org.au

The Cardiac Society of Australia and New Zealand

http://www.csanz.edu.au

VirtualAnaesthetics

http://www.virtual-anesthesia-textbook.com

World Anaesthesia

http://www.nda.ox.ac.uk

World Health Organization

http://www.who.int

Standardization

The Systeme Internationale d'Unites (SI system) is the standard against which to measure length in metres, mass in kilograms, and time in seconds, pressure in pascals, work in joules, volume in cubic metres and so on. Non-standard units are still widely used and include millimetres of mercury, litres, degrees Fahrenheit. It will be sometime before we drink 0.180×10^{-3} cubic metres instead of a tumbler (or glass) of water, or say today's temperature is 300 Kelvin (not 'degrees' Kelvin).

Factors

See Table A3.1 for a list of factors.

Table A3.1 Factors

Factor	Prefix	Symbol
10^6	mega	M
10^3	kilo	k
10^{-1}	dec	d
10^{-2}	centi	c
10^{-3}	milli	m
10^{-6}	micro	μ
10^{-9}	nano	n
10^{-12}	pico	p

Conversion table for solution strengths

By definition a 1 per cent solution contains 1 gram of substance in every 100 ml of solution. This can also be written as 1:100 or 10 mg/ml (Table A3.2).

Table A3.2 Dilution table

Dilution	Solution (%)	mg/ml
1:200,000	0.0005	0.005 mg/ml
1:100,000	0.001	0.01 mg/ml
1:10,000	0.01	0.1 mg/ml
1:5000	0.02	0.2 mg/ml
1:1000	0.1	1 mg/ml
1:500	0.2	2 mg/ml
1:200	0.5	5 mg/ml
1:100	1	10 mg/ml
1:50	2	20 mg/ml
1:10	10	100 mg/ml

Length

SI unit is the metre.

1 metre = 100 centimetres = 1000 millimetres
= 1,000,000 microns = 1,000,000,000 nanometres

1 foot = 30.48 cm = 304.8 mm

1 inch = 2.54 cm = 25.4 mm

Volume

SI unit is the cubic metre.

1000 millilitres = 10 decilitres = 1 litre

1 teaspoon = 4.5 ml

1 tablespoon = 15 ml

1 teacup = 120 ml

1 tumbler = 240 ml

1 pint = 568 ml

1 fluid ounce = 28.42 ml

Temperature

When heat energy flows from body A to body B, then body A is at a higher temperature than body B. Temperature is measure of thermodynamic activity.

SI unit is the Kelvin (not 'degrees Kelvin')

Centigrade means the same as Celsius.

Fahrenheit is a temperature scale used in the USA (see Table A3.3).

Water forms ice at 0° Celsius and boils at 100°C.

Water forms ice at 32° Fahrenheit and boils at 212°F.

Water forms ice at 273 Kelvin and boils at 373 K.

Table A3.3 Centigrade and Fahrenheit conversion table

$C° = (F° − 32) × 5/9$

$F° = (C° × 9/5) + 32$

C°	30	32	34	35	36	37	38	39	40
F°	86.0	87.8	93.2	95.0	96.8	98.6	100.4	102.2	104.0

Pressure

Pressure is the force per unit area exerted by a substance perpendicular to its boundary with another substance.

SI unit is the pascal. A kilopascal is 1000 pascals.

Some places measure pressures in kilopascals (kPa), whereas others measure it in millimetres of mercury (mmHg). See Tables A3.4 and A3.5.

7.6 mmHg = 1 kPa

1 mmHg ≈ 13 Pa

Occasionally pressure is measured in centimetres of water.

1.32 mmHg = 10 cm H_2O

Table A3.4 Conversion table for kPa and mmHg

SI unit	Old unit	Old to SI	SI to old
kPa	mmHg	× 0.133	× 7.60
	cm H_2O	× 0.098	× 10.20
	lb per inch²	× 6.894	× 0.145

mmHg	kPa	mmHg	kPa	mmHg	kPa	mmHg	kPa	mmHg	kPa
1	0.13	21	2.76	41	5.39	61	8.03	81	10.66
2	0.26	22	2.89	42	5.52	62	8.16	82	10.79
3	0.39	23	3.03	43	5.65	63	8.29	83	10.92
4	0.53	24	3.16	44	5.79	64	8.42	84	11.05
5	0.66	25	3.29	45	5.92	65	8.55	85	11.18
6	0.79	26	3.42	46	6.05	66	8.68	86	11.32
7	0.92	27	3.55	47	6.18	67	8.82	87	11.45
8	1.05	28	3.68	48	6.32	68	8.95	88	11.58
9	1.08	29	3.82	49	6.45	69	9.08	89	11.71
10	1.32	30	3.95	50	6.58	70	9.21	90	11.84
11	1.45	31	4.08	51	6.71	71	9.34	91	11.97
12	1.58	32	4.21	52	6.84	72	9.47	92	12.11
13	1.71	33	4.34	53	6.97	73	9.60	93	12.24
14	1.84	34	4.47	54	7.11	74	9.73	94	12.37
15	1.97	35	4.60	55	7.24	75	9.87	95	12.50
16	2.11	36	4.73	56	7.37	76	10.00	96	12.63
17	2.24	37	4.87	57	7.50	77	10.13	97	12.76
18	2.37	38	5.00	58	7.63	78	10.26	98	12.89
19	2.50	39	5.13	59	7.76	79	10.39	99	13.03
20	2.63	40	5.26	60	7.89	80	10.53	100	13.16

Blood pressure

Blood pressure is the force per unit area exerted by blood at right angle to its direction of flow.

Table A3.5 Typical pressures in mmHg

Pressures in mmHg	Range	Comments
Central venous pressure (CVP)	0–7	Zero reference at isophlebotic point
Right atrium	0–8	Mean = 5
Right ventricle	22/0	
Pulmonary artery	22/8	Mean = 14
Pulmonary artery wedge	2–8	Mean = 5
Left atrium	7	

Weight

1,000,000 microgram = 1000 milligram = 1 gram = 0.001 kg
1 ounce (oz) = 28.35 g
1 pound (lb) = 0.4536 kg
1 stone = 14 lb = 6.35 kg

Average blood requirement

Average blood requirement is the amount of blood usually needed for these operations (see Table A3.6). These figures help you work out whether the patient has received roughly the correct amount of blood for their operation, or that there is enough available to cover future needs. Smaller patients require relatively larger amounts of blood than more muscular people. For instance a 90 kg man would probably not need any blood for a total knee replacement, while a 50 kg old woman may need at least one unit.

Table A3.6 Blood cross-match estimates for common surgical procedures

Operation	Blood cross-match in 450 ml units
Abdominal lipectomy	2
Abdomino-perineal resection	3
Adrenalectomy	2
Amputation—above knee	Group and hold (G+H)
Amputation—below knee	G+H
Anterior resection	2

Table A3.6 (Continued)

Operation	Blood cross-match in 450 ml units
Aortic aneurysm—elective	3
Aorto-femoral bypass	4
Aorto-iliac bypass	4
Appendicectomy	Nil
Apronectomy	2
Arthroscopy	Nil
Bowel resection	2
Burns debridement	Lots
Caesarean section	G+H
Carotid endarterectomy	G+H
Cholecystectomy—laparoscopic	G+H
Cholecystectomy—open	G+H
Colostomy	G+H
Cystectomy	4
Cystoscopy	Nil
D&C ± hysteroscopy	Nil
Ectopic—ruptured	4
Ectopic—simple	G+H
Femoral-popliteal bypass	2
Gastrectomy	2
Gastric—high reduction	G+H
Gastric stapling	G+H
Gastrostomy	G+H
Haemorrhoidectomy	Nil
Harrington's rods	4
Hepatectomy—partial	6
Hiatus hernia—transthoracic	2
Hiatus hernia repair	G+H
Hip replacement	3
Hysterectomy—radical	2
Hysterectomy—abdominal	G+H
Hysterectomy—vaginal	G+H
Ileal conduit	4

(*Continued*)

Table A3.6 (Continued)

Operation	Blood cross-match in 450 ml units
Ileostomy	G+H
Ilio-femoral bypass	2
Incisional hernia	G+H
Infra-inguinal vascular redo	2
Inguinal hernia	Nil
Inguinal hernia—laparoscopic	G+H
Ivor Lewis oesophagectomy	4
Knee replacement	1
Laminectomy	G+H
Laminectomy + fusion	4
Laparoscopy	G+H
Lumbar sympathectomy	G+H
Lung lobectomy	2
Mammoplasty—reduction < 1 kg	G+H
Mammoplasty—reduction > 1 kg	2
Mastectomy—radical	2
Mastectomy—simple	G+H
Mastectomy + axillary clearance	2
Meniscectomy	Nil
Myomectomy	G+H
Nephrectomy—simple	2
Nephrectomy for cancer	4
Nephrolithotomy—open	4
Nephrolithotomy—fibreoptic	G+H
Oesophagectomy	4
Ovarian cystectomy	G+H
Pancreatectomy—partial	4
Pancreatectomy—total	6
Pancreatic cyst	2
Parotidectomy	G+H
Pelvic clearance	4
Pleurectomy	2
Pneumonectomy	4

(*Continued*)

Table A3.6 (Continued)

Operation	Blood cross-match in 450 ml units
Portocaval shunt	4
Prostatectomy—open	2
Pyelolithotomy	2
Pyeloplasty	G+H
Renal artery repair	3
Salpingoplasty	G+H
Shoulder-arthroplasty	G+H
Spinal fusion	2
Splenectomy	2
Splenectomy for ITP	4
Synovectomy—knee	G+H
Termination of pregnancy	G+H
Thymectomy	2
Thyroidectomy—simple	G+H
Thyroidectomy for cancer	G+H
Thyroidectomy for goitre	G+H
Tubal ligation	G+H
TURP	G+H
Ureto-lithotomy	G+H
Vaginal repair	G+H
Varicose veins	G+H
Vulvectomy—radical	4
Vulvectomy—simple	2
Whipple's operation	4

Drugs entering breast milk

See Table A3.7.

Factors to consider include:

- Older infants are less susceptible to drugs in breast milk than neonates or premature babies.
- Premature babies' ability to metabolize and excrete drugs is less than older infants.
- Consider other factors, such as liver or renal disease, which impair a baby's ability to deal with drugs.

Table A3.7 Drugs entering breast milk

Drug	In breast milk	Recommendation
Atenolol	Yes	Safe in short term
Atracurium	Unknown	Avoid where possible
Atropine	Yes	Safe as a single dose
Bupivacaine	Yes	Safe for 36 hours
Cisatracurium	Probably	Avoid where possible
Clonidine	Yes	Safe as a single dose
Codeine	Yes	Probably safe as a single dose
Dalteparin	Yes	Wait 2 days before restarting feeding
Desflurane	Trace	Probably safe
Diamorphine	Yes	Best avoid
Diazepam	Yes	Safe in single dose
Diclofenac	Trace	Safe in short term
Dolasetron	Probably	Avoid
Droperidol	Yes	Best avoid
Enoxaparin	Unknown	Safe in anaesthetic setting
Ephedrine	Yes	Safe as a single dose
Ergometrine	Yes	Safe as a single dose
Esmolol	Unknown	Best avoid
Fentanyl	Yes	Safe in anaesthetic setting
Flumazenil	Yes	Avoid where possible
Furosemide	Yes	Postpone breastfeeding
Gentamicin	Yes	Probably safe
Glycopyrronium bromide	Yes	Probably safe
Granisetron	Unknown	Best avoid
Hydrocortisone	Unknown	Safe as a single dose
Insulin	Unknown	Safe
Isoflurane	Unknown	Considered safe
Ketamine	Yes	Safe in short term
Lidocaine	Yes	Considered safe as a single dose
Mannitol	Unknown	Best avoid
Metoclopramide	Yes	May cause infant diarrhoea
Metronidazole	Yes	Withhold feeds for 4 hours after single dose
Midazolam	Yes—small	Considered safe

(Continued)

Table A3.7 (Continued)

Drug	In breast milk	Recommendation
Morphine	Trace	Considered safe in normal doses
Naloxone	Yes	Safe as a single dose
Naproxen	Yes	Avoid
Neostigmine	Negligible	Safe as a single dose
Ondansetron	Yes	Avoid
Oxycodone	Yes	Considered safe
Pancuronium	Trace—possibly	Safe in anaesthesia
Paracetamol	Yes	Safe—analgesic of choice
Pethidine	Yes	Morphine safer
Prochlorperazine	Unknown	Avoid
Propofol	Trace	Considered safe
Ranitidine	Yes	Avoid—use famotidine instead
Salbutamol	Yes	Considered safe in low dose
Sevoflurane	Unknown	Considered safe
Temazepam	Yes	Considered safe in single dose
Tetracaine	Yes	Avoid—significantly toxic
Thiopental	Yes	Considered safe in one dose
Tramadol	Yes	Avoid
Vecuronium	Unknown	Considered safe

Surgery grades
Major procedure (highly invasive surgery)

- expected to take more than 60 minutes;
- involves extensive tissue mass and trauma;
- major disruption to body physiology persists after 24 hours;
- requires a blood transfusion;
- involves a patient of ASA III grade or higher;
- all vascular surgery;
- major joint replacement;
- open abdomen or thorax including laparoscopy;
- intracranial or spinal operations;
- is an emergency.

Examples: aortic aneurysm repair, bowel resection, thoracotomy, major joint replacement.

Minor procedure (moderately invasive surgery)

* expected to take 30–60 minutes;
* some tissue trauma;
* minor disruption to body physiology persists after 24 hours;
* patient is intubated;
* no blood transfusion;
* laparoscopic surgery;

Examples: inguinal hernia repair, laparoscopic cholecystectomy, prostatectomy.

Minimal procedure (minimally invasive surgery)

* expected to take less than 30 minutes;
* minimal tissue trauma;
* no disruption to body physiology persist after 24 hours.

Examples: arthroscopy, D&C, cystoscopy.

Postsurgical classification

Postsurgical classification ranks patients according to how incapacitated they are, and allows resources to be allocated to suit the situation.

Stable

Patients who are to return to the ward who:

* had observations that remained within normal limits during their stay in the recovery room;
* are receiving no more than maintenance intravenous fluids;
* whose biochemistry and haematology results were normal.

Labile

Patients who are to return to the ward:

* after an invasive procedure whose stay in the recovery room was uneventful, but who now require more than routine observations. For example if they have an epidural catheter.
* who, while in the recovery room, developed an abnormal observation that is explainable and is unlikely to need intervention or to deteriorate.
* who, while in the recovery room, were found to have an abnormal biochemical or haematology result.

Unstable

Patients who are to return to the ward who:

- have undergone an invasive procedure, but whose recovery is not proceeding as expected;
- while in the recovery room had abnormal observations that responded to corrective measures;
- have worsening abnormal biochemical or haematological results;
- required additional unexpected intervention, e.g. insertion of a thoracic drain for a pneumothorax.

Critical

Critical patients are discharged to a high care unit. They remain in Stage 1 recovery.
These patients include those who, while in recovery room, have:

- worsening abnormal observations despite corrective intervention;
- been classified as unstable emergency cases;
- abnormal observations and the diagnosis remains obscure.

How to assign risk

In 1941 the American Society of Anesthesiologists developed a scale to quantify surgical and anaesthetic risk. It subsequently became known as the ASA scale. This scale has withstood the test of time; it is easy to remember and has over the years proved reliable in predicting postoperative trouble.

Not only does the ASA status provide a useful way of quickly conveying how sick a patient is, but also it correlates well with mortality, theatre cancellations, and unplanned emergency operations, and is useful when you are developing protocols. The ASA status's grave disadvantage is that it makes no assessment of the magnitude of surgery; a wart can be removed from an ASA IV patient without problems, but a hip replacement may kill them.

The ASA PS Class (American Society of Anesthesiologists' Grading of Physical Status) is ranked in order of how severely the patient is incapacitated, and the numbers are easy to remember (see Table A3.8):

ASA I—fit
ASA II—minor diseases
ASA III—major disease
ASA IV—life threatening disease
ASA V—near dead

If the case is an emergency append an E to the physical grade, e.g. IV E.

Table A3.8 A more detailed classification

ASA class	Disability	Mortality rate (est)
Class I	The patient is perfectly fit for their age. The patient has no organic physiological, biochemical or psychiatric disturbance. The surgical site is localized, and surgery does not entail systemic disturbance.	< 0.08%
Class II	The patient has a condition which does not limit their day-to-day activity. Mild to moderate systemic disturbance caused either by the surgical condition or by the pathophysiological process. For example: mild organic heart disease, non-insulin-dependent diabetes, mild hypertension (diastolic < 100 mmHg), anaemia, old age, mild obesity, mild asthma.	0.08–0.42%
Class III	The patient has a condition which limits their day-to-day activity. Severe systemic disturbance or disease from whatever cause, even though it may not be possible to define the degree of disability with any finality. Includes obesity (BMI > 35), angina (exercise- or emotion-induced but stable), healed myocardial infarction, insulin-dependent diabetes, peripheral vascular disease, cardiac failure (moderate systolic or diastolic dysfunction), moderate hypertension (diastolic 100–115 mmHg), severe asthma, warfarin therapy.	0.4–4.3%
Class IV	The patient has a condition which severely limits their activity and is a constant threat to life. Severe systemic disturbances that are already life threatening and not necessarily correctable by surgery. This includes marked obesity (BMI > 40), cardiac insufficiency (diastolic or systolic dysfunction), Hypertension with diastolic blood pressure ≥ 115 mmHg, persistent, frequent or unstable angina, active myocarditis, recent CVA or TIA (within last 16 weeks), advance pulmonary, renal or endocrine, or hepatic insufficiency.	4.4–23%
Class V	Moribund. Little chance of survival with or without surgery, but submitted to operation in desperation.	24–51%
Class VI	Brain dead patient whose organs are being harvested	100%

Source data from Owens, W.D., Felts, J. A., Spitznagel, EL Jr. ASA physical status classification: a study of consistency of ratings. *Anesthesiology*, 1978; 49: 239–243.

Emergency surgery

Add an E after the grade if the operation is an emergency.

Glossary

2,3-DPG 2,3-diphosphoglycerate. This biochemical molecule is normally found nested in a little hollow at the core of the haemoglobin molecule. 2,3-DPG lowers the force of attraction between haemoglobin and oxygen so that an oxygen molecule can escape more easily once the pressure of oxygen in the surrounding fluid falls.

Acetylcholine A neurotransmitter in the peripheral nervous system where it stimulates voluntary muscle fibres to contract, and in the parasympathetic nervous system, where it attends to house-keeping functions of the body, and in the central nervous system where it helps regulate memory. In the parasympathetic nervous system and central nervous system it has **muscarinic activity**, whereas in the peripheral nerve serving voluntary muscle it has **nicotinic activity**.

Acids Substances that donate hydrogen ions to chemical reactions.

Action potentials Action potentials occur when neurons are activated. A wave of electrical charge tumbles along the membrane of the neuron as ions enter through special ion channels. This temporarily reverses the electrical charge of the inside of the membrane from negative to positive. When the wave hits the end of the nerve it releases a **neurotransmitter**, and then the wave disappears. In muscles the action potential stimulates the muscles to contract.

Activated partial thromboplastin time (aPTT) tests the integrity of the intrinsic coagulation system, and common coagulation pathways. For most laboratories the normal range is 36–34 seconds (or < 6 sec above normal control values). Interpret this test cautiously. There is a poor correlation between the aPPT and a clinically significant coagulopathy. aPPT also rises with any inflammatory disease.

Acute coronary syndrome (ACS) A collection of signs and symptoms that suggest the patient has just had, or is about to have, a heart attack. ACS includes problems such as accelerating angina, ST changes on the ECG, rise in troponin or creatinine kinase (CK-MB) and ischaemic arrhythmias.

Acute pain Pain of recent onset and expected to have limited duration.

Acute tubular necrosis The end result of renal hypoxia or poisoning with toxins. The dying cells lining the kidney tubules swell to occlude the lumen of the tubule. Distressed endothelial cells lining the intra-renal blood vessels pile up on one another obstructing blood flow.

Adrenal cortex is an endocrine gland that secretes **corticosteroids**. These steroids are used for a wide range of long-term metabolic responses that help restore homeostasis. Cortisol is secreted in large amounts just before dawn to help the body prepare for the day. Aldosterone aids in the reabsorption of sodium from the kidney, androgens for male sexual development, and oestrogens for female sexual development.

Adrenal medulla is an endocrine gland that secretes adrenaline and some noradrenaline. The adrenaline circulates in the blood stream to activate a **sympathetic response**.

Adrenaline is the hormone of exercise. In the USA it is called **epinephrine**. Adrenaline prepares the body for exercise and helps sustain exercise once it starts. In physiological amounts it increases cardiac output, increases the blood flow to skeletal muscle, and mobilizes stored glycogen to glucose in the liver to provide energy for exercise. Adrenaline in pharmacological amounts is used as a vasoconstrictor in local anaesthetics, in the treatment of anaphylactic reactions to increase the blood pressure, and as an **ionotrope**.

Adrenergic drugs stimulate the sympathetic nervous system. **Sympatheticomimetic** drugs mimic the effects of noradrenaline or adrenaline; and include ephedrine, metaraminol, phenylephrine, dopamine, and dobutamine.

Adrenergic receptors Receptors for the two catecholamines adrenaline and noradrenaline. Some of their important functions are to regulate the blood flow through arterioles, and modulate blood pressure and cardiac output.

Aeration means to fill with ambient gas. Ambient means whatever the patient is breathing. It may be air, or air supplemented with oxygen.

Afferent and **efferent** arterioles. Afferent means to 'flow into', and efferent means to 'flow out of'.

Afterload is the pressure the heart needs to overcome to eject its stroke volume.

Agonist An agonist is a neurotransmitter, a drug or other molecule that stimulates receptors on the outside of cell membranes to change the chemical reactions inside a cell.

Alcohol-based hand rub designed to rub on the hands to reduce the number of viable micro-organisms. The 60% solutions in a water-based emollient work better than the 90% solutions, because the proteins in **microbes** are not denatured in the absence of water.

Aldosterone A steroid hormone produced by the adrenal cortex. It acts on the distal tubules in the kidney, triggering them to reabsorb sodium and water. The effect on a person is similar to a saline infusion.

All-or-none response With this response either nothing happens, or the maximal outcome occurs. Nerve fibres either conduct an impulse or they do not. Another useful term for this response is a ballistic response.

Allodynia is pain caused by a stimulus that would not normally provoke pain.

Allogeneic means a tissue that is genetically dissimilar and therefore potentially immunologically incompatible with other members of the same species. In other words, an allogeneic transfusion is a blood transfusion from a person who is not an identical twin. It comes from a donor. Note the spelling allogeneic, not allogenic.

Allogenic describes some event causing pain.

Amino-acid transmitters These are the most prevalent neurotransmitters in the brain and spinal cord. They include glutamate and aspartate which excite (or stimulate) neurons into action, or glycine and gamma hydroxybutyric acid (GABA) which inhibit neurons from passing on an **action potential**.

Aminoglycosides are bactericidal antibiotics used predominately against Gram-negative bacteria. They have to be given by injection because they are not absorbed from the gut. They have two major disadvantages: in higher doses they damage kidney tubules, and cause deafness.

Anaemia is either a low haemoglobin concentration or a low total red cell mass. Iron deficiency, or chronic bleeding usually causes microcytic anaemias, while the macrocytic anaemias are caused by liver or bone marrow disease.

Anaerobic means in the absence of oxygen.

Anaerobic metabolism are metabolic processes that can proceed in the absence of oxygen.

Analgesia is the absence of pain in response to a stimulus that would normally produce it.

Android obesity Represented by the typical male beer-gut. The man has skinny legs and looks like an apple on two matchsticks. Android obesity carries a high risk of cardiovascular disease, stroke, and diabetes, as well as deep vein thrombosis.

Angiotensin-converting enzyme (ACE) is found in the lungs. It converts angiotensin I into angiotensin II. Angiotensin II is the most powerful vasoconstrictor of all.

Angiotensin-converting enzyme inhibitors These are a first choice treatment for certain types of hypertension. They stop angiotensin I being converted to angiotensin II by the angiotensin converting enzyme (ACE) in the lungs.

Angiotensin-receptor blocking drugs (ARBs). These are a group of drugs—the sartans, e.g. irbesartan and candesartan—that block the effect of angiotensin II, and so prevent arterioles constricting. The ARBs are used when ACE inhibitors are causing unacceptable side-effects.

Angiotensinogen is a prohormone produced in the liver.

Anions are negatively charged ions. Usually they are formed from non-metals such as chloride (Cl^-), but may be more complex ions such as bicarbonate (HCO_3^-)

Anion gap The anion gap reveals the presence of ions in plasma that are not normally picked up on routine biochemistry. For example lactate ion, carrying a negative charge, is not included in the routine electrolyte tests; but a low anion gap may reveal its presence. Anion gap = (Na + K) − (Cl − Bicarb) normally lies within the range of 7–27 mmol/L.

Antagonist An antagonist is a drug or molecule that occupies a **receptor** so that an **agonist** cannot latch on to it to trigger a response.

Antidiuretic hormone (ADH) is also called **vasopressin**. It is a nine-peptide hormone released from the posterior pituitary gland. ADH makes the collecting tubules in the kidney permeable to water so that water is retained.

Apnoea The complete absence of breathing.

aPTT see **Activated partial thromboplastin time**.

Arachidonic acid is an unsaturated fatty acid, an essential component of cell membranes, which is a precursor for the production of prostaglandins.

Arginine vasopression see **Vasopressin.**

Arrhythmias are abnormalities in the heart rate or rhythm.

Aspartate An amino acid derivative used in the central nervous system as a neurotransmitter.

Asystole means the heart has stopped (a cardiac arrest). The ECG shows a straight or gently undulating base line with no electrical activity.

Atrial ectopic beats occur when the impulse arises in odd places within the atria and not in the SA node.

Atrial fibrillation (AF) occurs where the atrial excitation wave is uncoordinated and atria ceases to contract. No P-waves can be seen on the ECG and the ventricles contract irregularly. If the chest is opened the atria look as though they are shivering or writhing like a bag of worms.

Atrial flutter occurs where the atria are contracting ineffectively fast. It is seen as a saw-toothed picture between each QRS complex.

Autoantibodies are antibodies that occur naturally in people. They do not need an anti-genic stimulus to produce them. Examples are naturally occurring antibodies against blood groups, and **cold agglutinins**.

Autonomic nervous system (ANS) is part of the peripheral nervous system. It regulates the activity of internal organs. Traditionally the ANS was divided into **sympathetic** and **parasympathetic nervous systems**. More recently the term **sympathetic response** has been replaced by addressing its components: a **noradrenergic response** (mediated by **noradrenaline**) and an **adrenergic** response (mediated by **adrenaline**). In contrast, the term *parasympathetic response* is now more often called a *cholinergic response*, because it is mediated by the neurotransmitter *acetylcholine*.

Autoregulation is the ability of an organ to regulate its blood flow to keep it constant despite changes in the blood pressure. The kidneys autoregulate their blood flow to keep it constant between mean arterial blood pressures of 80–160 mmHg.

Axial and **non-axial airways** Between the lips and the terminal respiratory units the air-ways branch approximately 22 times. Most airways branch gently from the line of air-flow and are called axial airways. While other branches leave the main pathway at sharp angles and are called non-axial airways, because air does not readily divert from its natural course to flow through them. Air flowing down airways tends to take the line of least resistance preferring to flow through the axial airways. This preferential flow is the reason why the lower parts of the lungs are better aerated than the upper lobes.

Axons are the long fibre-like extensions leading to or from a neuron's cell body. Myelinated axons are covered in an insulating sheath made of Schwann cells and carry nerve impulse rapidly. Unmyelinated axons are naked, and transmit information more slowly.

Bacteraemia occurs where living bacteria can be isolated from blood's plasma. **Primary bacteraemia** occurs where there is no identifiable focus of infection. **Secondary bacteraemia** occurs where there is an identifiable focus of infection. Bacteria do not have to be present in the blood stream to activate the massive inflammatory response in severe sepsis. Fewer than 50 per cent of septic patients have a bacteraemia, the rest have a focus of infection somewhere outside the bloodstream.

Bacteriocidal substances kill bacteria.

Bag and mask A commonly used expression that means to use a resuscitation bag (such as a Magill circuit) and an anaesthetic mask to ventilate a patient who is not breathing.

Baroreceptors Sensors that detect stretching of the walls of blood vessels. The ones in arteries are called *high-pressure baroreceptors*, while those in veins are the *low-pressure baroreceptors*.

Barotrauma refers to lung injury caused by gas delivered under too much pressure causing structures to rupture, tear and burst.

Basal ganglia are a cluster of neurons deep in the forebrain. They play an important part in controlling movement, and include structures such as the caudate nucleus, putamen, globus pallidus, and substantia nigra. If certain cells in the substantia nigra die, the person gets Parkinson's disease.

Basement membranes Thin layers of collagen matrix on which a single layer of endothelial or epithelial cells lie. The basement membrane anchors these sheets of cells in place, and acts as a barrier to substances escaping through to the underlying tissue. Providing the basement membrane is not disrupted, epithelial and endothelial cells can regenerate and then migrate across the membrane to repair damage.

Bases Substances that accept hydrogen ions and in so doing release water.

Benzodiazepines A group of psychoactive drugs that depress the brain's arousal systems by potentiating the inhibitory effects of the neurotransmitter GABA. Midazolam is the most common one used for sedation and amnesia in anaesthesia. Their effect may take many hours to wear off, particularly in elderly patients. They may have paradoxically stimulant effects in some patients who can become abruptly violent in the recovery room. Taken over the long term they are drugs of dependence with severe withdrawal effects.

Beta lactams A group of antibiotics that include penicillins and cephalosporins. A beta lactam ring contains three carbon atoms and one nitrogen atom.

Bier's block is a form of regional anaesthesia. The arm is emptied of blood with an elastic bandage, an arterial tourniquet applied to the upper arm, and the arm veins filled with 40 ml of 0.5% prilocaine. This block gives excellent analgesia for up to 40 minutes, although the tourniquet can become intolerably uncomfortable unless an intercostobrachial nerve block is also inserted.

Body water is an imprecisely defined term often used informally to mean all the fluids in the body, both outside and inside the cells. Strictly speaking these fluids are not water, but are isotonic solutions of dissolved salts or **ions**.

Bougie A bougie is a long thin flexible rod that can be passed through an endotracheal tube to enable the tube to be moulded to a shape that can be guided through the laryngeal opening. They are made of gum-elastic, or occasionally silicon-coated stiff wire.

Bradycardia A heart rate less than 50 beats per minute.

Bradykinins are group of peptides found in the blood and tissue fluid that provoke inflammation. They are produced when special enzymes split globulins in the blood.

Brainstem The brainstem is like the stalk on a mushroom where the forebrain spreads out at the top of the stalk. Everything passing through the spinal cord to, and from, the forebrain passes through the brainstem. The brainstem also contains, among other things, the vital centres of respiratory and cardiovascular control.

Breathing is the mechanical act of moving air in and out of lungs. Strictly used the term breathing is different from the term *respiration*.

Buffers are compounds in a solution that resist a change in hydrogen ion concentration when an acid or an alkali is added to the solution. It is a sort of chemical storage box that can either hold hydrogen ions or release them to keep their concentration in the surrounding fluid constant. When you add a hydrogen ion to the solution the box accepts one into storage. If you take a hydrogen ion away, then the box releases one into the solution to take its place.

Bundle branch blocks are defects in the left or right major branches of the conducting system of the heart that impede the spread of the cardiac impulse.

Calcium channels Gates in the cell membrane through which calcium can flow. **Candela** (cd) The SI base unit of luminous intensity.

Capillary return time (CRT) The time taken for blood to flood back into a fingertip, or nailbed, once you stop squeezing on it. Ideally it should be about 1 second. It is a sign of poor peripheral perfusion if the CRT takes more than 3 seconds. CRT is particularly useful in neonates and small children.

Carboxyhaemoglobin Forms when the poisonous gas carbon monoxide (CO) binds to haemoglobin and displaces oxygen. Under certain circumstances carbon monoxide is generated in the anaesthetic machine if soda lime reacts with some of the volatile agents.

Cardiac failure Occurs when the heart does not function properly.

Cardiac impulse A small electrical current that washes like a wave over the surfaces of cardiac muscle cells causing them to depolarize. Depolarization triggers the cardiac myocytes to contract.

Cardiac index (CI) Allows cardiac output to be compared between people of different sizes and weights. It is the standardized cardiac output relative to body surface area. The normal CI at rest is 3000 ml/m²/min.

Cardiomyopathy Means there is something wrong with heart muscle. Many things damage heart muscle, such as congenital malformations, chronic ischaemia, alcohol, infiltrations with amyloid, fat, or iron, viral infections, or simply working too hard and wearing out (as occurs with hypertension).

Cardiopulmonary unit Refers to the heart and lungs functioning together to supply oxygen to, and remove carbon dioxide from, the tissues.

Carina The anatomical landmark that marks the bifurcation of the trachea into right and left main bronchi. It is easily seen on a chest X-ray.

Catabolism Involves the breakdown of tissues to provide the body with the energy it requires. The essential feature is that more energy is expended faster than it is replaced and tissues simply waste away. Frequently after surgery this amounts to a muscle protein loss of up to one kilogram a day. Feeding the patient slows, but does not halt, the process.

Catalysts Molecules, including enzymes, which speed up chemical reactions, but do not become part of the final product. They can be used over and over again.

Catecholamines Amine derivatives of a basic chemical structure called catechol. They include adrenaline, noradrenaline, dopamine, and isoprenaline. They include a group of three neurotransmitters: dopamine, adrenaline (USA = epinephrine) and noradrenaline (USA = norepinephrine). They activate both the peripheral nervous system and the brain. These three molecules have similar structures and are part of a larger class of neurotransmitters called the monoamines. They are all involved with the sympathetic nervous system.

Cations Positively charged **ions**. Usually they are ions formed by metals such as potassium (K^+), sodium (Na^+), but they may be more complex ions such as ammonium (NH_4^+).

Ceiling effect Means that even if you give a higher dose of the drug, it has no further effect.

Central sleep apnoea see **Sleep apnoea**.

Cerebral cortex The outermost layer of the cerebral hemispheres of the brain. It is responsible for all the conscious experiences that go into making you who you are and what you feel. The cortex receives data from your senses, and assembles the electrical impulses into facts or observations you can deal with. It pulls together facts into knowledge, processes them, and stores them as memories. The cortex generates emotions and allows you to reason. Emotions are autopilot responses to complex situations. It takes longer for the cortex to integrate knowledge into understanding (much of this happens while you are asleep). Eventually your experiences and understanding coalesce into insight and finally wisdom. With insight you can plan, invent and create things to give you some control over your environment, and with wisdom you can anticipate, analyse and avoid bad things happening to you.

Cerebral hemispheres The two halves of the forebrain. The left hemisphere is specialized for speech, writing, language and sequential reasoning such as calculation or following a map; the right hemisphere is specialized for spatial abilities, face and shape recognition, and the perception of music and patterns.

Cerebral perfusion Refers to the adequacy of cerebral blood flow (CBF). The CBF is the volume of blood passing through the brain every minute. Usually this is about 15% of the cardiac output, or 750 ml/min. Cerebral blood flow is autoregulated, and thus remains constant with mean blood pressures between 70 and 170 mmHg. If cerebral perfusion is stopped for more than 15 seconds the patient loses consciousness.

Cerebrospinal fluid (CSF) About 150 ml of colourless fluid that bathes, supports and protects the brain and spinal cord. It is held in a container formed on the outer side by the dura mater, and on the inside by the arachnoid mater. The CSF regulates the brains extracellular fluid, containing ions and buffers, but almost no protein.

Chronic kidney disease (CKD) is a term given to degenerative or pathological disease, which causes either a reduction in the glomerular filtration rate, or the inability of the kidney to concentrate urine. CKD is graded into five stages.

Chylothorax Occurs when lymph leaks into the thorax. Lymph is usually a clear amber colour, but after a meal it may be milky from the absorbed fat.

Cleaning A process that removes micro-organisms and biohazardous materials from the surface of an object.

Clearance That volume of plasma from which a drug is completely removed in a given time. Note the drug is extracted from **plasma** and not blood. Its units are expressed as millilitres per minute (ml/min). Clearance is really the sum of all the processes that eliminate a drug from the body. Clearance depends on how efficiently the kidneys and liver metabolize and excrete a drug. Clearance of a drug, or other substance, is decreased if a patient has renal or liver disease.

Clinical pathways (chemoreceptors are specialized cells that respond to changes in the chemical composition of body fluids) A roadmap of every aspect of patients' care from the time they first attend the hospital to the time they finally return to the care of their local doctor. Good clinical pathways document a treatment goal, define the intended objectives at any instant, and review whether the targets have been achieved. The clinical pathway includes a nursing plan, necessary medical interventions, documentation and communication strategies, psychological support of patients and their families, and a discharge plan. In a surgical case the pathway includes the patient's preoperative medical and nursing assessment, psychological preparation, education, perioperative and postoperative care and review after discharge from hospital.

Cold agglutinins *are* **Autoantibodies** that occur in some people (especially if the patient is septic). The autoantibodies cause red cells to burst (haemolysis) if their body temperature falls below 35.5°C.

Colony-forming units Bacteria are cultured on special agar plates kept in an incubator. Each bacterium rapidly replicates to become visible dots on the plate. The number of these colony-forming units gives an estimate of the number of bacteria present at the site where the sample was gathered.

Coma A state of unresponsiveness where patients have their eyes closed, and do not respond when their name is called, or when shaken by the shoulder. This may seem a strange definition, but some people with severe brain damage who are deeply unconscious, will react with a dramatic reflex rigidity (*opisthotonos*) to painful stimuli, and some otherwise unresponsive patients may spontaneously open their eyes or smack their lips.

Complement is a proteolytic enzyme system in plasma that punches holes in certain bacteria causing them to rupture.

Complete heart block Occurs where none of impulses generated by the sino-atrial node reach the ventricles. The atria are beating independently of the ventricles.

Compliant Refers to the ease at which the lungs can be inflated. Compliant lungs are more readily inflated than incompliant lungs.

Cor pulmonale Occurs when pulmonary hypertension causes right heart failure.

Core temperature The temperature of the blood in the pulmonary artery and reflects the temperature of the major central organs: the brain, liver, kidneys, heart and lungs.

Creatinine Formed from phosphocreatine at a more or less constant rate as muscle protein is turned over. The kidney steadily removes the creatinine from the blood, and excretes it in the urine. As the GFR slows creatinine accumulates in the blood. A raised serum creatinine indicates renal dysfunction. Once filtered creatinine stays in the urine, where it can be collected to measure GFR.

Creatinine clearance is a crude measure of the **glomerular filtration rate (GFR).** Creatinine clearance has been replaced with an *estimated glomerular filtration rate (eGFR).*

Critical pathways see **Clinical pathways**.

Cyanosis A blue tinge to the skin or mucous membranes. It is usually a sign of severe hypoxaemia, but can also be caused by other agents. For hypoxaemia to cause cyanosis at least 30 g/L of haemoglobin must be in its deoxygenated form.

Cytokines Biochemicals produced by nucleated cells that allow cells them to 'talk' to each other. Cells produce cytokines whenever their welfare is in danger. The stimulus can be sepsis, trauma, ischaemia, or anything causing inflammation. After surgery patients are a stew of circulating cytokines produced by injured cells to signal white cells to come to help clean up the damage.

Dalton's law of partial pressure States that in a mixture of gases the partial pressure of a particular gas is the pressure that gas would exert if it alone occupied the space available to it.

Day case procedure A procedure done in one day and does not require the patient to stay overnight or longer. Sometimes non-invasive investigations such as colonoscopy are referred to as day procedures.

Decontaminate hands means using an antiseptic hand-rub to reduce the bacterial counts on the hands.

Dehydration Imprecise jargon, which usually means loss of water, but not isotonic fluids, from the body. A term that is better avoided.

Delirium is an acute confusional state. The patients do not know where they are, cannot concentrate enough to remember what you have just told them, and will not consistently obey commands. You cannot reason with a delirious patient. For instance, they take off their oxygen mask having, just a moment before, agreed to keep it on. They may hallucinate, talk in a garbled manner, or become belligerent.

Demand pump is one that changes its output to match the oxygen demands of the tissues. When we exercise our tissues demand more oxygen, so our cardiac output rises to meet it.

Denatured To structurally change or destroy proteins.

Depolarization Occurs as the electrical voltage across a myocyte or nerve cell membrane abruptly reverses. In muscle the change in voltage causes an electric current to flow, and this current triggers the muscle fibre to contract. The voltage change occurs as charged ions flood back and forth through special ion channels in the cell membrane. Many of the channels require energy to pump the ions, while other in other channels the ions simply flow back and forth without help.

Desmopressin A synthetic analogue of the hormone **vasopressin**.

Detergents Compounds which, when added to water, penetrate grease and oils and cause them to go into solution.

Dextrose The name used in the USA for glucose. It is a cyclical 6-carbon monosaccharide.

Diaphoresis A pompous word meaning sweating (or perspiring).

Diastole The phase of the cardiac cycle of contraction and relaxation when the heart relaxes.

Diastolic dysfunction Characterized by a stiff non-compliant ventricle which needs to be stretched before it will contract properly. Once stretched it contracts harder. So for a few beats at the beginning of each inspiration positive pressure ventilation helps distend the ventricle, making it contract harder.

Diastolic pressure The minimum blood pressure in the arteries during the cardiac cycle.

Disseminated intravascular coagulation (DIC) Occurs when the clotting system is so deranged that microscopic clots start forming spontaneously throughout the circulation. Unless treated it is usually fatal.

Dissociative anaesthesia Occurs when the cortex is chemically isolated from the brain's lower centres. Ketamine is the only dissociative anaesthetic used clinically.

Diuresis To produce urine at a rate exceeding 1.3 ml/kg/hr or for an adult 100 ml/hr.

Dynamic equilibrium Occurs when a process that is forming something is exactly balanced by a process that is undoing the same process. It generally refers to chemical reactions, however an analogy is adjusting the rate of water flowing into the top of a bucket to exactly balance the rate at which water drains out a hole in the bottom of the bucket.

Dyslipidaemia A term covering a wide range of abnormal lipid concentrations in the serum. The term includes high cholesterol levels, and also abnormalities in the balance between high-density lipoproteins (HDL) and low-density lipoproteins (LDL).

Dysphoria means the patient outwardly appears calm and tranquil, but inwardly feels jittery, agitated, and fearful. Colloquially it is known as the 'heebie-jeebies'

Dyspnoea Describes what patients feel when they cannot get their breath. Health care workers call it dyspnoea, while patients say they are breathless.

ECG is the accepted abbreviation for electrocardiogram. This device measures the tiny electrical currents generated by the muscles of a beating heart.

Echocardiogram Two-dimensional echocardiography which uses high-frequency **ultrasound** to measure the movement of the anterior and posterior walls of the ventricles. It calculates the stroke volume by assuming the ventricle is ellipsoid in shape (which is not always the case). Three-dimensional echocardiography gives better results.

Ectopic means 'out of place'.

Ectopic cardiac beats Those arising from parts of the heart that normally would not initiate a beat.

Ectopic pregnancy occurs when the embryo implants somewhere outside the uterine cavity.

Efferent see **Afferent**.

Ejection fraction The proportion of blood ejected from the ventricle with each contraction. In a healthy heart it should be more than 50% of the volume of blood in the ventricle at the end of diastole.

Electroencephalograph (EEG) A device measuring the electrical activity of the brain.

EKG is a variant (usually used in Europe) of the abbreviation ECG.

Elastin is the connective tissue of youth and suppleness; it is coiled like a spring. As we age, elastin gradually uncoils to become collagen. Collagen is stiff fibrous non-elastic connective tissue. Young skin has a lot of elastin in it—hence no skin wrinkles. The elastin in the lung is responsible for its natural springiness.

Electromechanical dissociation (EMD) Occurs where a formed wave can be seen on the ECG, but there is no detectable peripheral pulse. Always check that the patient has not bled. If the patient is not hypovolaemic then EMD is usually fatal. EMD is now called pulseless electrical activity.

End-organs Organs that are at the end of an arterial supply, such as kidney, spleen and brain, but not organs which blood flows through on its way to somewhere else, such as the heart, lungs or gut.

Endogenous Something that is manufactured inside a person's body which does not come from somewhere else.

Endorphins are a group of naturally occurring chemical compounds synthesized in the body that interact with opioid receptors in the central and peripheral nervous system.

Endotoxins are lipopolysaccharide peptide complexes produced by Gram-negative bacteria. All Gram-negative bacteria produce similar endotoxins which in absolutely minute amounts damage **basement membranes** all over the body, causing protein-rich fluid to ooze out of the bloodstream into the tissues. Clinically this is most apparent in the lungs where it causes low pressure pulmonary oedema.

Energy is the capacity of a system to do **work**.

Enzymes Proteins that clamp biochemical molecules together to produce a bigger compound, or tear compounds asunder into their components. They do this without the enzyme being damaged in the process. Enzymes are biochemical **catalysts**.

Epidural space Also called the extradural space or peridural space.

Epinephrine see **Adrenaline**.

Exposure-prone procedures Procedures where there is a risk of injury to a health care worker (HCW). This injury can be caused by needles, sharp instruments or sharp tissues (teeth and spicules of bone) piercing the HCW's gloves, and allowing their blood to bleed back into the patient. The definition includes procedures where the operator's hands cannot be seen at all times. This would apply to surgeons, or those people working under drapes, but does not necessarily prevent workers affected by blood-borne viruses from taking blood samples.

Extracellular fluid (ECF) is the fluid bathing all the tissues in the body. There are two main compartments: the blood (whose volume is 80 ml/kg), and the interstitial fluid (which accounts for 15 per cent of body weight).

Exudates Outpourings of fluid as a result of inflammatory processes. They contain more than 30 grams of protein per litre of fluid.

Facilitate To enhance or make easier.

Fat-soluble hormones see **Hormones**.

Feedback Using the output of a system to control its input. Positive feedback reinforces the output. A well-known example is in a public address system where the microphone picks up the output from the loudspeaker and amplifies it producing a howl. Negative feedback weakens the output. If the temperature in your refrigerator falls to low, then the refrigerator stops cooling, until the temperature has risen to a preset range.

Filtrate Sometimes called **ultrafiltrate**, this is the fluid that enters the urine after the blood has passed across the glomerular sieve.

Force In 1685 Sir Isaac Newton elegantly pointed out that something at rest, such as a brick, will remain at rest until some sort of force causes it to move; while on the other hand if it is moving it will continue to move (in a straight line) until some force stops it or changes the direction in which it is moving. If the stationary brick moves, then a force is accelerating it from rest to its final velocity, and the force needed to do this can be calculated by the equation: Force = mass × acceleration. The SI unit of force is appropriately the **newton**, which is the amount of force necessary to increase the velocity (accelerate) a mass of one kilogram at one metre per second every second.

Frailty Frailty is defined as a state of decreased physiological reserve. It gives a holistic sense of how a set of conditions affects a patient's level of function.

Functional residual capacity (FRC) is the volume of air left in the lungs at the end of quiet expiration. At FRC the pressures distending the lungs equal the forces tending to collapse them. The FRC in a young adult is about 2.8 litres. It is a useful store of air that enables us to speak or hold our breath.

GABA is the acronym for the inhibitory neurotransmitter gamma-amino butyric acid.

General power outlet (GPO) is the formal name for that electric power outlet in the wall, which you plug devices into and then switch on.

Generic A generic drug is one where the name identifies its ingredients rather than its brand name. Generic names remain constant all over the world, whereas brand names tend to change from country to country. For instance, aspirin is a generic name recognized worldwide, whereas its brand names vary from place to place.

Glitazones are a group of drugs used to treat type 2 diabetes. They regulate the genes involved with fat and glucose metabolism.

Glomerular filtration rate (GFR) The volume of filtrate entering the collective proximal tubules every minute. Of this volume almost all is reabsorbed by the kidney tubules.

Glomerulus Forms the kidney's sieving mechanism. It is an invaginated bulb at the entrance to the nephron, which houses a tuft of about 20–40 capillaries.

Glucocorticoids are steroid hormones involved with metabolism and which have anti-inflammatory actions.

Glutamate An amino-acid derivative used by the central nervous system as a neurotransmitter.

Glyceryl trinitrate Also known as nitroglycerin, a potent vasodilator. Because it dilates arterioles by relaxing their smooth muscle, it reduces the force the heart needs to produce to eject its stroke volume. It may also vasodilate coronary vessels improving the blood flow through them.

Gold standard A term used to describe the most practical and most accurate way to obtain a clinical measurement. A benchmark is the standard or reference point against which things can be measured, but it may not be practical.

Gynaecoid obesity The typical woman's pattern with most of the fat around her bottom and upper thighs. Think pear-shaped. It is not as hazardous as android obesity.

Haematocrit (HCT) Similar to packed cell volume. As blood is centrifuged the heavier red cells sink to the bottom forming a layer underneath the plasma. The proportion of red cells when compared to the total volume is called the haematocrit. It is usually expressed as a percentage. The normal haematocrit is about 45%. In patients who have been resuscitated with colloids or crystalloids the haematocrit tells whether there are enough red cells in the blood. Once the haematocrit falls below 35% the patient is said to be anaemic.

Haemolytic crisis Occurs when red blood cells burst, releasing their haemoglobin into the blood stream. Free haemoglobin clogs up the glomerulus in the kidney causing renal failure.

Half-life The half-life of a drug is the time taken for the blood concentration of a drug to fall by half. *Context-sensitive half-life* is how long it takes for half the drug's effects to wear off.

Heart blocks Defects in the conduction of the cardiac impulse from the atria to the ventricles. You can see this on an ECG where P-waves are further away from the QRS complex than normal. They might be a constant distance from the QRS complex (serious) or they may vary in distance (dangerous).

Heat A form of energy. The amount of heat produced, or lost, is measured in either kilo-calories (Kcals) or kilojoules (KJ). If you extracted the heat from a litre of boiling water it would contain just over 1000 useable kilocalories before it turned to ice. A normal person uses about 1800–2000 kcal a day to live their humdrum sedentary lifestyle. A breastfeeding mother or manual labourer may use 3500 kcal or more each day.

HELLP Haemolysis, elevated liver enzymes and a low platelet count.

Hemiblocks Defects in the lesser branches of the conducting system of the heart that impede the spread of the cardiac impulse. The most common is a left anterior hemiblock. A left posterior hemiblock is more serious and suggests extensive cardiac disease.

HEPA masks High-efficiency particulate air-filtering masks.

Heparin-induced thrombocytopenia A life-threatening immune-mediated destruction of platelets. With exposure to heparin, antibodies are formed against platelet factor IV. It is associated with increased propensity to form clots, and may cause strokes, limb ischaemia, bleeding or death. Worry if the platelet count drops by 30–50% about 4 days after exposure to heparin.

Hepatic impairment Not well defined. Arbitrarily it occurs when one or more of the liver enzymes (ALT, AST or GGT) exceed three times its normal levels. Dying hepatocytes release these enzymes into the circulation. The liver is remarkably resilient, and at any age will repair itself if the noxious stimulus is brief, and the damage not excessive.

Hepatitis A generic term for inflammation of the liver. The inflamed liver cells release marker enzymes into the bloodstream, which can be detected on liver function tests. The most common cause of liver inflammation is alcohol, followed by prescribed medication.

Heterogenicity is a term used in statistics. When grouping things together for statistical **meta-analysis** (that is, analysing data from many diverse sources) you must group apples with apples, and oranges with oranges. This is called homogenicity. If you try to lump apples and hamsters together then you will have problems with heterogenicity.

High-pressure baroreceptors see **Baroreceptors**.

High-pressure pulmonary oedema see **Pulmonary oedema**.

Homeostenosis A condition whereby the physiological response to stress is impaired in the elderly

Hormones Chemical messengers secreted by endocrine glands. They regulate the activities of their target organs. There are two functional groups of hormones: *water-soluble hormones*, which in tiny amounts act rapidly and then quickly disappear such as **anti-diuretic hormone** (ADH), and fat-soluble hormones ones which are produced in much greater amounts, and act over long periods such as oestrogen, testosterone and thyroxine to guide the development of the organs.

Humidity A measure of the **mass** of water vapour in gas. Humidification is the process of increasing the moisture content of air, and a humidifier is the device that does this.

Hypercarbia Occurs when the arterial $PaCO_2$ > 44 mmHg (> 5.79 kPa). It is the result of **hypoventilation**. Physicians generally use the term hypoventilation rather than hypercarbia.

Hyperchloraemia The concentration of chloride ion in the ECF is higher than the normal range of 95–105 mmol/L.

Hyperexcitable state Occurs when nerves fire with a trivial stimulus that would normally not cause any response.

Hyperventilation The arterial $PaCO_2$ is below the lower limits of normal (< 36 mmHg) (< 4.75 kPa)). Hyperventilation is not the same thing as breathing. To use the term hyperventilation correctly requires that either you know the end-tidal CO_2 or the $PaCO_2$.

Hypocarbia Occurs when the arterial $PaCO_2$ < 36 mmHg (< 4.75 kPa). It is the result of **hyperventilation**. Physicians generally use the term hyperventilation rather than hypocarbia.

Hypokalaemia Occurs when the serum potassium levels fall below 3.5 mmol/L. It becomes severe if it falls below 3 mmol/L and will eventually cause cardiac arrhythmias.

Hypothalamus A complex structure nestling deep in the underside of the brain at the upper end of the brainstem. It regulates the activities of the internal organs, monitors information from the autonomic nervous system, and controls the pituitary gland.

Hypoventilation Failure of the lungs to eliminate carbon dioxide. It is measured by a rise in the partial pressure of carbon dioxide in the arterial blood.

Hypovolaemia A term that is not well defined. Hypovolaemia usually means an insufficient blood volume, which if untreated leads to shock. In contrast dehydration usually means insufficient body water.

Hypoxaemia Occurs when the arterial PaO_2 is < 60 mmHg (< 7.79 kPa). It reflects what is going on in the bloodstream. Severe hypoxaemia causes **hypoxia**.

Hypoxia Occurs when there is not enough oxygen to allow the cells to carry out their normal function. Oxygen-deprived tissues release lactic acid into the bloodstream. Blood gas analysis reveals a *metabolic acidosis*. It reflects what is going in the tissues. A patient can be hypoxaemic without being hypoxic, such as with opioid-induced respiratory depression. Or, more rarely is hypoxic without being hypoxaemic, such as with severe anaemia.

Idioventricular rhythms occur when all the heart's higher pacemakers are suppressed, and the ventricle contracts at its intrinsic rate of 25–35/min.

Infarction means the blood supply to a tissue has been cut off for so long that the tissue has died. Infarction is the end result of ischaemia.

Inotropes Drugs such as adrenaline and dopamine, which increase the strength of cardiac contraction.

Insensible fluid losses include those that we do not routinely measure; for instance: sweat, and water lost by the lungs. In a normal environment they amount to about 750 ml of fluid each day.

International Normalized Ratio (INR) This test is the same as the prothrombin time (PT) except that the test has been standardized so that all laboratories give consistent results. The normal INR is 1. INR is used to monitor warfarin therapy. For elective surgery the INR should be less than 1.5.

Interstitial nephritis is an acute allergic inflammatory reaction to drugs concentrating in the kidneys. The inflammation causes a damaging exudate into the area, usually around the glomerulus.

Ion channels are tailor-made pores or pumps in the cell membrane that only allow specific ions to pass.

Ions Atoms or molecules that have lost or gained one or more electrons. This means the atoms now carry either a positive (such as Na^+) or negative charge (such as Cl^-).

Ischaemia Means there is not enough blood supply to maintain tissue metabolism. If a tissue remains ischaemic for long enough it will *infarct*.

Isophlebotic point A point on the skin that is level with the right atrium.

Isotonic means a fluid has the same osmotic pressure as extracellular fluid.

Kernicterus occurs when unconjugated bilirubin leaks into and damages neonates' brains.

Korotkoff sounds Generated by turbulence as blood flows through arteries partially compressed by a blood pressure cuff. You can hear them with a stethoscope.

Laparoscopy Using a laparoscope is to directly visualize the contents of the peritoneal cavity. In gynaecology it is used to inspect the ovaries, the outside of the Fallopian tubes and uterus. A laparoscope is an instrument, somewhat like a miniature telescope, with a built-in fibreoptic system to bring light into the abdominal cavity.

Lapses see **Slips**.

Laryngeal oedema Swelling of the mucosa in the larynx. There is a grave danger this will obstruct airflow.

Laryngospasm The reflex contraction of the muscles serving the vocal cords so that they shut tightly. Its function is to prevent foreign material entering the lower airway. It sometimes occurs when the larynx is irritated by something such as infection or an endotracheal tube.

Lean body mass The mass in kilograms of the richly perfused tissues of the vital organs, skin and muscle, but excluding poorly perfused fat. If we dosed obese patients on their total body mass, we would overdose them because the drugs do not enter the poorly perfused fat tissue readily. For people over the height of 150 cm: Lean body mass for men = height in centimetres − 100 kg: Lean body mass for women = height in centimetres − 102 kg

Limbic system A group of brain structures including the amygdala hippocampus, and basal ganglia that work together to generate and regulate emotion, process memory and coordinate fine movement.

Lipoxygenases A group of enzymes that breakdown *arachidonic acid* into *leukotrienes*. These, and a number of other biochemicals initiate and sustain inflammatory responses.

Low-pressure baroreceptors see **Baroreceptors**.

Low-pressure pulmonary oedema see **Pulmonary oedema.**

Lymph Extracellular fluid with added white blood cells. The lymphatic system is similar to an agricultural drainage system used to drain swampy land. Lymph vessels drain all tissues except the brain, and finally end up in the body's main drain, called the *thoracic duct*. Lymph fluid in the thoracic duct usually is clear, but becomes milky after a fatty meal.

Macrocytic anaemia see **Anaemia.**

Mannitol A non-toxic alcohol made from the sugars fructose or mannose. The body cannot metabolize mannitol: 20% mannitol solution is hypertonic, and exerts an **osmotic pressure** equivalent to four times that of 5% glucose or 0.9% saline. It is excreted unchanged by the kidneys taking with it a large volume of water.

Mapleson circuits In 1954 William Mapleson classified semiclosed anaesthetic circuits into five types, of which the Mapleson A (the original **Magill circuit**) and C circuits are the two still in common use. In some places the Mapleson C circuit is also called the Magill circuit.

Mass A measure of the amount of matter in a body. Unlike weight it is not affected by gravity. The SI unit of mass is the kilogram.

Maximal sterile barrier precautions are a high level of aseptic technique. They require face mask, sterile gloves and sterile gown, and a large sterile drape to isolate the patient.

Mean A statistical term that describes the average of a range of values. There are a number of ways to describe how numbers are distributed over a range of numbers. Consider the numbers: 4, 4, 6, 8, 28. To get the mean value we add them up (sum them) and divide by 5. The mean value therefore is 50/5 = 10. The *median value* is the number in the middle of the range, in this case 6, and the *modal value* is the most common number; in this case 4.

Mercury-filled manometers An environmental and occupational health hazard. They have been removed from most clinical areas.

Metabolism The sum of all the physical changes and chemical processes that take place within an organism, including all the tiny steps where energy is transformed from one form to another inside cells. For instance chemical energy is transformed into electrical energy, or movement, or heat. Metabolism is the process of taking in a nutrient on a drug, breaking it down and reassembling it to repair and build body structures, and eliminating the wastes. Metabolism is the signature of life.

Methaemoglobinaemia occurs when the ferrous (Fe^{++}) ion in haemoglobin is oxidized to the ferric (Fe^{+++}) form. Oxygen, which binds loosely to ferrous ion, binds far more tightly to the ferric form so that it cannot escape from the haemoglobin. The blood becomes chocolate brown coloured, and the tissues may become hypoxic. The commonest cause of methaemoglobinaemia is an overdose of the local anaesthetic prilocaine. Ferric haemoglobin can be converted back to the ferrous form by methylene blue.

Micro-atelectasis Refers to the collapse of the smallest airways and alveoli in the lungs. It usually occurs when the terminal respiratory units fail to produce sufficient **surfactant**.

Microbes are living organisms that are too small to be seen with the naked eye. They include bacteria, yeasts, protozoa, and viruses. They do not include prions.

Microcytic anaemia see **Anaemia**.

Milli-osmol/kg Milli-osmols per kilogram of water is a measure of the osmolality of the solution. Osmolality represents the number of osmotically active particles in a kilogram of water.

Minute volume (MV) is the volume of air moved into or out of the lungs in one minute. $MV = RR \times TV$.

Mishaps see **Slips**.

mol Reflects the weight of a molecule. Molecules are very very small. Since we can't easily measure the weight of a single molecule physicists lump 6.023×10^{23} (602,300,000,000,000,000,000,000) of them together and measure the weight of the whole lot in grams. The weight of a mol of sodium is 23 g and the weight of a mol of chlorine is 35.5 g so that the molecular weight (or one mol) of sodium chloride (NaCl) is $35.5 + 23 = 58.5$ g.

Multifocal premature beats Sign of a very irritable myocardium.

Muscarinic activity describes the effects of stimulating the parasympathetic nervous system: bradycardia, bronchosecretion, bowel movement, bronchospasm, and pupillary constriction. Muscarine is a biochemical found in some fungi, which if ingested in sufficient quantities causes the bowels to contract expelling their contents at both ends, the lungs to fill up with mucus so that the person drowns, and their heart to slow down and stop. A similar effect can be caused by excessive release of acetylcholine or an overdose of neostigmine (and some nerve gases). Atropine blocks the effect of muscarine (and neostigmine and nerve gases).

Myocardial contractility The force with which the heart contracts during systole.

Myogenic Smooth muscle in the walls of arterioles will contract when they are stretched. This elastic band-like reaction is called a myogenic response.

Naive A term sometimes used to describe patients who have not been previously exposed to a drug. For instance, benzodiazepine-naive patients are usually sedated far more readily with lower doses of diazepam than those who take it regularly.

Nanomole This is one billionth of a **mol** (or one-millionth of a **millimole**). It is written as 10^{-9} mol. This small amount is roughly equivalent to finding one single pea in a cubic metre of peas, or roughly one pea in a pile of peas 30 metres high.

Narcotic An old imprecisely defined term indicating that a substance induces narcosis or sleep. It was a term applied to the opioids.

Neonates Babies in the first month of life.

Nephron The basic functional unit of the kidney. It is composed of a **glomerulus**, with its afferent and efferent arterioles, and the renal tubule.

Nephropathy Kidney disease where either the cause or its exact effect are unclear.

Neuroaxial block A block using local anaesthetics given into or around the spinal cord. This is a collective term for spinal and epidural anaesthetics.

Neuropathic pain Arises from damage to nerves along some part of their pathways from their origin in the periphery, to their integration in the CNS. It is caused by nerve damage due to compression, inflammation or direct trauma.

Neurotransmitter is a chemical released by neurons (such acetylcholine or noradrenaline) at synapses and neuromuscular junctions. It allows the effects of an **action potential** to be passed on to the next cell.

Newton not in (symbol: N) is a unit of force. It is the amount of force needed to accelerate a mass of one kilogram at one metre per second squared. One newton is roughly the amount of force exerted by gravity on an apple.

Nicotinic activity Acetylcholine is the neurotransmitter released at the neuromuscular junction in voluntary muscles, which makes them contract. In sufficient quantities nicotine (the same drug is in tobacco) causes similar effects. Excessive nicotine causes violent spasms of voluntary muscles. Muscle relaxants used during anaesthetics such as atracurium and vecuronium block the effects of acetylcholine (and nicotine) on voluntary muscle.

Nociceptors Pain receptors at the end of sensory nerves. They transduce the signal of pain. This means that they turn a painful mechanical stimulus into an electrical nerve action potential.

Nocioceptors detect pain arising from tissue damage, mediated by inflammatory biochemicals.

Nodal rhythms Occur where the AV node triggers the beat instead of the SA node. The pulse rate is usually 40–50 beats/min. The P-waves on the ECG are either absent (hidden in the QRS) or upside down.

Noise Occurs when an electronic signal is drowned out by unwanted stray signals from elsewhere. Examples of noise are muscle movement on an ECG, or 50-cycle AC hum from nearby mains current. To get a good trace you need as much signal and as little noise as possible.

Non-axial airways see **Axial airways**.

Noradrenaline One of the catecholamine-based neurotransmitters. It is secreted by sympathetic nerves to regulate blood pressure, and in the brain is involved in arousal, and reward stimuli. Noradrenaline regulates mood and sleep.

Noradrenergic response Part of the sympathetic response. As noradrenaline is released from sympathetic nerve endings it causes arterioles to constrict and the blood pressure to rise. The more life-threatening the event, the more noradrenaline is released. These events include hypoxia, hypovolaemia, sepsis, major tissue damage, and especially brain injury.

Normal The term normal has a number of different meanings. The most common meaning is average. A normal patient is a typical patient; one that does not deviate from the usual. A normal distribution curve is a graph which is distributed symmetrically about the average (or **mean**) value. Similarly normal biochemical results cover a range that applies to 95 per cent of healthy individuals.

Normal saline One that contains one gram of sodium chloride per litre; 0.9% normal saline therefore contains 900 mg of sodium chloride per litre.

Normovolaemia Implies the blood volume and the volume of the extracellular fluid are normal.

Nosocomial infections Infections acquired in the hospital.

Noxious stimulus One that damages tissue.

Obstructive sleep apnoea see **Sleep apnoea.**

Obtunded mental state A state of semi-consciousness where the patient only rouses when stimulated, or they are not fully conscious and cooperative.

Oedema Oedema fluid is a form of transudate. It collects in the interstitium of the ECF outside the cells.

Off-label drugs Registered drugs that are used in a way that has not yet been approved. Usually they are being used for a different indication than originally intended, or are given by a different route, or at a different dose to that recommended by the manufacturers. Using clonidine for pain relief, or **vasopressin** to support blood pressure are examples of off-label drug use, but so is crushing drugs to form a suspension to pass down a nasogastric tube. When using drugs off-label the prescriber may have some liability should anything go wrong. The legal implications of this practice are unclear.

Ondine's curse A property peculiar to opioid drugs where although conscious the patient forgets to breath. Opioids depress the central response to a rising $PaCO_2$, which is one of the main physiological triggers to breathe. Ondine was an immortal water nymph in Teutonic mythology. She laid a curse on her wayward and mortal lover that he would have to remember to breathe. When he fell asleep, he died. Neither she, nor her lover, lived happily ever after.

Opiate An outdated term referring to the alkaloids derived from the opium poppy (*Papaveretum somniferum*). Morphine, codeine and heroin are still produced from poppies.

Opioids A diverse group of natural and semisynthetic alkaloid derivatives of opium. This definition includes endogenous peptides that interact with opioid receptors.

Orthopnoea Occurs when patients get short of breath when they lie down.

Osmotic pressure The pressure (energy) that forces water to diffuse across a semi-permeable membrane (such as the cell membrane). Water tends to spread uniformly throughout a solution, so that its concentration is the same everywhere. It will pass through cell membranes to achieve this end.

Osmoreceptors are specialized cells that detect changes in osmotic pressure. They occur in the hypothalamus and in the kidneys and help regulate the body's fluid balance.

Packed cell volume Measured by spinning a sample of blood in a centrifuge so that the red cells pack down to the bottom while the plasma remains on the top. Normally the packed cells occupy about 45% of the volume (PCV = 0.45) and the plasma makes up the remaining 55%. Once the bleeding in young people has reduced the red cells to 22% (PCV = 0.22) they need a blood transfusion to prevent tissue hypoxia. The haematocrit is the same as the packed cell volume though it is quoted as a percentage not as a decimal fraction.

Paradigm Simply a different way of thinking about something. It involves a genuine change of attitude, or perspective. For example: orthopaedic surgeons wanting their patients to take aspirin preoperatively. This would have been unthinkable a few years ago.

Parasympathetic nervous system regulates housekeeping functions such as bladder and bowel control. Its neurotransmitter is **acetylcholine**.

Pascal (Pa) The SI-derived unit for pressure. It is equivalent to a force of one newton per square metre. A pascal is a tiny pressure; it as about the same pressure a grain of rice exerts on your hand. This unit is far too small to use in clinical work, so we measure pressure in units of 1000 pascals, which is a kilopascal (kPa). One kilopascal corresponds to about 1% of atmospheric pressure at sea level.

Peptides Strings of two or more amino-acids. Peptide chains join together to make proteins.

Peripheral shutdown A term used loosely by clinicians to describe a situation where the skin blood supply is poor. Patients with peripheral shutdown have cold hands, and poor capillary return. Their skin may be mottled or pale. It is a sign of excessive noradrenergic discharge.

pH A logarithmic scale used to measure the acidity or alkalinity of a solution. At 25°C a neutral solution, where the chemical and thermodynamic activity of the acid and alkali is equal, has a pH of 7.0. pH = 1 highly acidic and pH = 14 highly alkaline. The absolute extreme range for human life is pH 6.8–7.8.

Phantom limb pain A form of chronic intractable pain that occurs if acute pain has not been treated properly in the past. Severe unmodified pain causes neuronal wind-up in the dorsal horn of the spinal cord. The synapses transmitting pain become hyperexcitable so that the slightest stimulus triggers a huge response.

Phenothiazines A group of tricyclic drugs with anti-psychotic, major tranquillizing, and anti-emetic properties. They are competitive antagonists of dopamine (particularly D_2) receptors in the central and peripheral nervous systems. They also have anti-muscarinic activity (causing dry mouth, and urinary retention), antihistamine (sedation, anti-itch) and alpha-1 adrenergic blockade (causing hypotension). Drugs include chlorpromazine (a neuroleptic) and prochlorperazine (an anti-emetic).

Phospholipids A group of compounds formed by chains of fatty acids and glycerol bound to phosphates. They have a fat (hydrophilic) head and a long stringy (hydrophobic) tail.

Plasma What is left behind when all the cells are removed from blood. Blood is normally composed of 45% cells and 55% plasma.

Plasma cholinesterase deficiency Used to be called pseudocholinesterase deficiency. This glycoprotein enzyme breaks down certain drugs, such as suxamethonium, mivacurium and remifentanil. It is congenitally deficient or absent in about 1:1000 people.

Plasminogen A proenzyme in the blood. When activated to *fibrinolysin* it helps dissolve stray clots, and in doing so sometimes causes excessive bleeding. Fibrinolysin is the new name for *plasmin*.

Polycythaemia Occurs when there are excessive red blood cells circulating. The blood may become so viscous that the blood fails to flow properly though the microcirculation, and becomes prone to clotting.

Polypharmacy Taking many drugs. It is a major cause of morbidity in the elderly. As a rule if a patient is taking more than seven different medications it is highly probable they will have a problem with adverse effects. Then it becomes a vicious cycle, as they take one medication to offset the side effects of another; for instance amitriptyline causes constipation, so they need a laxative, or an NSAID causes stomach pain and aggravates peripheral oedema so they take a diuretic and a protein pump inhibitor.

Pons An identifiable swelling in the brainstem that, along with other structures, controls breathing, and regulates heart rate and blood pressure.

Positive fluid displacement (PFD) valve Attached to a central venous catheter to maintain a sterile closed system. They prevent tiny blood clots from plugging the tip of the catheter. When you disconnect a syringe after flushing the CVC a small quantity of fluid is forced through the catheter evicting any blood that might remain in the tip to form a clot. Unused lumens with these PFD valves need to be flushed only once a week; this greatly reduces the chance of bacteria colonizing an offending blood clot.

Positive pressure Pressure that is above the pressure of the surrounding atmosphere. Ventilators blow air into the patient's chest and in doing so exert a positive pressure in the lungs.

Positive end expiratory pressure (PEEP) A way of ventilating a patient so that at the end of their expiration the pressure in their airways remains above atmospheric pressure, usually by 2–5 cm H_2O.

Postoperative cognitive disorder (POCD) Cognitive function is about how well people solve problems, remember things, and anticipate events. Technically cognitive impairment is a blend of aphasia (language disturbance), apraxia (impaired ability to carry out motor activities despite intact motor function), agnosia (failure to recognize or identify objects despite intact sensory ability), and disturbance in the ability to plan, organize, sequence, and abstract. POCD is a real phenomenon affecting surgical patients over the age of 60 years (particularly men), 25 per cent of whom will have subtle impairment of their cognitive function 7 days after surgery, and 14 per cent will still be impaired at 3 months and 10 per cent at 2 years. Little is known about POCD—or its prevention. It is worse with longer anaesthetics. There is some evidence that periods of hyperventilation during the anaesthetic may contribute.

Postoperative nausea and vomiting (PONV) Customarily defined as nausea or vomiting occurring within 24 hours of anaesthetic. This is an unsatisfactory definition because anaesthetically induced nausea and vomiting usually occur almost immediately and certainly within 4 hours of anaesthetic. Vomiting occurring more than 12 hours after the last anaesthetic drug (including opioids) has been administered usually has a surgical cause such as gastric stasis or ischaemic gut.

Postural drop A useful way of telling whether a patient's vascular volume is adequately filled. Measure the patient's systolic blood pressure. Now cautiously ease the patient into a semi-sitting (*Fowler's*) position. Measure the blood pressure again. If the systolic pressure falls by 20 mmHg or more then this is termed a postural drop. This is a reliable sign of hypovolaemia.

Postural hypotension Occurs when a patient's blood pressure falls as they stand or sit up. The magnitude of the fall in blood pressure is measured as **postural drop**.

Pre-excitation Means that a part of the heart has been stimulated before it should have been.

Preload The length of a cardiac myocyte at the end of diastole. This depends on how far it has been stretched by blood flowing into the ventricle.

Premature atrial contraction Occurs when the atrial beat does not arise in the SA node, but somewhere else in the atria. Sometimes it is the result of a wave in the AV node taking a U-turn.

Premature excitations Ectopic beats arising from many different sites in the ventricles. It needs urgent treatment.

Pressure The force per unit area exerted by a substance perpendicular to its boundary with another substance. It is measured in newtons per square metre. The SI unit is the **pascal** which is a pressure of one newton per square metre. Atmospheric pressure is roughly 1000 Kpascals.

Primary bacteraemia see **Bacteraemia**.

Prion An abnormal form of abnormal host-encoded (PrP) protein found in the brain. Prions crumple adjacent normal protein (PrP) and turn it into another prion. Prions are not alive. They are responsible for variant Creutzfeldt–Jakob disease (vCJD) the most common human form of bovine spongiform encephalopathy (BSE), also known as mad cow disease. No method of sterilization inactivates vCJD (except heating the object to red-heat). The abnormal proteins gum up the brain eventually causing dementia. There is no cure.

Pro-arrhythmias Drug-induced arrhythmias. They occur in about 10 per cent of patients on antiarrhythmic agents.

Procoagulant states Individuals with procoagulant states (**thrombophilia**) are prone to perioperative deep vein thrombosis (DVT), venous thromboembolism (VTE) and pulmonary embolism (PE). Thrombophilia is inherited, and 12 per cent or more of the Caucasian population are at risk.

Prostaglandins A large group of compounds derived from essential fatty acids in our diet. They are incorporated in the phospholipids that make cell membranes waterproof. When cell membranes are damaged they are released into the tissue fluid where they are turned into *inflammatory mediators* and other local messengers by COX enzymes.

Protamine A basic peptide derived from fish testes, which combines with acidic heparin forming a stable compound, thus inactivating the heparin. Protamine sulfate 1 mg neutralizes 100 units of heparin. Give it slowly—no faster than 50 mg in 10 minutes—because it causes systemic hypotension and severe pulmonary hypertension. Excess protamine acts as an anticoagulant in its own right.

Proteolytic enzymes Break down proteins into smaller bits.

Prothrombin time (PT) tests the internal coagulation pathway. In its standardized form it is called the INR (**International Normalized Ratio**) which is used to adjust the dose of warfarin, and guide the peri-operative use of drugs that modify clotting factors. The INR (and PTT) are prolonged in some bleeding disorders such as disseminated intravascular coagulation (DIC).

Pulmonary oedema Occurs when fluid accumulates in the interstitium or alveoli in the lung. It can be classified into two types: *high-pressure pulmonary oedema* occurs when the pressure in the pulmonary capillaries exceeds the oncotic pressure of blood forcing fluid into the interstitium and eventually the alveoli. This oedema occurs if the capillary vascular pressure exceeds 25 mmHg. *Low-pressure pulmonary oedema* occurs when the alveolar–capillary membrane is damaged in some way allowing fluid from the circulation to transudate into the alveoli. The pulmonary capillary pressure is normal.

Pulse oximeter An electronic device that measures oxygen saturation in the haemoglobin inside red blood cells (erythrocytes).

Pulse pressure The difference in pressure between the systolic and diastolic blood pressures. Pulse pressure = systolic pressure – diastolic pressure.

QTc The corrected QT interval on the ECG adjusted to the patient's heart rate.

Radiocontrast media Special dyes that are opaque to X-rays. They are injected to define blood vessels during radiological procedures. Some types contain iodine which may provoke an allergic response in susceptible individuals.

Receptor A cell or part of a cell, which is specialized to detect a stimulus or a change in its environment.

Recovery position The posture in which to place comatose patients to protect fluid or secretions entering their airway. Patient should be positioned on their side in such a way that their mouth is dependent and fluid can drain out freely. The position must be stable with no pressure on the chest to impair breathing. You need to be able to access the patient's mouth and nose should it become necessary.

Recovery—stages of see **Stages of recovery**.

Recruitment To summon help or aid.

Reflex An automatic response to stimulus. The same stimulus always produces the same response.

Remifentanil A new potent synthetic opioid rapidly broken down by nonspecific enzymes in the blood and tissues. This gives it an ultrashort terminal half-life of less than 10 minutes which means its effects do not extend into the recovery room.

Rescue breathing used to be called mouth-to-mouth resuscitation (the kiss of life).

Resistance The resistance of the blood vessels to the forceful pumping of the heart is determined by their elastance and their diameter. The elastance is a measure of their ability to stretch with each pulse and then resume their previous shape.

Respiratory failure occurs when the patient becomes either hypoxaemic or is hypo-ventilating.

Respiratory rate (RR) The number of breaths taken each minute.

Re-uptake A conservation process whereby nerve cells reuse their neurotransmitters by absorbing them back into the neuron.

Rhabdomyolysis Occurs when damaged muscle releases myoglobin into the blood. Myoglobin, being almost exactly the size of the holes in the kidney's sieve, soon blocks it. The myoglobin, which escapes into the urine, turns it brown. Myoglobinuria can be mistaken for haemoglobinuria.

Ringer's solution Formulated by a British physiologist, Sydney Ringer in the 1880s. Alex Hartmann added lactate to Ringer's solution to make it more suitable for children.

R-on-T phenomenon occurs when the R-wave on the ECG snuggles right up next to, or even inside the T-wave. This is a dangerous sign as the patient may flip into ventricular fibrillation, or a ventricular tachycardia. Treat this urgently.

Root cause analysis A method used in risk management of identifying a single cause for an adverse event. This is a bad concept, because there is very rarely, if ever, a single root cause of anything.

Saline overload and **saline depletion** are (for want of a better word) useful shorthand terms to describe the status of all the osmotically active ions in the extracellular fluid (ECF) volume. The ECF is composed of fluid containing the **cations** sodium, potassium, and calcium, and the **anions** chloride, bicarbonate, lactate and a little phosphate. This fluid is *isotonic* with the fluid inside cells. If patients have excessive ECF (saline overload) they become oedematous. If the patient has ECF depletion (saline deficit) they are 'dry', have a low urine output and develop **postural hypotension** if they sit or stand up.

Secondary bacteraemia see **Bacteraemia**.

Sensitization A process that produces an acute hyperawareness of an otherwise minor stimulus; for instance a slap on a sunburnt back.

Sepsis The term sepsis tends to be used loosely to mean localized or generalized infection. More strictly, it is the presence of an infection and the subsequent physiologic responses to that infection including activation of the inflammatory cascade. Unchecked sepsis leads to the *systemic inflammatory response syndrome (SIRS)*. Severe sepsis causes end-organ dysfunction.

Series Blood flowing in series means that it flows sequentially down a single path from one point to the next. In contrast, if blood vessels are set in parallel, as they are in the lungs, then blood follows along a number of different paths to get from one point to another.

Serotonin A monoamine neurotransmitter that plays a crucial part in events such as temperature regulation, sensory perception, alarm mechanisms, emotion and the onset of sleep.

SI unit An abbreviation for *Systeme internationale d'unites* or International System of Units which defines units used in measurement such as mass, length, time, ampere, mol, candela and so on.

Sick sinus syndrome (SSS) Refers to a collection of diseases arising inside the sino-atrial node. SSS does not affect the conduction of impulses through the atrial muscle. The characteristic ECG feature is an irregular pulse with normal PR interval. The SA node may stutter along firing intermittently, or alternatively it may speed up and slow down (**tachycardia-bradycardia syndrome**).

Sigh Every few minutes we take a deeper breath, a *sigh*, to re-expand collapsing terminal respiratory units. Ventilators too need this provision to prevent **micro-atelectasis**.

Sinus arrhythmia Occurs in young fit people where the heart rate slows on inspiration and speeds-up on expiration. In patients over the age of 55 years an alternating heart rate is more likely to be **sick sinus syndrome**, in which case it will have no correlation with breathing.

Sinus rhythm Occurs when the sino-atrial node dictates the heart rate at a regular rhythm between 50–100 bpm.

Sinus tachycardia A heart rate greater than 100 bpm. The P-waves and QRS waves are normal.

Sleep apnoea *Obstructive sleep apnoea (OSA)* occurs especially in elderly obese men. Their airway collapses during deep sleep causing obstructive apnoea and frequently severe hypoxaemia. Some patients may have more than 30 episodes a night. There is a significant correlation between sleep apnoea and hypertension, dementia, cardiac failure ischaemic heart disease, stroke, and type 2 diabetes. *Central sleep apnoea* syndrome is the loss of respiratory drive when a susceptible individual is in deep sleep—they simply stop breathing until the noradrenergic nervous system is alerted. Usually their PaO_2 falls to damagingly low levels before this happens. These people are particularly susceptible to opioid-induced respiratory depression.

Slips, lapses and **mishaps** Slips and lapses are caused by human error, and mishaps are events that occur by chance. Slips occur because of system errors, inattention, fatigue, or inexperience. Lapses occur because procedures and protocols are, for whatever reason, not followed. Mishaps are inevitable, unpredictable (but not necessarily unforeseen) events such as an anaphylactic reaction.

Somatic pain Comes from superficial structures such as muscles and skin, and is perceived through the spinal nerves. It is described as sharp, well localized, stabbing and is usually localized by one finger pointing at the source.

Specialist perioperative nurses (SPN) Sometimes known as clinical nurse consultant (CNC) or specialist perioperative practitioners (SPP). Others, rather than being confined to one surgical specialty cover many disciplines; for example, integrated cancer coordinators (ICC) who care for cancer patients.

Spino-thalamic tracts Bundles of nerves passing from the spinal cord to the thalamus in the brain.

Squames Little flakes of shed skin. Like dust, they can float about in the air, and allow micro-organisms to hitch-hike from one place to another.

Stages of recovery Used to guide the care of patients in the recovery room, and determine their fitness to be discharged.

Stage 1 recovery Patients who need Stage 1 recovery are those who are physiologically unstable, or who potentially may become so.

Stage 2 recovery At this stage the patients are conscious, fully able to care for their own airways, and within the physiological limits defined by their preoperative evaluation.

Stage 3 recovery Following day procedures patients can be discharged into the care of a competent and informed adult who can intervene in the case of untoward events.

Stress Occurs when the body's homeostatic mechanisms deviate from normal. A strain is the event causing the stress.

Stroke volume The volume of blood ejected with each heart beat.

Subluxation Occurs where spinal joints are loose, and move relative to one another and in doing so may press on the spinal cord.

Substance P A peptide released from injured tissue. The P is an abbreviation for pain.

Substantia gelatinosa Part of the dorsal horn in the spinal cord where first-order sensory neurons synapse with second-order nerve cells passing to the brain. It works like a gate directing impulses either to the brain or back along reflex arcs.

Supraventricular arrhythmias arise in the atria.

Supraventricular tachycardia (SVT) A heart rate of between 150 to 250 bpm. On the ECG P-waves are usually, but not always, still visible. There are a number of causes.

Surfactant A complex phospholipid detergent produced by cells in the alveolus that prevents surface tension causing the alveolus to collapse. Premature neonates who do not produce enough surfactant get neonatal respiratory distress syndrome.

Suxamethonium A short-acting depolarizing muscle relaxant principally used for intubating patients. It is sometimes called simply 'sux'.

Sympathetic nervous system (SNS) Roused into action by threats to homeostasis such as hypovolaemia, hypoxia, fear and pain.

Sympathetic response is to raise the blood pressure, increase the heart rate and cardiac output. It makes the person hyperalert and vigilant.

Sympatheticomimetic A tongue-twisting word that means mimicking the effects of the sympathetic nervous system. Sympatheticomimetic drugs imitate the actions of adrenaline or noradrenaline.

Synapse A gap between two nerve cells. When stimulated by an **action potential** the end of one nerve cell releases a **neurotransmitter**, which drifts across the synapse, latches on to a **receptor** on the next nerve to trigger an action potential in the next nerve cell.

System Describes a group of interacting elements organized into a complex functioning whole. Systems can be closed to outside influences, or open to them. Your hospital is a system, and the recovery room is a subset of that system.

Systolic heart failure Characterized by a dilated floppy ventricle where the actin and myosin filaments do not overlap adequately. Therefore any increase in intraventricular pressure just stretches the filaments further, so cardiac output falls, especially at the beginning of inspiration.

Systolic pressure The maximum blood pressure in the arteries during the cardiac cycle.

T3 Triiodothyronine—a potent form of thyroid hormone.

T4 Thyroxine.

Tachycardia A heart rate greater than 100/min.

Tachycardia–bradycardia syndrome see **Sick sinus syndrome**.

Tachyphylaxis Occurs where patients develop an acute tolerance to a drug over minutes or hours. This means patients require progressively higher doses to achieve the same effect.

Tamponade To dam-up or squash. Cardiac tamponade means the heart is squashed by fluid pressure in the pericardial sac.

Temperature Difficult to define. Temperature is a physical measurement used to determine whether two bodies are in thermal equilibrium. If two bodies, A and B are placed next to each other, and heat energy moves from A to B then the temperature of A is higher than the temperature of body B.

Terminal respiratory units Functional clumps of alveoli and the terminal airways served by a common pulmonary arteriole. They are about the size of a match head.

Thalamus A collection of nerves shaped like two pigeon's eggs sitting deep in the brain. It lies above the hypothalamus right on top of the brainstem at the core of the brain. It is the key relay station for sensory information flowing to the brain. From the constant mass of information pouring in, and like a protective secretary, it only passes on immediately relevant information.

Therapeutic index Reflects the difference between the blood concentrations of a toxic dose of a drug, and its therapeutic levels. The therapeutic blood level of theophylline is only a whisker away from its toxic dose.

Thermistors Measure temperature. A thermistor is a tiny electrical device made from metal oxides semiconductors moulded together. A current passed through the wires varies exponentially with the temperature.

Thermodynamic activity The total kinetic and potential energy of a substance that could be converted into heat. It excludes electromagnetic and nuclear energy. Atoms and molecules vibrate and jiggle about according to their temperature, the hotter they are they faster they jiggle. The more they jiggle the more space they occupy. That is why things expand as they are heated. Thermodynamic activity is a measure of this vibration. At −273°C (absolute zero) they stop jiggling, stay quite still and have no thermodynamic activity.

Third space fluid Fluid that has been sequestrated in the bowel, peritoneum or pleural spaces because of either transudation or exudation. If the surgeon handles the bowel extensively during abdominal surgery, fluids will transudate into the lumen over the next 2–3 days. This can cause hypovolaemia, even though no fluid has been lost to the outside world. Although third space fluid forms part of the **total body water**, it is not available to boost the plasma or ECF volume.

Threshold potential A level of stimulus at which something becomes perceivable.

Thrombophilia The tendency to form spontaneous blood clots. It can be either inherited or acquired.

Thromboxane (TXA2) A powerful chemical made by platelets that causes them to stick together (aggregate) and causes vasoconstriction. It works hand in hand with a prostaglandin produced by vascular endocytes called PGI2 to help form blood clots and stop bleeding.

Tidal volume (TV) The amount of air moved into or out of the lungs with each breath.

Tolerance Tolerance to a drug is the progressive need for higher doses to achieve a consistent effect.

Tonicity is a measurement that compares the osmotic pressures of two solutions. The tonicity of a solution determines how water flows across cell membranes. Formally it can be defined thus: if two solutions are separated by a membrane only permeable to water, and water flows from one solution to the other, then the latter has a higher tonicity than the former. In practice, this means hypertonic solutions drag water out of cells, while hypotonic fluids allow water to flow into cells. If the solutions are **isotonic** then no fluid moves across the cell membranes.

Torsades de pointes (twisting of the points) A very fast and particularly lethal poly-morphic ventricular tachycardia. Each impulse arises in a different place in the vent-ricles so that the rapidly changing QRS trace on the ECG looks as though it is rotating about a baseline.

Total body water The total amount of fluid containing water in the body. It does not only include water, but also extracellular fluid, intracellular fluid, and cerebrospinal fluid. The volume of total body water is about 60% of lean body mass.

Tranexamic acid A drug (similar to amino-caproic acid) that inhibits plasminogen acti-vation and fibrinolysis. It is rapidly excreted by the kidneys. The dose is 0.5–1 g tds IV slowly.

Transducer A transducer is a device for converting one form of energy into another. For instance a pressure transducer converts pressure energy into electrical energy that a monitor can process. Unless carefully calibrated, transducers introduce inaccuracies and errors into measurements.

Transfusion threshold A nominated trigger point at which to give blood. In fit young people a **haematocrit** of 25% is the usual transfusion threshold, but in older and sicker patients it may be 30% or more.

Transient ischaemic attack (TIA) These transient attacks of cerebral ischaemia are caused by micro-emboli lodging in the small vessels in the brain causing symptoms that by definition resolve within 24 hours. The tiny clots often arise from the walls of the left atria in patients with atrial fibrillation. To prevent the formation of these micro-emboli, patients in atrial fibrillation usually take the anticoagulant warfarin.

Trans-oesophageal echocardiography (TOE) A technique where the patient swallows an ultrasound probe which does an echocardiogram from about two-thirds of the way down the oesophagus.

Transudate Fluid that has leaked across membranes. It is lower in protein content, than **exudate**. Exudate is protein-rich fluid produced by inflammation.

Trifascicular block A combination of an atrioventricular block, a right bundle branch block, and a left anterior hemiblock. Trifascicular blocks are high-grade blocks indicating extensive myocardial damage. If they are causing symptoms the patient requires a temporary pacemaker for major operations.

Triglycerides The body stores fat in fat cells (lipidocytes) in two forms: triglycerides and glycerol. These are easily broken down by enzymes called lipases into free fatty acids (FFAs). FFAs act as fast food for the heart and liver where they are degraded by β-oxidation to form energy. The proper name for triglyceride is triacylglycerol (but almost nobody uses it).

TURP syndrome occurs if the fibrous capsule around the prostate gland is breached during a *transurethral resection of the prostate* (TURP). The irrigation fluid used to dilate the bladder can leak into the circulation. It is possible for large amounts of water to dilute the electrolytes in the plasma to cause the typical symptoms of water overload.

Ultrafiltrate see **Filtrate**.

Uraemia The clinical and biochemical effects of an abnormal accumulation of waste products in the blood. It is a descriptive term describing the signs and symptoms of a patient with renal failure.

Urine The end-product of the renal tubules filtering, reabsorption, secretion, and concentration of tubular filtrate.

Vasopressin Also called **arginine vasopressin** (AVP). Another name for **antidiuretic hormone** (ADH).

Venothromboembolism (VTE) An umbrella term used to describe abnormal blood clots that are fixed in one place (**thromboses**) or those that have moved elsewhere (**emboli**).

Ventricular fibrillation (VF) In VF the cardiac impulse is chaotic and incapable of organizing coordinated ventricular contraction. If the chest is open you can see the heart muscle writhing like a bag full of earthworms, and there is no cardiac output.

Ventricular premature beats (VPBs) Wide, bizarre QRS complexes with a down-sloping ST segment, not preceded by a P-wave. They indicate an irritable myocardium, where the ventricle has contracted without the usual triggering sequence. Sometimes these are known as ventricular ectopics, or ventricular extrasystoles (VEs), or even premature ventricular contractions (PVCs). Suspect myocardial ischaemia—or too much coffee.

Ventricular tachycardia (VT) occurs when there are runs of more than three VPBs together.

Visceral pain comes from deep structures such as the gastrointestinal tract, bladder and other organs. It is difficult to localize with one finger, and is described in terms such as aching, nauseating, dull, or boring.

Vital centres The brainstem contains the grey matter neural connections responsible for controlling blood pressure, heart rate, the pattern and rate of breathing, temperature, plasma osmotic pressure, carbon dioxide levels, vomiting, thermal regulation, sweating, and the adrenergic and noradrenergic responses. The vital centres mostly interact with the autonomic nervous system.

Vital signs traditionally involve the measurement of blood pressure, pulse rate, respiratory rate and conscious state. In contrast *observations* seems to mean the addition of measurement of temperature and perhaps urine output. Neither term has a formal definition. They are often used interchangeably as a verbal short hand. Should 'observations' include oxygen saturation? Almost certain in the recovery room, the answer is yes.

Volume depletion Jargon for a loss of fluid from the body. Usually it refers to blood loss, but it may also refer to loss of extracellular fluid (ECF) or even intracellular fluid depletion. It is a better term than **dehydration**.

von Willebrand's disease A term that covers four subgroups of the most common inherited bleeding disorders. It is caused by a defect in the production of von Willebrand's factor (vWF) by the endothelium lining blood vessels. Unlike haemophilia it affects men and women equally.

Water intoxication occurs after prolonged irrigation with hypertonic fluids during urological surgery, or hysteroscopy. The patient becomes acutely water overloaded (*hyponatraemic*) and their brain cells swell. It can be fatal, particularly in premeno-pausal woman and children.

Water-soluble hormones see **Hormones**.

Whistle-tip catheters Made of soft silicon-plastic, they have holes on their side, and a moulded tip that will not damage delicate mucosa.

Wind-up The process by which a nerve cell becomes far more sensitive to stimuli that would previously have not had much effect.

Wolff–Parkinson–White (WPW) syndrome is one of the congenital syndromes, where the ventricle becomes prematurely activated when the cardiac impulse takes a shortcut through an accessory pathway to bypass the AV node. Consequently the PR interval is short (0.1–0.2 seconds), and there is a wider QRS complex.

Work is a physical measurement. Work (W) is done when a force (F) moves a mass (m) through a distance. Work = F × D. Its SI unit is the newton metre.

Abbreviations

Abbreviations are frequently used by medical and nursing staff. They are sometimes specific to a particular area, and are a mystery to outsiders, but many are in common use. To avoid errors and mishaps use only abbreviations approved by your hospital. Even approved abbreviations can be misunderstood if they are not written clearly, and clear script is not a virtue of many doctors. Always explain abbreviations if there is the possibility they have more than one meaning, for example, DOA could mean dead on arrival, or date of admission; ARF could mean acute respiratory failure or acute renal failure; and Cx could mean cervical spine or cervix.

This is a list of common abbreviations used in many hospitals.

Never act on an abbreviation unless
you are absolutely sure what it means.

#	fracture		μ	Greek letter, mu (pronounced mew)
#	number		μ	micro
%	per cent		μgm or less clearly μg	microgram
α	Greek letter alpha			
β	Greek letter beta		μmol	micromol
γ	Greek letter gamma		5-HT	5 hydroxytryptamine (also called serotonin)
π	Greek letter pi (pronounced pie)			
/	per or each (breaths/min)		a.c.	before food is given; it applies to medication.
@	at			
[X]	concentration of substance X		a.m.	before noon
[Na+]	concentration of sodium ion		ABG	arterial blood gases
<	less than		AC	alternating current
>	greater than		ACE	angiotensin-converting enzyme
±	plus or minus		ACEI	angiotensin-converting enzyme inhibitor
«	much less than			
»	much greater than		ACLS	advanced cardiac life support
Δ	Greek letter upper case delta used to describe differences		ACS	acute coronary syndrome
			ACTH	adrenocorticotropic hormone
≤	less than or equal to		ADH	antidiuretic hormone
≥	greater than or equal to		AE AED	atrial ectopic beats automated external defibrillator
®	registered name			
™	trademark		AED	automatic external
°	C degree centigrade		AF	atrial fibrillation
°	C degrees Celsius		AIDS	acquired immune deficiency syndrome
°	F degree Fahrenheit		AIMS	Australian Incident Monitoring System

AMI	acute myocardial infarction
ANP	atrial-naturetic peptide
ANS	autonomic nervous system
APACHE	acute physiology and chronic health evaluation
aPPT	activated partial thromboplastin time
APS	acute pain service
aPTT	activated partial thromboplastin time
AR	aortic regurgitation
ARB	angiotensin receptor blocker
ARDS	acute respiratory distress syndrome
ARDS	adult respiratory distress syndrome
ARF	acute renal failure
AS	aortic stenosis
ASAP	as soon as possible
Assist	assistants
AST	alanine aminotransferase
ATLS	advanced trauma life
ATN	acute tubular necrosis
ATP	adenosine triphosphate
AUC	area under curve
AV	node atrioventricular node
AV	shunt arteriovenous shunt
AV	atrioventricular
AVB	atrioventricular block
AVP	arginine vasopressin
AXR	abdominal x-ray
b.d.	twice daily
B.S.	blood sugar
BA	bowel action
BAN	British Approved Names
BBV	blood-borne virus
BCC	basal cell carcinoma
BCG	Bacille Calmette–Guérin
Bd	twice daily
BF	breast fed
BIP	bisthmus iodine paste
BiPAP	bi-level positive airway pressure
BKA	below knee amputation
BLS	basic cardiac life support
BLS	basic life support
BMR	basal metabolic rate
BP	blood pressure
bpm	heart rate in beats per minute
BUN	bound urinary nitrogen
BVM	bag valve mask unit
Bx	biopsy
C5	fifth cervical vertebra
Ca	carcinoma
Ca^{++}	calcium ion
CABG	coronary artery bypass graft
CABG	coronary artery bypass surgery
CAD	coronary artery disease
CAM	complementary and alternative medicine
CAN	cardiac autonomic neuropathy
CaO$_2$	arterial oxygen content
CAPD	ambulatory peritoneal dialysis
CAVDH	continuous arterio-venous haemodialysis
CBF	cerebral blood flow
CCF	congestive cardiac failure
CDH	congenital dislocation of the hip
CE	continuing education
CETT	cuffed endotracheal tube
CFU	colony-forming units
CGRP	calcitonin gene-related peptide
CI	cardiac index
CJD	Creutzfeldt–Jakob disease
CK	creatinine kinase
CKD	chronic kidney disease
CKMB	creatinine kinase isoenzyme–muscle band
Cl$^-$	chloride ion
cm	centimetre
CMV	cytomegalovirus
CNS	central nervous system
CO$_2$	carbon dioxide
COAD	chronic obstructive airway disease
COPD	chronic obstructive pulmonary disease
COX	cyclo-oxygenase
CPAP	continuous positive airway pressure
C-PAP	continuous positive airway pressure
CPK	creatinine phosphokinase
CPR	cardiopulmonary resuscitation
CRF	chronic renal failure
CRI	cardiac risk index

CRT	capillary return time
CSF	cerebrospinal fluid
CT	computed tomography
CTZ	chemoreceptor trigger zone
CVA	cerebrovascular accident
CVC	central venous catheter
CVD	cerebrovascular disease
CVL	central venous line
CvO_2	mixed venous oxygen content
CVP	central venous pressure
CWMS	colour, warmth, movement, sensation
Cx	cervical spine
Cx	cervix
CXR	chest X-ray
D&C	dilation and curettage
D5W	5% glucose (dextrose) in water
DB&C	deep breath and cough
DC	direct current
DCR	direct current cardioversion
DIC	disseminated intravascular coagulation
DNA	deoxyribose nucleic acid
DO_2	oxygen delivery
DOA	dead on arrival
DOB	date of birth
DPG	diphosphoglycerate
dTC	tubocurare
DVT	deep vein thrombosis
Dx	diathermy
E/o	excision of
EACA	epsilon amino caproic acid
EBP	evidence-based practice
ECF	extracellular fluid
ECG	electrocardiogram
ECT	electroconvulsive therapy
ED	emergency department
EDTA	ethyl diamine tetra acetic acid
EEG	electroencephalogram
EF	ejection fraction
eGFR	estimated glomerular filtration rate
EKG	electrocardiograph (alternative abbrev.)
ELISA	enzyme-linked immunosorbent assay
EMB	early morning breakfast
EMLA	eutectic mixture of local anaesthetics
ENT	ear, nose and throat enzyme
EPAP	expiratory positive airway pressure
EPP	exposure-prone procedures
ER	emergency room
ERAS	enhanced recovery after surgery
ERCP	endoscopic retrograde cholangiopancreatography
EREM	extended-release epidural morphine
ERSF	end stage renal failure
ESKD	end stage kidney disease
ESR	erythrocyte sedimentation rate
ESU	electrosurgical unit (diathermy in the UK)
ESWL	extracorporeal shock wave lithotripsy
ETA	estimated time of arrival
ETT	endotracheal tube
EUA	examination under anaesthesia
FB	foreign body
FBA	foreign body aspiration
FBC	fluid balance chart
FBE	full blood examination
FDA	Federal Drug Authority—a USA agency
FDA	Food and Drug Administration (USA)
FDP	fibrin degradation product
FES	fat embolism syndrome
FEV_1	forced expiratory volume in one second
FF	free fluids
FFP	fresh frozen plasma
FHx	family history
FiO_2	fractional inspired oxygen concentration
FIx	for investigation
FNAB	fine-needle aspiration biopsy
FNH	febrile non-haemolytic reactions
FNHTR	febrile non-haemolytic transfusion reaction
FRC	functional residual capacity
FS	frozen section

FSH	follicle stimulating hormone
FSPs	fibrin split products
FVC	forced vital capacity
FWD	full ward diet
FWT	full ward test of urine
G	gauge
g	gram
GA	general anaesthesia
GABA	gamma aminobutyric acid
GAMP	general anaesthetic, manipulation and plaster
GCS	Glasgow Coma Scale
GFR	glomerular filtration rate
GGT	gamma-glutamyltransferase
GOK	goodness only knows
GTN	glyceryl trinitrate (preferred abbrev.)
Gyn	gynaecology
H^+	hydrogen ion
H_2O	water
HAFOE	high airflow oxygen entrainment masks
HAV	hepatitis A virus
Hb	haemoglobin
HBV	hepatitis B virus
HCO_3^-	bicarbonate ion
HCT	haematocrit
HCV	hepatitis C virus
HCW	health care workers
HDU	high dependency unit
HFV	high-frequency ventilation
Hg	mercury
HIC	head injury chart
HIT	heparin-induced thrombocytopaenia
HIV	human immunodeficiency virus
HME	heat and moisture exchanger
HNPU	has not passed urine
HOCUM	hypertrophic obstructive cardiomyopathy
HPV	hypoxic pulmonary vasoconstriction
hr	hour
hrly	hourly
HRT	hormone replacement therapy

HSV	herpes simplex virus
HT	hypertension
HTLV	human T cell lymphotrophic virus
Htn	hypertension
HTR	haemolytic transfusion reactions
Hx	history
i.d.	internal diameter
I.U.	international units
I/M	intramuscular
IBP	invasive blood pressure monitoring
IBW	ideal body weight
ICC	intercostal catheter
ICF	intracellular fluid
ICP	intracranial pressure
ICU	intensive care unit
IDDM	insulin-dependent diabetes mellitus
IgA	immunoglobulin A, (others are M, E, and G).
IHD	ischaemic heart disease
IM	intramuscularly
IMV	intermittent mandatory ventilation
INR	international normalized ratio (see PTT)
IPAP	inspiratory positive airway pressure
IPC	intermittent pneumatic compression
IPPV	intermittent positive pressure ventilation
ISO	International Standards Organization
ISQ	in status quo (meaning 'unchanged')
ITP	idiopathic thrombocytopenic purpura
ITS	iontophoretic system
IU	international units
IUD	intrauterine device
IV	intravenous
IVI	intravenous injection
JVP	jugular venous pressure
K^+	potassium ion
Kcal	kilocalorie
KCl	potassium chloride
kg	kilogram
kPa	kilopasacal

L	litre		MRSA	meticillin resistant *Staphylococcus aureus*
L3–4	interspace between 3rd and 4th lumbar vertebrae		ms	millisecond
LA	local anaesthesia		MS	multiple sclerosis
Lac	laceration		MSOF	multisystem organ failure
LAHB	left anterior hemiblock		MTBF	mean time between failures
LBBB	left bundle branch block		MUA	manipulation under anaesthetic
LBM	lean body mass		mV	millivolt
LDH	lactic dehydrogenase		MVA	motor vehicle accident
LIF	left iliac fossa		MVPS	mitral valve prolapse syndrome
LMA	laryngeal mask airway		MVR	mitral valve regurgitation
LMWH	low molecular-weight heparin		N	normal (as in 0.9% Normal saline)
LOC	loss of consciousness		N/G	nasogastric
LOE	levels of evidence		N/S	normal saline
LP	lumbar puncture		N_2O	nitrous oxide
LUQ	left upper quadrant		Na^+	sodium ion
LVF	left ventricular failure		NAD	nothing abnormal detected
m^2	square metre		NBP	non-invasive blood pressure
MAC	minimum anaesthetic concentration		Neg	negative
mane	in the morning		NFO	no further orders
MAO	mono-amine oxidase		NFR	not for resuscitation
MAOI	mono-amine oxidase inhibitor		NHS	National Health Service (UK)
MAP	mean arterial pressure		NIBP	non-invasive blood pressure
MAT	multifocal atrial tachycardia		NIDDM	non-insulin dependent diabetes mellitus
MBA	motor bicycle accident		NIOSH	National Institute of Occupational Safety and Health
MCA	motor car accident			
MDRTB	multiple drug-resistant tuberculosis		NMBD	neuromuscular blocking drugs
MEAC	mean effective anaesthetic concentration		NMDA	N-methyl-D-aspartic acid
			nmol	nanomole
MET	metabolic exercise tolerance		NMS	neuroleptic malignant syndrome
mg	milligram		NNH	number needed to harm
MG	myasthenia gravis		NNT	number needed to treat
Mg^{++}	magnesium ion		NO	nitric oxide
MH	malignant hyperthermia		nocte	at night
MHAH	micro-angiopathic haemolytic anaemia		NOF	neck of femur
			NPA	nasopharyngeal aspiration
MI	myocardial infarction		NRL	natural rubber latex
MIC	minimum inhibitory concentration		NSAID	non-steroidal anti-inflammatory drug
min	minute			
mm	millimetre		NTG	nitroglycerin (see GTN)
mmHg	millimetre of mercury pressure		NYO	not yet ordered
mmol	millimole		O/A	on admission
mOsm	milli-osmol		O/call	on call
MRI	magnetic resonance imaging		O_2	oxygen

OD	overdose
OPD	out-patients department
OR	operating room
Ortho	orthopaedics
OSA	obstructive sleep apnoea
OT	operating theatre
OTC	over the counter
OXI	pulse oximetry
P	partial pressure as in PO_2
p.c.	after meals
PA	pulmonary artery
PACE	postoperative adverse cardiac events
$PaCO_2$	partial pressure of carbon dioxide in arterial blood
PACU	post anaesthetic care unit
Paed	paediatrics
PAG	periaqueductal grey matter
PaO_2	partial pressure of oxygen in the arterial blood
PAP	pulmonary artery pressure
PAT	paroxysmal atrial tachycardia
PAWP	pulmonary artery wedge pressure
PCA	patient-controlled anaesthesia
PCEA	patient-controlled epidural analgesia
PCI	percutaneous intervention
PCNL	percutaneous nephrolithotomy
PCO_2	partial pressure of carbon dioxide
PCTA	percutaneous transluminal angioplasty
PCV	packed cell volume
PD	peritoneal dialysis
PDE	phosphodiesterase
PDQ	pretty darned quick
PE	pulmonary embolism
PEA	pre-emptive analgesia
PEA	pulseless electrical activity
PEEP	positive end expiratory pressure
PERLA	pupils equal and reacting to light and accommodation
PFD	positive fluid displacement
PFR	peak flow rate
pH	inverse logarithm of the hydrogen ion activity

PHx	past history
PICC	peripherally inserted central catheter
PINDA	pain indicator and assessment
PM	post mortem
pm.	after midday
PND	paroxysmal nocturnal dyspnoea
PO_2	partial pressure of oxygen
PONV	postoperative nausea and/or vomiting
POP	plaster of Paris
PORC	postoperative residual curarization
Pos	positive
PPF	plasma protein fraction
PPI	proton pump inhibitor
ppm	parts per million
PR	per rectum
PRBC	packed red blood cells
Premed	premedication
prn	when necessary (*pro re nata*)
PS	pressure support
PT	prothrombin time (also see INR)
PTB	pulmonary tuberculosis
PTH	post-transfusion hepatitis
PTSD	post-traumatic stress disorder
PUD	peptic ulcer disease
PUO	pyrexia of unknown origin
PV	*per vagina*
PVB	premature ventricular beat
PVC	premature ventricular contraction
PVR	pulmonary vascular resistance
QD	once daily (use of this is discouraged)
QID	four times daily
RAS	reticular activating system
RBBB	right bundle branch block
RBF	renal blood flow
RCT	randomized controlled trial
Resps	respirations
RIA	radio-immuno assay
RIB	rest in bed
RIF	right iliac fossa
rINNs	recommended International Non-Proprietary Names
RNA	ribonucleic acid

ROP	retinopathy of prematurity
RPAO	routine post anaesthetic orders
RUQ	right upper quadrant
RVF	right ventricular failure
S/B	seen by
S/C	subcutaneous
SA	node sino-atrial node
SA	sino-atrial
SAED	shock advisory external defibrillator
SAL	sterility assurance level
SaO$_2$	haemoglobin's oxygen saturation
SAP	systemic arterial pressure
SBE	subacute bacterial endocarditis
SBP	systolic blood pressure
SCD	sequential compression devices
sec	seconds
SG	specific gravity
SG	substantia gelatinosa
SIADH	Syndrome of inappropriate antidiuretic hormone secretion
SLE	systemic lupus erythematosus
SMR	submucosal resection
SNP	sodium nitroprusside
SNS	sympathetic nervous system
SOF	shaft of femur
SOOB	sit out of bed
Sp/A	spinal anaesthesia
SPN	specialist perioperative nurses
SR	sinus rhythm
SSG	split skin graft
SSRI	selective serotonin reuptake inhibitors
SSS	sick sinus syndrome
stat	*statum* (immediately)
STD	sexually transmitted disease
STOP	suction termination of pregnancy
STP	sodium thiopental
sux	suxamethonium chloride
SVR	systemic vascular resistance
SVT	supraventricular tachycardia
SWMA	systolic wall movement abnormality syndrome
T3	triiodothyronine
T4	thyroxine
T6	sixth thoracic vertebra

Tabs	tablets
TAH	total abdominal hysterectomy
TAP	transversus abdominis block
TB	tuberculosis
TCP	transcutaneous pacemaker
tds	three times a day
TENS	transcutaneous electrical stimulation
TENS	transcutaneous nerve stimulation
THR	total hip replacement
TIA	transient ischaemic attacks
TIVA	total intravenous anaesthesia
TMJ	temporo-mandibular joint
TMOA	too many obscure abbreviations
TOF	train-of-four with a nerve stimulator
TOP	termination of pregnancy
TPN	total parenteral nutrition
TPR	temperature, pulse and respiration
TRALI	transfusion-related lung injury
TRU	terminal respiratory unit
Ts &	As tonsillectomy and adenoidectomy
TT	thrombin time
TTN	transient tachypnoea of the newborn
TURBT	transurethral bladder tumour resection
TURP	transurethral resection of prostate
U&E	urea and electrolyte
UH	unfractionated heparin
URTI	upper respiratory tract infection
UTI	urinary tract infection
UTT	up to toilet
UWSD	under-water sealed drainage
V	volt
VAPS	visual analogue pain scale
VC	vital capacity
VC	vomiting centre
VE	ventricular ectopics
VEs	ventricular extrasystoles
VF	ventricular fibrillation
VO$_2$	oxygen consumption
VPBs	ventricular premature beats
VRE	vancomycin-resistant *Enterococcus*

VT	ventricular tachycardia
VTE	venothromboembolic disease
VVs	varicose veins
vWD	von Willebrand's syndrome
WHO	World Health Organization
WNL	within normal limits
WPW	Wolff–Parkinson–White syndrome

wt	weight
WYSWYG	What you see is what you get (a computer term).
XDP	fibrin d-dimer
X-match	cross-match blood
Yr	year

Index

PSYCHOSOCIAL ASSESSMENT

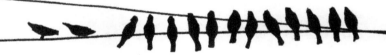

IN MENTAL HEALTH

Sara Miller McCune founded SAGE Publishing in 1965 to support the dissemination of usable knowledge and educate a global community. SAGE publishes more than 1000 journals and over 800 new books each year, spanning a wide range of subject areas. Our growing selection of library products includes archives, data, case studies and video. SAGE remains majority owned by our founder and after her lifetime will become owned by a charitable trust that secures the company's continued independence.

Los Angeles | London | New Delhi | Singapore | Washington DC | Melbourne

PSYCHOSOCIAL ASSESSMENT

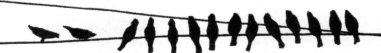

IN **MENTAL HEALTH**

EDITED BY

STEVE TRENOWETH

AND **NICKI MOONE**

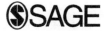

Los Angeles | London | New Delhi
Singapore | Washington DC | Melbourne

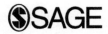

Los Angeles | London | New Delhi
Singapore | Washington DC | Melbourne

SAGE Publications Ltd
1 Oliver's Yard
55 City Road
London EC1Y 1SP

SAGE Publications Inc.
2455 Teller Road
Thousand Oaks, California 91320

SAGE Publications India Pvt Ltd
B 1/I 1 Mohan Cooperative Industrial Area
Mathura Road
New Delhi 110 044

SAGE Publications Asia-Pacific Pte Ltd
3 Church Street
#10-04 Samsung Hub
Singapore 049483

Editor: Becky Taylor
Assistant editor: Charlène Burin
Production editor: Katie Forsythe
Proofreader: Philippa May
Indexer: Adam Pozner
Marketing manager: Tamara Navaratnam
Cover design: Wendy Scott
Typeset by: C&M Digitals (P) Ltd, Chennai, India
Printed by CPI Group (UK) Ltd, Croydon, CR0 4YY

First published 2017

Disclaimer

This book is intended to support and not replace clinical decision-making. Before undertaking an assessment you must ensure that you are competent to do so. Organisational policies for conducting (and acting upon) psychosocial and/or risk assessments must be followed and legal advice sought before proceeding if necessary.

You must follow guidance issued by your respective professional regulatory body. Neither the authors, editors nor the publisher take responsibility for any consequences of any action taken as result of information contained in this book.

Library of Congress Control Number: 2016953840

British Library Cataloguing in Publication data

A catalogue record for this book is available from the British Library

ISBN 978-1-4739-1283-0
ISBN 978-1-4739-1284-7 (pbk)

CONTENTS

ABOUT THE EDITORS AND CONTRIBUTORS

About the editors

Steve Trenoweth qualified in 1991 and has worked in a wide variety of mental health care settings before entering higher education in 2003. He is currently a senior lecturer at Bournemouth University. He has authored several chapters, articles and books in nursing and health care and is an editorial board member of the *British Journal of Mental Health Nursing*. He is a trustee of Project Nurture, a Dorset-based charity committed to enhancing and enriching the natural and built environment for those who are suffering the effects of social exclusion and mental health difficulties.

Nicki Moone is an experienced mental health nurse who works as a lecturer practitioner in Berkshire Healthcare NHS Foundation Trust and the University of West London. As a mental health practitioner Nicki has been involved in developing and delivering services to families and carers for many years. She established a Family Intervention service in Berkshire in 2002, before moving to a lecturer practitioner post in 2009. She is a senior lecturer and the course leader for the BSc, Pg Cert, Pg Dip and MSc in Psychosocial Interventions for Psychosis-Thorn accredited course. Her broad experience as a mental health nurse has led to her specialising in community based mental health care and the use of evidence-based practice. Nicki is currently undertaking a professional doctorate looking at ways to maintain well-being at work amongst mental health practitioners.

About the contributors

Caroline Attard is an inpatient mental health nurse consultant currently working in Berkshire Mental Health Care Trust in the UK. Her career and expertise spans over 18 years. Caroline has worked in her native country, Malta, and in the United Kingdom. She specialises in inpatient mental health nursing and quality improvement. Her work consists of education, clinical leadership, research and service improvement. Caroline teaches at under and post graduate level mental health nursing programmes at various universities. She also develops and facilitates various in-house training programmes on a variety of subjects including suicide prevention, risk training and psychosocial interventions. She has developed a preceptorship programme for newly qualified mental health nurses which focuses on resilience and uses methods such as action learning sets and quality improvement methodology. Caroline has a passion for working with carers and facilitates family work in her own Trust. She is involved in several research projects from using sports with people who have severe and enduring mental health problems to CBT and sleep in inpatient mental health wards, and her expertise in service development has been utilised successfully in various areas on inpatient mental health wards.

Susan Bowman is semi-retired and currently works as a Community Psychiatric Nurse in the South Belfast Recovery Team. Starting her nursing career in 1972, she completed her training in mental health nursing in 1975. She went on to complete her general nursing and midwifery training. She has always focused her career in mental health nursing and started community psychiatric nursing in 1991. Since then she has been a member of multidisciplinary teams working in the recovery setting. Completing Thorn training in 1997, she worked with early intervention teams. She has a particular interest in working with families and has established strong links with CAUSE, who provide carer advocates and are an invaluable resource within Northern Ireland. She has also worked as a teaching assistant at Queens University Belfast, mainly with the Thorn training and also pre-registration courses.

Dr Teresa Burdett works at Bournemouth University as a lecturer in Integrated Care. She teaches on both undergraduate and post graduate programmes in integration, interprofessional and health promotion arenas. She is also the professional lead for Interprofessional Learning and Education. This involves promoting, arranging and delivering inter professional education between various disciplines such as the different branches of nursing, social work, nutrition, physiotherapy and paramedic science students and faculties. She has also co-initiated, designed and delivered the Foundations of Integrated Care programme. This programme has been very well received with some very positive qualitative data and comments, and has been successfully extended, becoming more person-centred and receiving accreditation. She has also successfully bid for research grants nationally and has presented at conferences both nationally and internationally. She is also part of two regional groups in the NHS which are forging ahead to enhance the integration agenda to improve patient services and standards. She works closely with a variety of stakeholders and partners, including trusts both locally and nationally, to continue to advance the level of services offered to individuals. Her nursing career has spanned adult health, health visiting and mental health in both inpatient and community settings.

John Butler is an experienced mental health nurse, former consultant nurse (Acute Mental Health & Psychosocial Intervention) and Head of Practice Development for a large NHS Trust, and former honorary chairperson of the Luton-based charity, Caraline. John joined University of Central Lancashire as a senior lecturer in mental health in January 2013. He is currently the Course & Mental Health Field Lead for the MSc Pre-Registration Nursing, and Course Lead for the Grad Cert Psychosocial Mental Health Care. Having undertaken specialist training in cognitive behavioural, behavioural family and mental health medication management interventions, which formed the focus of his clinical practice, John has been involved in facilitating educational workshops, short courses and university programmes for mental health practitioners and student mental health nurses since 1997. John has contributed a number of publications and conference presentations on a range of topics, which have included: the assessment and management of risk in mental health practice; the interface between primary care and specialist mental health teams; understanding generalised anxiety disorder and the anxiety disorders; collaborative approaches to managing depression; service improvement initiatives (including the Productive Mental Health Ward programme, caseload management, and protected therapeutic and engagement time); and the implementation of psychosocial intervention.

Alison Elliott is an experienced mental health nurse and senior manager. She joined University of Central Lancashire as a senior lecturer in mental health in September 2012 and is currently the course leader for the BSc(Hons) Psychosocial Mental Health Care, and Year 2 lead for pre-registration mental health nursing. Alison spent the majority of her career working in secure mental health and learning disability settings, but has also worked in community and adult and older adult inpatient settings, has undertaken specialist training in psychosocial interventions, and was involved in teaching whilst still in clinical practice, often with service users, in relation to a variety of topics. Alison has maintained an honorary contract with a local NHS Trust, and is involved in research activity in relation to Mindfulness Behaviour Therapy (MBT) for personality disorder.

Dr Mick Fleming is the Associate Professor for mental health at Edinburgh Napier University. He is a mental health nurse who is very experienced in delivering psycho-social interventions in clinical practice and has received national nursing awards for this work. For the last 15 years he has worked in academia, training and supervising mental health practitioners to deliver psychosocial interventions to people with psychosis. He has completed and published research into schizophrenia.

Mark Gillespie is a programme leader and nurse lecturer at the University of the West of Scotland. He has been involved in mental health care for over 30 years, working across a variety of clinical specialisms in both inpatient and community settings. Currently a doctoral student, his thesis investigates the role of assistant grade staff on the clinical development of student mental health nurses and previous research has investigated other aspects of student nurse learning. His current role includes coordinating a masters level programme in mental health care, with pathways available for the development of therapeutic skills, leadership or educational abilities. He has authored several journal articles and is keen to promote publication of the impressive materials generated by students. He has an interest in the Spanish Civil War and has authored a short book on the subject.

Jackie Glenister has been a mental health nurse for several years in a range of posts. She has a particular commitment to working with people using evidence-based approaches and developing these skills within the workforce. She has worked in most mental health services in her career and her special areas of interest are working in community settings and developing services within the community as an alternative to hospital admission. She is a joint service manager for a large urban community mental health team with particular interest in developing the skill mix of the team with a focus on; encouraging practitioners to undertake psychosocial interventions that will enhance service user experiences of mental health services. She strongly believes that mental health practitioners in a clinical setting are in a position to make a genuine difference to their clients in the journey towards recovery by using a considered and systematic approach to care delivery. Her current focus is to support practitioners to understand the importance of a systematic approach when drawing together assessment information to help the client make sense of their experiences.

Tracey Kearns is a lecturer in the School of Nursing working in the mental health division at The University of Central Lancashire. She is involved in teaching on a number of modules for the Pre-Registration Degree and Masters in Nursing. She also provides teaching on the BSc (Hons) & Grad Cert Psychosocial Mental Health Care. Tracey has provided clinical supervision to students in the clinical setting studying the BSc (Hons) Psychosocial Mental Health Care. She also gained experience in lecturing working as a lecturer-practitioner for 12 months on a part-time secondment at University of Central Lancashire before commencing her current full time position. An experienced mental health nurse and former Specialist Practitioner for Psychosis for a large NHS Trust, Tracey worked with individuals and their families with severe and enduring mental health illnesses and completed additional training to deliver specific family intervention. Tracey has completed additional continuing professional development studies including Brief Solution Focused Therapy and Mentorship and is currently working towards her Post Graduate Certificate in Education. Tracey's main areas of professional interest are: schizophrenia and psychosis, psychosocial intervention, recovery and family interventions.

Fiona Martin is a lecturer in the School of Nursing and Midwifery, Queen's University Belfast and has been active in developing the mental health profile within the School since the early 2000s. Co-production has been an important aspect of her teaching, which she finds brings an authenticity to the learning environment. More recently Fiona was awarded a Florence Nightingale Foundation travel scholarship to explore 'Open Dialogue', a mental health systems approach originating in Finland.

Vicky Naidoo is an occupational therapist who graduated from the University of Southampton in 2007. She is currently working as a clinical lead within the Slough Community Mental Health Team (CMHT) Recovery Team. Vicky is extremely passionate about the recovery approach within mental health services and promotes recovery in all that she does both clinically and academically. She has most recently been responsible for developing a recovery college within her CMHT and the first year of its launch has been very successful. She has worked in mental health services for the duration of her career and completed a PG Dip and then later an MSc in Psychosocial Interventions for Psychosis this year, which focused on carers support groups in particular. Vicky found that specialising within this particular area of mental health was very important in developing her knowledge of the most up-to-date evidence-based practices to support people with severe and enduring mental health conditions. Vicky is currently in the process of publishing her MSc dissertation and hopes that this will be completed early next year.

Mary O'Toole is qualified in both adult and mental health fields of nursing. She has worked in a variety of mental health and general health settings, and has a particular interest in psychosis, medicines management, drug and alcohol addiction and self-management of long-term mental health conditions. She has published a number of articles and book chapters. Mary is a lecturer in mental health nursing at Plymouth University, teaching on both undergraduate and post graduate nursing programmes.

Reuben Pearce is a senior lecturer in mental health nursing at the University of West London leading and teaching on a wide range of courses including BSc/PG Dip pre-registration nursing programmes, independent and supplementary nurse prescribing, crisis intervention and suicide prevention. He has a broad experience working as a mental health nurse with a career spanning over 20 years. He continues to maintain a strong presence in practice through involvement in various initiatives with NHS Trust partners, in particular, skills development in areas of communication skills underpinning systematic assessment, risk assessment and suicide prevention. Reuben is currently undertaking a doctorate exploring educational techniques that improve communication skills in mental health nurses.

Alicia Powell is a senior nurse practitioner. She began her nursing career at West London Mental Health Trust in 2003 after emigrating from Australia. Prior to this she graduated with a Bachelor of Behavioural Science in Psychology from Griffith University, Brisbane in 2000. In the UK, Alicia began as a health care assistant working in secure forensic units at St Bernard's Hospital, Ealing. This was followed by a 3 year secondment to undertake student nurse training at Thames Valley University where she graduated in 2008 with first-class honours. As a registered mental health nurse she initially worked as a staff nurse in an acute ward before moving into community-based mental health services. She has extensive community experience including working within integrated community teams as well as within a dedicated assessment service. In 2016 Alicia helped in the development and delivery of a new Single Point of Access service providing a streamlined entry point into mental health services and 24 hour access to crisis support for service users and their family and friends. Alicia has particular interests in recovery and social inclusion, health promotion, student development and education.

Brian Thomson comes from a background as a community psychiatric nurse and cognitive behavioural therapist, and moved into academia in 1999 to teach CBT and mental health nursing, eventually becoming Course Director for the Masters programme in CBT at the University of Hertfordshire. In 2013 he moved to Paisley where he has developed the Post Graduate Programme in CBT at the University of the West of Scotland. Brian developed the "nine box model" for Formulation as part of his PHD studies and has demonstrated its use both in class and at conferences over the past two years.

Francis Thompson registered as a mental health nurse in 2003, graduating from Southampton University. Francis has worked in a variety of clinical areas across inpatient and community services including older adults services, the National

Psychosis Unit and addictions services. Francis has also spent time as a charge nurse, a community dual diagnosis specialist, a practice development nurse and in education as a lecturer in mental health at King's College London. He has also worked in a number of senior management roles: as the lead for nursing development at Oxleas NHS Foundation Trust and the head of nursing education and standards at West London Mental Health Trust. He joined Plymouth University in August 2014 as an associate professor where he currently leads the mental health nursing team.

Alison Toner has been in nursing for 30 years working in both adult and mental health fields with experience in urology, learning disabilities, older adult, addictions, acute mental health care and education. She is a lecturer in mental health nursing at the University of the West of Scotland and currently the programme leader for the BSc Mental Health Nursing course covering 4 campus sites within the largest school of health, nursing & midwifery in Scotland. Before joining the higher education sector she was the charge nurse of an inpatient dual diagnosis unit. She has 14 years of experience working with pre-registration and post registration nurses both in designing and delivery of programmes. Her main areas of interest are ePortfolio, skills development for mental health student nurses, comorbity and physical health care of people experiencing mental health issues. Current research interests as part of her Professional Doctorate study relate to resilience in student nurses and student teachers. She is registered with the NMC and is a Fellow of the Higher Education Academy.

FOREWORD

STEPHEN TEE

Mental health care in the UK, and in some other parts of the world, has been through radical transformation over recent decades. There has been a growing awareness of the potential for recovery and new systems of service delivery and coordination that emphasise achievement of a fulfilling life, with those who use services having a greater role in self-determination.

Transformation of this scale will only be sustained by a workforce who understand and embrace the value-set of hope and recovery that enables people to achieve positive life choices. It is therefore perfect timing for a book such as this that focuses on a collaborative and emancipatory approach to psychosocial assessment, the cornerstone to effective mental health practice.

This book is a highly informative and welcome addition to the mental health practitioner toolkit and a 'must have' text for anyone working in modern mental health practice. It is not, however, just a 'how to?' book of useful techniques, although these are there in abundance, but something much deeper than that, for it explores the contemporary mental health discourse enabling readers to situate their practice within a sound philosophical framework, developing a positive professional identity, which is enlightened, purposeful and transformative.

The move to a socially inclusive, recovery-oriented philosophy is a long way from the overly paternalistic and oppressive approaches of a bygone era, but unless practitioners appreciate the significance of the journey travelled, practice can easily regress. This book not only embraces an overtly psychosocial philosophy but enhances our understanding by relating complex concepts such as normalisation, resilience and psychosocial stress to a practical context so that readers can see the application to real life scenarios. This is further enhanced through helpful exercises and reflective points to deepen understanding.

I would strongly argue that where this book's key strengths lie is in its engaging and accessible prose rooted in the extensive expertise of the multidisciplinary group of highly experienced health professionals and academics. The depth and scope of clinical knowledge of each of the authors speaks to both existing practitioners and those who are developing their skills and knowledge in preparatory nursing, occupational therapy and other mental health programmes. It is also interspersed with service user quotes that emphasis salient points and make explicit the focus on doing 'with' rather than doing 'to'.

As someone who has worked extensively in mental health care and education I am acutely aware that what practitioners often want is clarity about their role identity and the tools and techniques to engage with service users, and work purposefully toward some shared meaningful goals. This three-part book has been structured in a considered way that directly addresses these needs. For instance an important element of professional identity is to understand the policy and psychosocial context of practice that guides our stance as practitioners. The first few chapters of Part 1 helpfully spell out UK policy development tracing its origins from the recovery narrative of the 1980's and the need for collaborative and jointly negotiated understanding of needs, wants and wishes, as well as strengths and abilities.

Achieving this is often easier said than done and so in Part 1 the reader is taken on a journey that examines the dimensions and holistic nature of psychosocial assessment. The aim ultimately is to develop a sophisticated case conceptualisation, which is examined in much more detail in Part 3. The authors admit that this can be a complex process but never shy away from their goal to provide clarity and help the reader navigate the challenges they are likely to encounter along the way.

Importantly there is consistency throughout all chapters on emancipatory and empowering approaches and the skills and values that facilitate assessments in partnership with service users. In practice there has been a tendency to resort to the use of rating scales to measure change without fully understanding their use and value. Whilst extremely useful, it is recognised that training in their use is required and so the authors provide helpful tips for achieving competence.

Part Two of the book looks more deeply into the process of psychosocial assessment and on understanding the person's history, their social and interpersonal world as well as their performance and confidence within it. There are always risks that any 'process' can become mechanistic and dehumanised and I found in reading this book there is consistency in the emphasis on the end goal, namely an accurate case conceptualisation. I particularly like the suggestion that the different elements of a full psychosocial assessment can, in themselves, be used as a therapeutic tool for building engagement, developing understanding and fostering hope. In other words, practitioners should never underestimate the opportunity that psychosocial assessment can bring.

A key tenet of the recovery approach is the emphasis on hope and I found this tone reflected throughout the book. One particular example was the examination of satisfaction and happiness and those techniques that can enable individuals to flourish and achieve meaning and purpose. Perhaps one of the most challenging aspects is effective risk assessment and resultant safety planning, in the areas of suicide and self-harm, self-neglect and violence. This is comprehensively addressed examining factors that reduce longer-term risks. Such risks are often exacerbated in the presence of alcohol and drugs and the chapter on substance misuse provides further useful guidance.

It was particularly pleasing to see an oft-neglected area being addressed, namely physical health. Those working in mental health have been criticised in the past for not attending to the physical health needs of people that use mental health services and there is welcome emphasis on health promotion factors that may undermine physical health, such as a lack of exercise, poor diet and smoking.

The need for positive and purposeful engagement is captured in Part 3 which reflects the culmination of the whole process, namely to identify goal statements that are personalised and meaningful and monitored and reviewed within a collaborative and creative relationship. The authors help the reader navigate the process of analysis and integration, case formulation, strengths and needs statements and goals that ultimately seek to make sense of the service user's experiences.

Whenever I am seeking a new text to recommend to my students, I have three basic requirements: is it written by experts who understand contemporary mental health care? Is it underpinned by evidence from research? Is it strongly rooted in recovery-oriented philosophy that reflects modern mental health care?

In this book the editors Steve Trenoweth and Nicki Moone have created a resource that easily meet all these requirements and captures the essence of effective psycho-social assessment. This text will assist mental health practitioners everywhere, to work alongside people with mental health problems in more deliberate, informed and purposeful ways.

PREFACE

As mental health practitioners we are charged with supporting people on their journey towards recovery. Regardless of our area of practice, we are committed to ensuring that service users are empowered to achieve optimal wellbeing and that services offer timely and effective care. As mental health practitioners by nature, we strive to ensure a person-centred approach that reflects a belief in the uniqueness of every person that we work with.

It has long been expected that we offer evidence-based practice to our service users and their families. The combination of clinical skill and best evidence available ensure that we are able to guarantee that service users are offered services to meet with expectation. Comprehensive assessment facilitates good-quality mental health care. Recent developments in mental health care advocate genuine collaboration with service users and their families with an emphasis on hope and optimism. Within the reality of the ever changing mental health care arena, comprehensive assessment is surely the building block upon which all care should be delivered.

In writing this book, we aim to illustrate how the principles, knowledge and techniques of psychosocial assessment in mental health care can complement the specialist skills and knowledge of mental health practitioners to deliver the best possible care.

Scope of this book

This book is intended to introduce psychosocial assessment in mental health. There are many books available on the use of psychosocial interventions in mental health but none that focus specifically on the process of assessments that will inform evidence-based interventions. As mental health practitioners we decided to explore this area in more detail to highlight the necessity of a robust assessment process to underpin and inform decision-making about how best to proceed. We have decided to focus on the service user journey from contact with services through to goal setting to guide the reader through a systematic approach to the assessment process. Although mental health practitioners are well rehearsed in the skill of broad mental health assessment, a challenge faced by many is developing an assessment process that makes best use of the evidence and uses a range of approaches to identify service user strengths and needs. Therefore, as the book progresses it will explore the assessment process from broad mental health assessment through to clarifying assessment strategies to provide the most accurate reflection of the service user's experience. The final chapters of the book will discuss how the information gathered during the assessment process can be drawn together to develop a case conceptualisation. The case conceptualisation helps develop a working hypothesis of the service user's experience, strengths and needs and is used to inform the plan of evidence based interventions.

To set the context of the book, the initial chapters provide an overview of assessment in mental health care and explore the approaches and methods that can be used to develop a robust assessment process. This section also includes the principles that underpin the selection of rating scales and assessment tools to ensure best use of the evidence available and to encourage critical understanding of the processes that underpin clinical decision making. Throughout the book we have tried to ensure that the text is clear and concise and we hope this will ensure that practitioners are more easily able to translate content into the real world of practice. To facilitate this further, we have included opportunities at the end of each chapter to explore and reflect on practice. We hope that by completing exercises at the end of each chapter, this will provoke exploration and adoption of different ways to undertake each phase of the assessment process.

The main body of the book focuses on psychosocial assessment in mental health care. The aim here is to build on the reader's existing understanding of the key concepts that underpin assessment. Simply put – to guide a path from presenting problem towards a comprehensive assessment that reflects collaboration with service users to facilitate their recovery journey. This section is drawn together by exploring mental well-being and strengths and is line with the philosophical underpinning of the book; the value that is placed on the uniqueness of the individual and an intention to promote optimal well-being.

The final section of the book explores methods to facilitate the process of analysing and integrating the information gleaned during the assessment process. These chapters use a case scenario to help guide the reader through the process of making sense of the wealth of information gathered and explores how to make best use of this to inform evidence-based interventions in line with service user priorities. It is hoped that the final chapters will help assimilate the knowledge garnered throughout previous chapters to develop a clear understanding of how and why a systematic approach to assessment can inform optimal treatment and intervention plans.

Foremost this book has been developed to be a practical guide for practitioners to add to their existing knowledge and skills in conducting mental health assessments. Our intention is to encourage critical appraisal of existing methods of mental health assessment and promote commitment to develop a systematic evidence-based approach to the assessment process. Throughout, the focus is on working in collaboration with a service user using a range of clinical skills and methods. Throughout the book attention has been given to language used to ensure that it reflects the real world of practice. Time and attention has likewise been given to ensure the accessibility of the book, no matter the clinical area of the mental health practitioner. In principle this book is a straightforward text which provides a practical guide to psychosocial assessment in mental health care.

Who is this book for?

This book is intended to be a core textbook for mental health practitioners who are both pre and post registration. Mental health care is delivered in a range of settings and our intention is that the book will meet with expectation of mental health practitioners in all settings and act as a guide to best practice. Each chapter provides an opportunity to explore the content within the reader's area of practice and it is hoped this will promote both reflection and transfer of new skills and knowledge to practice.

The material in the book is most relevant to mental health practitioners but may also act as a resource for allied health professionals working with service users who have mental health issues to provide an overview of areas that may need consideration.

This book provides an overview of the central concepts and techniques of psychosocial assessment in mental health care as relates specifically to use in practice. Its applied approach is designed to ensure that both pre and post registration mental health practitioners will be able to use the content to enhance and develop their practice.

How to use this book

This book outlines how to develop a systematic approach to psychosocial assessment in mental health care. The principles and methods that underpin practice are explored and opportunities are afforded in each chapter to explore the content within the context of practice. Each chapter builds on the last in order to provide you with a full understanding of the assessment process. However, if you have a particular interest in a chapter topic, that chapter may be read independently as you will be directed to related content in others which will enhance your understanding.

Each chapter uses a similar approach to helping you make sense of the content and has been written to ensure that application to practice lies at the core. The learning activities at the end of each chapter have been written specifically to encourage you to think more critically about your practice and to assimilate what you have learnt. Each chapter starts with a set of learning objectives detailing the knowledge you will gain from reading it. Chapters end with a simple summary of the main points for revision and a reflection activity to help you to apply your new knowledge to your practice.

The final section of the book uses a case scenario to highlight how to make best use of the assessment process. The case scenario illustrates the development of a case formulation and subsequent formulation of goals and treatment plans. You are also encouraged to consider how you can make best use of the information gathered during assessment in your own area of practice.

Technical words are highlighted in the text in **bold,** the definitions of which can be found in the glossary at the end of the book.

ACKNOWLEDGEMENTS

We would like to thank the many contributors to this book and in particular to the service-users who have offered their invaluable insights. We would also like to thank all at SAGE who have been unfailingly supportive.

Publisher's Acknowledgements

The publishers would also like to thank the following lecturers for their invaluable feedback on the proposal and draft chapters:

Ian Beech, University of South Wales, UK

Angie Chadwick, University of Salford, UK

Keith Ford, Northumbria University, UK

David Gaylard, University of Chichester, UK

Ian Mckay, UEA, UK

The authors and publishers are grateful to the following for their kind permission to reproduce material:

Table 1.1: National Institute for Health and Clinical Excellence (2011) *Service User Experience in Adult Mental Health Services*. Manchester: NICE. Available at: www. nice.org.uk/guidance/qs14

Table 11.2: VIA Classification of Character Strengths is copyright VIA Institute on Character, 2004–2017. Used with permission. All rights reserved. www.viacharacter.org

Table 11.3: Ed Diener, Robert A. Emmons, Randy J. Larsen and Sharon Griffin as noted in the 1985 article 'The Satisfaction with Life Scale', *Journal of Personality Assessment*, 49 (1): 71–5.

PART 1

THEORY AND PRACTICE OF PSYCHOSOCIAL ASSESSMENT IN MENTAL HEALTH CARE

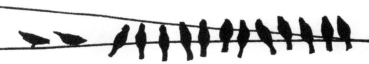

1

OVERVIEW OF ASSESSMENT IN MENTAL HEALTH CARE

STEVE TRENOWETH AND NICKI MOONE

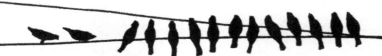

CHAPTER OVERVIEW

This chapter:

- Gives a contextual overview of psychosocial assessments in mental health care.
- Explores how psychosocial assessments can contribute to quality mental health care.
- Identifies the central features of, and professional skills needed for, a comprehensive assessment approach.
- Highlights how the **recovery approach** should underpin assessments by working in partnership and collaborating with service users and clients, an important aspect of contemporary mental health practice.

Introduction

Comprehensive assessment facilitates good-quality mental health care. Without knowing what a person's strengths and needs are, or at least might be, one is not in a position to offer appropriate help and support. In recent years, our ideas about how mental health care and support should be offered have been seen within the context of the recovery approach (National Institute for Mental Health in England, NIMHE, 2005). It is no longer acceptable to do *to* – we must now do *with*. This has considerable implications for any assessment process in terms of not only *what* is assessed but also actually *how* any assessment is conducted. The recovery approach emphasises the importance of a hopeful, optimistic positive approach to mental health care and treatment and of supporting people to live a life of personal value and worth. It also stresses the necessity for active involvement, collaboration and partnership working with mental health service users throughout all care processes, including assessment, in the context of a supportive and **empathic** professional relationship. It values negotiation and shared decision-making between service users and health care professionals, with the aim of supporting self-determination, self-advocacy and self-management by the development of resilience, self-esteem, optimism, a sense of mastery and control of one's life. In the context of psychosocial assessment, the recovery approach stresses a holistic view of the person and focuses on user-defined perceptions of their own strengths, needs and **goals**, recognising that individuals have personal strengths and abilities as well as needs (Department of Health, 2001; Future Vision Coalition, 2008; Jenkins et al., 2008).

EXPERT VOICE

❛ The challenge for the mental health practitioner is trying to meet the competing demands of the service with the expectations of service users and their families. In practice, we develop strategies that help us to manage large amounts of information and very quickly make decisions on how best to proceed. It is this ability that often comes at the cost of developing a systematic approach to assessment. In reality, we often complete a brief assessment based on minimal information and then move swiftly to intervention. Therefore, there is not enough detail to develop a shared understanding of what strengths, needs and priorities are. Without understanding these challenges, the mental health practitioner is likely to develop their own plans of care on behalf of an individual in line with what they believe should be the priority. ❜

The origins of the recovery approach can be found in the early writings of Patricia Deegan (1988) and the social recovery model described by Warner (1985). More recently, the work of the Centre for Mental Health (see, for example, the excellent *Making Recovery a Reality* by Shepherd et al., 2008) and the mental health service user movement in general have also been influential in the development of the approach.

There have also been a number of strategic policy initiatives that have endorsed the principles of the recovery approach, such as the now defunct NIMHE *Guiding Statement on Recovery* (2005), which have set the context for contemporary mental health care in England.

In 1999, the New Labour government set out its policy in the Department of Health's (1999) document, the *National Service Framework for Mental Health* (NSFMH), which sought to identify national service standards for mental health as part of an overall modernisation agenda, including: mental health promotion; access to primary care; delivering of effective services for people with severe mental illness; caring about carers; and preceding suicide (ibid.). Effective assessment and screening was seen as vital in ensuring that people were referred to appropriate services for advice, treatment and care and that the national standards were met. The strategy outlined the criteria that should be used in an effective, holistic assessment:

> Assessment should cover psychiatric, psychological and social functioning, risk to the individual and others, including previous violence and criminal record, any needs arising from co-morbidity, and personal circumstances including family or other carers, housing, financial and occupational status [and] physical health needs. (Ibid.: 43)

The NSFMH also recognised that mental health and social care services should be culturally competent and that assessments are enhanced in a multi-professional context and where a partnership exists between health and social care staff. The need for prompt assessments and subsequent treatment with vulnerable groups (such as prisoners and young people with the first signs of a psychotic illness) was also recognised (DH, 1999).

The replacement for the NSFMH proposed by the New Labour government, prior to the election of the Coalition government in 2010, was *New Horizons: Towards a Shared Vision for Mental Health* (DH, 2009). These proposals sought: to emphasise the need for preventing mental ill health, building individual and community resilience and promoting mental health; to integrate physical health and mental wellbeing; early intervention; to tackle stigma and promote social inclusion; and the delivery of personalised care with a focus on recovery and ensuring that care is based on an individual's wishes and needs (ibid.).

In 2011, the Coalition government built on the proposals outlined in *New Horizons* in their mental health strategy for England, *No Health without Mental Health* (DH, 2011). The strategy takes a **life-course approach**:

> recognising that the foundations for lifelong wellbeing are already being laid down before birth, and that there is much we can do to protect and promote wellbeing and resilience through our early years, into adulthood and then on into a healthy old age. (Ibid.: 2)

The strategy also seeks to empower mental health service users – 'no decision about me without me' (ibid.: 3) – to have more of a say about their care and treatment, including choice of provider. Emphasis is also placed on measurable quality outcomes (rather than process targets) and on the freedom for mental health services to innovate and improve the quality of services.

The role of the National Institute for Health and Care Excellence (NICE) is strengthened in the 2011 strategy, as, too, are the quality standards developed by NICE to support the delivery of care, inform commissioning decisions and underpin service inspection (DH, 2010, 2011). For example, the recent NICE Clinical Guideline (CG136) *Service User Experience in Adult Mental Health: Improving the Experience of Care for People Using Adult NHS Mental Health Services* (NICE, 2011) outlines a number of quality statements as listed in Table 1.1. Emphasis in these standards is placed on collaborative working with service users, and on shared decision-making. During the assessment phase, this collaboration should reveal a joint and negotiated understanding of the service user's perceived needs, wants and wishes, and also details of their strengths and abilities.

Table 1.1   Quality standards developed by NICE, 2011

	Quality Statements
1	People using mental health services, and their families or carers, feel optimistic that care will be effective.
2	People using mental health services, and their families or carers, feel they are treated with empathy, dignity and respect.
3	People using mental health services are actively involved in shared decision-making and supported in self-management.
4	People using community mental health services are normally supported by staff from a single, multidisciplinary community team, familiar to them and with whom they have a continuous relationship.
5	People using mental health services feel confident that the views of service users are used to monitor and improve the performance of services.
6	People can access mental health services when they need them.
7	People using mental health services understand the assessment process, their diagnosis and treatment options, and receive emotional support for any sensitive issues.
8	People using mental health services jointly develop a care plan with mental health and social care professionals, and are given a copy with an agreed date to review it.
9	People using mental health services who may be at risk of crisis are offered a crisis plan.
10	People accessing crisis support have a comprehensive assessment, undertaken by a professional competent in crisis working.
11	People in hospital for mental health care, including service users formally detained under the Mental Health Act, are routinely involved in shared decision-making.
12	People in hospital for mental health care have daily one-to-one contact with mental health care professionals known to the service user and regularly see other members of the multidisciplinary mental health care team.
13	People in hospital for mental health care can access meaningful and culturally appropriate activities 7 days a week, not restricted to 9 a.m. to 5 p.m.
14	People in hospital for mental health care are confident that control and restraint, and compulsory treatment including rapid tranquillisation, will be used competently, safely and only as a last resort with minimum force.
15	People using mental health services feel less stigmatised in the community and NHS, including within mental health services.

Acknowledgement: National Institute for Health and Care Excellence, *Service User Experience in Adult Mental Health: Improving the Experience of Care for People Using Adult NHS Mental Health Services*. Manchester: NICE, 2011. Available at: https://www.nice.org.uk/guidance/qs14

What is a Psychosocial Assessment for?

A psychosocial assessment in mental health care seeks to illuminate and clarify the strengths and needs of an individual as a prelude to setting personally meaningful goals. This will, in turn, support the negotiation of individualised care plans, bespoke intervention and treatment options and of measuring the success of such interventions in meeting an individual's **personal recovery outcomes** (see, for example, Ion et al., 2013).

As we have seen from the discussion above, an assessment is an activity that must be done *with* an individual – that is, in keeping with the recovery approach, it must be a person-centred and collaborative process. To this end, the NICE Clinical Guideline 136 (2011; and Table 1.1) highlights another important feature of modern mental health care, that of self-management. By this, we mean the process by which individuals are empowered and supported to take charge of their own care and to recognise when care and treatment may be needed. This is a central feature of crisis management – people recognising an impending emergency and then taking steps to mitigate its impact. In order to facilitate this, mental health assessments should be clear, transparent and instructive. This will help individuals to learn from their experience and recognise both their needs and also their strengths (and how to identify them) in overcoming issues and capitalising on their abilities.

SERVICE USER VOICE

An assessment should be a shared understanding of what is happening for the service user and should be between them, the practitioner, family and anyone else who is involved with the service user. It is crucial that the service user is helped to build on their strengths and that the practitioner understands the different ways that this can be done and in light of the service user's own learning styles. Assessment is not a solitary piece of work, completed and never seen again. Assessment can be used repeatedly to reiterate and determine areas of need and strengths and skills. It is part of a process and not an activity. My understanding is that assessment is often the first step that should help develop meaningful plans; you cannot decide what is the most important thing to concentrate on if you have not looked at everything that affects you. Finally, recovery means different things to us all: perhaps thinking about recovery as a way of acknowledging difficulties and being able to live your life and fulfil your dreams is what we all strive for.

The recovery approach is also about moving beyond the medical/biological dimension of the person, important though this is, to an understanding of the *whole* person. As a consequence, in contemporary mental health care, assessments should be *holistic* and *comprehensive*, encompassing all dimensions of the *self* – from the physical, to the psychological and emotional, to the social and spiritual. This is, indeed, a complex process, as there will also need to be a consideration of the interplay between each of these dimensions.

There are, of course, important elements of shared expertise in this assessment approach (DH, 2001). While service users, their families and carers will have considerable expertise in the experience of the individual, mental health professionals will need to use their clinical expertise and must also be equipped with the latest evidence base. This is an important resource to be drawn upon when negotiating understandings about an individual's current problems, and when collaborating with other members of the multi-professional team on decisions about the way forward in helping the person improve the quality of their lives.

The Assessment Process

While a holistic and comprehensive assessment is likely to be complex, the process itself should be systematic. That is, the assessment process should start off by exploring the current issues that a person is facing (see Chapter 4), before moving on to develop a deeper, shared understanding of the problem(s). This deeper understanding will encompass a number of key areas (see Figure 1.1 and Chapters 5 through to 11 for further information) and there is no particular order in which they should be conducted:

- *Presenting Problem*: the **presenting problem** will include an initial understanding or conceptualisation of the person's current issues (stressors that may have triggered the problem, factors which have aggravated and maintained the problem, along with factors which help to alleviate the problem) and a review of current treatments. It is vital that the assessment captures the service user's understanding of their current troubles.
- *Social and Environmental Context*: Including the person's family life, current relationships, working relationships, and overall social and vocational functioning. This also includes consideration of the environmental and community context of the individual.
- *Physical Health*: Co-morbid physical health problems should be considered, along with the impact of the mental health need on the individual's current functioning.
- *History*: The person's history may have increased their vulnerability to mental distress and needs to be understood by the assessor, as this may contribute to the ongoing difficulties the service user might be experiencing. Central to this theme is the consideration of factors which may also have previously assisted and supported the client which can be used in the present to support their individual journey to their recovery.
- *Mental State Examination*: A mental state examination will be needed and this will include an individual's appearance and behaviour; speech and language; emotional and mood state; thought and thinking processes; cognition; and the individual's ability to organise and regulate information, along with their insight, problem-solving, decision-making, judgement and planning.
- *Risk Assessment*: Safety is a vital part of assessments in mental health care. A risk assessment for adults must cover, as a minimum, the most common types of risk in mental health care, namely violence, suicide, self-harm and self-neglect.

- *Substance Use*: The possibility of a co-morbid and concurrent substance misuse issue must also be considered in any assessment. An assessment must catalogue the individual's pattern, and extent, of their usage (if any), and possible links to risks must be considered.
- *Strengths and Abilities*: Psychosocial assessments must consider not only the difficulties that a person may be facing in their lives, but also the skills, talents, abilities and assets that help them to cope and manage their current troubles. Assessments must consider the individual's mental well-being and overall satisfaction with life.

It is likely that a variety of different assessment approaches, techniques and methods will be used in the assessment process (including interview, direct observation, questionnaires, **psychometric tools** and rating scales, **self-report** measures, clinical screening and physiological assessments and so on (see Chapters 2 and 3 for more details) in order to explore and gain a deeper and triangulated understanding of the need. However, it is unlikely that all the information required for a comprehensive assessment will be obtained in one session.

There is an associated challenge for mental health professionals here – that is, how to render meaningful the large quantity of assessment data which is likely to be accumulated in this process. The process of analysing assessment information is complex. This includes how to organise and make judgements about assessment data, and

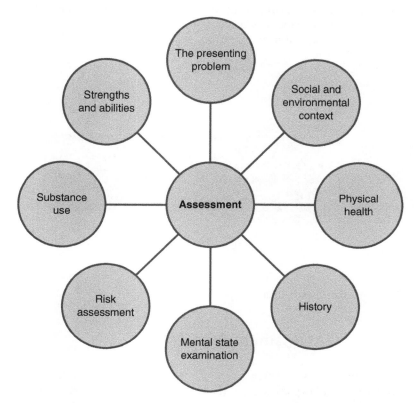

Figure 1.1   An overview of psychosocial assessment in mental health

identifying themes and conceptualising needs in order to build a coherent story of the service user's current experiences. People may present with multiple and complex needs, which may be interrelated, and one of the most important challenges here is to be able to understand and clarify not only the needs but also their strengths and abilities. This process is known as a **case conceptualisation,** where mental health professionals offer structured feedback in order to facilitate a shared understanding and develop a working hypothesis of the need (see Chapter 12 for further information). A case conceptualisation summarises assessment information with an aim of developing a clearer understanding of the issue(s) in order to identify and prioritise needs. This is especially helpful where there are many multiple and complex issues. Crucially, this process helps to collate, organise and summarise information in a way that facilitates communication with service users and other members of the multi-professional team.

A **needs statement** is formulated to clearly illuminate an aspect of the service user's current troubles but it is also important to identify strengths, talents and abilities, which protects the person from harm and which the person can draw on to support their recovery (see Chapters 11 and 13 for further information). This facilitates discussion and affords agreement and shared understandings with the service user. Once a need has been clearly identified, then action can be taken to identify ways to address issues.

These actions are summarised in a **goal statement** (see Chapter 14 for further information). Goal statements are those that clearly identify, prioritise and define personal goals and how any potential obstacles may be identified and overcome. In supporting the achievement of a goal, mental health and non-mental health resources (such as friends, contacts and organisations) may be identified that are supportive of, and relevant to, the achievement of an individual's goals.

The process is summarised in Figure 1.2.

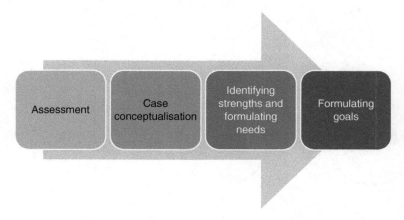

Figure 1.2   The assessment process

Supporting the Assessment Process

The assessment process is complex and there needs to be support for the assessor at both the individual and organisational level. Assessors should have access to clinical supervision, where they can discuss assessments they have undertaken, so as to check for accuracy and to discuss complex cases and resolve therapeutic stalls in the process. There will also need to be organisational and management support for the sort of assessment discussed above, through the use of policies and ring-fenced time and space. Comprehensive and holistic assessments, grounded in a recovery approach, are likely to be more involved and time-consuming than a medical, symptom-based assessment. However, such assessments are also likely to be more revealing and more helpful in identifying an individual's needs and wishes, and thus more supportive of their personal journey to recovery.

SERVICE USER VOICE

‘ Mental health care is changing all the time: the idea of recovery has replaced the older approaches of just looking at symptoms and not thinking about living life. The recovery approach is based on giving the service user a sense of hope and supporting someone to have a quality of life which is meaningful to them and their family. Recovery is the service user's journey, in which the aim is to reach their full potential and be able to live, cope with and manage their illness and mental health conditions. Recovery will have a different meaning to each individual. For some, recovery will be being completely symptom free, where for others, recovery may be being able to get out of bed in the morning or being able to return to work.

Mental health practitioners need to understand what the service user thinks their recovery is and also share how they, as the practitioner, will help and support this. There is a lot of focus on recovery at the moment and this needs to be more about words: some practitioners still seem to not really understand the recovery philosophy. ’

Chapter Summary

In this chapter, we have given a contextual overview of comprehensive and holistic assessment in mental health care. Psychosocial assessments in mental health care should be collaborative, recovery-focused and person-centred. Personal and professional skills of rapport-building and engagement facilitate the assessment process. Assessments must be comprehensive, holistic and systematic, and are likely to take into consideration a number of factors, including: the presenting problem; social and environmental factors; physical health; history; mental state examination; risk assessment; substance use; and strengths. This facilitates the shared understanding of development of a case conceptualisation, bringing clarity to the person's need(s) and strengths statements, and the setting of goals.

Assessments must contribute to quality care and we have identified the central features of, and professional skills needed for, a comprehensive and collaborative assessment approach. The recovery approach should underpin psychosocial assessments by working in partnership and collaborating with service users and clients, an important aspect of contemporary mental health practice.

EXERCISE

1. Using the references at the end of this chapter, explore how mental health policy has influenced care delivery. Read *No Health without Mental Health* (DH, 2011; available at: www.gov.uk/government/uploads/system/uploads/attachment_data/file/213761/ dh_124058.pdf) and then consider the impact that this strategy may have on how contemporary mental health assessments should be undertaken.

CONSIDERATIONS FOR PRACTICE

1. How should the recovery approach influence the assessment process?
2. What preparation does the assessor need to undertake prior to beginning the assessment process?
3. How might the assessor engage with an individual who appears reluctant to collaborate on an assessment?

Further Reading

Barker, P. (2004) *Assessment in Psychiatric and Mental Health Nursing: In Search of the Whole Person*. Cheltenham: Nelson Thornes.

A comprehensive book that clearly makes the case for holism. Barker reminds us that, while technical knowledge and skills in mental health care are important, it is the interpersonal nature of professional caring relationships that facilitates the assessment process.

Nelson-Jones, R. (2014) *Practical Counselling and Helping Skills*, 6th edn. London: Sage.

An excellent and comprehensive guide to counselling and helping skills. Nelson-Jones reminds us of the core skills which are needed to relate to and understand an individual during the assessment process, and as a prelude to offering interventions and support.

Rogers, C. (1951) *Client-Centered Therapy*. London: Constable.

An important and still relevant book that establishes the humanistic nature of the professional helping relationship in mental health care. Rogers reminds us that the goal of helping is not the data that we accumulate through the assessment process, but that this is a means to support the personal road to their recovery, and it is the support of the individual which is the ultimate aim of mental health care.

Shepherd, S., Boardman, J. and Slade, M. (2008) *Making Recovery a Reality*. London: Sainsbury Centre for Mental Health.

An excellent and key resource that outlines, clearly and concisely, the principles and practice of the recovery approach. This work also identified the barriers and resistance to the implementation of this approach and how they may be overcome.

References

Deegan, P.E. (1988) 'Recovery: the lived experience of rehabilitation', *Psychosocial Rehabilitation Journal*, 9 (4): 11–19.

Department of Health (1999) *National Service Framework for Mental Health*. London: DH.

Department of Health (2001) *The Expert Patient: A New Approach to Chronic Disease Management for the 21st Century*. London: DH. Available at: http://webarchive.national archives.gov.uk/+/www.dh.gov.uk/en/Publicationsandstatistics/Publications/Publications PolicyandGuidance/DH_4006801 (accessed 10 January 2016).

Department of Health (2009) *New Horizons: Towards a Shared Vision for Mental Health*. London: DH.

Department of Health (2010) *Equity and Excellence: Liberating the NHS*. London: DH.

Department of Health (2011) *No Health without Mental Health: A Cross-Government Mental Health Outcomes Strategy for People of All Ages*. London: DH.

Future Vision Coalition (2008) *A New Vision for Mental Health*, Discussion Paper. Available at: www.centreformentalhealth.org.uk/publications/future_vision_for_mh.aspx?ID=673 (accessed 10 January 2016).

Ion, R., Monger, B., Hardie, S., Henderson, N. and Cumming, J. (2013) 'A tool to measure progress and outcome in recovery', *British Journal of Mental Health Nursing*, 2 (4): 56–60.

Jenkins, R., Meltzer, H., Jones, P., Brugha, T., Bebbington, P., Farrell, M., Crepaz-Keay, D. and Knapp, M. (2008) *Foresight Mental Capital and Wellbeing Project: Mental Health: Future Challenges*. London: Government Office for Science.

National Institute for Health and Care Excellence (NICE) (2011) *Service User Experience in Adult Mental Health: Improving the Experience of Care for People Using Adult NHS Mental Health Services*, NICE Clinical Guideline 136 [CG136]. Available at: http://publications.nice. org.uk/service-user-experience-in-adult-mental-health-improving-the-experience-of-care-for-people-using-cg136 (accessed 2 February 2016).

National Institute for Mental Health in England (NIMHE) (2005) *NIMHE Guiding Statement on Recovery*. London: DH. Available at: http://studymore.org.uk/nimherec.pdf (accessed 10 January 2016).

Rogers, C. (1951) *Client-Centered Therapy*. London: Constable.

Shepherd, S., Boardman, J. and Slade, M. (2008) *Making Recovery a Reality*. London: Sainsbury Centre for Mental Health.

Warner, R. (1985) *Recovery from Schizophrenia: Psychiatry and Political Economy*. London: Routledge and Kegan Paul.

2

ASSESSMENT APPROACHES AND METHODS

STEVE TRENOWETH, REUBEN PEARCE AND NICKI MOONE

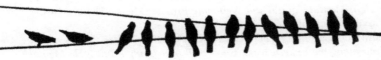

CHAPTER OVERVIEW

This chapter:

- Gives an overview of the different approaches to comprehensive and holistic assessment in mental health care.
- Explores how assessments can contribute to quality care.
- Identifies the central features of, and professional skills needed for, a comprehensive assessment approach.
- Shows how the recovery approach should underpin assessments by working in partnership and collaborating with service users, an important aspect of contemporary mental health practice.

Introduction

The purpose of any assessment approach is to help the individual convey and narrate their current experiences. There are, of course, many challenges with this and however we may try, psychosocial assessments in mental health care are not neutral or objective. They reflect the experiences, understanding, motivations and biases of the mental health service user and, in turn, the experiences, understanding, motivations and biases of the assessor. And we can never really fully or completely appreciate another's experience as if we were that person – the best that we can hope for is an understanding that is a close approximation of their experience. Assessments, then, must be approached with a degree of humility and an understanding that such assessments can never be considered definitive. They must be revisited and revised over time, particularly when new information or insights into a person's experience come to light.

Skills and Values Needed for Assessment

Assessment is a skilled process, requiring considerable technical knowledge and skill that aims to support a person to convey a meaningful narration of their experience. There are therapeutic skills that are needed to ensure a person-centred approach, and' to promote engagement and develop rapport, and to facilitate and guide discussions. These encompass core skills of agenda setting, communication, **active listening**, using reflective statements, questioning, boundary setting, affirmation and summarising (see below). The assessor will also need attention to detail, and be able to analyse and synthesise complex information. Skills of negotiation and collaboration with service users and the multi-professional team will also be needed.

SERVICE USER VOICE

'In order to ensure that the service user is able to feel that they are an essential part of the process of assessment they will need support in managing their current difficulties and in living a fulfilling life. It is my experience that not all practitioners have the same skills or interest in the assessment process and the information that can be derived. Sometimes practitioners' priorities can come into play, ranging from pressure from the organisation, their feelings towards the service user, through to their own stress and difficulties. Practitioners need to understand the issues that affect their judgement and be honest about this. By doing this, the focus can remain on what should be focused on and a genuine commitment to collaborative work with the service user can be had. Service users should also be self-aware and if this is not possible, the practitioner should gently help facilitate this.

There are also personal skills and qualities that the mental health professional needs to demonstrate as part of the assessment process. The assessor will need to have warmth, patience and perseverance and demonstrate a willingness to hear the person's story. They should convey a hopeful and optimistic attitude and be both personally reflective and **reflexive**. Rogers (1951) identified a person-centred approach to counselling, and the qualities needed to facilitate this process. In particular, he identified three central features:

- **Empathy** –Developing an understanding of the service user's point of view.
- **Congruence** – Being a genuine person.
- **Unconditional positive regard** – Acceptance and being non-judgemental.

EXPERT VOICE

❝ To be a mental health practitioner in health care services today requires a range of values, skills and attributes which enable a person to be able to provide the highest standard of care. Traditional nursing values, including being caring, compassionate and empathetic, are the core qualities that a mental health practitioner should possess. To be able to care for people with mental health issues should be seen as a privilege, and those in this role should embody values such as respect and inclusion of all people, irrespective of their religious, cultural and ethnic group, gender and age. In an ever-changing health care service, those in mental health settings should also be able to serve as a visionary for the future, to improve practice and service provisions, to be part of innovations in order to help change services for the better and to be able to provide ❞ a high standard of care.

There are also professional values that are needed to underpin any helping relationship in modern mental health care, and these are guided by ethical codes and guidelines issued by relevant professional bodies. Such values will include empathy and compassion, ethical values and moral principles and the requirement to treat people with dignity and respect. Crucially, the assessor must: approach an assessment with an open mind; possess a desire to reflect on their own practice; have a degree of self-awareness, and a willingness to recognise how their own biases and misunderstandings may lead to subjectivity in the assessment process.

Essential Communication Skills for Assessment

Undertaking an assessment in mental health care requires an ability to communicate effectively. Without effective communication, it is unlikely that any collaborative discourse will occur. Poor communication can hinder the formation of a therapeutic alliance, of which assessment is a crucial part. In fact, poor communication alongside a lack of self-awareness can even lead to a misinterpretation of someone's experiences. So, the skills needed in order to be an effective assessor are: excellent facilitative communication skills; a desire and an ability to develop positive relationships with service users and their families and friends; and a degree of self-awareness through reflective and reflexive practice.

A practitioner who is demonstrating high-quality active listening skills can sometimes begin to help someone who is distressed to feel better based on the use of those skills alone (Kagan and Evans, 1995). Active listening demonstrates to the person that you can appreciate what their difficulties mean to them as an individual. Active listening is more than just demonstrating patience and hearing. It involves a range of skills that can be developed by the practitioner's toolkit for communicating and

relating. Appropriate use of body language, minimal verbal interaction and the art of using the power of silence where appropriate are key components to active listening.
There are three essential active listening skills:

- Appropriate use of silence.
- Minimal verbal interruption.
- Demonstrating active listening through body language.

Such skills, effectively demonstrated, can provide the person with a safe emotional space to think and talk (McCabe and Timmins, 2013). As Rollnick et al. argue: 'A few words carefully chosen, delivered slowly and respectfully, are worth more than many mouthfuls of busy talk' (1999: 33). That is, there is a value to choosing words carefully and in a considered way that facilitates, rather than hinders, the person's narration of their experience. It also provides the practitioner time to reflect and consider their verbal interaction so that it is appropriate, constructive and person-centred. Silence can make the practitioner uncomfortable and feel the need to fill the silence with words which can often be unnecessary and be more about the uncomfortable feeling with the silence, rather than what the person experiencing distress is feeling (Stein-Parbury, 2005).

Types of Assessments

Often, when we are meeting someone for the first time, or when we do not have a clear understanding of the person, we will need to undertake a broad and holistic scoping of the person's current experience. This is the start of what is frequently referred to as a **funnelling approach**, where one starts with initial, broad, opening questions before moving on to probe a specific issue in more depth through detailed questioning. It is vital that, at first, a complete, wide-ranging and holistic assessment is undertaken to enable a full understanding of each individual. If we focus too early on the specific areas, the individual's experience may become 'fractured' and the global picture is lost. As such, other areas that may impact on, or be related to, the perceived primary need may be unknown, ignored or go unmet.

Global Assessments

Global assessments provide an initial framework for a broad understanding of the person's current experiences and encompass all aspects of the biological, social, psychological and even spiritual self. Any health care problem, whether this is primarily psychological or physical in nature, can impact on our holistic health and functioning. Global assessments must reveal the person's subjective understanding of their current difficulties and how this interconnects with, and subsequently affects, the totality of their lives.

For example, a problem we are facing can impact on our personal and interpersonal world and our experiences within it, from our social life (such as our personal and intimate relationships, finances, work, leisure and so on) to our psychological health (such as our perceptions of our on **self-efficacy** and confidence, and beliefs about our selves and others, including our self-esteem). This can impact our emotional well-being as the person may experience fear, stress, distress and uncertainty about the course that their disorder may take (Sin and Trenoweth, 2010). That is, it is important to understand the individual's perception of their own health, particularly that which is ongoing, long term or resistant to treatment.

There are many examples of such global assessments – one is undertaken by asking a simple question: 'How are you?' or 'How are you feeling today?' Other examples of more structured assessments of health and social care needs use rating scales (such as the Camberwell Assessment of Need; see Phelan et al., 1995) or global assessments of symptomatology – such as the **Brief Psychiatric Rating Scale (BPRS)** (Overall and Gorham, 1988; also see Chapter 3).

Clarifying Assessments

Once an issue or area of need has been identified from the global assessment, this can be clarified and explored more fully by careful and elaborative questioning so as to pursue the topic or line of thinking in more detail. This is known as a **clarifying assessment**. This also reinforces the issue and encourages contemplation.

There are many questioning techniques that can be used to encourage elaboration and to clarify the person's current needs. For instance:

- Asking for a specific example (e.g. 'for example', 'such as …').
- Asking for clarification (e.g. 'how much', 'when', 'in what way?').
- Use verbal and non-verbal prompts (e.g. 'anything else?', 'what else?', 'can you tell me more about that?').

Specific rating scales can also be used to clarify a person's meaning and to explore their experiences in greater depth (see Chapter 3). For example:

- Beck Depression Inventory (BDI-II) (Beck et al., 1996)
- Beck Anxiety Inventory (BAI) (Beck et al., 1993)
- **Beliefs About Voices Questionnaire (BAVQ)** (Chadwick et al., 2000)
- Positive and Negative Symptom Scale (PANSS) (Kay et al., 1987)
- **Social Functioning Scale (SFS)** (Birchwood et al., 1990)

The Assessment Interview

Whatever approach is taken, all assessments need to be facilitated within the context of an interview. Interviewing is a complex and highly skilled task that is designed to help the person to share their experiences verbally. In structuring an assessment interview, a number of key issues need to be considered (see Figure 2.1).

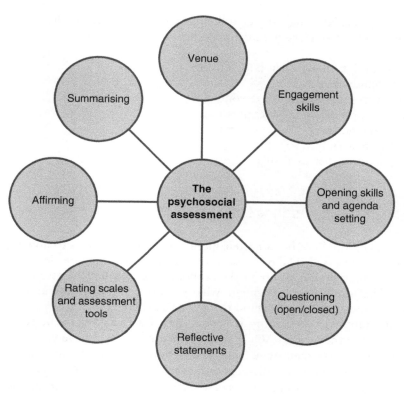

Figure 2.1   The psychosocial assessment

Venue

Before any assessment, consideration needs to be given to the arena within which it will take place, that is, the venue. The venue should be a comfortable and welcoming environment, private and quiet, free from distractions, as this is conducive to developing a collaborative therapeutic alliance. Consideration must be given to the safety of both the service user and assessor, in line with service policies and practice.

Engagement Skills

The best interviews are conversational in style, and seek to put the person at ease. The interviewer should be supportive and reassuring, adopting a quiet, curious tone to encourage talk. Time must be taken to establish a psychologically safe environment within which the person is open and willing to share their experiences without fear. It is important to consider how one's dress, grooming and appearance impact on engagement.

Nelson-Jones (2003) suggests the following to demonstrate to others that you are ready and willing to engage with them in a helping relationship:

- Adopt a relaxed and open body posture.
- Lean slightly forward.
- Use appropriate gaze and eye contact.
- Convey appropriate facial expressions.
- Use 'good' gestures.
- Use touch sparingly.
- Be sensitive to personal space.

Opening Skills and Agenda Setting

Introductions should not be forgotten, along with clarification as to how the person wishes to be addressed. The purpose of the assessment should be clearly explained to the individual. Be honest about the agenda. Explain what the assessment is and how it will be administered. Highlight what you hope to understand and how it will help health care staff to understand the person's experience.

It is important to stress that this is a collaborative activity and the person must feel fully involved in the process. While you, as the assessor, will have your agenda, the service user may have their own, equally important, agenda and you must establish if there is anything that the individual wishes to discuss first. Questions or concerns about the assessment should be answered clearly and directly. Permission to talk and to undertake the assessment should be sought, along with reassurances that the person can bring the interview to a close whenever they wish. A time limit for the assessment should be clearly established and strictly adhered to.

For example:

- 'Hello, my name is Simon. Is it OK if I chat to you? ...'
- 'I have something I would appreciate the chance of talking to you about. It would take about 20 minutes. Would that be OK?' ...'
- '... is there anything you feel we should talk about first? ...'
- '... I would appreciate the opportunity of discussing with you what you feel your current needs are. I have an assessment tool which will help us. I wonder if we could talk about this?'
- 'If it's not convenient to talk to you now, could I have a chat with you later?'

Questioning

Questioning is another key skill that you must develop in order to facilitate successful assessments. Questioning is the main way of getting the information we need. It is important to strike a balance between asking enough questions so that the service user is feeling listened to, but not so many that an intervention begins to feel like an interrogation.

Interviews vary in terms of the amount of structure. Commonly, semi-structured questioning is used to structure an assessment interview. Thought should be given to the phrasing and sequencing of the question, and the interviewer needs to be attuned to the emotional impact of the questions on the individual and the degree to which the questioning makes the person feel comfortable. Checking for understanding and clarifications should be sought on both sides in order to minimise the possibility of misunderstandings.

Throughout an assessment interview, appropriate communication skills should be used to encourage the individual to 'tell their personal story'. While it is likely that specific questioning will form an integral part of any interview, it is also vital to ensure that people are able to present their problems as stories and that this has led to a 'narrative-based approach', which helps the person to describe (and the interviewer to understand) their experiences (Launer, 2002). One such useful approach, used in **motivational interviewing** (Miller and Rollnick, 2012), facilitates and structures the individual's sharing of their frame of reference and is that of the 'typical day' strategy. Here, the service user is asked to conversationally describe a usual or common day in their life, and to annotate how their health status, problem/ need or condition impacts on this (Rollnick et al., 1999).

Typically, questions used in interviews are *open* or *closed*.

Open Questions

Open questions are very important, particularly in the initial stages of an interaction. An example of a good open question to begin an interaction could be (after initial introductions): 'Can you tell me what has brought you here today?' An open question will very often start with a 'Can you tell me about' or 'How', 'What', 'Where', 'When', 'In what way.' These questions are not at all specific, giving the service user the opportunity to respond in a variety of different ways. Open questions give the service user the opportunity to tell their story and can provide a lot of information that can easily be missed if closed 'yes' or 'no' questions are used straightaway (Dickson and Hargie, 2006). An open question provides the service user with the opportunity to talk about their own individual experience of the issue, rather than it becoming about the practitioner making their own subjective interpretation. This can reduce the practitioner's influence on the direction of the service user's response and can also demonstrate that they have time to listen, which can help in building rapport.

Open questions can provide broad information around the information required. The practitioner can then clarify points and elicit some specific information based on some of the content in the broad response from the service user. The practitioner can then move on to using slightly more focused open-ended questions. An example of this might be that a service user, when responding to the practitioner's open questions, mentions that they have had a lot of difficulty with relationships. The practitioner might ask a focused question such as: 'You mentioned that you are having some difficulty with relationships, can you tell me a bit more about this?'

Closed Questions

Closed questions are used to get a very specific response. This might be to gain a crucial piece of information once a service user has talked openly. For example, in trying to understand a person's feelings prior to a recent suicide attempt, the practitioner might ask them whether they intended to end their own life or not. Another example might be in the case of the service user who is depressed, malnourished and has said that they are lacking appetite, the practitioner might then ask: 'When did you last eat?', 'Did you manage to finish your meal?' or 'Have you ever felt like this before?'

Closed questioning can be extremely useful in interactions when the person is unable to engage for any length of time due to their current mental state. Service users who are struggling to process their thoughts may find it easier to respond to simple 'yes' or 'no' questions. At the other extreme, closed questioning may be helpful with someone who is excitable and over-stimulated and who may find it difficult to concentrate on, or respond to, open questions because their thoughts are racing.

EXPERT VOICE

'If you reflect on many of your own interactions, you can probably assume that you make a lot of decisions over whether you like someone or not very quickly, often within seconds or minutes of meeting them. This demonstrates how much first impressions count and it is therefore important that you work hard on those initial rapport-building stages of your interactions with people who are emotionally distressed. When a person is mentally distressed, some basic communication skills that people value when they meet people for the first time can be lost – such as a warm smile and non-verbal acknowledgement. This may be due to personal anxiety about how to manage the situation. Setting the scene for an interaction is crucial when working with mental distress. Remembering to introduce yourself, your role, why your are there, offering a warm smile, offering eye contact and giving careful consideration to your opening statement can really make the difference to the success of the intervention. Remember to be reading for verbal/non-verbal communication cues as you enter into the room to greet the person. 'How are you today?' with a big smile may not always be an appropriate greeting for somebody who is extremely depressed, agitated or angry! In this case, it may be more appropriate to start the consultation with an empathic statement such as: 'I can see that you are very distressed, thanks for taking the time to see me.' You can also introduce yourself and verbalise your observation by saying: 'I can see that you are very upset. I am here to see if there is something I can do to help you.'

Reflective Statements

Simple reflective statements can be very powerful in encouraging and supporting talk. It also encourages the person to consider and pursue a particular line of thinking when sharing their experiences. There are three core types of reflective statements: repeating, rephrasing and paraphrasing.

Repeating

That is, simply repeating what the service user has said. For example:

Service User:　'I'm so angry at being in this state. Nobody ever listens to me ...'
Interviewer:　　'You are angry that nobody ever listens to you ...'

Rephrasing

Expressing the remark in a slightly different way using synonyms. For example:

Service User: 'I'm so angry at being in this state. Nobody ever listens to me ...'
Interviewer: 'It seems to you that no one hears what you are saying ...'

Paraphrasing

The meaning of the service user's remark is inferred and reflected back. A good para-phrase can provide reflections, and underlying meanings/emotions, that are clearer and more succinct than the original statements (Nelson-Jones, 2003). However, a paraphrase should not be a guess, but a statement based on a deep understanding of the person's current position. It should be expressed tentatively, and the service user should be given the opportunity to confirm or deny the paraphrase. For example:

Service User: 'I'm so angry at being in this state. Nobody ever listens to me ...'
Interviewer: 'You feel that you would like to be able to make more decisions about your life ...'

It is also possible to use reflective statements *selectively*. This technique involves focusing on a significant aspect of the person's behaviour and reflecting this back, using selective repeating, rephrasing or paraphrasing. This encourages the pursuit and clarification of a particular line of thinking. For example:

Service User: 'I worry that I drink too much. It helps me cope with my pain.'
Interviewer: 'Your drinking worries you'.
Service User: 'Yes, it does worry me. It's probably time I stopped. I'm still in pain, anyway.'
Interviewer: 'You feel alcohol is not controlling your pain. This worries you and you feel that it's time that you gave up drinking.'

Rating Scales and Assessment Tools

Rating Scales and assessment tools are another way of assessing an individual's expe-rience (see Chapter 3). Typically, they are questionnaires or inventories (or psychometric tests) and are often used to quantify a person's experience. They ask a series of questions, usually in survey form, about a general or particular experience, and ask the rater(s) to assign a value to it. In this way, rating scales are structured ways of asking people to give specific responses to predetermined questions. Examples include symptom-focused rating scales of mental state as mentioned above, such as Beck Depression Inventory (Beck et al., 1996); assessments of physical health, such as pain inventories (e.g. Cleeland, 2009); and personality assessments (e.g. Minnesota Multiphasic Personality Inventory (MMPI); see Hathaway and McKinley, 1940).

Data gathered from such numerical rating scales or tests can be **ordinal** (which refers to the rank ordering of data, such as establishing preferences amongst a choice of options); nominal (a fixed number of categories or possibilities, such as 'yes' or 'no', gender, ethnicity, blood type); ratio (where each unit of a scale is equivalent but where there is not a meaningful zero point, such as a Likert rating scales, which allows people to express how much they agree or disagree with a particular statement); or interval (as with interval data but with a zero point, such as height).

Affirming

Affirming statements are a way of demonstrating an empathic understanding, recognition and acknowledgement of the difficulties the person is experiencing or has experienced. Such statements are a means of providing direct, genuine support and encouragement but they can sound insincere or even patronising if you are not being genuine. This is a core element of a **normalising rationale** (see Chapter 4). Examples of affirming statements include:

- 'That must have been very difficult for you ...'
- 'I think if I were in your position, I would also find that very difficult.'
- 'You certainly have had a lot to cope with – more than most people, perhaps'.

Summarising

Summarising is repeating what someone else has said in your own words. In order to do this, a practitioner will need to have been listening carefully. Summarising demonstrates to the service user that they have been listened to and the practitioner is interested in what they are saying. It is also a useful way of drawing a conversation to a close.

Summarising prevents misunderstandings and misinterpretation of information (Moss, 2008) and is an open and non-judgemental technique (Rogers, 1959). The practitioner can view this as an opportunity to share their thoughts about what they have been told and to clarify their own understanding of the service user's experience – a way of checking with the service user that they have correctly understood.

For example:

'I'd like to pull together some of the things that you have said so far. Let me know if I have misinterpreted something or if I have missed something out. So, you feel that ...'

'... is that a fair summary? Have I left anything out?'

Assessment Issues

Remote Assessment

In recent years, there has been an increase in the use of *telemedicine*, that is, *digital* and *remote technologies* (such as telephonically, videotelephony and teleconferencing, email and mobile technologies via tablets and smartphones) to assess, diagnose, monitor symptoms and treat a range of illnesses and health care problems. For example, **telephone triage** can be used to offer health care advice and guidance, whilst **remote patient monitoring (RPM)** can raise the alarm if a vulnerable person has a fall at home, whilst specialised equipment can monitor a range of vital signs, including weight and blood glucose, at home sending data directly to health care practitioners. This is convenient, and has increased access and availability of general and specialist health care advice, support and treatment, whilst reducing travelling time and costs. However, telemedicine has added a level of complexity for the assessor and awareness of factors that may impact on the **reliability** and **validity** of remote assessments is vital for any assessor. This seems particularly true for **telemental health (TMH)**. Luxton et al. (2014), for example, highlighted the following challenges for remote assessments:

- The lack of an in-person physical presence may mean that the establishment of rapport is compromised or that subtle non-verbal cues (such as body posture, facial expressions, body language and so on) may be missed, along with more overt clinical observations, such as hygiene, self-neglect and use of alcohol.
- Technological issues, such as the quality of connections, bandwidth and equipment, which may mean that remote images are of poor quality, subject to picture break-up or to time delays.
- Service user acceptance of, satisfaction with, and comfort with technology.
- Procedural and ethical issues, such as confidentiality and the possibility that remote assessments may be overheard, or if the person becomes distressed or there are concerns about safety.

In 2012, the Mental Health Foundation (MHF) set up an inquiry to consider the nature of mental health care in the UK in the next 20 to 30 years (MHF, 2013). The outcome recognised that new technology may bring improvements in the delivery of mental health care, but they were cautious, adding:

> One-to-one human contact, a smile and kind words have a timeless benefit to people with mental health problems ... Many people will continue to need active support to gain equal benefit from new technology, and this support must be available from within the future mental health workforce. (Ibid.: 5)

Recovery-Focused Assessments

In order for an assessment to be a collaborative exercise, it can be very useful for the service user to be involved in collecting information about themselves. Some rating scales and tests are by nature self-report, but there are many other ways in which the service user can be an active participant in the process, and these include keeping journals and diaries about their thoughts, feelings and experiences.

There are also a number of recovery-focused assessments that can be used to help the person consider their current needs and the progress they are making towards their goals and improving their quality of life. For example, personal **timelines** are ways of helping the person to chronologically capture, narrate and review significant events, both positive and negative, successes and failures that have occurred over their life. This can be visual, such as via a river of life (see: www.kstoolkit.org/River+of+Life), which uses the representation of a river as the course of a person's life experiences.

Other recovery-focused assessments include the Mental Health **Recovery Star**™ (see www.outcomesstar.org.uk/mental-health/ for further information). This is a tool for supporting and measuring change when working with adults of working age who are accessing mental health support services. It is designed to support individuals in understanding where they are in terms of recovery and the progress they are making. It identifies and measures 10 core areas of life:

- Managing mental health
- Self-care
- Living skills
- Social networks
- Work
- Relationships
- Addictive behaviour
- Responsibilities
- Identity and self-esteem
- Trust and hope

The star also helps to identify any difficulties that people using services are experiencing in each of these areas and how far they are towards addressing them and moving on (in terms of whether the person is currently 'stuck'; or whether they are accepting help; or is believing that their life could be better; or whether the person is learning about themselves and working towards their goals; or whether they are, ultimately, self-reliant and taking control of their lives). In this way, it provides both the service user and the health-care worker a shared language for discussion of mental health and well-being.

Chapter Summary

In this chapter, we have considered the various approaches that may be used in undertaking comprehensive and holistic assessments in mental health care. We have also explored the skills and values that are needed by mental health practitioners to facilitate assessments and have shown how the recovery approach should underpin assessments by working in partnership and collaborating with service users.

EXERCISE

1. Take a close look at the Mental Health Recovery Star™ (available at: www.outcomesstar. org.uk/mental-health/) and consider how you might use this to structure a recovery-focused conversation to help identify the person's goals, needs and strengths.

CONSIDERATIONS FOR PRACTICE

1. What skills and values do you bring as a practitioner to the assessment process?
2. What assessment approaches might you use with people who are difficult to engage with?
3. Imagine that you are going to assess a person for the first time. How will you plan the initial assessment process?

Further Reading

Nelson-Jones, R. (2016) *Basic Counselling Skills*, 4th edn. London: Sage.

A clearly written book that outlines core therapeutic engagement and communication skills to underpin the therapeutic process. Nelson-Jones is an excellent communicator and his book is highly recommended.

Phelan, M., Slade, M., Thornicroft, G., Dunn, G., Holloway, F., Wykes, T., Strathdee, G., Loftus, L.P., McCrone, P. and Hayward, P. (1995) 'The Camberwell Assessment of Need: the validity and reliability of an instrument to assess the needs of people with severe mental illness', *British Journal of Psychiatry*, 167 (5): 589–95, and doi 10.1192/bjp.167.5.589.

The Camberwell Assessment of Need is used throughout the world as a way of structuring conversations about a person's global health and social care needs. This article shows that the tool is a valid and reliable assessment instrument. It has the benefit that it can be learnt easily and quickly by practitioners from a range of professional backgrounds.

References

Beck, A.T. and Steer, R.A. (1993) *Beck Anxiety Inventory Manual*. San Antonio, TX: Psychological Corporation.

Beck, A.T., Steer, R.A. and Brown, G.K. (1996) *Manual for the Beck Depression Inventory–II*. San Antonio, TX: Psychological Corporation.

Birchwood, M., Smith, J., Cochrane, R., Wetton, S. and Copestake, S. (1990) 'The Social Functioning Scale: the development and validation of a new scale of social adjustment for use in family intervention programmes with schizophrenic patients', *British Journal of Psychiatry*, 157 (6): 853–9, and doi 10.1192/bjp.157.6.853.

Chadwick, P., Less, S. and Birchwood, M. (2000) 'The revised Beliefs About Voices Questionnaire (BAVQ-R)', *British Journal of Psychiatry*, 177 (3): 229–32, and doi 10.1192/bjp.177.3.229.

Cleeland, C.S. (2009) *The Brief Pain Inventory: User Guide*. Available at: http://tinyurl.com/nqfyqo9 (accessed 21 March 2016).

Dickson, D. and Hargie, O. (2006) 'Questioning', in O. Hargie (ed.), *The Handbook of Communication Skills*. London: Routledge.

Hathaway, S.R., and J.C. McKinley (1940) 'A multiphasic personality schedule (Minnesota): I. Construction of the schedule', *Journal of Psychology*, 10: 249–54.

Kagan, C. and Evans, J. (1995) *Professional Interpersonal Skills for Nurses*. London: Chapman & Hall.

Kay, S., Fiszbein, A. and Opler, L. (1987) 'The Positive and Negative Syndrome Scale (PANSS) for schizophrenia', *Schizophrenia Bulletin*, 13 (2): 261–76, and doi 10.1093/schbul/13.2.261.

Launer, J. (2002) *Narrative-Based Primary Care: A Practical Guide*. Abingdon: Radcliffe Medical Press.

Luxton, D., Pruitt, L. and Osenbach, J. (2014) 'Best practices for remote psychological assessment via Telehealth Technologies', *Professional Psychology: Research and Practice*, 45 (1): 27–35, and doi 10.1037/a0034547.

McCabe, C. and Timmins, F. (2013) *Communication Skills for Nursing Practice*, 2nd edn. London: Palgrave Macmillan.

Mental Health Foundation (MHF) (2013) *Starting Today: The Future of Mental Health Services*. Available at: www.mentalhealth.org.uk/sites/default/files/starting-today.pdf (accessed 3 May 2016).

Miller, W. and Rollnick, S. (2012) *Motivational Interviewing: Helping People Change (Applications of Motivational Interviewing)*, 3rd edn. New York: Guilford Press.

Moss, B. (2008) *Communication Skills for Health and Social Care*. London: Sage.

Nelson-Jones, R. (2003) *Basic Counselling Skills: A Helpers' Manual*. London: Sage.

Overall, J.E. and Gorham, D.R. (1988) 'The Brief Psychiatric Rating Scale (BPRS): recent developments in ascertainment and scaling', *Psychopharmacology Bulletin*, 24: 97–9.

Phelan, M., Slade, M., Thornicroft, G., Dunn, G., Holloway, F., Wykes, T., Strathdee, G., Loftus, L., McCrone, P. and Hayward, P. (1995) 'The Camberwell Assessment of Need: the validity and reliability of an instrument to assess the needs of people with severe mental illness', *British Journal of Psychiatry*, 167 (5): 589–95, and doi 10.1192/bjp.167.5.589.

Rogers, C. (1951) *Client-Centered Therapy*. London: Constable.

Rogers, C. (1959) *On Becoming a Person*. Boston, MA: Houghton Mifflin.

Rollnick, S., Mason, P. and Butler, C. (1999) *Health Behaviour Change: A Guide for Practitioners*. Edinburgh: Churchill Livingstone.

Sin, J. and Trenoweth, S. (2010) 'Caring for the mind', in C. Margereson and S. Trenoweth (eds), *Developing Holistic Care for Long-Term Conditions*. London: Routledge.

Stein-Parbury, J. (2005) *Patient & Person: Interpersonal Skills in Nursing*, 3rd edn. Sydney: Elsevier Churchill Livingstone.

3

PRINCIPLES OF SELECTING RATING SCALES AND ASSESSMENT TOOLS

MARK GILLESPIE, ALISON TONER AND MICK FLEMING

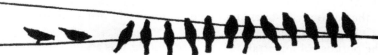

CHAPTER OVERVIEW

This chapter:

- Gives a contextual overview of the principles of selecting psychosocial and mental health assessments.
- Identifies and explains psychometric considerations, including concepts such as validity and reliability.
- Reviews the practical factors that need to be addressed when selecting a method and process of assessment.

Introduction

As assessment is considered the bedrock that supports subsequent treatment choice (Coombs et al., 2013), it is important to understand the options available and the scope of deliberation needed in order to inform a safe, effective and appropriate choice of how best to complete a mental health assessment.

The use of psychosocial and mental health assessments are indicated within several clinical treatment guidelines, adding weight to the efficacy of the use of such assessments in order to ensure that the best treatment is offered to the person. The National Institute for Health and Care Excellence (NICE, 2013) highlight that the aim of psychosocial assessments are to identify personal factors which may explain issues such as self-harm, and can also be an effective way to begin the therapeutic relationship and the journey to recovery for the service user. In addition to inclusion within several of the NICE guidelines (e.g. NICE, 2014), psychosocial assessment is also indicated in many of the guidelines published by the Scottish equivalent of NICE – the Scottish Intercollegiate Guidelines Network (SIGN) (e.g. NHS Quality Improvement Scotland, 2007, 2008; Health Improvement Scotland, 2013) – thus supporting the idea that a robust assessment is a requirement for the treatment that is subsequently delivered.

Psychosocial assessments in mental health care often involve the use of rating scales and assessment tools. Practitioners must select the best scales, meaning those that are: well designed and constructed; the most relevant and effective for the information that needs to be gathered; and the most helpful to the individual to share their experiences. Subsequent information which we gather from people must ultimately be of value to them, and to us. However, unless we are careful, this can become more of a tick-box exercise so that we can evidence that the person has been thoroughly 'assessed'. Moreover, the importance of selecting the 'right' assessment must be of benefit to the person whilst helping to gain sufficient information to support discussions of the best treatment plan.

So, what then is the purpose of undertaking any assessment? It is an information-gathering and structuring exercise so that, as practitioners, we can use our skills and knowledge to help people share and narrate their experiences with the aim of supporting them to move towards recovery. As we saw in Chapter 2, by using interpersonal skills, we begin therapeutic engagement to empower and enable the person to work towards recovery once both parties have a clear idea of the issues to be addressed and the support and abilities that the person has available to them.

What are Rating Scales?

Rating scales can capture people's experiences of both physical and mental health conditions, ranging from depression, brain injury, cancers, cardiovascular disease and chronic long-term conditions, and allows structured investigations of issues such as severity of symptoms, social function, beliefs and experiences. Rating scales are tools that can be used to obtain a clearer idea about the person's condition, current problems or needs, or an aspect of those problems or needs. They provide structure to an assessment. They may ask people for their agreement with particular statements or 'items' or ask people if they have particular experiences (often by ticking a box marked either 'yes' or 'no'), and, if so, to then rate the extent of such experiences (often by using an ordinal scale). For example, the Satisfaction with Life Scale (SWLS; Diener et al., 1985; also see Chapter 11 and Table 11.3) is a 5-item self-report scale, which respondents rate on a 7-point ordinal scale their agreement with particular statements, where:

1 = Strongly Disagree

2 = Disagree

3 = Slightly Disagree

4 = Neither Agree nor Disagree

5 = Slightly Agree

6 = Agree

7 = Strongly Agree

Having a numerical score can be useful to compare an individual with a population mean (to see how far a person's experiences might deviate from the average or general population), and also to compare an individual's score over time – to see if there has been an improvement or deterioration in an aspect of their experience.

Rating scales can be self-report (which are completed by the service user) or **clinician-administered**, where the practitioner asks a series of questions and completes the appropriate form or interview schedule. This, in effect, becomes a way of structuring an interview.

Later on in this chapter, we will discuss specific issues about how the scales are constructed – suffice it to say that before they are published, a number of techniques are used by the authors to ensure that they are fit for use. For example, if a rating scale was used to try to establish the extent of a person's low mood, then the tool must be able to measure that (known as 'validity'). It should also measure this aspect of a person's experience consistently (known as 'reliability'). After publication, it is not uncommon to see other researchers subsequently testing the claims made by the original authors to see if they can also demonstrate the validity and reliability of the tool, or to make suggestions or modifications to the tool so as to ensure that it continues to be appropriate to use.

Choosing a Rating Scale or Assessment Tool

There are many issues to consider when choosing the appropriate rating scale or tool to use in an assessment. In order for a scale or tool to be effective, there must be a cohesive link between a variety of factors. As outlined in Figure 3.1, the choice of assessment is influenced by: the purpose of the service within which the interaction takes place; the purpose of the assessment in relation to the processes within that service; the documentation used by, and available to that service; the theoretical influences guiding the assessment; the expertise of the practitioner; and by service user need, preferences and capabilities.

In short, for an assessment to be effective, consideration must be given to its *appropriateness*, *availability* and *usability*. The details of these requirements are explored below in order to identify the key considerations required around the factual and practical influences on the assessment process.

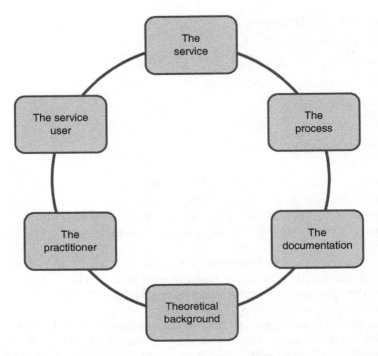

Figure 3.1   Influences on the selection of an assessment format

Appropriateness

A tool can be considered appropriate if it allows us to discriminate between those that have a particular health condition and those that do not have the health condition, or to evaluate and assess the effectiveness of treatment programmes or to predict changes in health conditions (Portney and Watkins, 2009). Practitioners draw inferences from the data collected and will often base clinical decisions on their interpretation of this data. Rating scales or tools are designed to provide structure, consistency and meaning to the process of measurement within clinical practice.

An important aspect of selecting the appropriate assessment tool is to have some indication at the outset of what the psychosocial and mental health difficulties broadly are, and this is often achieved by completing a global assessment (see Chapter 2). This enables the assessor to select the most relevant tool that will ensure that the information-gathering process is a succinct one because, when the assessment is being carried out, the person may be cognitively impaired or in some distress. In a study by Bradford and Rickwood (2012), the authors suggested that most people aged 12 – 25 years preferred pen-and-paper format or verbal disclosure, whereas younger people found self-administered assessments more acceptable. This possibly indicates a generational shift in the understanding of who is responsible for the individual's health. Such individual factors must be taken into account to maximise the accuracy of the assessment. If we use a format that the individual is not familiar with, then will the results of the assessment be a true reflection of the individual's psychosocial functioning? A further study by Bradford and Rickwood (2014) outlined how, by engaging with relevant stakeholders at the conceptualising stage of development of psychosocial assessment, this ensured person-centred design and a self-reporting tool that was acceptable to users. Selection may also be influenced by a number of factors that do not include which tool is the most relevant. Other considerations include: cost, availability, service preference and skills and qualifications of the practitioners to undertake the assessment because many tools involve pre-administration training (see below and Chapter 2).

Mental health practitioners collect assessment information over time (longitudinally) in order to investigate changes in measured variables such as symptoms, functioning and quality of life, and evaluate the meaning of these changes for treatment. At the same time, the reality of team-working also means that more than one practitioner may undertake and interpret the assessment of the same service user.

Factors Affecting Consistency

A further significant problem with any rating scale or test is that the outcome can be exaggerated or minimised by the rater. This means that the results can be influenced by an individual's personal motivations and goals – a person is free to 'fake good' or 'fake bad'. The way in which the test is administered can also have an impact. For example, if a person is watched when completing the test, then the results are likely to be different than if completing it in private. That is, social expectations are likely to influence a person's responses.

These issues can significantly affect the accuracy of the assessment process as there needs to be consistency in the way in which service users are assessed each separate time, and there needs to be consistency in the way in which each separate practitioner assesses the same service user over time. Meaningful comparisons of measures taken over time require stability in the findings, which relies on the consistency of the assessment (Portney and Watkins, 2009). For rating scales and tools to be consistent, they must demonstrate that they can produce the same values for the same service user each time they are used for assessment purposes. This should be the case, even when the assessment instrument is used by different practitioners (Coolican, 2009). Without this consistency, comparisons are meaningless and any changes found may occur as a consequence of the lack of consistency, rather than real changes in the measured variable caused by treatment interventions.

Design of the Rating Scale

The wording of the questions used in assessment instruments, the structure and the scoring system can mediate the accuracy and credibility of those instruments. If the wording of questions does not comprehensively capture the meaning and true definition of the construct being measured, then the assessment instrument will not measure the actual construct and the assessment findings become invalid. The meaning of words can be misunderstood, or a variety of meanings can be applied by different groups of people from different countries, continents and cultures. The consequence of this is that assessment instruments can produce different assessment findings in different groups of people. Again, this may influence the accuracy of the assessment and clinical decision-making based on the evidence from the assessment instrument.

Properties of the Rating Scale

Practitioners need to be aware of the potential for inaccurate assessment when selecting assessment instruments for use in their clinical work. In order to ensure that the findings that accrue from an assessment instrument are meaningful, consistent, accurate and trustworthy, instruments are evaluated against a scientific criterion. This criterion is made up of a series of rules and conventions based on statistical techniques, and the term that is applied to this scientific method is known as 'psychometrics'. Psychometric validation is the process by which these rules and conventions are applied to assessment instruments to check their robustness and to test their accuracy (Bowling, 2004). It is important for practitioners to be confident in the quality and accuracy of the evidence that they have collected from assessment instruments as this forms the basis for clinical decisions, case conceptualisation and treatment planning.

Practitioners reviewing the psychometric properties of rating scales or tools with a view to selecting an appropriate instrument for use should consider simple contextual factors. The design of measurement instruments is based on a theoretical model of a construct (Portney and Watkins, 2009). For example, the Positive and Negative Syndrome Scale (PANSS; see Kay et al., 1989) is based on a dichotomous model of two distinct sub-types of **schizophrenia** (positive and negative symptoms). This model is reflected in the structure of the PANSS, which has a positive symptoms domain made up of seven items (delusions, conceptual disorganisation, hallucinatory behaviour, excitement, grandiosity, suspiciousness/persecution and hostility) and a negative symptoms domain made up of seven items (blunted affect, emotional withdrawal, poor rapport, passive/apathetic social withdrawal, difficulty in abstract thinking, lack of spontaneity and flow of conversation and stereotyped thinking). Each measurement instrument should reflect the theoretical underlining of the construct that it alleges to measure.

Psychometric properties of rating scales and tools such as reliability and validity are related to the population and context in which they are used (Portney and Watkins, 2009). That is, rating scales and tools can perform differently in different groups or populations, and practitioners need to consider this when reviewing the suitability of an instrument for clinical use. Consulting the literature reporting testing of rating scales in specific groups is a prerequisite for all practitioners selecting a suitable measurement instrument. The discussion on cultural and age-related considerations elsewhere in this chapter indicates how these factors can influence the application of assessments.

Reliability

Another issue when considering the appropriateness of a tool is 'reliability'. Simply put, reliability refers to the consistency with which a scale reveals its results. Coolican (2009) makes a distinction between two types of reliability: **internal** and **external reliability**.

'Internal reliability' is the consistency within the measurement instrument itself. As with all psychometric principles, internal consistency is a single continuum with low internal consistency at one end, which indicates that service users have answered the questions that relate to each other in an inconsistent manner. At the other end of the continuum, there is high internal consistency, which would indicate that service users have answered the questions that relate to each other in a consistent manner. There are a number of factors that can influence the consistency with which service users answer questions on an assessment instrument. One of those factors may be the wording and understanding of the questions being asked. It is important that practitioners are aware of how consistent the service user answers have been when the assessment instrument has been used. Many psychometric studies that have tested the internal consistency of assessment instruments studies report a statistic that provides a numerical value relating to the internal consistency of the instrument. This numerical value allows practitioners to make an informed decision about whether an instrument has sufficiently high internal consistency to use in clinical practice.

The most commonly cited value is the Cronbach's alpha, which provides a value of 0.0–1.0. Values closer to 0.0 indicate low internal consistency, whilst values closer to 1.0 indicate high internal consistency (Brace et al., 2009). An alpha value of 0.7 or above is considered to be good enough for use in clinical practice (ibid.). Another statistical test for internal reliability is the split-half method – whilst the test uses a different method for calculation, the values provided (0.0–1.0) and a value of 0.7 indicating acceptability for clinical use are the same as those for the Cronbach's alpha (Brace et al., 2009).

'External reliability' relates to consistency over time and between different raters using the same instrument. Within clinical practice, measurement instruments are used several times over a period of time, particularly over the period of treatment. In situations where the aim is to evaluate the efficacy and effectiveness of treatments, practitioners will be required to measure pre- (baseline) and post-treatment and then compare the findings from the two measures to see the extent of differences between the two measures. The length of time between pre- and post-measures depends on the type of treatment being evaluated, for example if it is the effects of anti-depressant medication, the time between measures may be weeks. However, if the treatment is family intervention with a family, where there is a member with a diagnosis of schizophrenia, the time between measures may be 6–9 months. At other times, practitioners may monitor trends and changes in functioning, mood, symptoms and quality of life to evaluate longer-term outcomes of psychosocial treatments.

In both of these cases, the measurement instrument needs to provide consistent and stable results over a specified period so that any comparison is meaningful. If there is any inconsistency over time, then the comparison will be meaningless and any clinical decision based on this comparison will also be meaningless. Psychometric testing of measurement instruments often takes account of test-retest reliability, especially where instruments are likely to be used longitudinally or to take measurements across time. Researchers will report test-retest figures after taking at least two measurements from the same sample in the form of correlations. Kappa figures between the values of 0 and 1 are used when the data in the measurement is ordinal level and Pearson's correlation coefficient where the data in the measurement is interval level (Bowling, 2004). Values closer to 1 indicate a larger magnitude of consistency between the two measurements; conversely, values closer to 0 indicate weaker strength of consistency between the two measurements. Values of 0.75–0.8 or above would indicate a good enough level of consistency for the measurement instrument to be used in clinical practice (Coolican, 2009).

There may be an issue in cases where measurements of the same service user with the same instrument is made by different practitioners. Although measurement instruments are made up of standardised questions and response options, others rely on observation and interpretation of responses to standardised questions. Where there is interpretation required as part of the assessment/measurement, there is an increased risk for variations and inconsistency between the ratings of practitioners. 'Inter-rater reliability' is the term used to describe consistency between different raters. Psychometric studies will often report the findings in relation to inter-rater reliability or the level of agreement between raters in terms of correlations, which indicate the strength of agreement or association between the raters. Where ordinal data is collected, Kappa figures are used to indicate poor (<0.59), fair (0.60–0.74), good (>0.80) levels of agreement. Where the instrument collects interval data, Pearson correlation coefficient is used to indicate the level of agreement, with values of >0.70–0.80 indicating a good level of consistency in agreement for the measurement to be used in clinical practice (Bowling, 2004; Clark-Carter, 2010).

Validity

When applied to measurement instruments, validity refers to whether a rating scale or test measures what it is supposed to measure. Bowling (2004) notes that instruments have to be exposed to repeated rigorous and satisfactory testing before validity can be claimed. It is the responsibility of practitioners to consult the reports of these validation studies and consider the findings as part of the selection process. There are four types of validity that practitioners need to consider:

- *Face validity*: Is a basic form of validity and is an intuitive and subjective evaluation of the acceptability, relevance, suitability and appropriateness of the appearance, structure of the measurement instrument and the questions and rating criteria. Face validity needs to be established for both the practitioners – to ensure that the findings are accurate and meaningful – and for those being assessed because an instrument needs to be acceptable and understandable.
- *Content validity*: Is more rigorous than face validity and relates to the extent and breadth to which the content of a measurement instrument measures the aspects of the construct it alleges to measure. Content validity can refer to an instrument's inadequacy in covering sufficient aspects of the construct, the rigour and weighting with which the construct and its domains are covered by the instrument and/or the inclusion of irrelevant items that do not relate to the construct.
- *Construct validity*: Relates to the ability of the measurement instrument to measure the theoretical underpinning constructs from which the instrument was designed. Using the example of the PANSS, construct validity would be a

measure of the ability of the PANSS to measure the positive and negative symptoms of schizophrenia. The process of testing construct validity involves comparison with related and relevant measures. This allows researchers to evaluate the level of association between items representing the theoretical construct on the measurement instrument and related items that represent the theoretical construct on other measures or instruments.

- *Criterion validity*: Is commonly reported in psychometric studies and relates to the extent to which a measurement instrument produces the same findings as an established and already validated instrument, usually a 'gold standard'. If, through comparison with an established and already validated instrument, another measurement instrument is found to produce the same findings, then this measurement instrument fulfils the requirement of criterion validity. The process involves identifying the magnitude of association (correlation) between participant responses to items on the measurement instrument and participant responses to items on the 'gold standard'. The use of statistical values provides a useful method for comparison of the performance of the two instruments. One of the assumptions underlying this comparative process is that the 'gold standard' instrument should be relevant to both the phenomena being measured and to the measurement instrument being tested (Portney and Watkins, 2009). There are two forms of criterion against which measurement instruments are tested/compared: where a measurement instrument produces the same findings as the 'gold standard' instrument then the measurement instrument is said to have **concurrent validity**; where the measurement instrument accurately predicts an event or phenomena such as changes in, e.g., psychotic symptoms, relapse, recovery, self-harm or the development of a specific condition, then the instrument fulfils the criterion for **predictive validity** (Clark-Carter, 2010).

A thorough exploration of reliability and validity of psychological tests is outside the scope of this book (for a comprehensive overview see, for example, Fernandez-Ballesteros, 2003).

Sensitivity and Specificity

Within clinical practice, practitioners need a measurement instrument to be sensitive – that is, the instrument is capable of accurately identifying people with a condition, particularly any new cases. **Sensitivity** is the 'true positive rate' – that is, it is a measure of how many people the rating scale or test have accurately identified as experiencing the phenomena of interest (the percentage of people who are correctly identified as being depressed or anxious and so on). Similarly, instruments should be capable of accurately discriminating those that do *not* have a specific condition. Measurement instruments that are capable of accurately discriminating are said to have **specificity**. This is the 'true negative rate' and is a measure of people who are correctly identified as *not* experiencing the phenomena of interest (that is, the percentage of people who are correctly identified as not being depressed or anxious and so on).

Cultural Diversity

The interviewer needs to take into consideration any issues of diversity which may impact on the assessment. These include issues relating to race, culture, religion, gender, disability, sensory impairments, age, sexuality and so on. A considerable level of sensitivity and understanding of the diverse nature of individuals within society is needed in the assessment process, which requires us to be aware of our own beliefs and attitudes and how this may colour our perceptions.

Understanding the service user's individual and cultural background is key in gauging the appropriateness of an assessment format, and in determining the need for adaptation of that format to suit. Consider the impact, then, of asking how many friends a socially isolated adolescent has, or when the last time a devout Muslim woman went nightclubbing. Bernstein et al. (2014) identify barriers to Korean Americans accessing mental health services in the USA which include a culturally held understanding of mental distress based around energy flows, and mental distress being perceived as a sign of weakness and/or emotional strain. As these beliefs can strongly conflict with the illness-based perceptions that underpin much of Western mental health care, so we can understand why some groups avoid accessing mental health services, why some commonly used assessment formats may not be particularly productive across all of today's multicultural society, and why choice and flexibility are important in selecting and applying an appropriate assessment.

Availability

Copyright and Fees

Some rating scales or tests are copyrighted and this means that you cannot use them without the express permission of the copyright holder. The production of an effective assessment tool is a lengthy and complicated process that requires significant effort on the part of the developers. Recognition for their efforts is often presented in the copyrighting of the approach and the subsequent control over access and possible financial reward that this facilitates. To use such a tool, therefore, frequently requires both payment and involvement within a training or preparation programme which ensures a fidelity to the developer's original model. Breach of copyright is serious and leaves the miscreant open to public and private prosecution and it is, therefore, imperative that the copyright status of any assessments are confirmed prior to use. Assessment tools will often display standard information around copyright, showing statements such as: 'All rights reserved,' 'Permission granted to be used for educational and personal use only' or even the simple © symbol (see the Copyright Licensing Agency, n.d., for more information on what each of these statements actually means). If you are unsure about the copyright status of the tool and no information is available, you should consider contacting the original authors for clarification.

You should also be aware that a fee is sometimes charged for the use of a test, and occasionally you may be required to pay for the forms. The record forms for the BDI-II, for example, are currently charged at £54.50 for 25 forms (see: www.pearsonclinical.co.uk/Psychology/AdultMentalHealth/AdultMentalHealth/BeckDepressionInventory-II(BDI-II)/BeckDepressionInventory-II(BDI-II).aspx).

You should always assume that a test is copyrighted, unless the authors have clearly stated that it is in the public domain. If you are in doubt, you should always seek permission from the authors, who may wish to monitor the usage of their scale.

Usability

Training

It is vital that you have sufficient training and experience to use a rating scale or test. That is, you should always ensure that you are capable to safely apply any rating scale or tool within a specific practice setting before using them with a service user/family. This preparation could involve observation of a more experienced practitioner, role rehearsal to try the approach in a practise scenario, receiving feedback from others on your performance and reflecting on how best to use the approach. You should never read an assessment tool as you apply it for the first time.

For example, the American Psychological Association (APA) identifies a three-tiered system based on levels of qualification that are required in order to use particular tests (the BDI-II, for example, requires at least Qualification Level B, as described below).

Qualification Level A

There are no special qualifications required.

Qualification Level B

Tests may be used by individuals with one of the following:

- A Master's degree in psychology, education, occupational therapy, social work, or in a field closely related to the intended use of the assessment, and formal training in the ethical administration, scoring and interpretation of clinical assessments.
- Certification by, or full active membership in, a professional organisation that requires training and experience in the relevant area of assessment.
- A degree or license to practice in the health care or allied health care field.
- Formal, supervised mental health, speech/language and/or educational training specific to assessing children, or in infant and child development, and formal training in the ethical administration, scoring and interpretation of clinical assessments.

Qualification Level C

Tests with a C qualification require a high level of expertise in test interpretation, and can be purchased by individuals with one of the following:

- A doctorate degree in psychology, education or closely related field with formal training in the ethical administration, scoring, and interpretation of clinical assessments related to the intended use of the assessment.
- Licensure or certification to practice in a field related to the test.
- Certification by, or full active membership in, a professional organisation that requires training and experience in the relevant area of assessment.

However, you must always be guided by the legal and ethical codes of your own profession, and you must not use any scale or test without prior thought and/or preparation and training.

Intended Use

Rating scales and tools will always clearly state its intended use. If, for example, a tool is designed to be used with an adult population (aged 18–65), then it is not suitable for use with children. This can give misleading results that can affect the quality and accuracy of an assessment. Also, you should not modify any scale or tests without the express permission of the authors.

Accessibility

It is important to determine the accessibility of any assessment format before use. With a large-scale UK government study recently suggesting that 17 per cent of the population of England had what they termed low proficiency in literacy, and that 18 per cent had similar difficulties with problem-solving (Department for Business Innovation and Skills, 2013), it is imperative that we consider the cognitive and reading abilities of those being assessed when selecting an appropriate assessment format. With many mental health conditions causing or contributing to cognitive impairment and the average reading ability in the UK being compared with that of a nine-year-old (See a Voice, 2010), thought and effort needs to guide the selection and adaptation of assessments, and some of the more commonly used word-processing programmes have inbuilt facilities that will grade the readability of documentation.

Linguistic complexity is not the only factor influencing comprehension, though. Within the UK, there are currently somewhere between 200 and 300 languages spoken, with the most common of these originating from places as diverse as Africa, Europe and the Indian Subcontinent (British Council, 2013). We should never assume, therefore, that the service user's grasp of English will accommodate comprehension of documentation, which is often densely packed with obscure phrases that originate from a specialist medical, psychological or research setting. Even for those for whom English is understandable, there are cultural and generational nuances influencing interpretation, both in the assessor and in those being assessed. It is suggested that higher levels of cultural dialect use equate with lower levels of understanding of mainstream language (Edwards et al., 2014), further emphasising the need for deliberation around the service user's abilities and, indeed, the abilities of the assessment to meet those needs.

Overload

The chance of getting the perfect-fit assessment poses some challenges, given the wide choice of formats available. It is essential that we consider the *assessee*, who must feel as though they spend a considerable amount of time in the midst of a crisis, with a variety of health professionals who appear to ask exactly the same questions, over and over. If we consider a person who is experiencing such a crisis involving their mental health: they are often initially seen by their GP, who refers them to hospital, where they are assessed by a junior doctor and then a nurse, social worker, occupational therapist, dietician and so on. As most of these professionals will be asking the same questions, to get to know the person and their story, and to develop information for their records, this means that the assessment process is driven by the needs of the health professionals, rather than being efficiently tailored to suit the person's needs. Conversely, as health professionals, we are duty-bound to manage issues such as risk – issues that are most effectively managed when we have as much information as possible. There is a balance, therefore, between accessing relevant and current information and potentially harassing the person. As assessment relies on the person responding truthfully on how they are feeling or thinking or around what has happened to them, so must we endeavour to develop the collaborative working relationship that will facilitate this sharing of information. This will be best accommodated through tailoring the assessment process to suit the individual.

The practitioner is responsible for providing a clear explanation of the assessment and its purpose, and for identifying a strong rationale for the use of such an approach. This is not always the experience for service users, though: in a study by Hunter et al. (2013), some participants indicated that they thought that psychosocial assessment was an exercise to protect staff. Therefore, it is essential that the person is at the heart of the assessment and not merely a participant of a tick-box exercise that has limited benefit to them.

Format

As improvements in technology advance, assessments that may in the past have been undertaken in a traditional pen-and-paper format may now be delivered electronically, however what practitioners need to consider around this is that this format appears more relevant to younger people, who are generally more computer literate. We need to remember, then, that the format of the psychosocial assessment used may be driven more by availability and custom, rather than by need of the person.

A study by Gies et al. (2014) discusses assessing the needs of caregivers who have a relative with Alzheimer's disease, using a web-based psychosocial assessment, which is less time intensive and may fit around the caring responsibilities of the carer. However, for it to be effective, it is necessary that the practitioner is proficient with the technology being used, and can also develop a rapport with the carer, in circumstances where face-to-face interaction may not take place. Accessibility will dictate whether an electronic assessment will be used, rather than a paper format. One factor that we must take into account where multi-formats are available is the impact on engagement. It is important to remember that, whilst as practitioners we have a purpose to ensure that a thorough assessment is carried out for the person, this may be a limited opportunity for engagement with someone. Thus, we have two people with differing agendas, hoping for the right outcome.

Self-Report or Clinician-Administered

It is vital to consider how the originators of a rating scale intended it to be used. Sometimes, this can be given to the service user for their completion, either within an interview or at a later date. Sometimes, the rating scale or test is clinician-rated. As such, the tests act as a prompt or guide to a clinical conversation. In order to build and maintain trust, thought must be given to how this is administered and explained to the service user and how the results of the test may subsequently be shared with them.

Chapter Summary

The selection of an appropriate and effective assessment process or tool is key to the development and maintenance of a positive therapeutic relationship, and provides a vehicle through which a detailed and comprehensive understanding can emerge of a service user and of the factors that influence their health and well-being. As the information arising from the assessment provides the foundation for all subsequent interactions with that service user and their family, it is imperative that the assessment process is well planned and includes consideration of the individuality of the service user, and balances this with the requirements and capabilities of the assessment format. A well-chosen and well-delivered assessment will underpin a collaborative approach to care delivery and will in itself provide therapeutic benefits.

Practitioners working within settings where mental ill health influences service user outcome should familiarise themselves with the scope of assessment formats suitable for their service user group and plan, apply and refine their ability to incorporate such assessments successfully within their routine practice.

EXERCISE

1. Choose a rating scale that you would like to explore in more depth. Using search terms relevant to the measurement instrument you want investigate (e.g. Positive and Negative Syndrome Scale) and other related words (e.g. psychometric, reliability, validation), access relevant academic databases (e.g. PubMed, MEDLINE, CINAHL and PsycINFO) to search for research papers relating to your chosen instrument. Consider how this tool has been/could be used in your clinical practice.
2. How reliable is your chosen rating scale?
3. What steps have been taken to demonstrate the validity of your chosen rating scale?

CONSIDERATIONS FOR PRACTICE

1. Outline the stages that you would follow when selecting a rating scale.
2. Reflect on a time when you have been undertaking assessments in practice:

    a) Did you use an assessment tool?
    b) If so, to what extent did the person have a choice in the selection of the assessment tool?
    c) In future practice, how can you maximise the opportunity for the person to have a choice in the assessment tool and the format used?

3. What factors do you take into account when considering the format of an assessment?

Further Reading

Simmons, J. and Griffiths, R. (2014) *CBT for Beginners*, 2nd edn. London: Sage.

This book provides the underpinning theory that guides much of our current assessment practice and explains the factors influencing choice within specific assessment processes.

Smith, G. (2012) *Psychological Interventions in Mental Health Nursing*. Maidenhead: Open University Press.

This book connects the assessment process with available interventions across a range of common mental health conditions.

References

Bernstein, K.S., Cho, S., Roh, S., Nguyen, M.H.T., Chen, D., Chiu, Y. and Bang, H. (2014) 'Development and psychometric testing of the mental health service barrier assessment instrument', *Journal of Theory Construction and Testing*, 18 (2): 40–9.

Bowling, A. (2004) *Research Methods in Health: Investigating Health and Health Services.* 2nd edn. Milton Keynes: Open University Press.

Brace, N., Kemp, R. and Snelgar, R. (2009) *SPSS for Psychologists*, 4th edn. Basingstoke: Palgrave Macmillan.

Bradford, S. and Rickwood, D. (2012) 'Psychosocial assessments for young people. a systematic review examining acceptability, disclosure and engagement and predictive utility', *Adolescent Health, Medicine and Therapeutics*, 3: 111–25.

Bradford, S. and Rickwood, D. (2014) 'Electronic psychosocial assessment tool: concept development and identification of barriers to successful implementation', *Journal of Technology in Human Services*, 32 (4): 275–96.

British Council (2013) *Languages for the Future: Which Languages the UK Needs Most and Why.* Available at: www.britishcouncil.org/sites/britishcouncil.uk2/files/languages-for-the-future-report.pdf (accessed 5 June 2015).

Clark-Carter, D. (2010) *Quantitative Psychological Research*, 3rd edn. Hove: Psychology Press, Taylor and Francis.

Coolican, H. (2009) *Research Methods and Statistics in Psychology*, 5th edn. London: Hodder-Education.

Coombs, T., Curtis, J. and Crookes, P. (2013) 'What is the process of comprehensive mental health nursing assessment? Results from a qualitative study', *International Nursing Review*, 60: 96–102.

Copyright Licensing Agency (n.d.) Copyright information. Available at: www.cla.co.uk/copyright_information/copyright_information (accessed 26 May 2015).

Department for Business Innovation and Skills (2013) *The International Survey of Adult Skills 2012: Adult Literacy, Numeracy and Problem Solving Skills in England.* London: Department for Business Innovation and Skills.Available at: www.gov.uk/government/uploads/system/uploads/attachment_data/file/246534/bis-13-1221-international-survey-of-adult-skills-2012.pdf (accessed 5 June 2015).

Diener, E., Emmons, R.A., Larsen, R.J. and Griffin, S. (1985) 'The Satisfaction with Life Scale', *Journal of Personality Assessment*, 49 (1): 71–5.

Edwards, J., Gross, M., Chen, J., MacDonald, M.C., Kaplan, D., Brown, M., and Seidenberg, M.S. (2014) 'Dialect awareness and lexical comprehension of mainstream American English in African American English-speaking children', *Journal of Speech, Language and Hearing Research*, 57: 1883–95.

Fernandez-Ballesteros, R. (2003) *Encyclopedia of Psychological Assessment.* London: Sage.

Gies, C., Pierce, L., Steiner, V., van der Bijl, J. and Salvador, D. (2014) 'Web-based psychosocial assessment for caregivers of persons with dementia: a feasibility study', *Rehabilitation Nursing*, 39: 102–9.

Health Improvement Scotland (2013) *Scottish Intercollegiate Guidelines Network 131: Management of Schizophrenia.* Available at: www.sign.ac.uk/guidelines/fulltext/131/ (accessed 3 May 2016).

Hunter, C., Chantler, K., Kapur, N. and Cooper, J. (2013) 'Service users perspectives on psychosocial assessment following self-harm and its impact on further hope seeking: a qualitative study', *Journal of Affective Disorders*, 145: 315–23.

Kay, S., Opler, L. and Lindenmayer, J. (1989) 'The Positive and Negative Syndrome Scale (PANSS): rationale and standardisation', *British Journal of Psychiatry*, 155: 59–65.

National Institute for Health and Care Excellence (NICE) (2013) *News & Features: Psychosocial Assessments Can Help Tackle 'Hidden Problem' of Self-Harm.* Available at: www.nice.org.uk (accessed 26 May 2016).

NICE (2014) *Psychosis and Schizophrenia in Adults: Prevention and Management.* Available at: www.nice.org.uk/guidance/cg178/chapter/1-recommendations#first-episode-psychosis-2 (accessed 20 May 2016).

NHS Quality Improvement Scotland (2007) *Scottish Intercollegiate Guidelines Network 94: Cardiac Arrhythmias in Coronary Heart Disease.* Available at: www.sign.ac.uk/guidelines/fulltext/94/ (accessed 20 May 2016).

NHS Quality Improvement Scotland (2008) *Scottish Intercollegiate Guidelines Network 106: Control of Pain in Adults with Cancer.* Available at: www.sign.ac.uk/pdf/SIGN106.pdf (accessed 20 May 2016).

Portney, L.G. and Watkins, M.P. (2009) *Foundations of Clinical Research: Applications to Practice*, 3rd edn. Upper Saddle River, NJ: Prentice-Hall.

See a Voice (2010) *Readability.* Available at: www.see-a-voice.org/marketing-ad/effective-communication/readability/ (accessed 5 June 2015).

PART 2

PSYCHOSOCIAL ASSESSMENTS

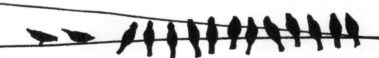

THE PRESENTING PROBLEM

SUSAN BOWMAN AND FIONA MARTIN

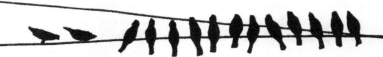

CHAPTER OVERVIEW

This chapter:

- Identifies the core components of a presenting problem.
- Discusses how to structure and undertake an initial meeting.
- Guides the reader through a framework in order to understand the person's presenting problem.
- Discusses how to develop an **initial conceptualisation** so as to make sense of the service user's presenting problem, based on a shared understanding of the individual's presenting strengths and needs.

Introduction

The concept of the 'presenting problem' is often not clearly defined in the health care literature. However, Owen et al. (2014) suggest a definition of the presenting problem as essentially getting the answer to the question: 'Why has this person presented in this way at this point in time?' Sadock et al. (2014) and Morrison (2014) use the term 'chief complaint' in place of 'presenting problem', describing it as why the person has come or been brought for help. Hamkins (2014), a supporter of narrative inquiry, describes the presenting problem as the initial reason for which a person seeks help, as well as their efforts and successes in overcoming it. Seikkula and Arnkil (2006) use more ordinary language to describe what we understand as the presenting problem, and suggest that it is finding out: 'What has happened?' or 'What has changed?'

Whichever way it is defined, any psychosocial assessment must begin with a broad, general understanding or sketch of the person's presenting problem, leading to a preliminary initial conceptualisation, which, in turn, becomes the foundation for the later, more detailed, assessment.

The Initial Meeting

At the initial meeting, it is impossible to know how long the person will need to talk about what is worrying them. That is because the person does not always know what exactly is wrong, and may describe what is troubling them as unpleasant physical experiences, emotions or frightening thoughts. What is known is that one of the significant ways through which individuals make sense of, and give meaning to, their experiences is to organise them in a narrative form (Mishler, 1986).

It takes courage to confide in others, but it is done in the hope of a compassionate response. Meeting with service users in a way that is unconditional and respectful will facilitate the start of the service user's narrative about their source of distress/presenting. For this to happen, it is essential that the practitioner communicates very quickly to the individual, and that they remember that taking time to listen and to develop a shared understanding are the most important objectives of the first meeting. A situation where a professional is in a hurry is more likely to produce a rapid solution that is not in the best interest of the person in distress or their immediate support network (Seikkula and Arnkil, 2006). The initial goal for practitioners is to psychologically engage with the service user, while holding an attitude of acceptance, empathy and authentic collaboration (Rogers, 1980). These fundamental values have been echoed by the Francis Public Inquiry, which urges that 'Patients/clients must be the first priority by ensuring that, they receive effective care from caring, compassionate and committed staff' (The Mid Staffordshire NHS Foundation Trust Public Enquiry, 2013: 3).

Using a Normalising Rationale

A 'normalising rationale' is a way of validating an individual's experience(s). It aims to reduce distress by enabling the individual to make sense of their present experiences and by conveying an understanding that their response is understandable. Kingdon and Turkington (1991) first introduced the use of a normalising rationale to help reduce the distress caused by auditory hallucinations. For example, while hallucinations are typically associated with psychosis/schizophrenia, they can also occur in the realm of everyone's experiences such as when we have a very high temperature (pyrexia); sometimes when an excessive amount of alcohol is taken, or when psychotropic drugs are used. Hallucinations are also not uncommon as an aura before a seizure; following a head injury; when we are deprived of sleep/stimulation; or after bereavement. A normalising rationale describes how a person's experience is very reasonable and very understandable, considering recent events/experiences; and also that their response to the distress may be very reasonable. A normalising rationale aims to reassure people that they are not alone in their distress. While normalising the distress might not significantly change the reality of the situation that is causing the distress, it can be an effective way of decatastrophising the experience and of providing hope for the future. It can focus on any experience, not solely hallucinations, and provides a useful reflection and reminder for the service user that they are not alone in their distress and difficulty.

Practitioners have different competencies in using this particular skill. The potential to deepen understanding and demonstrate empathy is significant and this is why a normalising rationale is a very useful and effective skill. However, there is always the potential to be seen to minimise or discount a person's experience or distress using a normalising rationale and practitioners need to be sensitive to the service user's reaction and not assume that everyone will find it useful.

The Presenting Problem Interview

At your first meeting with a service user, you will need to help the person set the scene by cataloguing what has gone wrong in the person's life and also what has gone well. This will involve developing a shared understanding of the person's strengths as well as needs. A collaborative, inquiring style of opening question should be adopted. This allows the person freedom to talk about what is important to them. It also helps to build rapport and promote a relaxed style early in the interview, which can enhance the quality of information gathered. Open questioning is the best way to develop an initial, broad and general understanding of the person's situation, by asking such questions as:

- I understand you have been to see your GP recently. Can you tell me about that?
- I know it might be difficult for you to talk about why things might have been distressing for you recently, but it would be an idea for us to talk about this so we can both make a bit more sense of what is happening recently.
- What has changed in your life?
- Please tell me, in your own words, what you see as the problem?
- What do you feel have been some of the good things that have happened to you recently?
- What do you think your family/friends think about your current situation?

These initial opening questions have qualities that will affect the information you will receive. It is worth taking time to help the person consider these issues as it helps to let the person know that you want to help them. It also provides the practitioner with an opportunity to gain a shared understanding of the meaning the person gives to their experiences. When gathering information about the presenting problem, the service user is the most important source of that information: *there is no room for guesswork, jumping to conclusions or making assumptions.*

The focus and interaction is person-centred, working collaboratively with the individual, but remember that the person's family/personal network will have invaluable knowledge to share in this process. The majority of people presenting in distress are living with their family, or have close contact with them, and they can often assist in developing a knowledge base of the individual's strengths and attributes as a person. For this reason, the family/personal network is always relevant. Families know the individual and how they were before illness. They can remember details, help with timelines and can often help with identifying anything that may have increased the individual's vulnerability to illness. The presenting problem is also a time to mobilise supportive resources for the service user and the family.

The mental health professional should be able to engage with families/personal network in ways that are meaningful to them and the service user. Authentic engagement with families/personal networks require that you:

- Have a genuine desire to want to listen and understand.
- Work through a spirit of negotiation and collaboration.
- Validate concerns, take their concerns seriously.
- See the family/personal network as experts in their experiences.
- Resist the urge to jump to conclusions based on your beliefs.
- Understand that the majority of families are doing, or trying to do, their best.
- Understand the impact of illness on the family's life/routine/plans/aspirations.

Often, there can be more than one presenting problem, therefore it is essential that you:

- Identify all problems by encouraging the service user to talk freely about their understanding of why they are there.
- Ask the service user if they have other concerns.
- All problems should be individually listed, collaboratively with the individual and their family/support network.
- Problems should be listed in order of severity – starting with the most distressing. (Aquilina and Warner, 2004; Kinsella and Kinsella, 2015)

After setting the scene, it is important to develop a more focused understanding of the current presenting problem (which will help develop your initial conceptualisation). A structured approach makes best use of the service user's and family's time with you. It can prevent the service user/family feeling overwhelmed; help maintain focus on what is important; enhances feelings of certainty; and ensures that everyone is involved.

In developing your initial conceptualisation, it would be useful to structure the conversation by considering a number of factors (see Figure 4.1).

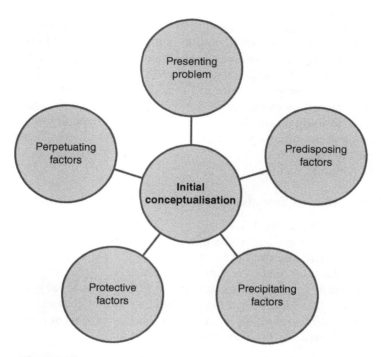

Figure 4.1   The initial conceptualisation

Presenting Problems

These are factors that impact on the person's difficulties, and their current health and functioning. They include psychiatric symptoms, emotions, bodily sensations, problem behaviours. Changes in somatic functioning such as sleep pattern, appetite, cognitive ability, sexual functioning should also be noted. Here, in exploring the presenting problem, current risk factors also need to be considered.

People are usually referred to specialist mental health services from primary care (such as GPs) and there will usually be accompanying referral information, which will contain important details about the person's current presenting problems. It can help provide some context for the current problem. Likewise, the family/personal network may also provide background detail to the person's present problem. However, it is crucial to capture the service user's own idea about what might be happening for them (in their own words) – this will provide a valuable insight into the perspective of the service user (Carlat, 2004). Because of the nature of mental and emotional distress, the service user's statement may differ greatly from the family, carer or referrer's assessment of the situation and may be at odds. This does not mean that the service user's perspective should be discounted, but it is important to note that there are different perspectives and interpretations of the person's current presenting problems. It can sometimes be useful to offer the concerns raised by a family member, carer or referrer (such as the GP) and allow the service user to comment on other people's perspective of their current concerns.

The current presenting problem, and the history of the presenting problem, may be difficult to separate, especially in more complicated cases. However, what is important is that you get a good account of what is troubling the service user and thoroughly investigate any associated symptoms (Buckley et al., 2005). In some cases, for example, someone may not feel that there is a problem, or may feel that the problem is caused by other people and is beyond their control to resolve. It is still important to explore any issues and record the information from their perspective. It is also an initial opportunity to observe the individual's actions, body language and speech.

Questions here may include:

- Could you tell me a little about how you have been feeling recently?

    o   What has your mood been like?
    o   Have you been feeling unusually sad? Or happy?
    o   Have you had any strange experiences?
    o   Have things not seemed real to you at times?
    o   Have you been doing anything that you feel is unusual for you?
    o   Have you been doing anything that has been out of character?
    o   Have you had any strange ideas that have been worrying or even frightening?
    o   Have you had any problems with your thoughts?

- Have you been having difficulties with your family, friends or work colleagues or other people? In what ways?
- What impact has this had on your daily life and everyday functioning?

    o   Have you been unable to do anything that you could usually do?
    o   Has this impacted on your social life?
    o   Has this affected your work?
    o   Has the problem changed the way in which you care for yourself? Are you able to keep yourself clean?
    o   Have their been changes to your eating habits?

- Have you been having any physical health problems? Do you think they might be connected to how you feel at the moment?
- Do you think it is likely that you might harm other people or yourself? Do you worry that you might harm other people or yourself?

If a problem or issue has been identified, it is useful to consider with the person how much of a problem it is for them. Here, you may wish to clarify this initial problem a bit more by asking:

- How often do you experience this? How many times a day, for example?
- When you do experience it? How intense/bad does it seem to you?
- When you do experience it? For how long does it last each time?
- Is the problem/symptom there all the time? Does it come and go?
- Does it seem to be improving or getting worse?

Predisposing Factors

Issues which may have led the person to be more vulnerable to developing mental health problems are **predisposing factors**, e.g. attachment history, early upbringing, their core beliefs and underlying assumptions about themselves, the world and their future. A defining condition of being human is our urgent need to understand and order the meaning of our experiences, and to integrate this with what we know. Frequently, things appear to happen as a bolt out of the blue, but quite often the person in the midst of the distress cannot see the connections to their previous experiences or events.

Concepts of vulnerability to illness can be traced back to when psychiatry began to evolve into a scientific discipline. For example, in 1977, Zubin and Spring argued for a 'new view of schizophrenia' that sought to explore how stressors could lead to a breakdown of coping in people vulnerable to schizophrenia. They argued that we all have a degree of vulnerability which can be *inborn* (for example, due to a person's genetic profile) and/or *acquired* (for example, the influence of disadvantageous early life experiences, traumas, perinatal complications and formative life events), which due to the interaction and presence of challenging circumstances (or **exogenous stressors**) may provoke a crisis for a person's mental health. Zubin and Spring (ibid.) argue that such stressors include background, ambient day-to-day stresses and crises brought about by significant life events (such as bereavements, marriage, divorce) that require a degree of coping and readjustment in the person's life. Vulnerability, therefore, may be seen as an inability to cope and adapt to stresses that may place their mental health under strain and increase the likelihood of mental ill health or relapse.

Questions, which may help to understand a person's vulnerability, include:

- Could you tell me a little about your background?
- How long have you felt/been feeling like this?
- When was the first time you noticed this?
- When you think back, is there anything you think might have contributed to how things are for you now?

Precipitating Factors

There are recent events that might have contributed to the onset of the person's current difficulties, such as recent life events and stressors. It is difficult to be precise about the exact time frame for considering those factors that may have precipitated the current situation as this is likely to be different for each person. We suggest that a time frame of the previous eight weeks should be considered.

In identifying **precipitating factors**, you are, in effect, taking a recent history of presenting problem as a chronologic account of the events leading up to the current contact with the mental health professional. It includes a description of the evolution of the service user's symptoms that covers onset, duration and changing of symptoms over time. Exacerbating factors of the current distress should be explored, and the practitioner should precisely describe factors that may have precipitated the current distress (Aquilina and Warner, 2004). Stress can arise from events which may be seen as both negative (for example, bereavement, divorce, job loss) and positive (such as getting married, job promotion).

Zubin and Spring (1977) defined vulnerability as an individual's threshold for tolerating stress, where stress was defined as either ambient/everyday stress or life-event stress. It is now almost universally accepted that the stress, which will cause major illness in one individual, will cause barely a ripple in another. Put another way, this means that a crisis will either be contained homeostatically or lead to an episode of illness/ill-health, depending on the individual's resilience/**protective factors** and vulnerability.

The basis of the Stress Vulnerability hypothesis is that everyone varies in their capacity to remain well in the face of personal and environmental stressors (ibid.). People who are predisposed to have a low threshold for tolerating stress are more vulnerable to the effect of ambient and life-event stress. What might be perceived as slight changes in a person's life may be sufficient to increase their vulnerability to becoming unwell or to experiencing a relapse. Thus, whilst getting a clear picture of the presenting problem, the practitioner needs to accurately identify, if possible, all of the changes that have occurred in the service user's life circumstances.

Questions that may be helpful in understanding precipitating factors include:

- What do you make of how things have been going for you recently?
- How would you describe your life over the recent number of weeks?
- Have you experienced any stress recently? Have there been any crises?
- Any problems with your family or social circles? How is work?
- What has led up to your current difficulties?
- Would you say that your problems have been continuous or intermittent over this time?
- When was the last time you felt well?
- How did the condition develop? Is this a long-standing problem? Or has it developed suddenly, gradually, over a period of time?
- How have you been coping? What have you been doing to help you cope?

A timeline is another way of helping the person share recent previous experiences that may impact on the presenting problem. A timeline can be a textual narrative and/or graphical depiction of key events and responses in a person's life ordered chronologically (Kirk, 1994). It can help the person see how a series of apparently unconnected events are, more often than not, connected. It can organise confusing experiences; help the person recognise their strengths and vulnerabilities; and identify recurrent themes and patterns. Some people find written accounts, diagrams or charts easier to follow (e.g. Table 4.1) than listening to verbal explanations.

Table 4.1 Example of a timeline

Event	Time	Response
Announcement of redundancies at work	30 May 2016	This was such a shock. I was frightened that I was going to lose my job and income. I thought they were trying to get rid of me.
Asked to speak to my manager about my fears of losing my job. Manager refused to talk to me about this.	1 June 2016	I felt that I was already being targeted. Anxious that I would lose my job. How will I pay the mortgage? Felt that I have not been performing well and that's why they wanted to get rid of me.
Received a letter telling me I was 'at risk' of losing my job. Needed to attend a redundancy interview for my job on 4 July 2016.	2 June 2016	Increasingly anxious. Losing sleep. Couldn't eat. Felt sick. Didn't want to talk to anyone. Kept myself to myself. Having arguments with family. Feeling angry with everyone.
Sick leave	25–30 June 2016	Couldn't go to work. Too tired. Exhausted and feeling the world is against me. Drinking too much alcohol.
Day of the redundancy interview	4 July 2016	Phoned in sick and cancelled the interview. Had not slept well for days. Lost weight. Couldn't stop thinking about the interview and losing my job. Felt that I was worthless.
Attended GP appointment	5 July 2016	GP feels I might be depressed. Wants me to be seen by a mental health professional. Worried that if work find out, they will make me redundant.

EXPERT VOICE

The way I complete a timeline is to literally draw a straight line across one or two large pieces of paper and, through a collaborative process between the practitioner, service user and family member(s), as appropriate, encourage them to think back and tell you their life story to date. Be aware that this may be a very painful process for some people due to the fact that, most commonly, people who have a psychotic illness will have experienced trauma or abuse in their past, which you are encouraging them to talk about. Ensure that this session is not rushed and that you have allowed enough time to complete it with them. For example, that you don't have back-to-back service users booked in on that day. This exercise may also take more than one session but, generally, the most useful and accurate timelines work best when not rushed.

Protective Factors

Protective factors include personal strengths and coping abilities, resilience, helpful beliefs, positive relationships, situations where the person feels better, skills, functional coping skills and so on.

As mentioned above, a timeline, and discussions about precipitating factors, can help to identify significant factors in a person's life that underpin the current problem. This can also be helpful in establishing the person's resources and ability to cope. *Helpful coping strategies* – such as talking things through with a confidant, doing something pleasurable, having a laugh, getting out and about – are often protective to the person's psychological health. Affirmative feedback (see Chapter 2) should be offered when a person has devised elaborate, novel, sophisticated or ingenious ways of coping with the distress caused by their problems.

Questions include:

- How have you coped?
- Has anything helped you to cope over this time?
- Who has been helpful? In what ways?
- What are some of the good things in your life?

Perpetuating Factors

Factors that maintain the person's problem, such as unhelpful or dysfunctional coping skills, negative automatic thoughts and so on are **perpetuating factors**. Coping strategies, of course, can be both helpful and unhelpful. While *helpful coping strategies* may be seen as protective (see above), *unhelpful coping strategies* may perpetuate a current problem or prevent a resolution to ongoing difficulties. Such strategies include apathy, avoidance, denial, anxiety, fear, bursts of anger, and the misuse of alcohol and drugs. There is an opportunity here to acknowledge that such coping strategies are not likely to be very helpful in the long term and may ultimately cause additional stress and difficulties for the person.

Questions include:

- Has anything made the situation worse for you over this time?
- What has not been helpful?
- Is there any reason that you have not sought help up until now?
- Has anything happened to prevent the situation from improving?
- Have you done anything, such as using alcohol, to cope with or avoid the situation?

Initial Conceptualisation

An 'initial conceptualisation' uses a normalising rationale (Kingdon and Turkington, 1991) and factors discussed above (see Figure 4.1) to help the individual make sense of what has been happening. The practitioner's aim is to help translate the service user's narrative into an authentic shared understanding/conceptualisation (Persons, 2012). This helps the service user and practitioner to better understand what is often seen as a diverse set of unrelated problems and sources of distress (ibid.). The initial conceptualisation of the presenting problem also facilitates an understanding of the possible origin(s) of the difficulties against the backdrop of the service user's strengths/resilience and vulnerabilities/needs and enables the development to the next stage in the care planning process.

Sharing Your Initial Conceptualisation

Below is an example of how you might share an initial conceptualisation using the example of the timeline described in Table 4.1, but remember that this will be an initial sketch and further assessment discussion may reveal a deeper understanding of the problem(s) or issue(s):

- *Normalising rationale*: Coping with the threat of redundancy has been very difficult for you. It is not surprising that you have experienced problems with losing your appetite and not going to work. It is understandable that you have been worrying about losing your job – this is a concern that most people would also have.
- *Presenting problem*: You are losing weight and you feel very tired at the moment. You feel you can't concentrate on anything and you are quick to anger. You feel low in mood and have not been eating or sleeping well. You have been isolating yourself and having arguments with your family.
- *Predisposing factors*: You have told me that your situation reminds you of your father losing his job when you were at school and you feel that it led to his premature death. You are still angry as you feel that his employers took him away from you.
- *Precipitating factors*: You have described a number of current stresses for you. You are worried that you will be unable to provide for your family if you lose your job. You have money worries. Your mortgage is very high and you worry that you are not able to keep up payments, and you have no idea how you would cope if you lose your job. You have been worried that you are not performing as well in your job as some newer members of staff and that your manager wants to get rid of you.
- *Perpetuating factors*: You say you have been drinking heavily recently, and it is understandable that you have done this to help you cope, but this is likely to prove unhelpful if you were to continue in that way. It may lead to addiction and cause additional stresses for you and may prevent you from working on a resolution to the current situation. You feel distant from your wife and not able to talk to her about the situation and your fears. You feel she will blame you.
- *Protective factors*: You love your family and they are supportive of you and each other. You enjoy your job and you feel you have good working relationships with your colleagues. You are usually determined to succeed. You have kept on top of your work and usually know to seek out help when things are getting on top of you. You are keen to be proactive and want to look at ways of managing these stresses more effectively.

In sharing your initial conceptualisation, you should acknowledge the person's feelings, remaining empathic and hopeful. Be flexible: if the person does not agree with you, then provide them with the opportunity to discuss.

Above is an example of how you might share your initial conceptualisation conversationally. However, it would also be a good idea to provide this in written form
so that it can be revisited and reviewed later.

Seeking Feedback

It is very important that you check that the person can validate this initial conceptualisation and that you obtain feedback from the service user. This helps to ensure
your shared understandings and that any inaccuracies or misunderstandings can be
corrected. Helpful questions here might include:

- How do you feel about what I have said?
- Do you think what I have said accurately captures the situation for you?
- Is there anything I have left out or misunderstood?
- Is there anything else you would like to add?
- Do you have any questions?

Hypothetical Questions

In developing a shared understanding of the initial conceptualisation, the use of
hypothetical questions allows you to gauge how the person might act or what they
think about a possible situation moving forward. They are effective in getting a
person to think about and discuss new ideas or approaches to a problem from a
different perspective. Hypothetical questions can usually be perceived as less challenging than open questions. It is important to emphasise that, in this situation, we
are not suggesting that hypothetical questions are used to assess judgement and
reasoning, or to evaluate the person's response, but purely as an alternative to gaining an understanding of the presenting problem in a manner that may be less
stressful for the individual. For example:

- Tell me how things would be if everything was OK.
- How would things be different if you didn't have these concerns?
- If this continued, what do you think would happen?
- If you didn't manage to resolve this current difficulty, what do you think would
  happen?
- If these feelings/experiences didn't stop, what is the worst thing that might happen?

Difficulties with Understanding the Person's
Presenting Problem

Sometimes, of course, there is considerable difficulty in understanding the person's
presenting problem. This may be due to the fact that the service user is too distressed
or unwell to discuss the issues with you – or they might find it difficult to talk about

painful issues. You might also encounter difficulties in trying to make sense of the person's problem or in finding the words to accurately capture the complexity of the person's situation. This can be very frustrating but it is not uncommon. The skills and techniques we have described in this chapter require practice and you should always ensure that you have access to an experienced colleague with whom you can discuss your initial conceptualisation and who can help you to consider issues for your personal and professional development when using psychosocial techniques.

Chapter Summary

The presenting problem is just the beginning of appreciating what is causing the person distress. More detailed information needs to be gathered through a comprehensive assessment to develop a shared understanding of strengths and needs and to collaboratively develop an effective treatment plan. Throughout, the practitioner needs to be able to maintain a style that fosters collaboration and, in order to achieve this, they must have, or develop, the ability to engage the service user and family/personal network, expressing empathy and showing compassion.

A meeting between a service user and professional is a direct intervention in their lives, and a minimum requirement for such an encounter is that they leave this first meeting feeling more empowered and knowing that something can be done to lessen their distress (Seikkula and Arnkil, 2006).

EXERCISE

When new styles of therapeutic conversation are being entered into, it can take a considerable amount of time to become familiar with them and to become proficient in the skills. You may first want to test out your skills of questioning with a colleague to build your confidence:

1. Use the above framework to structure an initial presenting problem interview. It can be helpful to test out questions in a safe environment, so that you can stumble, reflect and repeat, as it is not unusual to find new ways awkward, unnatural or unspontaneous to use.

CONSIDERATIONS FOR PRACTICE

1. Asking helpful questions requires the practitioner to have current knowledge of mental health and mental ill health. How would you rate your knowledge and understanding of the impact of illness? How might you develop your subject knowledge?

(Continued)

(Continued)

2. How might you deal with the following challenges in interviewing:

   a) The person has difficulty organising his/her thoughts.
   b) They find open-ended questions too difficult to answer.
   c) They are struggling with voices, intrusive thoughts, overwhelming emotions.
   d) They seem fearful and unable to trust others.
   e) They are frightened and concerned of the consequences of sharing information.
   f) They are overwhelmed by negative past experiences.

Further Reading

Cooper, P. (ed.) (2012) *The Complete Overcoming Series*. London: Constable and Robinson.

This is a compilation of everything in the Overcoming Series, which uses a cognitive behavioural approach to understanding and treating very common causes of mental distress. The books successfully combine a person-centred and methodical approach to gaining a shared understanding of the individual's distress from presenting problem to successful outcome.

Filer, N. (2014) *The Shock of the Fall*. London: Borough Press.

This fictional novel could be used very easily as a parallel text to a psychiatry text. Each stage of the protagonist's (Matt Homes) journey from early resilience, to the emergence of psychosis is expertly ascribed to paper. In this book, Matt Homes narrates his experiences of mental illness. Filer deftly captures the authentic meaning of narrative.

Gawande, A. (2011) *The Checklist Manifesto: How to Get Things Right*. Croydon: Profile Books.

There seems to be no profession where a checklist might not help, health care included. There are good and bad checklists: the good checklists are precise, efficient, to the point and easy to use, and they provide reminders of the most critical and important steps. This is not to suggest that therapeutic conversations become formulaic or manual driven. We all refer to guiding ideas of some sort in the development of therapeutic conversations, but frequently they are invisible and unavailable to critical reflection. Gawande is very convincing in his argument that checklists work to guard against complacency in practice.

White, M. (2011) *Narrative Practice: Continuing the Conversation*. New York: W.W. Norton.

Michael White is one of the pioneers of narrative therapy. White's approach creates space for therapeutic dialogue that clears the way for narratives of hope, possibility and change. Via real therapeutic conversations with service users, he captures each of the five main areas of narrative practice and provides readers with an explanation of the practical implications of these conversations.

References

Aquilina, C. and Warner, J. (2004) *A Guide to Psychiatric Examination*. Norwich: Pastest.

Bruner, J. (1990) *Acts of Meaning*. Cambridge, MA: Harvard University Press.

Buckley, P., Prewette, D., Bird, J. and Harrison, G. (2005) *Examination Notes in Psychiatry*, 3rd edn. New York: Oxford University Press.

Carlat, D. (2004) *The Psychiatric Interview*, 2nd edn. Philadelphia, PA: Lippincott Williams and Wilkins.

Hamkins, S. (2014) *The Art of Narrative Psychiatry*. Oxford University Press.

Hawton, K., Salkovskis, P., Kirk, J. and Clarke, D. (1989) *Cognitive Behaviour Therapy for Psychiatric Problems*. New York: Oxford University Press: Oxford

Kingdon, D. G. and Turkington, D. (1991) 'Preliminary report. The use of cognitive behaviour therapy and a normalising rationale in schizophrenia', *Journal of Nervous & Mental Disease*, 179: 207–21

Kinsella, C. and Kinsella, C. (2015) *Introducing Mental Health: A Practical Guide*. 2nd edn. London: Jessica Kingsley.

Kirk, J. (1994) 'Cognitive–behavioural assessment', in K. Hawton, P. Salkovskis, J. Kirk and P. Clarke (eds) *Cognitive Behaviour Therapy for Psychiatric Problems*. Oxford: Oxford Medical Publications, pp. 13–51.

The Mid Staffordshire NHS Foundation Trust Public Inquiry (2013) *Report of the Mid Staffordshire NHS Foundation Trust Public Inquiry*. Available at: http://webarchive. nationalarchives.gov.uk/20150407084003/http://www.midstaffspublicinquiry.com/sites/ default/files/report/Executive%20summary.pdf (accessed 31 October 2016).

Mishler, E.G. (1986) *Research Interviewing: Context and Narrative*. Cambridge, MA: Harvard University Press.

Morrison, J. (2014) *The First Interview*. 4th edn. New York: Guilford Press.

Owen, G., Wessely, S. and Murray, R. (2014) *The Maudsley Handbook of Practical Psychiatry*. 6th edn. Oxford: Oxford University Press.

Persons, J. (2012) *The Case Formulation Approach to Cognitive-Behaviour Therapy*. New York: Guilford Press.

Powell, T. (2009) *The Mental Health Handbook: A Cognitive Behavioural Approach*, 3rd edn. London: Speechmark.

Rogers, C. (1980) *A Way of Being*. New York: Houghton Mifflin.

Sadock, B., Alcott-Sadock, V. and Ruiz, P. (2014) *Kaplan and Sadock's Synopsis of Psychiatry*. 11th edn. Philadelphia, PA: Lippincott Williams and Wilkins.

Seikkula, J. and Arnkil, T. (2006) *Dialogical Meetings in Social Networks*. London: Karnac.

Zubin, J. and Spring, B. (1977) 'Vulnerability: a new view of schizophrenia', *Journal of Abnormal Psychology*, 86: 103–26.

5

SOCIAL AND ENVIRONMENTAL CONTEXT

STEVE TRENOWETH

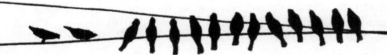

CHAPTER OVERVIEW

This chapter:

- Considers the quality of an individual's social life.
- Discusses factors relating to an individual's social and environmental context and those that impact on the social health and well-being of the individual.
- Highlights those factors that facilitate and support, or impede and undermine, the individual in their social and interpersonal functioning.

Introduction

In this chapter, we consider the issues that potentially affect how the individual is grounded within their community, society and wider environmental context. We will also consider issues relating to an individual's *social performance* or *competency*. This will inevitably consider issues such as the impact of social inclusion/exclusion, social and interpersonal stressors, stigma and stereotyping, community integration and social functioning but we will also consider the impact of the built and natural environment on the individual's well-being. Specifically, we will consider the individual's interpersonal and intimate relationships, family and work, but also activities which forge social and community engagement (**prosocial activities**), including the culture, language and identity, and the positive role that organised religion, social clubs and groups can play. A number of assessment approaches and rating scales are described to illustrate how we can help the person to share their social and interpersonal experience.

Psychosocial Stress

An individual's social context (their social circumstances and the environment in which they live) can have a profound impact on their mental health and well-being. The Stress Vulnerability model (Zubin and Spring, 1977; also see Chapters 4 and 11) reminds us of the factors which impact on our ability to cope with challenging circumstances in our lives. While the model originally considered an alternative view of the development of schizophrenia, it has, over time, been seen as a useful theoretical approach to explain the possible influences and interplay of social and environmental contexts on our biological mechanisms (Goh and Agius, 2010).

The model suggests that it is the exogenous stressors (such as bereavements, divorce, marriage, childbirth and so on) that may precipitate a crisis, and may pose challenges for an individual's ability to cope and adapt to such stresses and subsequently readjust their lives. One of the most widely cited scales used to capture the impact of such stressors on your social and interpersonal lives in research is the Social Readjustment Rating Scale (SRRS) (Holmes and Rahe, 1967), which seeks to capture the impact of life events on our health. The SRRS seeks to catalogue the impact that 43 stressors have on health and our chances of becoming ill as a consequence, such as: bereavements; changes in our social circumstances (such as moving house, having a child, divorce), work-related difficulties; and problems with family relationships. Interestingly, the scale highlights the psychosocial stress we experience from what we might consider positive experiences (such as an outstanding personal achievement, holidays and Christmas!). Each factor is weighted in terms of its psychological impact and stressors are considered to compound one another to which numerical values are assigned. For example, if a person experiences the death of a spouse (which on the SRRS is given a value of 100), with a concomitant major change in financial state (which scores 38), and a subsequent revision of their personal habits (which scores 24), then this person's overall score is 162 – which suggests a 50 per cent risk of developing a stress-related health problem over the next two years.

However, there have been criticisms of the major life-events approach, in that it does not consider the individual impact of each life-event stressor on our daily lives or factors that may mediate and protect us from psychological harm in the face of such events. It should also be remembered that not all events carry equal weight to individuals in terms of their psychological impact – that is, not everyone will necessarily experience a bereavement in the same psychological manner (Office for National Statistics, ONS, 2002). Kanner et al. (1981) suggest an approach that considers the psychological impact of daily 'hassles' (i.e. irritating, frustrating, distressing demands or practical difficulties) for the individual in their transaction with their environment. Such daily hassles can involve:

- Social (e.g. crowding, queuing, being ignored or talked over).
- Interpersonal (e.g. family problems, work-related conflict, arguments).
- Situational (e.g. traffic jams).
- Practical (e.g. accommodation problems, financial difficulties, debt).
- Environmental (e.g. noise, pollution).
- Any of the above in combination.

Kanner et al. (1981) further argue that everyone can expect to experience a number of hassles in their lives, but any impact of such stressors on an individual's physical and mental health will depend on, for example:

- The number of hassles.
- The repetition and frequency of hassles, particularly if the person remains in the same context (e.g. due to their routines, lifestyle choices and habits, work or marriage).
- The compounding effect of daily hassles during a rare occurrence, life event or a crisis, such as a serious injury, bereavement or the birth of a baby.
- Hassles that have particular psychological importance for the individual, such as receiving an unexpected bill when the person is already experiencing financial problems.
- The ability of the person to cope and manage hassles.

There are also a number of issues which may be very detrimental to a person's psychological well-being but which may not be accounted for within a life-stress inventory and/or may be given sufficient weighting. People who experience mental health problems, particularly psychosis, are disproportionately far more likely to suffer victimisation than the general population (ONS, 2002). The ONS survey of 2002 found that, amongst people diagnosed with a psychotic disorder: 47 per cent said that they had been bullied; 37 per cent had been subject to violence in the home; 34 per cent had run away from home; 31 per cent cited sexual abuse; 28 per cent had been homeless; and 11 per cent had experienced violence at work.

'Uplifts', on the other hand, involve positive experiences and help mitigate daily hassles, such as having a good night's sleep; engaging with nature; solving and overcoming challenges; shopping; getting good news and so on. Kanner et al. (1981) suggest that assessing the balance of hassles and uplifts may be a better approach to understanding the person's experience of, and ability to cope and adapt to, life stress. That is, in assessing the quantity and quality of an individual's daily hassles, an assessment would also be needed of what might be considered mitigating factors – namely, daily uplifts, that is, positive experiences such as relief at receiving good news, support from friends and colleagues and so on. (See Kanner et al., 1981, for further details of the 'Hassles' and 'Uplifts' Scale.)

Social Inclusion/Exclusion

Social exclusion is defined as: 'the phenomenon where particular people have no recognition by, or voice or stake in, the society in which they live' (Charity Commission, 2001: 2). For Maslow (1943), social inclusion, in the form of belongingness and love, were essential motivational needs. This included friendship, romance and intimacy, affection and love and from relationships from work colleagues, family and friends.

A sense of belonging, access to social networks and an affiliation to a community can bring significant psychological and practical benefits to individual citizens. While it is arguable that everyone is motivated in the same way to fulfil such social needs, social exclusion from a community (or communities) can drastically reduce access to services, facilities and amenities and their life chances (such as career prospects) and from participating fully in wider society. It can also, of course, significantly impact on their mental health and well-being.

Community affiliation occurs when an individual becomes attached to a group who share similar aims and ideals, and helps to create a feeling of belonging and group identification. This can take many forms, including membership of, for example:

- Organised religions: While for some people their religion is an important part of their spiritual lives, organised religion represents a set of shared beliefs and values between people that can also offer community support.
- Cultural and ethnic groups: Expressed through language, beliefs, national, ethnic and personal identities.
- Political organisations.
- Occupational groups.
- Associations and social clubs.

Such affiliations provide opportunities for engagement in social and recreational activities and prosocial behaviour (Birchwood et al., 1990).

There are many possible reasons why a person, group or community may be socially excluded (including self-exclusion, where people may remove themselves; see Charity Commission, 2001), such as:

- Unemployment.
- Financial hardship.
- Youth or old age.
- Ill health (physical or mental).
- Substance abuse or dependency, including alcohol and drugs.
- Discrimination on the grounds of sex, race, ethnic origin, religion, creed or sexuality.
- Poor educational or skills attainment.
- Relationship and family breakdown.
- Poor housing (i.e. housing that does not meet basic habitable standards).
- Crime (either as a victim of crime or as an offender rehabilitating into society).

Mental ill health may be just one factor for social exclusion, compounded by others, facing an individual, which further undermines their social inclusion.

Social exclusion often occurs following the stigmatisation of a person or group and people with mental health problems can be amongst the most excluded in society (ONS, 2002). Similarly, the fear of being stigmatised may lead to a reluctance to seek help and support, which may have an effect on the recovery rates (Norman and Malla, 2001). Stigma originally referred to a distinguishing mark that was burned or cut into human flesh (Goffman, 1963) to identify slaves or criminals so that others would know their status in society. The term today reflects societal attitudes towards people who are deemed by a group to be less valued or who are to be excluded in some way (Link and Phelan, 2001; Porter, 2004).

Stigma can result in marginalisation from society, oppression, distress, poorer prospects of training for employment and associated socioeconomic restrictions, loneliness, loss of self-worth and feelings of hopelessness, or in extreme cases deliberate self-harm or even suicide (Bracken and Thomas, 2005). There is evidence, too, which suggests that stigma may have a negative impact, not only on the onset of a person's mental health problems, but also on the trajectory and course of the condition (Penn and Wykes, 2003). Families and friends can also feel stigmatised by association, which can, in turn, negatively impact on family dynamics and relationships (Link et al., 2001).

It is important to help the person share their social and community experiences by asking questions such as:

- Do you feel a part of your local community? Tell me about this.
- Are you an active member of an organised religion? Do you feel a part of this community?
- What groups, clubs or societies do you belong to?
- What hobbies/social/sport/recreational activities do you enjoy? Do these involve other people? In what ways?
- Tell me about your culture. Do you feel a part of your community?
- How often do you visit (or are visited by) family and friends?

Work

Work potentially bestows a sense of personal development, growth and achievement along with financial independence, but in social terms it can offer a sense of team sprit and collegiate camaraderie that is both personally and interpersonally rewarding. However, it has long been recognised that people with mental health problems consistently find obtaining meaningful work challenging. The *Social and Economic Circumstances of Adults with Mental Disorders* survey (ONS, 2002), for example, found that about a third of respondents in the sample group (no disorder, alcohol dependency, dependency, neurosis or psychosis) were unemployed or economically inactive, but amongst those diagnosed with a psychosis this rate was more than double at 72 per cent. People with a diagnosed disorder were represented more in the manual social classes: 39 per cent in the no disorder group contrasted to 44 per cent of those with a diagnosed neurotic disorder, 52 per cent and 54 per cent of those with alcohol and drug **dependence** and 61 per cent of those with a psychotic disorder (ibid. p.x). However, people diagnosed with an alcohol or drug-related problem were more likely than others in the sample to work in skilled manual occupations (such as craft, metalworking, textile, vehicle maintenance and so on).

Any psychosocial assessment, then, needs to explore not only the person's occupational history (see Chapter 7), but also their training, talents, abilities, skills, opportunities and motivations to obtain current meaningful employment, for example:

- What is your current job?
- What skills, abilities and knowledge do you have that may be valuable in the workplace?
- Have you any occupational training?
- What job would you like to do? What are your ambitions?

Social Support and Relationships

An important part of any social assessment (see Figure 5.1) is that of capturing an individual's social support because there is evidence that people with mental health problems have a poorer social network than the general population (ONS, 2002). Likewise, there is much evidence that adults with a primary support group

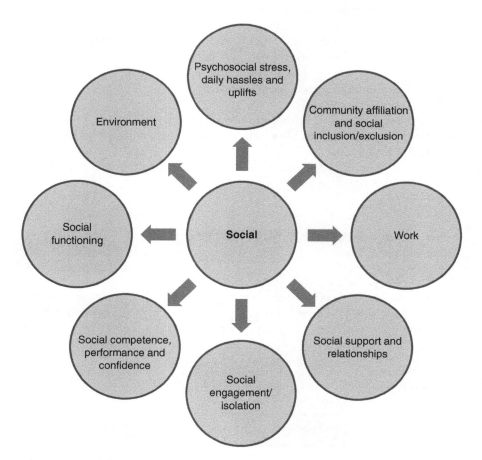

Figure 5.1 An overview of social assessments

(comprising close friends and relatives) of three people or fewer are at greatest risk of developing mental health problems (Brugha et al., 1993).

The ONS survey (2002) found that those with a diagnosed mental health problem are more than twice as likely to have a small primary support group of less than four people (9 per cent), compared to those with no mental health problem (4 per cent). The survey also found that 32 per cent of those people with a diagnosed psychotic disorder had a primary support group of three or fewer people.

There are a number of ways of capturing an individual's family and social networks. A **sociogram**, for example, is a graphical representation of a person's social networks, as illustrated in Figure 5.2 (we will be introduced to Emily in a later chapter).

There are a number of online tools for drawing, some free and some requiring a fee, (e.g. www.text2mindmap.com). A sociogram can be a powerful visual tool for helping the person to identify the quantity and quality of their social and interpersonal networks.

Likewise, a family tree is a visual representation of a person's ancestry and genealogical descent, and can be a helpful way of exploring the relationship(s) of all members of their family. This can be done very simply with a pen and paper but there are also some online tools that could be used (these, however, tend to be ancestry sites for which a charge is usually required).

There may also be a number of questions that you want to ask here to fully understand the person's social support network, for example:

- Do you feel you have a good social network?
- Tell me about your friends.
- Do you have a partner/children? How is that for you?
- Tell me about your parents. Do you have any brothers and sisters? Do they have families? Are you close?
- Do you feel able to talk freely to your friends and family about problems or issues you may have?

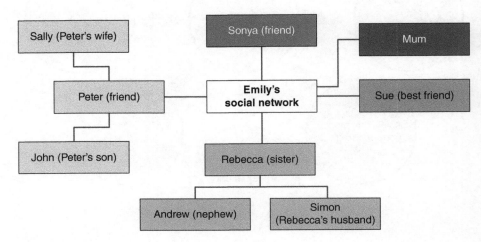

Figure 5.2   A sociogram of Emily's social network

Social Engagement/Isolation

People with mental health problems are more likely to experience social isolation, particularly people diagnosed with a psychotic disorder. The ONS survey (2002) found that amongst people with a psychosis, 10 per cent had seen no friends in the past week, compared to a rate of 4 per cent across the entire sample group (no disorder, alcohol dependency, dependency, neurosis or psychosis), and 45 per cent had only seen one or two friends, compared to an overall rate of 18 per cent.

Here, it is important to capture details about the person's level of social engagement or withdrawal. A number of questions might be helpful, such as:

- Tell me about how you structure your day? How much time do you spend by yourself?
- Do you feel socially isolated?
- Do you ever feel that you would like to avoid people or social situations?
- Do you enjoy occasions when you are alone?

Social Performance, Competence and Confidence

Birchwood et al. (1990) make an important distinction between a person's *competence* in social functioning (which refers to skills that have been lost or are absent) and the *performance* (which they see as the disuse or non-use of a skill). We may add that a person's social performance and competence is also a feature of how much *confidence* we have in ourselves. This may, in turn, be influenced by *internal factors* (such as our mood, fears, expectations, motivations and so on) and *external factors* (which may be situation-specific, such as the presence of people whom the individual finds intimidating, the number of people and other audience factors which may facilitate or inhibit social interactions, e.g. level of support or hostility).

In attempting to understand a person's interpersonal social performance and competence, it is likely that the practitioner will use their observation skills in assessing the quality of an individual's social skills. For example:

- Is the person able to establish eye contact?
- Do they initiate and/or sustain conversations?
- What is the quality of their communication?
- Are they monosyllabic or are they able to sustain a conversation?
- Is their communication clear and understandable?
- How is their body language?
- Do they use active listening?
- Do they follow social conventions, for example by saying 'hello' and 'goodbye'?

It is also important to ascertain the person's perception of their social performance, competence and confidence. Here, a number of general questions may be helpful to structure such a conversation, for example:

- Do you feel awkward in social situations?
- Do you find it easy to make conversation?

- In the past, did you used to find it easier to have conversations with people than you do now?
- How comfortable do you feel around people you don't know very well?
- Do you find yourself being annoyed or having arguments with other people?

Social Functioning

Social functioning can be broadly described as the ability to gain and maintain employment and interpersonal relationships, and generally to look after oneself (Erol et al., 2009). As such, our social functioning is an essential part of our ability to live, adapt to, and operate within, our social and interpersonal world. This is, of course, affected by our current mental state and other factors, such as our level of education, employment and financial status, and the amount of social support available to us (McDonald and Badger, 2002). Psychological factors also affect our social functioning such as memory, concentration, judgement, attention and executive and neurocognitive functioning, which are outside the scope of this book (see, for example, Erol et al., 2009). Here, we are concerned with those self-care, domestic and social skills necessary for community living and functioning.

There are a number of rating scales that can be used – such as Birchwood et al.'s (1990) Social Functioning Scale (SFS), as well as the Global Assessment of Functioning (GAF) scale and the Social and Occupational Functioning Assessment Scale (SOFAS) – to help structure conversations around social functioning. General areas for consideration when assessing social functioning are listed in Table 5.1.

Table 5.1   Areas for assessment of social functioning

Community living	Use of public transport, shopping, community orientation, knowledge and use of public amenities and council offices
Dealing with paperwork	Writing letters, sending cards or filling in forms
Financial	Budgeting, paying bills
Communication	Use of telephone, Internet
Vocational	Looking for a job, occupational skills and behaviour such as attendance, punctuality
Functional mobility	The ability to get around in the community independently; the physical ability to go shopping or visit local amenities

Environment

The environment in which we find ourselves can affect our physical and mental health (Evans, 2003). The built urban environment, for example, can have direct and indirect effects on our mental well-being. Some authors would go even further and argue that our mental well-being is affected by the apparent disconnection between ourselves and the natural world (Buzzell and Chalquist, 2009). It is further argued that we, as human beings, are part of a complex ecosystem. For example, in his Gaia hypothesis,

Lovelock (1979) suggests that the earth could be viewed as a self-regulating entity with interdependent component parts, including humanity. While this hypothesis has advocates and opponents (and further discussion is outside the scope of this book), it does draw our attention to the idea that we, as human beings, cannot be isolated from our environment (Sackett, 2010). The positive health effects of contact with the natural environment are becoming increasingly well recognised (Barton et al., 2012; Annerstedt and Wahrborg, 2011). Hartig et al. (2003), for example, found that spending time in a natural setting reduced blood pressure, stress levels and feelings of anger when compared with an urban setting, and Mitchell and Popham (2008) found that mortality rates were lowest in areas with the greatest exposure to green space.

The quality of our accommodation also has a significant bearing on our mental well-being. For example, cramped, high-rise housing and poor-quality housing appears to increase psychological distress (Evans, 2003). The *Social and Economic Circumstances of Adults with Mental Disorders* (ONS, 2002) survey found that those with a mental disorder were much more likely to be living in rented accommodation than those with no disorder (38 per cent compared to 24 per cent). Approximately 50 per cent of people with a diagnosed psychotic disorder were living in accommodation rented from a housing association or local authority. People with mental health problems are also more likely to live in accommodation that is in a poor state of repair and with a lack of space (ibid.). Other accommodation concerns are security and safety; financial problems in meeting rent; the lease or contract running out; domestic problems; and problems with the landlord or agent (ibid.). These are often conditions that are imposed on people and there may be little subsequent chance of home ownership. There is also a strong link between homelessness and poor mental health, with consistently reported high rates of people with mental health conditions and substance misuse among the homeless population (NHS Confederation, 2012).

Here, it is helpful to understand the person's perception of their environment by asking such questions as:

* Where do you currently live?
* Are you happy with the general environment where you live?
* Do you have any concerns about your living arrangements and accommodation?
* Are there any problems with the quality of your accommodation?

Chapter Summary

Our social and interpersonal environment is complex and can affect our mental health and well-being. Psychosocial stress arises not only from any number of life events but also from daily hassles, which may be mitigated by positive social experiences, social support and uplifts. Social inclusion, and a sense of belonging to a community, organisation and/or group, is important for our well-being, and being socially excluded can impact negatively on our personal identity, mental health, life chances and opportunities. In attempting to understand the person's social and interpersonal world, assessors also need to consider issues relating to an individual's working life; social performance, competency and confidence; and their social engagement and social functioning. The built and natural environment also have a potential impact on the individual's well-being, as do their accommodation arrangements.

EXERCISE

1. Draw a sociogram for your own social networks and a family tree to chart your family and ancestry.
2. When you are using this approach in an assessment, how might you introduce this activity? How might you subsequently use this to understand a person's helpful and not so helpful social relationships?

CONSIDERATIONS FOR PRACTICE

1. How might you involve the family/friends in understanding the person's social and interpersonal context? What are the challenges with this?
2. What can be done if the person's accommodation proves to be unsuitable for them?
3. How could the multi-professional team work together to support the person to share an accurate picture of their social functioning?

Further Reading

Birchwood, M., Smith, J., Cochrane, R., Wetton, S. and Copestake, S. (1990) 'The Social Functioning Scale: the development and validation of a new scale of social adjustment for use in family intervention programmes with schizophrenic patients', *British Journal of Psychiatry*, 157 (6): 853–9, and doi 10.1192/bjp.157.6.853.

A highly influential article which is essential reading for anyone wishing to undertake social assessments in mental health care. Clearly written and comprehensive.

References

Annerstedt, M. and Wahrborg, P. (2011) 'Nature-assisted therapy: systematic review of controlled and observational trials', *Scandinavian Journal of Public Health*, 39 (1): 371–88.

Barton, J., Griffin, M. and Pretty, J. (2012) 'Exercise-, nature-, and socially interactive-based initiative improve mood and self-esteem in the clinical population', *Perspectives in Public Health*, 132 (2): 89–96.

Birchwood, M., Smith, J., Cochrane, R., Wetton, S. and Copestake, S. (1990) 'The Social Functioning Scale: the development and validation of a new scale of social adjustment for use in family intervention programmes with schizophrenic patients', *British Journal of Psychiatry*, 157 (6): 853–9, and 10.1192/bjp.157.6.853.

Bracken, P. and Thomas, P. (2005) *Postpsychiatry: Mental Health in a Postmodern World*. Oxford: Oxford University Press.

Brugha, T.S., Wing, J.K., Brewin, C.R., MacCarthy, B. and Leasge, A. (1993) 'The relationships of social network deficits in social functioning in long-term psychiatric disorders', *Social Psychiatry and Social Epidemiology*, 28: 218–24.

Buzzell, L. and Chalquist, C. (2009) *Ecotherapy: Healing with Nature in Mind*. San Francisco, CA: Counterpoint.

Charity Commission (2001) *The Promotion of Social Inclusion*. Available at: www.gov.uk/government/uploads/system/uploads/attachment_data/file/359358/socinc.pdf (accessed 17 January 2016).

Erol, A., Keleş Unal, E., Tunç Aydin, E. and Mete, L. (2009) 'Predictors of social functioning in schizophrenia', *Turk Psikiyatri Derg.* 20 (4): 313–21.

Evans, G. (2003) 'The built environment and mental health', *Journal of Urban Health*, 80 (4): 536–55, and doi 10.1093/jurban/jtg063.

Goffman, E. (1963) *Stigma: Notes on the Management of Spoiled Identity*. New York: Simon and Schuster.

Goh, C. and Agius, M. (2010) 'The Stress-Vulnerability Model: how does stress impact on mental illness at the level of the brain and what are the consequences?', *Psychiatria Danubina*, 22 (2): 198–202.

Hartig, T., Evans, G., Jamner, L., Davis, D. and Garling, T. (2003) 'Tracking restoration in natural and urban field settings', *Journal of Environmental Psychology*, 23 (1): 109–23.

Holmes, T. and Rahe, R. (1967) 'The Social Readjustment Rating Scale', *Journal of Psychosomatic Research*, 11 (2): 213–18.

Kanner, A., Coyne, J., Schaefer, C. and Lazarus, R. (1981) 'Comparison of two modes of stress measurement: daily hassles and uplifts versus major life events', *Journal of Behavioral Medicine*, 4 (1): 1–38.

Link, B.G. and Phelan, J.C. (2001) 'Conceptualizing stigma', *Annual Review of Sociology*, 27: 363–85.

Link, B.G., Stuening, E.L., Neese-Todd, S., Asmussen, S. and Phelan, J.C. (2001) 'The consequences of stigma for the self-esteem of people with mental illnesses', *Psychiatric Services*, 52: 1621–6.

Lovelock, J. (1979) *Gaia: A New Look at Life on Earth*. Oxford: Oxford University.

Maslow, A.H. (1943) 'A theory of human motivation', *Psychological Review*, 50 (4): 370–96.

McDonald, J. and Badger, T.A. (2002) 'Social function of persons with schizophrenia', *Journal of Psychosocial Nursing and Mental Health Services*, 40 (6): 42–50.

Mitchell, R. and Popham, F. (2008) 'Effect of exposure to natural environment on health inequalities: an observational population study', *The Lancet*, 372: 1655–60.

NHS Confederation (2012) *Mental Health and Homelessness*. Available at: www.nhsconfed.org/~/media/confederation/files/publications/documents/mental_health_homelessness.pdf (accessed 23 May 2015).

Norman, R. and Malla, A. (2001) 'Duration of untreated psychosis: a critical examination of the concept and its importance', *Psychological Medicine*, 31: 381–400.

Office for National Statistics (ONS) (2002) *The Social and Economic Circumstances of Adults with Mental Disorders*. London: TSO.

Penn, D. and Wykes, T. (2003) 'Stigma, discrimination and mental illness', *Journal of Mental Health*, 12 (3): 203–8.

Porter, R. (2004) 'Is mental illness inevitably stigmatising?', in A. Crisp (ed.), *Every Family in the Land*. London: Royal Society of Medicine Press.

Sackett, V. (2010) 'Ecotherapy: a counter to society's unhealthy trend?', *Journal of Creativity in Mental Health*, 5 (1): 134–41.

Zubin, J. and Spring, B. (1977) 'Vulnerability: a new view of schizophrenia', *Journal of Abnormal Psychology*, 86 (2): 103–24.

6

PHYSICAL HEALTH

TERESA BURDETT

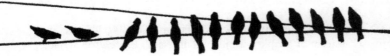

CHAPTER OVERVIEW

This chapter:

- Highlights the importance of physical assessment and physical health care to mental health practitioners.
- Offers a usable, flexible and supportive strategy of physical assessment to inform, educate and update mental health practitioners.
- Provides a variety of opportunities for the reader to critically reflect on their own present level of knowledge and setting.
- Suggests how the reader may enhance their level of knowledge of physical assessment and care that they provide in their own setting and share this knowledge with other practitioners.
- Demonstrates assessment of some commonly presenting conditions, including the interventions and strategies to undertake.

Introduction

Undertaking a physical health assessment with people experiencing mental health problems is vital. Appropriate assessment and care is fundamentally important as individuals with mental health issues are particularly at risk from physical health issues (Robson and Gray, 2007). This is particularly noticeable in individuals who have a diagnosis of schizophrenia or bipolar disorder, whose lifespan is on average 15–20 years shorter than the general population (Laursen et al., 2014; Miller and Bauer, 2014).

It is important that procedures to protect the service user and promote their health and safety are being applied appropriately and safely, including, for instance, appropriate infection control practices such as hand hygiene (National Patient Safety Agency, 2008; DH, 2008). In response to this, organisations will have their own specific policies and training in place to uphold these legislative and professional demands.

An Overview of Physical Assessment

Physical health has been sometimes overlooked in mental health care. Fewer than 30 per cent of all individuals with a diagnosis of schizophrenia have a yearly physical health screening (NHS England, 2016), despite their increased risks (Laursen et al., 2014; Miller and Bauer, 2014; Brown et al., 2010). Physical health assessments and subsequent care are vital to prevent long-term ill health and disability, which may exacerbate a mental condition. It is also crucial that physical illnesses are excluded before a mental disorder is suspected, as the symptoms of physical illness may appear superficially similar to a psychiatric presentation. For example, confusion arising from an acute urinary infection can mask an underlying cognitive impairment.

Conducting a Physical Health Assessment

Presented in this chapter are suggestions that may be useful for you to use when assessing physical health needs. However, whatever way you physically assess a service user, your approach needs to be: person-centred; suitable to capture all the relevant information; effective, safe, timely and responsive to the presenting issues; and appropriate to the service user and the environment in which they inhabit. The assessment needs to lead to a subsequent resolution of health concerns for the service user, such as treatment, referral and review.

You should, of course, explain what the physical health assessment entails and ensure that you have the person's consent to proceed. You should also consider where the assessment is taking place. For example, the venue should be comfortable and clean, and people should be able to discuss their symptoms privately.

Physical assessment incorporates a number of skills that we need to consider and practice each time we are involved with our service users. This includes care that is sensitive and it is vital that an assessor is able to adapt the physical assessment to accommodate the person's gender and cultural needs. This may mean, for instance, arranging non-urgent appointments so that they do not clash with days that have specific meaning for the service user.

You should also consider the use of a chaperone. This may be due to cultural or gender reasons or to the intimate nature of the assessment taking place.

Barriers to communication may involve language or communication difficulties, sensory impairment or the lack of understanding, which can impact and undermine the accuracy of the assessment made. Therefore, an interpreter may need to be arranged or information re-explained in a different format.

Initial Questions

Ensuring a collaborative dialogue is vital and your actions should work to make certain that this happens. For instance: ensure that hearing aids are working and in place; book and arrange an interpreter prior to the consultation.

It is important to start off with broad, open, global questions about how the person is feeling, for example:

- How can I help you?
- How do you feel today?
- What is causing you concerns?
- What brings you here today?

Such questions help to elicit what the person's concerns may be and will also allow you to understand their personal experience. Such a broad narrative will allow you to follow up with more direct, specific questioning so as to explore particular symptomatology. Broader questioning should also be used to gather information on a wide range of biographical data which may be of relevance in your assessment of physical health, such as:

- Age.
- Occupation.
- Previous medical history, e.g. allergies.
- Family health.
- Medication, e.g. dosage, usage, effects and side effects.
- Previous hospital admissions.
- Operations.
- Serious illnesses.
- Present conditions.
- Social activities and lifestyle factors, e.g. diet and exercise.
- Use of substances, e.g. alcohol, tobacco, drugs.

It is vital that you accurately record your consultation. Policies vary slightly in differing organisations but will require you to document the discussion, and recording your results ensures transparency of your actions and that you fulfil policy and professional obligations (Nursing and Midwifery Council, NMC, 2015). Practitioners can vary in the degree of skills to undertake physical health assessments but everyone should be able to notice if a person is experiencing symptoms which are out of the ordinary for them (either because this is reported by the person themselves or by their family/friends) and subsequently to refer the person on to someone who can undertake a more thorough assessment. Needless to say, you should not undertake any intervention for which you have not been adequately trained or prepared.

Signs and Symptoms

Physical assessment includes taking and recording baseline observations of a person's vital signs, including pulse, blood pressure, **oxygen saturation**, temperature and respirations. Mnemonics are commonly used tools to aid structuring the physical assessment and can be helpful in directing your questioning to gain a fuller picture of the presenting issue and the service user's signs and symptoms.

An example of mnemonic is **OLDCART** (Seidel et al., 2003), which refers to:

- Onset: When did it start?
- Location: Where is it? Is it all over? Can you point to it?
- Duration: How long has it lasted or is it continuous?
- Characteristics: What is it like? For example, is the pain sharp or stabbing or a dull ache?
- Aggravating factors: Are there other symptoms which you feel are connected? For example, do you feel hot and sweaty as well as having abdominal pain?
- Relieving factors: What makes it better? For example, is sitting more comfortable than standing?
- Treatment: What can I/we do to help to alleviate symptoms?

Utilising another mnemonic such as Morton's (1993) **PQRSTU** can also be helpful in directing your questioning to gain a fuller picture of your service user's signs and symptoms:

- Provocative or Palliative: What makes the symptom/s worse or soothes the symptoms?
- Quality or Quantity: Ask the person to describe and define the symptom – What is it like? How often do they experience it? How many times?
- Region or Radiation: Where it is?
- Severity: On a scale of 1–10, where 1 is 'no severity' and 10 is 'extremely severe'. Does the person feel that the problem is getting better or worse?
- Time: Time it started? How long has it lasted?
- Understanding: What does the person think about their symptoms?

Using these frameworks can greatly increase your knowledge about your service user's presenting issue and ensures that a person's physical and mental health needs receive equal assessment and appropriate treatment (British Medical Association, 2014). However, these are only tools, and your own professional knowledge, and your knowledge of your service user and/or setting, will also help to form the framework of your questioning.

Head-to-Toe Assessments

When assessing the person's physical health, you may take the **head-to-toe systems approach** (see below), which ensures a systematic comprehensive approach (Bickley2013). An overview of a head-to-toe assessment can be found in Figure 6.1.

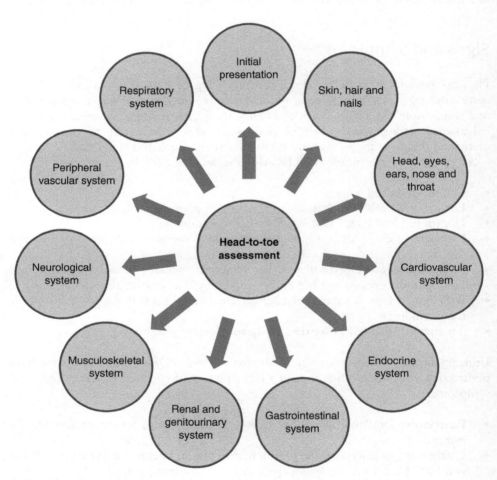

Figure 6.1 An overview of a head-to-toe assessment

Initial Presentation

Here, you will be using your observational skills to gain an initial impression of the person's physical health issue(s). There is much you can tell about the person's symptoms by their initial presentation. In asking questions, always ensure that any sensory aids that are required by the person (e.g. glasses, hearing aids) are worn so that they are able to respond. Consider, for example:

- Are there any obvious or suggestive signs of injury – such as bleeding, bruising?
- What is their facial expression like? Is it contorted or are they expressing pain?
- Are they agitated? Do they seem confused?
- Are they awake and alert? Or drowsy?
- How do they stand and hold themselves?
- What is their pallor and skin condition? Do they appear hot and sweaty? Or cold and clammy?
- Are their eyes clear or bloodshot?
- Do they appear to understand what you are asking or do they appear confused?
- What state is their clothing in – is it stained, if so, are they neglecting themselves?

Following on from the initial presentation, you may wish to consider the particular system which is first affected before moving on to consider which other systems may also be affected. Underpinning all of the assessment process is your own knowledge of the human anatomy and physiology system.

Skin, Hair and Nails

Skin review includes looking for rashes. If they are present, are they itchy? Rashes in the **flexures** could be indicative of **atopic eczema**. Larger patches or plaques on elbows and knees may indicate **psoriasis**. If moles or lumps are present, and are bleeding or have changed shape, this might be an early indicator of skin cancer.

Hair and nails are often reviewed with the skin. What is the person's hair condition like? Has there been recent hair loss? Changes in the hair and nails can often indicate illness, for example thinning hair is symptomatic of **hypothyroidism**.

Head, Eyes, Ears, Nose and Throat (HEENT)

Head

When reviewing the head, consider the size and shape, including measuring if appropriate. Has there been a history of a head injury, dizziness, light-headedness or headache? All may need further investigation or referral for a **CAT/CT** scan. For instance, a headache is a common neurological symptom, so assessment includes asking about its duration, type of ache or pain, and where in the head it is situated.

Eyes

Eyes may reveal a number of health-related issues. Physical assessment includes asking about the eye history of the service user and their family and making a visual assessment. If they use ocular aids, what are they for and when are they used? Has the person seen an optician recently and, if so, what was said?

Ears

Ears help with balance and hearing. When assessing, it is important to include asking about the person's ability to hear and if the person has noticed any changes?

Do they use aids and are they helpful? If the person has earache, then the mnemonic **OLDCART** is useful. If there is discharge, a sample may need to be taken, but on visual inspection, what does the discharge look like? What colour is it? Does it look infected or is there blood? The sample will need to be sent for analysis. This may aid with any subsequent treatment.

Nose

Have there been any nosebleeds recently or discharge? Is their breathing affected? Is there a nasal infection or upper respiratory tract infection evident?

Throat, Mouth and Neck

Are there any complaints of difficulty in swallowing? Is there any evidence of an allergic reaction? What is the colour and shape of the tongue like? Is it normal? Does the person wear dentures? Is there any dental pain? Is there swelling present in the neck? Is the person holding their neck in an unusual position (**torticollis**)? Are they complaining of pain?

The Cardiovascular System

Cardiovascular episodes or incidents are elevated as much as three times amongst individuals who have a diagnosis of schizophrenia when compared with the general population (Jindal et al., 2005; Robson et al., 2008; Chang et al., 2011). Cause for concern here may incorporate a wide variety of symptoms, including chest pain (which may indicate a **myocardial infarction** or **MI**), palpitations, **oedema** or shortness of breath, including **dyspnoea, orthopnoea** or **paroxysmal nocturnal dyspnoea**. All of these may be of concern and such presentations may be life-threatening, so be prepared to act swiftly if needed.

The Endocrine System

Endocrine glands secrete hormones directly into the blood and include the thyroid and pituitary. A number of symptoms may be evident in endocrine disorders. They may be diffused and have different onsets, some over many years. Taking a full medical history and investigating the presenting symptoms is paramount to make sense of what may otherwise be a random array of symptoms. Taking baseline observations may reveal changes. The pulse is often elevated (**tachycardia**) when **hyperthyroidism** (**thyrotoxicosis**) is present. **Hypertension** is present in **Cushing's syndrome**, recorded weight and height and extrapolating the **Body Mass Index (BMI)** may be helpful in indicating **polycystic ovary syndrome** (**PCOS**) and Cushing's syndrome. Weight loss may indicate hyperthyroidism and **diabetes mellitus**.

Urinalysis is an important initial observation and cannot be underestimated. It is a simple and inexpensive assessment (Krogsboll et al., 2015) and provides very useful diagnostic information about a person's health (Merenstein et al., 2006; Gronhoj Larsen et al., 2012). Urinalysis may, for instance, reveal **proteinuria** in hypertensive renal damage and **glycosuria** in diabetes mellitus. Further investigations may include blood tests to investigate specific complaints, for example calcium is high in **hyper-parathyroidism**; imaging, including **ultrasound** of the thyroid, parathyroid, ovary, testis and **Magnetic Resonance Imaging (MRI)** of the pituitary and pancreas, may be necessary.

Diabetes mellitus is an endocrine disorder and is more common in the mental health service user group (Sernyak et al., 2002; Smith et al., 2008). This can be either type 1 diabetes (where the person is dependent on insulin) or type 2 diabetes (diet-controlled, with or without medication). Assessment of diabetes consists of a routine approach, baseline observations and recording BMI, fluid assessment, input and output, urinalysis (Krogsboll et al., 2015) and blood tests. Common symptoms include **polyuria** and also **nocturia**. Signs of diabetes may include a relentless thirst as the person tries to consume more liquid. Recent weight loss may be suggested by a person's clothes being noticeably baggier and a reducing BMI.

Referral is required and both short- and long-term care and patient education is vital to reduce the secondary complications of diabetes mellitus. These include macrovascular disease (WHO, 2016) and sexual dysfunction (Phillips and Phillips, 2015).

Diabetes that is usually well controlled by the service user may become unstable in the event of deterioration in their mental state.

CASE SCENARIO 6.1   ADRIAN

Adrian is 27 years of age and has type 1 diabetes. Recently, he has been acutely unwell with a virus. There is danger that his blood sugar levels could become unstable. Adrian should be assisted to care for himself and maintain his own diabetes, depending on how he is feeling. Factors to control his diabetes include testing his glucose levels every 2–4 hours throughout the 24-hour period. Adrian should be encouraged to take glucose foodstuffs such as fruit juice and soup if he is finding eating difficult. His urine should be tested every time he voids for the presence of ketones, which are a product of fat-burning. As Adrian is taking fluids and his glucose levels are stable (6–15 mmol/l) and there is no presence of ketones in his urine, this demonstrates that his diabetes is being kept within manageable limits whilst he is unwell.

The Gastrointestinal System

The gastrointestinal system has a number of functions, including ingestion, digestion of food products and excretion of waste products. Symptoms of gastrointestinal disorders may include abdominal distension, abdominal or flank pain, altered bowel habits, heartburn, indigestion, nausea, vomiting and/or weight loss. Each symptom will need to be investigated and the use of the mnemonics (OLDCART or PQRSTU described above) may be useful here for a thorough approach.

Abdominal distension may be associated with obesity but if a person has lost weight and abdominal distension is present, it may be an indicator of a gastrointestinal disorder. Abdominal distension may also be due to **ascites** and this always requires further investigation.

Additional assessment requires recording bowel habits, taking a stool sample, assessing and recording dietary intake, BMI and monitoring weight. Urinalysis is an appropriate assessment as is assessing skin discolouration. The presence of **jaundice** is an indicator to act upon. Any acute abdomen symptoms require prompt referral and urgent review.

The Renal and Genitourinary System

The renal and genitourinary system includes the kidneys, urinary tract and reproductive organs. Signs and symptoms that may be cause for concern include pain, discharge from the penis or vagina and frequent voiding.

Sensitivity is required due to the nature of the areas being discussed, including taking a sexual history and/or examination. Ngwena (2011) suggests that individuals with mental health issues may have reduced awareness of sexually transmitted diseases and are therefore increasingly vulnerable to a genitourinary disorder. Hence the enhanced need for appropriate assessment by practitioners caring for, and providing support to, mental health service users.

Urinalysis is a fundamental assessment tool in a genitourinary disorder which may indicate changed kidney function, and the presence of blood in the urine or protein may indicate an infection or **glomerular disease**. Further investigations include abdominal X-ray, ultrasound scan, blood tests and investigation of any discharge. Flank or back pain may indicate kidney disease or urinary tract infection.

The Musculoskeletal System

The musculoskeletal system consists of bones, joints and muscles. Symptoms of a musculoskeletal disorder may include locking of joints, nodules, pain, stiffness, swelling and weakness. Assessment consists of a routine approach, including a full history as well as any trauma and history of injuries. Baseline observations need to be taken and recorded, including an X-ray of the painful area, assessment of pain and appropriate referral, for instance to a rheumatologist.

Urinalysis may detect protein, which may indicate **rheumatoid arthritis**, and X-rays may detect factures; **ultrasonography** may detect **effusion** or **synovitis**. Joint aspiration may detect raised **white cell count**, which may indicate infections.

The Neurological System

The neurological system is a complex system that may well require specialist assessment and treatment. Symptoms of neurological disorder may include cerebrovascular accident, dizziness and headache, loss of consciousness, loss of sensation, speech impairment, syncope (fainting), tremors and weakness. **Epilepsy** is one of the most common neurological conditions (Ogden, 2015).

A neurological assessment consists of completing baseline observations as described below. Physical assessment includes identifying areas of weakness or stiffness. Blood tests and **nerve conduction studies** may also be required. A CAT/CT brain scan may indicate **subarachnoid/intracranial haemorrhage.**

An assessment of the level of consciousness can be facilitated by using the AVPU scale, namely:

- **A:** Is the person awake or alert?
- **V:** Are they responsive to your voice and/or commands?
- **P:** Are they responsive to a pain stimulus?
- **U:** Are they **un**responsive?

In assessing orientation, it is common to consider:

- Person (knows their own name).
- Place (knows where there are).
- Time (knows the day and date).

Another level of orientation is that of *purpose* – does the person know that they are being examined and why you are examining them?

The role of the mental health practitioner includes being alert to the possibility of neurological disorders, responding to the service user's presenting issues, offering support and reassurance appropriately, and referral as appropriate once an issue has been identified.

The Peripheral Vascular System

Pain in the legs or cramping pains is not uncommon. Assessment consists of checking for swelling in the limbs, oedema, colour of the limbs, evidence of ulceration, temperature of the limbs and recent medical history such as surgery or bed rest which may have increased the likelihood of **deep vein thrombosis (DVT).** Deep venous thrombosis is relatively common, with one individual in every thousand being diagnosed with a DVT (Scottish Intercollegiate Guidelines Network, 2010). It is potentially life-threatening and the role of the mental health practitioner includes assessment, offering adequate pain referral and prompt referral. Subsequent medical actions may include checking for the presence of the pulse in the **femoral, popliteal dorsis pedi** and **posterior tibial artery** and conducting a **Doppler** ultrasound scan.

The Respiratory System

The respiratory system includes the upper respiratory tract and the lungs. Mental health service users are four times more likely to die from diseases of the respiratory system than the general public (Health and Social Care Information Centre, HSCIC, 2013).

People may present with symptoms including a cough, excess or discoloured sputum, pain, breathing difficulties and **cyanosis.** Assessment includes asking about their smoking and occupational history and baseline observations including respiration rate. A sputum sample may need to be taken and any cough over three weeks old needs referral: a **chest X-ray** is usually required.

Activities of Daily Living (ADLs)

Activities of Daily Living (ADLs) are those things we normally do in daily living, including any daily activity that we perform for self-care (see Table 6.1). The ability or inability to perform ADLs can be used as a practical measure of ability/disability whilst people are experiencing mental health problems and can be helpful in understanding the person's ability to care for themselves in the face of medical conditions or physical challenges (Barker, 2004).

Table 6.1 Activities of daily living

Personal appearance	Dressing oneself, cleanliness and appropriateness of clothing, ability to launder clothes
Personal hygiene	Bathing or showering, washing hair, dental hygiene, manages menstruation, use of toilet and toilet hygiene
Household	Housekeeping and domestic-living skills, cooking and food preparation, cleaning, tidying, gardening, decorating or doing household repairs
Functional mobility	The ability to undertake activities independently, such as getting in and out of bed or a chair; to undertake self-care actions (moving from one place to another while performing activities)
Eating and drinking	The ability to meet own dietary and fluid-intake needs
Sexual functioning	Changes in sexual expression; difficulties

Some helpful questions in understanding a person's ADLs include:

- What's your appetite like?
- How are you eating?
- Is there any change in your weight?
- How are you sleeping?
- What time do you get to sleep and what time do you wake up?
- Do you sleep right through or wake up in the night?
- After you've woken up, do you get back to sleep?
- What time do you eventually wake up in the morning?
- Is there any change in your interest in sex?
- Are you less interested in sex than usual?
- Is there any change in how often you have your bowels open?
- Do you experience constipation?
- Is there any change in your energy levels?
- Do you have more or less energy than usual?

Screening and Health Promotion

People with mental health problems are more vulnerable to physical ill health than the general population (HSCIC, 2013; Keyes et al., 2010). However, mental health service users often receive less health promotion advice than the general population (Hardy et al., 2013; DH, 2006). Parity of esteem, which was enshrined in law in 2014 by the Health and Social Care Act, will only be achieved between physical and mental health when such disparities are addressed. Hence the even greater need for health promotion to be offered to this population group.

In undertaking a physical assessment as part of an overall psychosocial assessment, it is likely that the opportunity to discuss health promotion will arise. This may, in turn, raise awareness of issues when considering a case conceptualisation and when formulating needs and goal statements.

There are a number of factors to consider when offering health promotion to individuals who have mental health issues. For instance, breast cancer rates are higher and bowel cancer rates are twice as high in individuals who also have a diagnosis of schizophrenia than in the general population (Disability Rights Commission, 2006). Also, when co-morbid physical conditions are diagnosed, care is often poorly managed (Lawrence and Kisely, 2010; Robson et al., 2008).

In mental health care, assessment of physical health tends to occur only when the person presents with specific symptoms or when a pre-existing complaint is known, but it is vital that a proactive approach is taken and that broader health promotion practices are routine. This may occur opportunistically, such as offering smoking-cessation advice when a person identifies a need to stop smoking. However, health promotion practices also need to be organised and arranged, including offering yearly health screening. All male service users should be offered health promotion information on testicular examination and prompt referral should be encouraged as required (NICE Guidance, 2014). This is important as, according to Prostate Cancer UK (2016), more than 10,800 men a year die of testicular cancer. All female service users need to be offered gender-specific health promotion information, for instance regarding breast care, breast self-examination, mammograms and cervical smears.

Annual Health Checks

To optimise the physical health of individuals with mental health illness, Robson et al. (2008) recommended annual health checks that should be inclusive and comprise physical assessment. However, there is still clear evidence that the physical health of the mental health service user population is below the general population, especially in individuals with long-standing mental health issues such as schizophrenia (Brown et al., 2010; Lawrence and Kisely, 2010). Nevertheless, some new initiatives in Cheshire (Cole, 2015) and Bradford (Dale, 2015) are demonstrating that, in some areas, this imbalance may be reducing. Cole (2015) demonstrates an increased uptake of health screening from 6 per cent to 94 per cent.

However, health promotion is not a once-a-year stand-alone venture. Health promotion needs to be offered, both routinely and as a bespoke service. Areas of health promotion to discuss may include activity and exercise, dental care, diet and nutrition, medication, sleep, sexual health, substance use and ocular health.

Activity and Exercise

There are significant physical and mental health benefits of being active and exercising (Reid et al., 2010). These benefits are of additional importance in individuals with mental health issues as they often have poorer physical health outcomes. Health promotion activities may include providing information on the benefits of physical exercises and also the potential additional risk to their health of being inactive. Guidelines suggest weekly 150 minutes of moderate intensity activity (UK Chief Medical Officers, 2011). Advising people of what is available to them in their community may enable them to achieve these suggested guidelines. Enhancing access to facilities and supporting the mental health service user's aims may play a significant part in increasing their own health, both physical and mental.

Dental Care

Dental care should be a service offered to all mental health service users as they tend to have higher levels of tooth decay than the general population (Kisely et al., 2015). Providing information about dental care and hygiene and ensuring access to dental services may reduce the discomfort of poor teeth and enhance an individual's self-esteem.

Diet and Nutrition

A healthy diet can improve both physical and mental health (NHS England, 2016). Hence, maximising opportunities to promote the diet and nutrition of mental health service users is vital as they tend to have a poorer diet than the general population (McCreadie, 2003). A poorer diet raises the risk of other health issues such as coronary heart disease (Emberson et al., 2003) and may also compound the impact of mental health problems (Peet, 2004). Such health-promoting activities may include offering education about an appropriate healthy diet and weight, recording BMI and recording dietary intake. Giving information about local services that help with, for instance, weight loss, is also useful, as is signposting available services and enabling access to them by the mental health service user.

Medication

Health promotion includes ensuring that mental health service users are informed about the purpose and benefits of their medication and the contraindications, too. There are also other risks to consider. For instance, there is a link between antipsychotic medication (such as olanzapine) and **hyperlipidaemia,** which increases by five times the risk associated with cardio- and cerebrovascular disease (Gatineau and Dent, 2011; Koro et al., 2002). Weight gain is also associated with the newer antipsychotics (Bak et al., 2014; Gatineau and Dent, 2011), which also increases the risk of physical disorders such as type 2 diabetes (Citrome and Yeomans, 2005). Therefore, promotion around eating healthily is of additional importance to mental health service users.

Sleep

Adequate sleep is a building block for good health (National Heart, Lung and Blood Institute, 2012). However, a poor sleeping pattern may impact on an individual's health (Luyster et al., 2012). Sleep may be disrupted by lifestyle actions such as television and computer use, medication being taken to improve mental health, or by cigarette smoking (Liu et al., 2013). Health promotion education, including a baseline assessment of the individual's sleep pattern as well as discussing the benefits of good sleep and sleep-enhancing strategies, may be beneficial. Such signposting for better sleep may well help mental health service users to sleep better and consequently function at a higher level.

Sexual Health

Health promotion requires sensitivity, tact and cultural competence (Leininger, 1999) and, due to the increased risks for mental health service users, the topic of sexual health needs to be discussed. The sexual health of the service user is often ignored (Volman and Landeen, 2007) and as psychiatric medication often alters sexual function, it has been identified that this is a factor behind non-adherence (Higgins et al., 2006). Psychiatric medication dampens sexual desire and impacts on erectile function. The weight gain associated with psychiatric medication causes physical health issues and reduces self-esteem. Antipsychotic medication has also been associated with an enhanced rate of osteoporosis in this group (Halbreich and Palter, 1996). Increased risk-taking and a reduced knowledge base leads to an increased risk of HIV and sexually transmitted disease (Ngwena, 2011). Signposting to services and referral and also offering support and education, for instance regarding breast care and monthly self-breast examination and testes examination, are vital and health education is therefore additionally beneficial to mental health service users.

Substance Use

The impact on mental health service users' physical health due to alcohol and drugs use is profound and up to 60 per cent of individuals diagnosed with schizophrenia may abuse substances (Citrome and Yeomans, 2005; also see Chapter 10). The use of drugs and alcohol may interact with neuroleptic medication that may lead to an increased risk of suicide and violent behaviour (Vose, 2000). Such usage may impact on physical health, and a loss of inhibition leads to increased risk-taking behaviour and enhanced risk of sexually transmitted disease and HIV (Ngwena, 2011).

Mental health service users tend to smoke more than the general population (McCloughen, 2003). The reasons for smoking are complex, including habit, addiction and relaxation (Robson and Gray, 2007). However, there is a significant amount of data that demonstrates the profound effect that smoking has on physical health and mortality (NICE, 2015; Ezzati and Lopez, 2003).

Health promoting actions consist of discussing the present situation with the mental health service user and including the potential impact that their actions are having on their physical health. It is also useful to assess the level of alcohol being consumed, the drugs being taken and the cigarettes being smoked and why. There are clear guidelines for the support strategies available, including referral and appropriate signposting, which can be tailored to the individual once a thorough assessment has been completed.

Ocular Health

Individuals' use of health services is affected by a variety of factors and the use of ocular services are no different (Donoghue, 1999). Promoting the ocular health of the mental health service user includes being aware of potential visual changes, signposting to ocular services, enabling access to ocular services and offering support and assistance. This may include encouraging the mental health service user to attend appointments, wear glasses and instil eye drops. However, mental health service users do have specific risks to their eye health, including an increased risk of cataract due to some antipsychotics which can cause a loss of vision (Marder et al., 2004). Chlorpromazine and prochloperazine, for example, have been identified as increasing the risk of developing cataracts (Ruigómez et al., 2000). Consequently, guidelines (Marder et al., 2004) suggest being aware of visual changes in mental health service users and acting on such changes, including asking yearly about blurred vision and the quality of distance vision. Mental health service users should have yearly ocular examinations if they are over 40 and every two years if they are under 40.

Chapter Summary

In this chapter, we explored how to conduct a general physical health assessment, but we also considered those specific areas where the physical health of the mental health service user may be particularly vulnerable. Strategies offered in the chapter to achieve this include person-centred assessment, reviewing symptoms, treating symptoms and conditions using mnemonics and a head-to-toe systems strategy. We have also highlighted factors which may undermine physical health (such as a lack of exercise, poor diet, smoking and so on) and the need for appropriate health promotion strategies in mental health care, whether opportune or planned.

EXERCISE

May is a 65-year-old woman being cared for at home by twice-daily carers and her family, and has become increasingly confused, agitated and distressed over a period of two days. She is complaining of pain in her pelvis and lower back. Her sleep has deteriorated and she is falling more frequently. Her family are exhausted but are under the impression that it was her mental health that was deteriorating. Consider:

1. How would you structure an assessment of May's physical health?
2. What physical health problems might May be experiencing?
3. Why might concerns over her mental health overshadow her physical health?

An outline answer is given at the end of this chapter.

CONSIDERATIONS FOR PRACTICE

1. Revisit the skills and knowledge contained in this chapter and reflect on the implications for your own personal and professional development. How might you address any deficits that you have highlighted? Are there any issues that you would like to include in your appraisal/personal development plan?
2. How might mental health services ensure that they routinely screen for physical health conditions? Is there anything else that your service could do to promote psychosocial health?

OUTLINE ANSWER TO EXERCISE (MAY)

In May's case, it is important to be open to the potential of a physical issue being the cause of her sudden deterioration. A head-to-toe assessment would be appropriate as she is presenting with issues affecting a number of systems (e.g. musculoskeletal, neurological). The use of OLDCART or PQRSTU to understand the overall experience of symptoms would be helpful.

The rapidity of onset of her confusion and agitation, along with pain in her pelvis, is suggestive of an infection (possible urinary tract) that needs exploring. It would be vital to assess her fluid input, urinary output, amount, frequency, colour and smell of her urine. A urinalysis should be conducted alongside a full physical health assessment. We should not assume that confusion and agitation is 'simply' due to May's age. Such a misdiagnosis can be due to a number of factors, such as ageist views about older people or to a lack of knowledge or experience about physical health on the part of the practitioner. It may also be due to diagnostic overshadowing, in which physical symptoms are interpreted in terms of existing mental health conditions or diagnoses (Jones et al., 2008).

Further Reading

Bickley, L.S. (ed.) (2013) *Bates' Pocket Guide to Physical Examination and History Taking*, 7th edn. New York: Wolters Kluwer/Lippincott Williams and Wilkins.

A comprehensive guide to physical examination and history taking and which is a handy size to carry around with you.

Douglas, G., Nicole, F. and Robertson, C. (2009) *Macleod's Clinical Examination*, 12th edn. London: Churchill Livingstone Elsevier.

A comprehensive guide to history taking and both general and systematic examinations within a variety of patient populations. This book is filled with useful photographs and diagrams to aid diagnosis and enhance assessment and care.

Marieb, E.N. (2014) *Essentials of Anatomy and Physiology*, 11th edn. San Francisco, CA: Pearson Education.

Anatomy and physiology can often be an area where mental health practitioners feel that their knowledge is deficient. This useful aid has an understandable writing style and use of tools to enhance learning.

Rushforth, H. (2009) *Assessment Made Incredibly Easy: Adapted for the UK*. New York: Wolters Kluwer/Lippincott Williams Wilkins.

The title says it all. A guide to the aspects of health assessment presented in a format that is easy to read and follow.

References

Bak, M., Fransen, A., Janssen, J., van Os, J. and Drukker, M. (2014) 'Almost all anti-psychotics result in weight gain: a meta-analysis', *PLoS One*, 9 (4): e94112.

Barker, P. (2004) *Assessment in Psychiatric and Mental Health Nursing: In Search of the Whole Person*, 2nd edn. Cheltenham: Nelson Thornes.

Bickley, L.S. (ed.) (2013) *Bates' Pocket Guide to Physical Examination and History Taking*, 7th edn. New York: Wolters Kluwer/Lippincott Williams and Wilkins.

British Medical Association (BMA) (2014) *Recognising the Importance of Physical Health in Mental Health and Intellectual Disability: Achieving Parity of Outcomes*. London: BMA. Available at: www.bma.org.uk/workingforchange/doctors-in-the-nhs/mental-health-parity-report (accessed 24 May 2015).

Brown, S., Kim, M., Mitchell, C. and Inskip, H. (2010) 'Twenty-five year mortality of a community cohort with schizophrenia', *British Journal of Psychiatry*, 196 (2): 116–21.

Chang, C., Hayes, R., Perera, G., Broadbent, M., Fernandes, A., Lee, W., Hotopf, M. and Stewart, R. (2011) 'Life expectancy at birth for people with serious mental illness and other major disorders from a secondary mental health care case register in London', *PLoS ONE*, 6 (5): e19590.

Citrome, L. and Yeomans, D. (2005) 'Do guidelines for severe mental illness promote physical health and wellbeing?', *Journal of Pharmacology*, 19 (6): 102–9.

Cole, D. (2015) 'Challenging people's ideas', *Nursing Standard*, 29 (52): 21–3.

Dale, K. (2015) 'Achieving parity of esteem', *Independent Nurse*, 17 August: 35–7.

Department of Health (2006) *Choosing Health: Supporting the Physical Health Needs of People with Severe Mental Illness Commissioning Framework*. London: DH. Available at: webarchive.nationalarchives.gov.uk/+/en/publicationsandstatistics/publications/publicationspolicyand guidance/dh_4138212 (accessed 17 November 2015).

Department of Health (2008) *Health and Social Care Act*. Available at: www.gov.uk/government/publications (accessed 18 November 2015).

Department of Health (2014) *Health and Social Care Act*. Available at: www.gov.uk/government/publications (accessed 18 November 2015).

Disability Rights Commission (2006) *Equal Treatment: Closing the Gap*. Available at: http://disability studies and Leeds.ac.uk/files/libraryDCR-Health-FI-main.pdf (accessed 6 February 2016).

Donoghue, M. (1999) 'People who don't use eye services: "making the invisible visible"', *Community Eye Health Journal*, 12 (31): 36–8.

Emberson, J.R., Whincup, P.H., Morris, R.W., et al. (2003) 'Re-assessing the contribution of serum total cholesterol, blood pressure and cigarette smoking to the aetiology of coronary heart disease: impact of regression distribution bias', *European Heart Journal*, 24 (19): 1719–26.

Ezzati, M. and Lopez, A.D. (2003) 'Estimates of global mortality attributable to smoking in 2000', *The Lancet*, 362 (9387): 847–52.

Gatineau, M. and Dent, M. (2011) *Obesity and Mental Health*. Oxford: National Obesity Observatory. Available at: www.noo.org.uk/uploads/doc/vod_102666_Obesity%20and%20mental%20health_Final_070311_MG.pdf (accessed 17 November 2015).

Gronhoj Larsen, C. Jorgensen, K.J. and Gotzsche, P.C. (2012) 'Regular health checks: cross sectional survey', *PLoS ONE*, 7 (3): e33694.

Halbreich, U., and Palter, S. (1996) 'Accelerated osteoporosis in psychiatric patients: possible pathophysiological processes', *Schizophrenia Bulletin*, 22: 447–54.

Hardy, S., Hinks, P. and Gray, R. (2013) 'Screening for cardiovascular risk in patients with severe mental illness in primary care: a comparison study with patients with diabetes', *Journal of Mental Health*, 22 (1): 42–50.

Health and Social Care Information Centre (HSCIC) (2013) *Mortality Rate Three Times as High among Mental Health Service Users than in the General Population*. Available at: www.hscic.gov.uk/article/2543/ (accessed 1 December 2015).

Higgins, A., Barker, B. and Begley, C. (2006) 'Sexual health education for people with mental health problems: what can we learn from the literature?', *Journal of Psychiatry and Mental Health Nursing*, 13 (6): 687–97.

Jindal, R., Mackenzie, E.M., Baker, G.B. and Yerangari, U.K. (2005) 'Cardiac risk and schizophrenia', *Journal of Psychiatry Neuroscience*, 30 (6): 393–5.

Jones, S., Howard, L. and Thornicroft, G. (2008) 'Diagnostic overshadowing: worse physical care for people with mental illness', *Acta Psychiatrica Scandinavica*, 118 (3): 169–71.

Keyes, C.L.M., Dhingra, S.S. and Simoes, E.J. (2010) 'Change in level of positive mental health as a predictor of future risk of mental illness', *American Journal of Public Health*, 100 (12): 2366–71.

Kisely, S., Baghaie, H., Lalbro, R., et al. (2015) 'A systematic review and meta-analysis of the association between poor oral health and severe mental illness', *Psychosomatic Medicine*, 77 (1): 83–92.

Koro, C.E., Fedder, D.O., L'italien, G.J., et al. (2002) 'An assessment of the independent effects of Olanzapine and Risperidone exposure on the risk of hyperlipidemia in schizophrenic patients', *Archives of General Psychiatry*, 59 (11): 1021–6.

Krogsboll, L.T., Jorgensen, K.J. and Gotzsche, P.C. (2015) 'Screening with urinary dipsticks for reducing morbidity and mortality', *Cochrane Database of Systematic Reviews*, 1: CDO10007.

Laursen, T.M., Nordentoft, M. and Mortensen, P.B. (2014) 'Excess early mortality in schizophrenia', *Annual Review of Clinical Psychology*, 10: 425–8.

Lawrence, D. and Kisely, S. (2010) 'Inequalities in health service provision for people with severe mental illness', *Journal of Psychopharmacology*, 24 (4): 61–8.

Leininger, M. (1999) 'What is transcultural nursing and culturally competent care?', *Journal of Transcultural Nursing*, 10 (19): 9.

Liu, J.T., Lee, I.H., Wang, C.H., Chen, K.C., Lee, C.I. and Yang, Y.K. (2013) 'Cigarette smoking might impair memory and sleep quality', *Journal Formos Medical Association*, 112: 287–90.

Luyster, F.S., Strollo, P.J., Zee, P.C. and Walsh, J.K. (2012) 'Sleep: a health imperative', *Sleep*, 35: 727–34.

Marder, S.R., Essock, S.M., Miller, A.L., et al. (2004) 'Physical health monitoring of patients with Schizophrenia', *American Journal of Psychiatry*, 161 (8): 1334–49.

McCloughen, A. (2003) 'The association between schizophrenia and cigarette smoking: a review of the literature and implications for mental health nursing practice', *International Journal of Mental Health Nursing*, 12 (2): 119–29.

McCreadie, R. (2003) 'Diet, smoking and cardiovascular risk in people with schizophrenia: a descriptive study', *British Journal of Psychiatry*, 183: 534–9.

Merenstein, D., Daumit, G.L. and Dowe, N.R. (2006) 'Use and costs of non-recommended tests during routine preventative health exams', *American Journal of Preventative Medicine*, 30 (6): 521–7.

Miller, C. and Bauer, M.S. (2014) 'Excess mortality in bipolar disorders', *Current Psychiatry Reports*, 16 (11): 499.

Morton, P. (1993) *Health Assessment in Nursing*, 2nd edn. North Wales, PA: Springhouse.

Nambiar-Greenwood, G. (2015) 'What is the real meaning of culturally appropriate care', *Nursing in Practice*, 85: 30–1.

National Heart, Lung and Blood Institute (2012) *Why is Sleep Important?* Bethesda, MD: National Heart, Lung and Blood Institute. Available at: www.nhlbi.nih.gov/health/health-topics/topics/sdd/why.html (accessed 7 January 2016).

NHS England (2016) *Commissioning Guidance for Rehabilitation* Available at: https://www.pmguk.co.uk/data/page_files/publications%20and%20reports/2016/NHS%20England%20Commissioning%20Guidance%20for%20Rehabilitation.pdf (accessed 31 October 2016).

NHS England (2016) *Improving the Physical Health of People with Mental Health Problems: Actions for Mental Health Nurses*. Available at: tinyurl.com/hdlnky4 (accessed 7 March 2016).

NICE Guidance (2014) *Prostate Cancer: Diagnosis and Management*. Available at: www.nice.org.uk/guidance/cg175 (accessed 7 January 2016).

NICE Guidance (2015) *Smoking: Reducing and Preventing Tobacco Use Quality Standard* [QS82] 2015. Available at: www.nice.org.uk/guidance/qs82 (accessed 28 October 2016).

National Patient Safety Agency (2008) *Clean Hands Save Lives*. Patient Safety Alert 0773. Available at: http://www.nrls.npsa.nhs.uk/resources/?entryid45=59848 (accessed 28 October 2016).

Ngwena, J. (2011) 'HIV/Aids awareness in those diagnosed with mental illness', *Journal of Psychiatry and Mental Health Nursing*, 18 (3): 213–20.

Nursing and Midwifery Council (NMC) (2015) *The Code*. London: NMC.

Ogden, C. (2015) 'Champions needed', *Nursing Standard*, 30 (3): 63.

Peet, M. (2004) 'Diet, diabetes and schizophrenia: review and hypothesis', *British Journal of Psychiatry*, 184 (47): s102–5.

Phillips, A. and Phillips, S. (2015) 'Recognising sexual dysfunction as an essential aspect of effective diabetes care', *Applied Nursing Research*, 28 (3): 235–8.

Prostate Cancer UK (2016) *About Prostate Cancer*. Available at: http://prostatecanceruk.org/prostate-information/prostate-cancer (accessed 4 January 2017).

Reid, K.J., Glazer Baron, K., Lu, B., Naylor, E., Wolf, L. and Zee, P.C. (2010) 'Aerobic exercise improves self-reported sleep and quality of life in older adults with insomnia', *Sleep Medicine*, 11 (9): 934–40.

Robson, D. and Gray, R. (2007) 'Serious mental illness and physical health problems: a discussion paper', *International Journal of Nursing Studies*, 44 (3): 457–66.

Robson, H., Trenoweth, S. and Margereson, C. (2008) 'Co-morbidity in physical and mental health', in J. Lynch and S. Trenoweth (eds), *Contemporary Issues in Mental Health Nursing*. Chichester: Wiley.

Ruigómez, A., Rodriguez, L.A.G., Dev, V.J., Arellano, F. and Raniwala, J. (2000) 'Are schizophrenia or antipsychotic drugs a risk factor for cataracts?', *Epidemiology*, 11: 620–3.

Scottish Intercollegiate Guidelines Network (2010) *Prevention and Management of Venous Thromboembolism Quick Reference Guide*. Available at: sign.ac.uk (accessed 7 January 2016).

Seidel, H., Ball, J., Dains, J. and Benedict, G.W. (2003) *Mosby's Guide to Physical Examination*, 5th edn. St. Louis, MO: C.V. Mosby.

Sernyak, M.J., Leslie, D.L., Alarcon, R.D., Losonczy, M.F. and Rosenheck, R. (2002) 'Association of diabetes mellitus with use of atypical neuroleptics in the treatment of schizophrenia', *American Journal of Psychiatry*, 159: 561–6.

Smith, M., Hopkins, D., Peveler, R.C., Holt, R., Woodward, W. and Ismail, K. (2008) 'First- v. second-generation antipsychotics and risk for diabetes in schizophrenia: systematic review and meta-analysis', *British Journal of Psychiatry*, 192: 406–11.

Stone, S., Teare, L. and Cookson, B., for the Hand-Hygiene Liaison Group (2001) 'Guiding hands of our teachers', *The Lancet*, 357 (9254): 479–80.

UK Chief Medical Officers (2011) *Start Active: A Report on Physical Activity for Health from the Four Home Countries*. Available at: www.gov.uk/government/publications/start-active-stay-active-a-report-on-physical-activity-from-the-four-home-counties-chief-medical-officers (accessed 4 January 2017).

Volman, L. and Landeen, J. (2007) 'Uncovering the sexual self in people with schizophrenia', *Journal of Psychiatry and Mental Health Nursing*, 14 (4): 411–17.

Vose, C.P. (2000) 'Drug abuse and mental illness: psychiatry's next challenge', in T. Thompson and P. Mathias (eds), *Lyttle's Mental Health Nursing*, 14 (4): 411–17.

World Health Organization (WHO) (2016) *Global Report on Diabetes*. Available at: who.int/diabetes/globalreport/en (accessed 18 June 2016).

7

HISTORY TAKING

REUBEN PEARCE

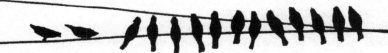

CHAPTER OVERVIEW

This chapter:

- Provides a contextual overview of recording a comprehensive history.
- Discusses the specific communication skills required to sensitively explore a service user's history.
- Demonstrates a systematic approach to exploring a history in partnership with the service user.

Introduction

It is vital that health care staff are able to understand how a service user's current presenting problem fits into their previous experiences. This chapter seeks to explore the person's history, which may have predisposed or increased vulnerability to mental distress and ongoing difficulties they might experience.

History taking is an important component in aiding development of a case conceptualisation and informing subsequent interventions with a service user. The history will normally be taken at an appropriate point at which the service user feels able to revisit their past. The purpose of taking the history is to gather the information necessary to better understand the lifetime of the service user and the impact of this on their biological, psychological and social functioning. Effective history taking is an important clinical skill to learn, most effectively developed by 'doing'.

SERVICE USER VOICE

' I have had both good and bad experiences of nurses discussing my history with me. The time it was bad was because I was feeling very anxious, having just been admitted to hospital for the first time. The nurse just kept firing questions at me and was reading the questions off a bit of paper. He was asking really personal stuff about my childhood and even my sex life. He didn't seem to pick up on my distress and appeared more interested in getting all the answers he wanted as quickly as possible. I noticed that he kept looking at his watch, too, I knew that the ward was busy and so decided just to tell him what I thought he wanted to hear. It actually left me feeling worse than I did before I saw him because it made me start thinking about how rubbish my life was at that time. On the following admission a few years later, I had a much better experience – the nurse really took their time and I could tell they actually cared as they went at my pace and picked up on the things that were particularly hard for me to talk about. The thing I think was most important was that they were genuinely interested in me, I knew they wanted to help me. '

The History-Taking Interview

The history-taking interview is a conversation with a deliberate purpose. It differs from a social conversation in that the practitioner is responsible for the content and flow of the interaction, while the service user is the focus of the discussion. The interview must take place within a specific time frame. The content and process of the interview will vary according to the emotional state of the service user and the context in which the interview takes place.

The aim of history taking is to obtain a comprehensive idea of the service user's experiences over their lifetime, with a focus on their biological, psychological and social functioning. The criteria to be addressed in a comprehensive history-taking session are summarised in Figure 7.1.

It is vital to get off to a good start when taking a history by making sure that the environment is comfortable and the service user has an idea of what to expect (Mackinnon et al., 2015). It is important to remain mindful that the discussion is likely to bring up a number of sensitive issues. Therefore, always remember that the well-being of the service user comes before your own need to gather the information you require.

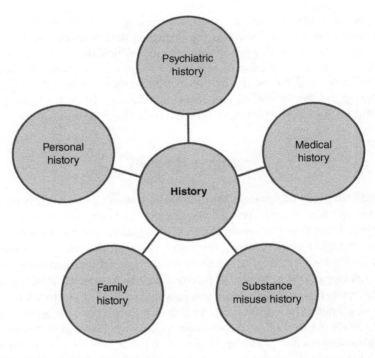

Figure 7.1   The comprehensive history

To aid the process, the following may be helpful to remember at the start of the session:

- Introduce yourself fully.
- Explain who you are and the purpose of the session.
- Put the service user at ease and build a rapport.
- Inform the service user of timings of the interview. How long will it take, roughly?
- Inform them that you may need to take notes.
- Explain confidentiality issues.

Psychiatric History

Information concerning past psychiatric conditions must be obtained in order to better understand the current episode and to aid case conceptualisation. Psychiatric conditions may be a single event, or there may be intermittent episodes, or the condition may be chronic and unrelenting, and the course of the illness may improve or deteriorate over time. Remember that the service user's understanding of their problem may be different from the formal diagnosis and it is important that you understand their perception of the condition and how they might have changed over time. This will then help shape any **psychoeducational** interventions that might be necessary in the future. Corroborative evidence such as previous notes can often be helpful, especially in cases of multiple episodes when it can be difficult to piece together a full picture.

It can be easy to get lost in long accounts of past admissions if these are frequent and this can take some time (Bowers et al., 2009). It may be useful to arrange another date to discuss issues around previous experiences with services if the service user so wishes and keep to the basic facts such as rough dates and length of admissions, treatment given and follow-up arrangements (Aquilina and Warner, 2004).

EXPERT VOICE

' It is important that you explore in detail any previous diagnoses or contact with any psychiatric or other mental health services. Record (as far as possible): dates of illness, symptoms, diagnoses, treatments, any hospitalisations, outpatient treatments, any compulsory treatment under the Mental Health Act 1983/2007:

- Don't forget to establish whether the service user has had episodes of illness for which they have sought help. '

Medical History

The practitioner should ascertain significant previous illnesses, injuries and treatments received (see Chapter 6). It is also important to ask about drug allergies and past and present side effects of medication. The service user's beliefs about their medication can give useful insight into what they believe is wrong with them. Remember to ask about side effects and adherence and bear in mind possible drug interactions (Bickley, 2013). It is important to ask, not just about current and previous prescribed medication, but also over-the-counter and other alternative therapies that the service user may have tried or may be currently using. Make a chronological list of all major physical illnesses, long-term conditions and treatments. There are many physical health conditions that can impact on mental health problems, for example head injuries and chronic pain are often likened to depression and low mood (Aquilina and Warner, 2004).

Substance Misuse History

Studies have shown high co-morbidity of mental ill health and alcohol or substance misuse. Cause is difficult to discern, as alcohol and drug misuse may precipitate an episode of mental illness or may represent a person's attempt to cope with a pre-existing mental health issue. The details here are vital and so, if a service user does disclose that they are using a substance, it is necessary to explore in depth their use and relationship to the substance (see Chapter 10; and Mackinnon et al., 2015). Remember to establish the duration, frequency, amounts and route they use to take the drug. Find out whether the amount/frequency is increasing, and how do they finance the activity? Establish whether they have had periods without using the drug. What are the person's own views on their drug usage? The practitioner should also obtain a history of the caffeine, alcohol and nicotine use. It is important to be aware that some drugs, such as nicotine, may impact on the efficacy of prescribed medication (Taylor et al., 2012).

Family History

Families play a huge role in the recovery process and so obtaining a comprehensive history of the family set-up is crucial. The family history should give you a good indication of the service user's family relationships. Find out which members of the family they have felt close to, and why. Equally, reasons for discord within the family should be explored. Bear in mind social, psychological and genetic risk factors for mental illnesses, and remember to ask about family psychiatric history (Jones, 2010). It can also be helpful when taking the family history to include some reference to cultural tradition, socioeconomic background, family interests and aspirations. When exploring family relationships, it can be useful to draw a family tree (see Chapter 5), recording age, health, occupation and quality of relationship. When exploring the history of psychiatric conditions in family members, don't forget to include alcohol and substance misuse, deliberate self-harm and suicide. An often overlooked area is domestic violence in the family: this can have a severe impact on the development and well-being of a person into adulthood. Finally, include important family events such as death, divorce, separation and the service user's feelings about these events (Mackinnon et al., 2015).

Personal History

The personal history is an account of the service user's infancy, childhood and adolescence through to adulthood. It may provide clues to the origin of current behaviours, for example childhood mental disorders, temperament and style of interpersonal relationships may have remained into adulthood. Personal history is important as it helps you to understand what has led to your service user becoming the person they are (Buckley et al., 2005).

SERVICE USER VOICE

❛ We had a lot of issues in my family growing up that we never talked about, my dad was depressed from when I was young, he never managed to hold down a job for long and had problems with alcohol. This meant that my mum was always working and we never got to do much as a family. I used to feel envious of my friends at school when they talked about holidays they had or going clothes-shopping with their mum. As we didn't have much money, I would be embarrassed of my clothes and got bullied quite a lot by other girls and had trouble getting to know boys. My dad once came to the school and had been drinking, he fell over in front of everyone and other parents were staring. I could see other children whispering to each other. I had never had the opportunity to talk about these things before I saw a mental health nurse following a period of anxiety and depression. Just being able to talk through them with someone who recognised how difficult it had been was a huge relief. What really made a difference was that they genuinely seemed to be interested in my story and wanted to help me work through my problems.

It is easiest to work through the personal history in chronological order, remembering that some of the information may have been gathered earlier on. The key areas to explore when taking a personal history are as follows (also see Figure 7.2).

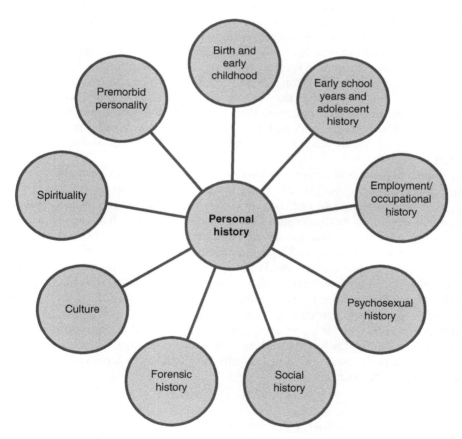

Figure 7.2 The personal history

Birth and Early Childhood

Difficulties in the early years of a child can have a huge impact on our ongoing development into adulthood. It is therefore important to explore all significant events from birth to adolescence. Birth complications, for example, can have an impact on those initial weeks with the mother and, in more severe cases, can cause lasting physical and neurological issues. Complications with the mother, such as post-natal depression, may have an impact on secure attachments being developed. It is important to remember, however, that all human beings respond differently to their environment and what may have a huge impact for one person may have had little impact on another. This is why it is crucial to remember to always view each case on its own unique terms (Aquilina and Warner, 2004).

To aid structure, it can be helpful to record the information chronologically. Work through the developmental milestones of the person from birth to the onset of the current illness. Begin with recording the date and place of birth. It can be helpful to establish what the family social, economic and emotional circumstances were at this time, including the parents' health and marital relationship. In terms of the birth, find out whether it was full term and normal. Also, try to establish whether the service user was breast- or bottle-fed and if feeding was normal.

Importantly, find out whether the service user met those early developmental milestones within the typical time frames – walking, talking, weaning and toilet training. Establish whether they are aware of any early infections that impacted on their development. Record whether they report on any bedwetting, night terrors, sleep walking, fingernail biting, thumb sucking or stuttering – please note that these are not necessarily diagnostic of mental ill health, however, combined together and with other patterns, they may demonstrate some level of anxiety/stress during the person's formative years.

It is rare that we will remember anything before our fourth year and so we are often calling on memories given to us by our parents for those very early years. The years between birth and school 0–5 are widely recognised as crucial in shaping our emotional development (Reder and Lucey, 2014). Establish whatever you can from the service user about their family circumstances, physical, emotional and social development as well as physical health. Find out how they got along with their siblings and other children their age. How did they remember the atmosphere in the home, what was their relationship with mum and dad? The aim is to have a detailed picture of those pre-school years, including any significant event that may have influenced their progress in growing up (Jones, 2010).

It is not uncommon for a service user to ask 'How are these questions relevant?' and so it can be helpful to explain how you want to get a full picture of their life from birth to the present day and how the very earliest experiences may have an impact on our life later on.

Early School Years and Adolescent History

Much like the early years, it is important to continue to get a detailed picture of the school years from age five years through secondary school and adolescence (Carlat, 2004). Work through in chronological order, recording events during the primary, secondary and further education years. Take into account relationships with family members, peers, friends and teachers at school. Did they experience bullying? Did they feel they 'fitted in' – if not, why? What were their achievements during this period – both personally through interests and hobbies and also academically? For example, were they high achievers at school/further education? Did they engage in the education system or did they dislike it – for example, could they be disruptive, have difficulty concentrating, play truant, were they in fights with peers? How were the circumstances at home through their adolescence (Reder and Lucey, 2014)?

SERVICE USER VOICE

' It was weird going through all my childhood and teenage years with the CPN (community psychiatric nurse). Initially, it felt a bit uncomfortable and I was wondering what it had to do with the problems I was seeing the CPN about. As the meeting went on, though, I actually found it really helpful, I had never really gone back through my life like that and we started to see certain patterns that had happened throughout my life. In meetings with my CPN afterwards, we were able to use the information to help me better understand myself and stop blaming myself as much for things that had happened in the past. I learnt that not everything that happened to me was my fault, and that there are some things that are out of your locus of control in your life. I feel **)** much more in control of my life now.

Employment/Occupational History

It is essential to establish the service user's past and present level of function in work. A sporadic or chaotic employment history may indicate emotional instability or frequent episodes of mental illness. It may also offer information in terms of occupational resilience and coping strategies. It is often useful to look at occupational history next to relationship history, for example it may demonstrate difficulties in establishing or maintaining relationships. Work-related stress may have precipitated the illness or high levels of stress at home may have impacted on work life. The impact of hospital admissions or other forms of treatment may have impacted on the service user's function at work or at school (Mackinnon et al., 2015). Furthermore, difficulty with employment, for example finding work, may further exacerbate low self-esteem and other components related to a sense of well-being and a happy home life, relationships and opportunities for fulfilment (DH, 2011).

Psychosexual History

A tactful approach must be employed when discussing the person's sexual history. It may be necessary in some circumstances for a person of the same gender to interview the service user, should they feel uncomfortable (Levine, 2006).

A sexual history is helpful for a number of reasons. First, it can indicate a service user's ability to make and maintain intimate relationships and capacity to love and be loved. It can also highlight the ramifications of the impact in the early years through childhood sexual abuse and other negative experiences.

Important areas to consider are the service user's onset of puberty, their first sexual encounter and their thoughts and feelings at the time in relation to this. The practice of safe sex, number of sexual partners and sexual preference are all areas to sensitively explore, if the service user feels comfortable in doing so. It is crucial as a practitioner that you are mindful of your own values and beliefs when asking about such personal subjects so that you are able to be clear in your own mind that you are not passing judgement (Aquilina and Warner, 2004). A service user will very quickly pick up on embarrassment, disapproval or cultural/religious judgement projected by you, which could then lead to distress in the service user. This is especially the case if a service user discloses that they have experienced childhood sexual abuse, rape or that they themselves have had sexual feelings towards children. In terms of sexual feelings towards children, there would be a number of risk factors to consider (Mackinnon et al., 2015), such as whether the person has the current intention of acting out such feelings and that children might be at risk. If so, you must follow relevant policies within your organisation to ensure that the appropriate people and/ or agencies are notified.

Social History

Larger social networks tend to promote recovery (see Chapter 5). The practitioner should inquire about the service user's family and household members. Explore whether the service user feels satisfied with their social role at this point in life. Determine the service user's wider previous social network, such as clubs and religious organisations they have belonged to, and how this might be different from their current social situation. Their living situation is also integral to the assessment, as many of life's most potent stressors are environmental in origin. It is often difficult to ascertain whether a person's social problems have precipitated or resulted from a mental illness (Jones, 2010). Consider homelessness – did mental health problems lead to the person becoming homeless, or did the homelessness subsequently cause or exacerbate a mental condition (Gonzalez and McLoughlin, 2014)?

Forensic History

A forensic history is concerned with establishing any recent or past offending behaviours. This can help in getting a clearer picture of triggers, events, links and patterns of behaviour which can aid assessment with regards to the person's current presentation (Aquilina and Warner, 2004). This is likely to be an area that the service user will have difficulty in disclosing and talking about. It can also be a difficult issue for you as a practitioner to ask about and so it will be useful to introduce the subject and why you are going to ask about it. An initial question might be something like: 'Have you ever done anything that could have got you into trouble with the police?' Should the answer be 'yes', then ask for details of actual arrests, charges and imprisonments as well as events where the person could have faced charges if they had been found out. If you only ask about whether someone has been in trouble with the police, then it may not capture regularly offending for which they have yet to be caught.

It is very possible, of course, that the person may not disclose this. Service users may be anxious about confidentiality for fear of being reported to the authorities. It is therefore good practice to explain how confidentiality works. This means that the service user is aware that you may have to contact relevant agencies should they disclose a serious past, present or potential future crime such as serious violence towards other people or sexual abuse of minors (Carlat, 2004).

Culture

Ethnicity, race, social class and language should be included in the cultural assessment. One's cultural upbringing can significantly influence the development and expression of mental disorders (Fernando, 2010). For example, members of certain groups are likely to present with more somatic complaints. The efficacy of different treatment modalities and beliefs regarding the cause and treatment of mental illness may also vary among cultures and must be considered when developing a treatment plan. However, the mental health practitioner must avoid stereotyping individual people on the basis of ethnic, racial or social group membership.

Spirituality

Spirituality is an often neglected aspect of a psychosocial assessment. However, a service user's lack of sense of spirituality may have a tremendous impact on illness and recovery (Mackinnon et al., 2015). If the service user declares that they do not follow an organised religion or are atheists, alternative sources of strength, hope, comfort and meaning in life should also be explored as part of the spiritual assessment. Some service users feel that spiritual expression, however that is manifested, decreases their sense of aloneness and despair. Gaining insight into the service user's religious beliefs and practices and any associated satisfactions and/or conflicts will be useful in planning interventions.

SERVICE USER VOICE

' I have had some awful experiences with mental health services over the years, especially when being admitted into hospital. I am 55 now, and have been diagnosed with schizophrenia since my early 20s. I never recognised until I was in my 40s that I had this illness and was maybe in denial or something. It helped when I moved to a new area and the mental health team there seemed a lot more culturally aware. Where I was before, they didn't seem to care much and could be very judgemental of my West Indian heritage – I saw them as not understanding me. I mean this in no disrespect but they was of a very middle England, Christian background, which I got nothing against but they were talking to me about things they had no idea about and trying to tell me what I should and shouldn't think about life. Where I am now, the nurses and doctors respect my values and also helped me to find ways of coping when the demons come.

I think what has helped is that they were actually interested in me as a person and valued what my beliefs on things were, in a way I think it has helped them, too, to better understand people like me and they have helped me understand what mental illness is and that it's not something to be ashamed of but something I need to manage to live a happier life. **'**

Premorbid Personality

Unless you have previous knowledge about what the service user is usually like already, it is difficult to fully understand how their illness or current problems have affected them. In asking about premorbid personality, the information from a family member or friend can be particularly helpful. Think about coping styles, interests and activities and how the person usually relates to other people (Aquilina and Warner, 2004). This, along with the rest of the history that you have recorded, will help build a better understanding of an individual's coping skills. Coping skills are mechanisms that people use to manage internal and external stressors. Discerning the service user's characteristic pattern of coping helps to identify the coping mechanisms that may be used in the current crisis situation and those that require further development. Coping skills may be 'adaptive' or 'maladaptive' (Carlat, 2004). Adaptive skills include the ability to engage social support systems and perform relaxation exercises in times of stress. Previous patterns in using alcohol or self-harm to cope in a maladaptive effort to cope with psychological pain should be explored.

Chapter Summary

The history-taking process should be collaborative, recovery-focused and person-centred. This chapter stresses the importance of positive engagement and being mindful that you will be exploring some potentially sensitive areas of an individual's life. The chapter moves on to discuss the skills involved in recording a person-centred, systematic and comprehensive history. Through this, we are better able to build a fully informed case conceptualisation in order to support our service users through the recovery process.

EXERCISE

Using the above information, catalogue your own personal history:

1. What are some of the challenges for you in doing this?
2. Consider what might be some of the challenges in taking a history from another person.

CONSIDERATIONS FOR PRACTICE

1. An assessment of a person's history can be a long and complex process. Consider how you might best achieve this. If the person is known to services, do you feel you need to revisit historical information that might have been well recorded (such as the person's place of birth, educational history, forensic history)?
2. Do you think you can ever truly obtain an accurate historical picture of a person's life? What might some of the barriers and biases be when looking back at a person's life?
3. How might you engage the person's family/personal network in building a historical picture of the person's life?

Further Reading

Aquilina, C. and Warner, J. (2004) *A Guide to Psychiatric Examination*. Norwich: Pastest.

Written with the help of tutors and students, this practical guide is invaluable for everyone working with people with mental health problems, and is an aid to conducting efficient and comprehensive psychiatric assessments. The book contains a detailed review of a general psychiatric assessment and has practical guides on assessments in 11 specific problems and four groups of people.

Fernando, S. (2010) *Mental Health, Race and Culture*, 3rd edn. Basingstoke: Palgrave Macmillan.

This book offers a unique analysis of the impact of race and culture on contemporary issues in mental health. Drawing on extensive international experience, the author challenges the traditional ideas that inform practice in clinical psychology and psychiatry in order to promote new and alternative ways of thinking.

Mackinnon, R., Michels, R. and Buckley, P. (2015) *The Psychiatric Interview in Clinical Practice*, 3rd edn. Arlington, VA: American Psychiatric Association.

This book presents the psychiatric interview in the context of the enormous and ongoing progress that has been made in biological and descriptive psychiatry. In addition, it emphasises the shift in the social relationship between service user and clinician, recognising that the therapeutic alliance has become the foundation of all medical treatment efforts and that service users are now better informed and seek active involvement in treatment decisions. The text reflects this growing equality and supports the clinician's efforts to nurture the relationship for optimum therapeutic outcomes.

References

Aquilina, C. and Warner, J. (2004) *A Guide to Psychiatric Examination*. Norwich: Pastest.
Bickley, L. (2013) *Bates' Guide to Physical Examination and History Taking*, 11th edn. Philadelphia, PA: Lippincott Williams and Wilkins.

Bowers, L., Brennan, G. and Winship, G. (2009) *Talking with Acutely Psychotic People: Communication Skills for Nurses and Others Spending Time with People Who are Very Mentally Ill.* London: City University.

Buckley, P., Prewette, D., Bird, J. and Harrison, G. (2005) *Examination Notes in Psychiatry*, 3rd edn. New York: Oxford University Press.

Carlat, D. (2004) *The Psychiatric Interview*, 2nd edn. Philadelphia, PA: Lippincott Williams and Wilkins.

Department of Health (2011) *No Health without Mental Health: A Cross-Government Mental Health Outcomes Strategy for People of All Ages.* London: DH.

Dickson, D. and Hargie, O. (2006) 'Questioning', in O. Hargie (ed.), *The Handbook of Communication Skills.* London: Routledge.

Fernando, S. (2010) *Mental Health, Race and Culture.* 3rd edn. Basingstoke: Palgrave Macmillan.

Gonzalez, R. and McLoughlin, P. (2014) 'Youth homelessness, mental health and complex trauma: implications for policy and practice', *Parity*, 27 (1): 56.

Jones, K. (2010) 'The unstructured clinical interview', *Journal of Counseling and Development*, 88 (2): 220.

Levine, S. (2006) 'How to take a sexual history (without blushing)', *Current Psychiatry, Evidence Based Reviews*, 5 (8): 16–25.

Mackinnon, R., Michels, R. and Buckley, P. (2015) *The Psychiatric Interview in Clinical Practice.* 3rd edn. Arlington, VA: American Psychiatric Association.

Reder, P. and Lucey, C. (2014) *Assessment of Parenting: Psychiatric and Psychological Contributions.* Hove: Routledge.

Taylor, D., Paton, C. and Kapur, S. (2012) *The Maudsley Guidelines in Psychiatry.* 11th edn. London: Wiley-Blackwell.

8

MENTAL STATE EXAMINATION

CAROLINE ATTARD

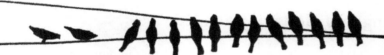

CHAPTER OVERVIEW

This chapter:

- Provides a detailed description of what a mental state examination (MSE) consists of and what skills and knowledge mental health practitioners need to conduct one.
- Explores how an MSE can contribute to therapeutic engagement with a service user.
- Provides examples of useful questions to use in an MSE.

What is a Mental State Examination?

A mental state examination (MSE) is an assessment of the mental state of a service user at a given time. It reflects the subjective report and experience of the person as well as the objective observations and impressions of the mental health practitioner at the time of the interview. Traditionally, an MSE uses a common format and language to record information, which may be understood across different services and professions (Gelder et al., 2012), but this may not be so meaningful or easily understood by a service user or their friends and family. The goal of an MSE is to help the person share their experiences of their mental health in order to ensure that appropriate assistance can be given and that any risks are addressed accordingly.

A mental state examination is used to:

- Establish a baseline of a person's current mental health and behaviour.
- Provide a platform for a shared understanding about the person's experiences about their mental health.
- Facilitate and evaluate changes in mental health over time.

In addition, the information obtained enhances the therapeutic alliance between the practitioner and service user. Like any skill, the MSE is one which is enhanced through practice, clinical supervision and constructive feedback.

An MSE involves the systematic appraisal of the appearance, behaviour, mental functioning and overall description of a person. It reflects a 'snapshot' of a person's psychological functioning at a given point in time. An MSE is an important component of the psychosocial assessment of a service user. Most mental health practitioners intuitively perform many parts of an MSE every time we interact with or observe others.

Rapport-Building in Undertaking an MSE

Taking the time to establish rapport with a service user before initiating an MSE is very important. Acknowledging the service user's feelings is both important for the success of the interview and for any ongoing engagement with treatment (Jordan Halter, 2014). Mental health practitioners need to listen closely to what the service user has to say and to ask for clarification or examples, if needed. Showing empathy to the service user's distressing thoughts and beliefs will help in working collaboratively with the service user towards developing a shared understanding of the problems and symptoms in question (Gamble and Brennan, 2006).

The Importance of Listening in an MSE

Listening is the ability to accurately receive and interpret messages in the communication process. Listening is key to all effective communication. Without the ability to listen effectively, messages and signals may be misunderstood, communication breaks down and the sender of the message can easily become frustrated or irritated (Harrison et al., 2004).

Of all the communication skills that a mental health practitioner should aim to master, listening sensitively and respectfully should be the top priority. There is an assumption that, as a mental health practitioner, one is already good at listening. However, service users and families have reported that they have been misquoted and misunderstood (DH, 2009). Many service users also report that mental health professionals repeat and duplicate assessments, which is frustrating for them (DH, 2011). Therefore, the service user should always be at the centre of an MSE examination, which should be coordinated between team members.

Listening means paying attention, not only to the person's narrative, but also the way in which it is told through the use of language and voice, and how the person uses his or her body. In other words, it means being aware of both the person's verbal and non-verbal messages (Clarke and Walsh, 2009). Your ability to listen effectively depends on the degree to which you perceive and understand these messages.

A good listener will listen, not only to what is being said, but also to what is left unsaid or only partially said. This is particularly important in an MSE. For example, a service user might answer the question 'How are you feeling?' with 'I am okay' but his non-verbal communication might suggest otherwise – looking down on the floor, minimal eye contact, looking particularly sad, worried or anxious. There is an incongruity (see below) here that clearly needs exploring. Effective listening involves observing body language and noticing inconsistencies between verbal and non-verbal messages.

How to Conduct an MSE

Psychiatric terminology and medical diagnostic classifications used in mental heath care can be daunting but it is not necessary for mental health practitioners to have a detailed knowledge of all of these in order to complete a baseline MSE. What is essential is for the practitioner to have an understanding of the basic concepts used in an MSE (see Figure 8.1). A key skill for the mental health practitioner is being able to notice and recognise the basic presentation of a service user, helping them to share their experiences.

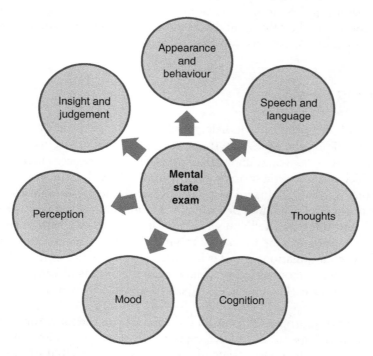

Figure 8.1   A framework for structuring a mental state examination

Open-ended questions are essential for gathering relevant information on a person's mental state (O'Carroll et al., 2007). For example, 'How are you feeling today, Emily?' is preferable to 'Is your mood still low, Emily?' This gives the service user a chance to talk about their experiences and concerns whilst allowing the practitioner an insight into the person's experience (Schultz and Videbeck, 2013).

It is important to note that the MSE should not be a series of questions but an evaluative process based on the mental health practitioner's observations and interactions with the service user. If broad mental health issues are identified during the course of an MSE, then more direct, clarifying and specific questioning about the service user's experience may be required. Moreover, the use of more in-depth evidence-based assessment tools (see Chapter 3) such as the Brief Psychiatric Rating Scale (BPRS) (Overall and Gorham, 1988) or Auditory Hallucination Rating Scale (Haddock, 1994) may be helpful to gather more focused information and, again, with the aim for a shared understanding.

Over time, the mental health practitioner will develop his or her own style of interviewing. It is important that the practitioner feels comfortable with the style that they have adopted so that questions do not seem awkward or forced and keep the service user at the centre whilst a therapeutic engagement is achieved.

Background to Taking an MSE

Taking an MSE is a core skill for mental health practitioners (Simms, 2015) and is best learned by practice and repetition. The MSE should be service user-focused and a common error is to see the assessment purely as an information-gathering exercise. Each step covered in the MSE should help the mental health practitioner make sense of what is going on for the service user.

Structuring an MSE

The framework in Figure 8.1 will help you develop the areas that you need to look out for whilst doing the MSE. The framework keeps the service user in the centre and aims to develop a greater understanding of their experience. There is no correct order in which to discuss these areas and it is most likely that the interview will not be sequential. It is best facilitated as a narrative, with the person sharing their experiences as they come to mind. For example, if someone has not been sleeping, this may be the first thing they tell you when you sit down to talk with them. This may be the most important issue for them at that time, so it is natural that they would want to draw your attention to it. It is important to take notice of this when it arises and, if you enquire about it later, acknowledge that it has already been said, for example: 'You said earlier you haven't been sleeping, can you tell me a bit more about that?'

It is not always appropriate to ask all the questions all the time. Sometimes, it can be better to leave gaps to fill in later, especially if service users are suspicious and paranoid or acutely distressed. Some of the MSE can be gathered from speaking to a family member or a friend.

Appearance and Behaviour

A person's appearance can provide valuable information about their mental state. Observations of the person's appearance and behaviour takes place from the first meeting and throughout the interview (Simms, 2015) and should be described whilst maintaining a non-judgemental approach and attitude. Mental health practitioners need to consider the person's:

- Eye contact and rapport: Is the service user able to maintain eye contact? Are you able to build a rapport?
- Clothing: Is attire appropriate for the context?
- Hygiene: Are there any indications that there may be problems with grooming or personal hygiene?
- Facial expressions: Are there signs that the service user is responding to the interview? Do expressions portray emotions?
- Movements: Are there any signs of movements being slow?
- Signs of arousal: Are there any signs of either panic or anxiety? Are they agitated or excited?
- Affect: Do they seem sad? Happy? Anxious? Worried? Are their emotional responses appropriate?

So, overall, how does the service user look? Consider the person's age, gender, race/ethnicity, build, hairstyle and colour, grooming, posture, level of hygiene, mode of dress and apparent level of health.

When we talk about a service user's *affect*, we are referring to how people convey their mood by their behaviour. A 'normal' affect, within reason, would be described as reactive and appropriate such as when a person laughs at a joke or cries when sad. However, it is imperative that the mental health practitioner documents this in an objective and non-judgemental manner in order to avoid bias and ensure that any record is accurate, fair and respectful.

An example of an objective report of a person's appearance is as follows: Mrs Smith is a 27-year-old Caucasian single woman who is slightly overweight for her height of approximately 5 ft, with minimal clothing of shorts (jeans), T-shirt and flip-flops – considering that it is cold outside – and a poor level of hygiene is also evident. During the interview, her eye contact was poor, with her constantly looking at the window. She seems in good health, however her clothes seem small for her stature and age.

Descriptions of appearance in an MSE should include any prominent or unusual physical characteristics (shaved head, tattoos, etc.), height and weight (obesity or thinness), posture, grooming, hygiene, level of eye contact, apparent age in relation to chronological age, facial expression in relation to thought content, and anything unusual such as clothing which is inconsistent with the time of day or season, or unusually applied clothing or make-up.

Appearance and behaviour during the interview can also provide valuable insights into the person's social and interpersonal functioning. It is therefore essential that consideration is given to the service user's attitude to both the mental health practitioner and to the assessment/interview processes itself. It is also important that you understand that this may influence your judgement and content of information obtained, and may pose special challenges. This is especially important during the development of the therapeutic relationship as this may impact on the ability to objectively report on the MSE findings. The service user's behaviour towards the practitioner may be described using terms such as cooperative, uncooperative, frank, deductive, defensive, evasive, guarded, hostile or threatening. Any changes in behaviour throughout the interview, as well as the level of rapport established, should also be recorded. For example, Mrs Smith seemed suspicious and angry towards me and asked, 'Why do you want to know everything?' and was at times uncooperative during the session and refused to answer some of the questions. At times, she asked rhetorical questions and insisted that I share personal information before she would proceed.

It is important that the assessment is culturally sensitive and that a person's appearance and behaviour is seen in the context of what, for the person, may be culturally appropriate behaviours (Simms, 2015). Judgements about mental state should also always consider the developmental level of the person and age-appropriateness of the noted behaviour(s) (ibid.).

In assessing psychomotor behaviour, the practitioner is observing the person's actions and coordinated activity involving the arms, hands, fingers and feet. This also includes all non-verbal behaviour evident during the interview, and this can reveal information regarding a person's mood, energy level, muscle strength, coordination, general medical condition and potential adverse effects of medication (Morrison, 2008). The documentation of activity and behaviour in the MSE should include abnormalities in the level of activity, any involuntary motor activity or behaviour, and any excessive, repeated or distinctive activity or behaviour. It is important to describe the actual behaviour shown, so, instead of recording 'appears anxious', it is important to be specific and a record of 'constantly wringing hands or tapping foot repeatedly' is therefore preferable.

Speech and Language

When assessing the *content* of speech, we are interested in what the service user actually says (see below). We are also interested in examining the *way* in which the person communicates. That is, how does the service user verbally express himself/herself?

In assessing the person's ability to communicate verbally, the assessor is noticing the rate, rhythm and fluency of speech, all of which may be affected by severe and enduring mental health problems (Simms, 2015). We should consider the person's speech pattern and examine, in particular:

- *Rate* – rapid, pressured (fast), slow, retarded (slow motion).
- *Volume* – loud, whispered, quiet, monotone, varied.
- *Rhythm* – clear, hesitant.
- *Tone* – angry, irritated, monotone.
- *Quantity of information* – poverty (lack of) or pressure of speech, mute/silent.
- *Quality* – stutter, slurring or any atypical qualities.

Consideration should also be given to the absence of speech or inability of the person to speak.

Thoughts

Thoughts can be considered in terms of *form* (that is, how one's thoughts are organised) and *content* (that is, what one is actually thinking about). Obviously, we cannot directly access the person's thoughts, and we can only understand what a person is thinking through their speech. Note that we all often edit our thoughts before expressing them in speech, although facial expressions and body language might betray what we are really thinking.

Form

The sequence of our thoughts may illustrate difficulties in the way in which our thoughts are organised (Mackinnon et al., 2006) and might suggest a breakdown of normal thought processes. For example:

- *Thought block*: The flow of thought stops abruptly. On occasions, it is possible to witness this where a person may stop what they are saying halfway through the sentence and be unable to continue for a period.
- *Flight of ideas*: Is particularly seen when a person is in an over-excited state, where there are rapid associations made by the person between each thought and where there is a shifting of ideas.
- *Incoherent/illogical*: Disorganised or senseless speech.
- *Derailment*: Unrelated or loosely connected ideas.
- *Tangentiality or loosening of association*: Unrelated or incomplete replies.

While the form of a person's thoughts may often be inferred by directly listening to their verbal communication, there are some helpful questions that you may wish to ask a person about the form of their thinking which may be particularly helpful, for example:

- Do your thoughts seem faster than normal?
- Do you ever have the experience of when your thoughts suddenly stop?
- Do you ever feel that your mind is suddenly wiped blank and you have no thoughts at all?
- Do you often start a sentence and then forget what you are going to say? How often does this happen?

Content

Here, we are interested in the content of a person's beliefs and, in particular, the experience of people who may experience *delusions*. A delusion is an unshakeable idea or belief that is out of keeping with the person's educational, cultural and social background and which is held with extraordinary conviction and certainty (Simms, 2015). This may not make any sense to the assessor, but we need to try to understand what these beliefs mean to the service user.

The most helpful response to a service user's delusional beliefs can be to address the emotion or feeling that is behind them (which can be terrifying or upsetting for the individual), rather than to the content. Sometimes, practitioners can worry about reinforcing delusions or strange ideas by asking about them. However, the role of the mental health practitioner is to develop a shared understanding of the service user's experience, rather than to pass judgement on the content.

Delusional beliefs can be extremely distressing to the individual and can present in many different ways, including beliefs of being persecuted, having bizarre strange thoughts which are out of keeping with the person's cultural background, grandiose ideas (where the person might feel that they are unduly important in some way), self-referential thoughts (that is, the tendency for people to believe that information is related to themselves), and delusions of control (the belief that other people are controlling their thoughts and/or actions or that external parties have manipulated their thoughts). Other examples include:

- *Thought withdrawal*: The experience of thoughts being removed by a third party. Does the service user feel that their thoughts are being taken away, wiped blank or that the thoughts are removed so that they are not there anymore?
- *Thought insertion*: The opposite to thought withdrawal, whereby thoughts are experienced as alien, not arising from oneself but being placed there by a third party.
- *Thought broadcast*: This is when the service user may experience their thoughts being communicated publicly by TV or radio, for example, or that anybody can hear their thoughts.
- *Passivity*: This is the sense that the person feels that they are being controlled by an external source to themselves, whether this is physically, emotionally or cognitively.

There are some helpful questions that you may wish to ask a person about the content of their thinking, for example:

- Has anything strange or unusual been going on?
- Do you feel that there is anything special about yourself that makes you different from other people?
- Are you sure that this is happening or do you feel that you might be imagining it?

We are also interested here in whether a person has any thoughts to harm themselves or others, which will be discussed more fully in Chapter 9.

Cognition

Cognition refers to the mental processes of attention, concentration, knowing and thinking, including aspects such as memory, awareness and reasoning. This could be inferred from their vocabulary, level of education and how easily they recall important personal information and dates. Unless you detect a problem, for most people you can briefly screen the following areas (Folstein et al., 1975):

- Orientation for time, person and place.
- Registration – Ability to repeat new information such as a name and address.

- Recall – Repeating the new information five minutes later.
- Concentration and attention – You can check this by asking the service user to spell 'WORLD' backwards or serial sevens or simply ask how their concentration is?
- General knowledge – Name of the prime minister, recent news items.

The purpose of asking the above questions is to ascertain whether or not the person is alert and orientated to time, person and place. You may be able to infer these during the interview and, in which case, do not ask the questions if it is obvious. Listen carefully to the service user to avoid unnecessary irritation or agitation of multiple questioning.

Mood

Our mood is reflective of our emotional state. Do people feel sad, happy, apathetic, anxious, angry, excited? In a mental state examination, the person should be encouraged to describe how they are feeling in their own words. If not spontaneously reported, the practitioner should ask about mood and whether how they are feeling is typical for them. It is also important to note when the service user's mood is relatively 'normal' to the situation, age and circumstances.

Simms (2015) states that a person's mood may be further characterised in terms of its 'stability', 'reactivity' and 'duration':

- *Stability*: Refers to the consistency of the mood, particularly over the course of the day. That is, does a person's mood fluctuate? Are they brighter in the morning or evening?
- *Reactivity*: Refers to whether or not a person's mood changes in response to external events or circumstances.
- *Duration*: Refers to the persistence of a particular mood, measured in hours, days, weeks, months or even years.

Some helpful examples of how to ask appropriate questions related to mood include:

- How do you generally feel most of the time?
- What is your mood like?
- How would you say you feel generally – happy, sad, frightened, angry?
- Is there any pattern to how your mood changes through the day?
- Is there any time of the day when you tend to feel better or worse?
- Do you tend to feel worse in the evening?
- Are you able to get enjoyment from anything?
- Do you still enjoy activities that you used to enjoy?
- If something nice happens, do you cheer up a bit?
- Do you find yourself crying a lot?
- Would you say that you're more cheerful than usual?
- What's your view of the future?
- Do you think that things will get better or worse?

- Do you hope that things might get better?
- Is there any possibility that things might get better?
- Do you see any possibility at all that things might get better, even a little bit?

Further questions about appetite, sleep and general functioning (see Chapter 6) can help in the screening for low mood, excitable states, and other issues such as psychosis. It also gives the practitioner a guide to the person's overall functioning and areas in which they may wish to have further help.

A service user's affective state consists of several components, which are objectively observed and cannot be elicited by direct questioning. It should be monitored throughout the interview, and its congruence with thought content should be noted. Gelder et al. (2012) explain that written description of affect in the MSE examination should be characterised in terms of its range, change pattern, intensity and appropriateness, as explained below:

- *Range*: A practitioner who is conducting an MSE assessment needs to refer to the variation in emotional expression observed throughout the interview. It is characterised as 'full' (normal variation in emotional expression) or 'constricted' (limited variation in emotional expression). 'Blunted' affect is a reduction in the intensity of an individual emotional response.
- *Change pattern*: Refers to the rate of change of emotional expression. It is characterised as 'stable' (normal rate of change) or 'labile' (rapid change in emotional expression, without external stimuli).
- *Intensity*: Refers to the strength of emotional expression. It is characterised as 'average', 'flat' (complete lack of emotional expression) or 'blunted' (reduced intensity of emotional expression).
- *Appropriateness*: Refers to congruence of affect and thought content, i.e. a happy thought tends to produce or reflect a happy mood. A service user's mood and affect should be congruent with each other. Incongruence can be observed when a person expresses an inconsistent emotion with what they are talking about (i.e. laughing when talking about a loved one's death).

Perception

Screening for perceptual disturbances is critical for detecting serious mental health problems such as psychosis, cases of severe anxiety and mood disorders. These include *hallucinations* and *illusions* in the case of psychosis, and *dissociative experiences* (see below), which may be experienced in trauma, substance abuse, anxiety and other emotional disorders (Gelder et al., 2012). Perceptual disturbances may be disturbing or frightening, so it is important for the mental health practitioner to be aware of them and notice related symptoms, as described below:

- *Dissociative experiences*:
  o Derealisation: Feeling that the world or one's surroundings are not real.
  o Depersonalisation: Feeling detached from oneself, or feeling that you are observing yourself from the outside.

- *Illusions*: The service user perceives things as different to usual, but accepts that they are not real, or that things are perceived differently by others.
- *Hallucinations*: These are sensory experiences in the absence of an external stimuli which seem absolutely genuine to the person.

Hallucinations are indistinguishable from 'reality' for the person and can affect all sensory modalities – sight (visual), smell (olfactory), touch (tactile), hearing (auditory) and taste (gustatory) – although auditory hallucinations are the most common (Carlat, 2005). Olfactory hallucinations can also be a sign of physical health problems (such as epilepsy) that may require investigation and, whilst visual hallucinations can occur amongst people who have been recently bereaved and people living with Lewy Body Dementia, they can also be present in delirium from organic causes, substance use and withdrawal.

Command hallucinations occur when the person experiences voices telling them to do something (Simms, 2015). These should be investigated carefully as this can be a significant risk issue because the service user may feel that they have to respond to the command. It is important that the practitioner notes the degree of fear expressed by the service user, whether they feel compelled to act on what they are hearing and how able they feel to ignore the instruction. *Third person hallucinations* are those where the service user may experience a running commentary on their actions and this can be very intrusive, for example: he is trying to sleep, he's making a cup of tea, he's trying to read a book.

Some helpful examples of how to ask appropriate questions related to perception include:

- Do you ever hear voices when there is no one else around?
- Do you ever hear things that other people don't hear?
- Do you ever hear anything strange?
- Where do you think the voices come from?
- Are the voices in your head or outside? Are these thoughts in your mind or sounds that you would hear with your ears?
- Do you recognise any voices?
- How many voices are there?
- Do they talk to you or do they talk to each other about you?
- Do they ever talk about what you are doing?
- Do they repeat your thoughts or comment on your thoughts?
- Do your thoughts ever sound loud, as if somebody next to you could hear them?
- Do the voices tell you to do things?
- Do you see things that other people don't see?
- Do things ever smell strange or taste strange?
- Do you ever feel things touching you?
- Do you feel things changing inside your body?

Insight and Judgement

During the MSE, the mental health practitioner should also consider if the service user has any *insight*. When we talk about insight, we are referring to the service user's capacity to recognise his/her own problems and mental state. When we talk about *judgement* in the MSE, we are referring to the service user's capacity to make sound, reasonable, reasoned and responsible decisions to maintain their health and protect their own safety and those of others (David, 1990).

Families and Friends

If during an MSE, a service user is found to be significantly unwell, it is recommended that they are asked if they would like a family member or another to be contacted for support and assistance. If it is assessed that a service user's judgement is significantly impaired (and they refuse any assistance from others), it may be appropriate to contact the service user's registered next of kin. If the service user refuses for you to speak to a family member due to confidentiality, you are bound not to give out any information, but there is no reason why you should not ask the person's family and friends about how the person's mental state has been recently.

Challenges with MSE

You may need to ask some questions which may be challenging, especially if you are not experienced in carrying out an MSE. You might find that the service user does not want to talk about a particular topic or glosses over things. Some skilful techniques you can use in these circumstances include:

- Normalising statements: 'Often, when people are that down, they feel like they can't carry on ... Have you ever felt like that?'
- Pointing out behaviours: 'You seem distracted and you keep on looking outside of the window, Mrs Smith, is there anything or anyone outside?'
- Reassuring statements: 'You seem very scared. Is there a reason and can I do anything to help?'

Sometimes, service users may be reluctant to be interviewed for a variety of reasons. It may be that their mental state makes them suspicious of your motives, or frightened to disclose information. In these circumstances, it is important for the mental health practitioner to emphasise that they want to help without giving false reassurances. Promises should not be made that cannot be kept, for example: 'Don't worry, I won't tell anyone.' The mental health practitioner needs to be mindful of his/her own safety, professional and legal obligations and trust their instincts. If the practitioner feels threatened, then it is best to remove themselves from the situation and seek help from a more experienced colleague or the team. It might help to leave a particular line of questioning for a time and move on to more neutral information-gathering until the service user feels more relaxed.

Another potential problem during an MSE is that of the over-inclusive patient, who wants to tell you details about every aspect of a situation, for example about the dress their sister wore at her wedding and the engraving on the groom's cufflinks. The practitioner may need, tactfully, to interrupt this monologue, and bring the service user back to the point, or change tack entirely if this fails. The practitioner can interrupt and be firm without being rude.

Think about good ways of phrasing difficult questions here, such as:

• Thanks for telling me about the wedding but I wonder if we could now focus on how your day was yesterday?

Chapter Summary

In this chapter, we have explored how to conduct an MSE in detail, making sure that the service user is at the centre of the assessment. We have looked at what skills and approach the mental health practitioner needs to have to successfully conduct an MSE. Mental health practitioners are in an excellent position to use the MSE towards a shared understanding of the problems presented and to develop a therapeutic relationship. Assessment can be a therapeutic tool when used skillfully: it can give the service user a real opportunity to talk about how they have been feeling, and the mental health practitioner can hope to increase their understanding of the service user's experience.

EXERCISE

In this chapter, we have consciously avoided using medical terminology and psychiatric diagnoses wherever possible. Our position is that we prefer to develop a shared understanding about people's experiences as part of a negotiated, meaningful case conceptualisation, rather than gather evidence for a diagnosis that is then applied to a person. There are some people who go further than this and believe that psychiatric diagnoses are 'dangerous' labels that disable and disempower the person. Others argue that diagnoses are 'desirable' and help to ensure that the person receives the best treatment:

1. Where do you stand?

CONSIDERATIONS FOR PRACTICE

1. Mental health practice in the UK is often medically dominated and the use of psychiatric terminology and diagnosis is widespread. How would you develop your knowledge in this area, should you wish to?
2. Assessing a person's mental state requires considerable skill and sensitivity. Consider what skills you may need to develop to support your practice.

Further Reading

Goffman, E. (1963) *Stigma: Notes on the Management of Spoiled Identity*. Englewood Cliffs, NJ: Prentice-Hall.

Written at a time when mental health services comprised large psychiatric institutions, Goffman's book is an essential read for sociologists and mental health practitioners alike. It remains relevant in the context of the ongoing debate about the place of psychiatric diagnoses in modern person-centred, mental health care.

References

Carlat, D. (2005) *The Psychiatric Interview*, 2nd edn. Philadelphia, PS: Lippincott Williams and Wilkins.

Clarke, V. and Walsh, A. (2009) *Fundamentals of Mental Health Nursing*. Oxford: Oxford University Press.

David, A.S. (1990) 'Insight and psychosis', *British Journal of Psychiatry*, 156: 798–808.

Department of Health (2009) *New Horizons: Towards a Shared Vision for Mental Health*. London: DH.

Department of Health (2011) *No Health without Mental Health: A Cross-Government Mental Health Outcomes Strategy for People of All Ages*. London: DH.

Folstein, M., Folstein, S. and Mchugh, P.R. (1975) '"Mini-mental state": a practical method for grading the cognitive state of patients for the clinician', *Journal of Psychiatric Research*, 12 (3): 189–98.

Gamble, C. and Brennan, G. (2006) *Working with Serious Mental Illness: A Manual for Clinical Practice*. London: Bailliere Tindall.

Gelder, M., Andreasen, N., Lopez-Ilbor, J. and Geddes, J. (2012) *New Oxford Textbook of Psychiatry*, 3rd edn. Oxford: Oxford University Press.

Haddock, G. (1994) *Auditory Hallucination Rating Scale*. Manchester: University of Manchester Press.

Harrison, M., Howard, D. and Mitchell, D. (2004) *Acute Mental Health Nursing: From Acute Concerns to the Capable Practitioner*. London: Sage.

Jordan Halter, M. (2014) *Foundations of Psychiatric Mental Health Nursing: A Clinical Approach*. St. Louis, MO: Elsevier Saunders.

Mackinnon, R., Michels, R. and Buckley, P. (2006) *The Psychiatric Interview in Clinical Practice*. Arlington, VA: American Publishing.

Morrison, J. (2008) *The First Interview*, 3rd edn. New York: Guilford Press.

O'Carroll, M., Park, A. and Nicol, M. (2007) *Essential Mental Health Nursing Skills*. Philadelphia, PA: Mosby Elsevier.

Overall, J.E. and Gorham, D.R. (1988) 'The Brief Psychiatric Rating Scale (BPRS): recent developments in ascertainment and scaling', *Psychopharmacology Bulletin*, 24: 97–9.

Schultz, J.N. and Videbeck, S.L. (2013) *Lippincott's Manual of Psychiatric Nursing Care Plans*, 9th edn. Philadelphia, PA: Lippincott Williams and Wilkins.

Simms, A. (2015) *Symptoms of the Mind: An Introduction at Describing Psychopathology*. London: Bailliere Tindall.

9

RISK ASSESSMENT

FRANCIS THOMPSON, STEVE TRENOWETH AND ALICIA POWELL

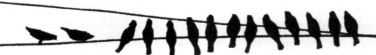

CHAPTER OVERVIEW

This chapter:

- Describes and defines risk assessment and emphasises the importance of risk assessment as a tool for enabling the management of risk through collaborative assessment and safety planning, rather than risk prediction.
- Reiterates the importance of engagement and service user involvement in the risk assessment process.
- Describes and discusses the need to consider risk in its broadest context, i.e. risks posed to the individual as a result of having a mental health problem, including physical health, stigma, social situation, employment and finance which need to be tackled to minimise long-term risk.
- Gives an overview of assessing risk in key risk areas, namely suicide/self-harm, violence and self-neglect.

Introduction

Risk assessment and management is a fundamental component of mental health care practice (DH, 2007). The majority of relevant literature addresses either the efficacy of risk assessment tools in predicting outcomes or the links between conditions and behaviours and risk, for example Brown and Langrish (2011), Daffern (2006), Singh et al., (2011) and Snowden et al., (2009). Much of the risk literature focuses on catastrophic risk – i.e. suicide, self-harm and violence – the prediction of this risk and its importance in deciding on both the treatment plan, and the level of care and restriction required to mange it (DH, 2007; Langan, 2010; Leitner and Barr, 2006).

Whittington and Logan (2011) argue that mental health services predominantly consider these catastrophic risks and that the view that these risks can be predicted and managed is the dominant paradigm. However, this is problematic. Langan (2010) argues that the aim of risk assessment should not be to attempt to see into the future and predict actual outcomes. The Royal College of Psychiatrists (RCP, 2008) concur, arguing that risk assessment has, even when skilfully conducted, limited value in predicting risk incidents. The Royal College of Psychiatrists argue that risk assessment should be seen as a part of an overall assessment of the person's current situation. Whittington and Logan (2011) feel that this disparity has led to conflict as to what risk assessment is, and how to balance risk management and treatment, with a tension between patients' freedom and rights and the protection of the individual and the public. They assert that viewing risk in terms of prediction and prevention has led to clinicians focusing on the risks that individuals present to themselves and others to the detriment of helping people to plan to minimise and control the risks they face in everyday life. The intent behind risk assessment may be to protect people, but the way in which this is carried out, they argue, stigmatises people and focuses on the negative (ibid.).

Despite clinical guidance (DH, 2007) emphasising the importance of collaboration with service users in risk assessment and management planning, Boardman and Roberts (2014) argue that organisations' approaches to risk management may at times be perverse, and actually getting in the way of an individual's recovery. Whittington and Logan (2011) suggest that suicide, self-harm and violence dominate the risk assessment process because these are the most anxiety-provoking. This, they argue, presents clinicians with a difficulty in engaging and empowering the service user to be collaboratively involved in the risk assessment process and in decision-making about care and treatment, and that this lack of engagement has a detrimental effect on the management of risk. The Royal College of Psychiatrists (2010) support this view, arguing that risk assessment has come to dominate practice and is based on an incorrect view that people's behaviour can be predicted and on what they refer to as the rise of a 'blame culture', which has led to a tick-box culture of defensive practice; and, while helping staff to feel protected, this ultimately takes time away from talking to and supporting service users.

This view is echoed by Leitner and Barr (2011), who argue that the clinician's primary task should be to work with service users in order to support their well-being, rather than framing their relationships in terms of risk, which they argue is detrimental to recovery.

Defining Risk Assessment

Safety is at the centre of all good health care. This is particularly important in mental health but it is also more sensitive and challenging. Patient autonomy has to be considered alongside public safety. A good therapeutic relationship must include both sympathetic support and objective assessment of risk. (DH, 2007: 3)

Risk assessments must consider what the risk factors may be in any given situation in a consistent, reliable way. It is important to note that, while we cannot predict and prevent all adverse incidents, we can – and still have a duty to – identify potential risks with service users and work with them and their families to manage and try to avoid potential adverse outcomes.

An overview of the factors that should be considered in a risk assessment, discussed later in this chapter, can be found in Figure 9.1.

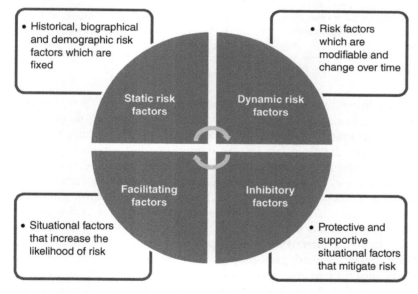

Figure 9.1 An overview of risk factors

Static and Dynamic Risk Factors

Best practice in risk assessment and management involves making decisions based on knowledge of the research evidence, knowledge of the individual service user and their social context, knowledge of the service user's own experience, and clinical judgement. (Department of Health, 2007: 5)

In any assessment of risk, consideration must be given to those variables (or factors) that increase (or, indeed, decrease) the likelihood and/or frequency that a risk may materialise. The Department of Health identifies a risk factor as: 'A personal characteristic or circumstance that is linked to a negative event, and that either causes or facilitates the event to occur' (ibid.: 13). Risk factors can help us to predict what types of risks are potentially present and may be categorised as *static* or *dynamic* (see Table 9.1).

Table 9.1 Static and dynamic risk factors

Static risk factors	Dynamic risk factors
These are factors that are known to be associated with increased risk which do not change. These include historical indicators, for example a history of suicide attempts, family history of completed suicide/suicide attempts, violence or childhood abuse. These factors will always be present, although their relevance will vary across individuals and over time.	These are factors that change over time, for example the misuse of alcohol or drugs. These factors may be aspects of the individual or of their environment and social context or indeed all of these. Examples of this are: attitude and beliefs of carers, financial status, living arrangements, social deprivation, and current mental state. These factors may change over time and are therefore more amenable to management. Dynamic factors may change slowly (stable factors) or rapidly (acute factors): the impact of these factors on the level of risk may be short lived or longer term.

Source: DH (2007)

There has traditionally been a focus on considering static risk factors in risk assessment, for example age, gender and history of risk incidents. While these factors are undoubtedly extremely important in the consideration of risk, they must be viewed in the context of dynamic factors. By definition, static factors will not change (although their meaning to the person may shift over time), and, yet, professionals often focus on these, from which the level of current risk for service users may be derived. Dynamic factors such as housing, finances, social situation and employment are often more amenable to effective interventions, and by interceding in these areas, health care professionals can work collaboratively with the service user and their friends and family to effectively manage potential risks and thus avoid harm.

However, in making a risk assessment, we are interested, not only in the type of risk factor(s), but also the frequency, magnitude, duration and likelihood of a risk event, and the extent and impact of potential harm (for the individual, for others, including vulnerable groups, and for the community), if the risk should materialise. This will, in turn, influence the nature and extent of risk management plans or, indeed, if any action needs to be taken – sometimes, it might be considered that an intervention by services might actually increase or precipitate a crisis, thereby leading to a risk event that may not have otherwise occurred. If it is decided that no direct action needs to be taken by mental health services, practitioners should consider whether any other services may be of assistance or should be informed, for example their GP, housing departments or adult social care.

Inhibitory (Protective) Factors

Inhibitory or protective factors are those variables that may inhibit or mitigate risk – either in terms of the magnitude, frequency, duration of the risk event or the likelihood that it may arise at all – and must be taken into consideration in any risk assessment. These factors are likely to include internal resources that an individual is able to draw on – such as coping abilities, insight, the person's belief in their abilities (self-efficacy), knowledge, hopefulness, motivation and so on – and external resources – such as support from communities, family and friends, engaging in prosocial activities, employment, sufficient income to satisfy needs and so on.

It is also vital for any risk assessment to consider the person's access to well-trained, motivated and compassionate health care staff who are easily accessible and responsive at a time of crisis for the individual and their family and friends.

Types of Risk Assessment

The *Best Practice in Managing Risk* (DH, 2007) guide identifies three types of risk assessment approaches. An 'unstructured clinical approach' takes the form of an unstructured conversation. It is not systematic and is therefore less reliable. This method is not recommended as the basis of a formal risk assessment, but may be helpful to open up initial discussions about the service user's experiences and possible areas to explore using more structured approaches.

An 'actuarial approach' tends to focus on static factors known to be statistically associated with increased risk. For example, statistically, people who have self-harmed in the past, are at a higher risk of suicide. Actuarial risk assessments apply mathematical/statistical modelling to look at trends of particular risk events within populations and is of value in placing people in particular risk categories for the likelihood of an adverse event happening. However, as they are based on *population* data – that is, the association of identifiable demographic and other static characteristics of individuals and circumstances with particular risk events – and do not take into account dynamic and personal factors, they are not sensitive in predicting that the event will or will not occur in an *individual* case.

A 'structured clinical approach' is the preferred method of assessing and subsequently managing risk because it combines the use of a structured method of assessing risk with the use of actuarial information in order to assess clearly defined risk factors, risk triggers and ameliorants of risk, and makes use of:

- Clinical experience and knowledge of the service user.
- The service user's view.
- The views of carers and other professionals.

Suicide

Suicide is a complex phenomenon representing 'the end point of a complex history of risk factors and distressing events' (HM Government/DH, 2012: 4). In 2014, the Office for National Statistics reported that there were 1775 road deaths in the UK; in the same period, 6122 people took their own lives (ONS, 2016).

Suicide is a leading cause of premature death in the UK and the UK suicide rate was 10.8 deaths per 100,000 population in 2014 (ibid.). The *National Confidential*

Enquiry into Suicide and Homicide (NCE) (University of Manchester, 2014) reports that between 2002 and 2012, out of the total suicides in England and Wales, 28 per cent were by people who had been in contact with mental health services in the 12 months prior to their death – an average of 1248 per year. In the mental health service user population, the most used methods of suicide are, in decreasing order: hanging (41 per cent), overdose (26 per cent) and jumping (15 per cent) (ibid.).

In 2016, the suicide definition was revised to include deaths from intentional self-harm in children aged 10 to 14. However, the number of deaths from suicide in this age group is very low (ONS, 2016).

Risk Factors for Suicide

Risk factors thought to be associated with suicide, some of which are discussed below, can be found in Table 9.2.

Table 9.2   Risk factors for suicide

Demographic factors	Male
	Middle age (especially those aged 45–49 years old)
	Low socioeconomic status
	Unmarried, separated, widowed
	Living alone
	Unemployed
Background history	Deliberate self-harm (especially with high suicide intent)
	Childhood adversity (e.g. sexual abuse)
	Family history of suicide
	Family history of mental illness
Clinical history	Mental illness diagnosis (e.g. depression, bipolar disorder, schizophrenia)
	Personality disorder diagnosis (e.g. borderline personality disorder)
	Physical illness, especially chronic conditions and/or those associated with pain and functional impairment (e.g. **multiple sclerosis**, malignancy, pain syndromes)
	Recent contact with psychiatric services
	Recent discharge from psychiatric inpatient facility
	Psychological and psychosocial factors
	Hopelessness
	Impulsiveness
	Low self-esteem
	Life event
	Relationship instability
	Lack of social support
	Co-morbid drug and/or alcohol misuse

Current context	Suicidal ideation
	Suicide intent
	Life stressors
	Suicide plans
	Availability of means
	Lethality of means

Source: Adapted from DH (2007) and ONS (2016)

Previous History

Features of the individual's previous history that may be associated with an increased risk of suicide are *static* risk factors (that is, not amenable to change). This historical context helps to establish the current baseline risk of suicide for the individual. These factors include:

- History of self-harm (people who self-harm have an increased risk of attempting suicide).
- History of suicide attempts, including recent incidents.
- History of mental disorder and admissions to mental health facilities.
- Personality traits.
- Childhood adversity.
- Family history of suicide.

It is very important to understand the nature and context of previous suicide attempts, if present, as there is evidence that people tend to repeat patterns when suicidal. Risk is increased where previous attempts have occurred. Here, the assessor should note:

- Triggers and context for previous attempts.
- The level of intent to commit suicide at the time and the person's subsequent view of this attempt (e.g. remorse, lack of emotion, sense of failure).
- Past methods for attempting suicide.
- Perceived and actual lethality of chosen method.
- Attempts to avoid detection.
- Any final acts (e.g. leaving a suicide note).

Risk is also increased in the context of escalating frequency and severity of self-harming behaviour, help-seeking behaviour (e.g. frequent presentation to services) and substance misuse.

Gender

Men complete suicide more frequently than women in a ratio of about 3:1 (University of Manchester, 2014); and, in 2014, it was recorded that 76 per cent of all suicides were males, compared to 24 per cent females (ONS, 2016). In 2014, the male suicide rate was 16.8 male deaths per 100,000, compared to 5.2 female deaths (ibid.). While the male suicide rate in the UK in 2014 decreased (from 17.8 to 16.8 deaths per 100,000 population), the female suicide rate has increased (from 4.8 to 5.2 deaths per 100,000 population) (ibid.).

Age

Middle-aged men are at the greatest risk from suicide (ibid.). Suicide rates in older men aged 60 to 74 years and those aged 75 and over have decreased steadily since 1981. In 2014, the highest suicide rate in the UK in 2014 was amongst those aged 45 to 59 (23.9 deaths per 100,000 for men, compared to 7.3 deaths per 100,000 population) (ibid.). Since 2007, the suicide rate in the 45–59 age group has been increasing. Suicides by 10–29-year-olds have consistently been the lowest rates.

Marital Status

There is a clear link between marital status and suicide, and being unmarried has consistently been found to be a risk factor for suicide, whereas marriage seems to have a beneficial effect (Griffiths et al., 2008). Lesbian, gay and bisexual people have an elevated risk of suicide (HMG/DH, 2012).

Ethnicity

There is no consistently clear evidence of the link between ethnicity and suicide risk (Hawton et al., 2005b).

Life Events

There is no doubt that current life-event stressors in our lives increase the likelihood of suicidal ideas and attempts. This has long been recognised, with the Holmes and Rahe's (1967) Social Readjustment Scale attempting to quantify the risk of such stressors and capturing the compounding nature of such stressors (see Chapter 5). The factors are *dynamic* variables and include:

- Psychosocial stress – such as relationship difficulties, conflict and marital break-up, employment and work-related stress, severe financial difficulties and debt, family relationships, role changes, accommodation troubles such as inability to make mortgage repayments, evictions.
- Social and community stresses – such as stigma, prejudice, harassment and bullying, can all contribute to increasing an individual's vulnerability to suicide.
- Recent losses – such as redundancies, bereavements and severe financial difficulties.
- Recent life events and anniversaries.
- Imprisonment.

Of the total number of people who killed themselves between 2008 and 2011, 45 per cent were unemployed (University of Manchester, 2014). Barr et al. (2012) provide evidence linking the recent increase in suicides in England with the financial crisis that began in 2008. English regions with the largest rises in unemployment have had the largest increases in suicides, particularly among men.

In general, there is no evidence that people who have served their country in armed conflict are at higher risk of suicide. However, people who leave the armed services in their early 20s seem to have an elevated risk of suicide (two or three times greater risk) compared with people who have not served (HMG/DH, 2012).

Mental Health Problems

People with mental health problems represent one of the most important high-risk groups for suicide. It is worth noting that almost all the patients in contact with special-ist mental health services are at increased risk compared with the general population. Current mental health problems are a significant factor in increasing risk of completed suicide (University of Manchester, 2014). Psychiatric conditions that can increase the risk of suicide include depression (Hawton et al., 2005a), bipolar disorders, schizophre-nia, personality and childhood disorders (McLean et al., 2008). Some psychiatric symptoms are particularly implicated such as insomnia, anorexia, low mood, negative cognitions (such as anergia, anhedonia, motivation, poor concentration, problem-solving deficits), agitation and psychomotor restlessness, psychotic symptoms including delusional beliefs and command hallucinations. However, Hawton et al. (2005a) found a lesser or reduced risk of suicide amongst people experiencing hallucination but there appears to be an elevated risk amongst people diagnosed with schizophrenia and per-sonality disorders at the initial diagnosis (McLean et al., 2008).

Other mental health-related issues that increase the risk of suicide include:

- Current suicidal ideation, intent and active plans (with access to means; see below).
- Feelings of hopelessness and helplessness.
- Recent admission and discharge to/from mental health services.

Substance misuse increases the risk of suicide attempts and subsequent death by suicide. The risk of suicide from alcohol misuse is greater among women than among men (ibid.), and the suicide risk is higher for those who use opioids and intravenous drugs than that for alcohol.

It also seems that fears of relapse and a deteriorating mental health and non-compliance with treatments plans – including any failure to attend appointments and the level of engagement – are also associated with an elevated risk of suicide (Hawton et al., 2005a).

A lack of hope for the future is a key predictor of suicide risk and an important aspect of assessing for the risk of suicide. Questions here include, for example:

- Do you have any hope for the future?
- Have you got anything to look forward to at the moment?
- Do you think you will get through this?

Physical Health

There is a well-documented link between suicide and long-term, chronic, debilitating and painful diseases (HMG/DH, 2012). Living with long-term conditions can also increase the risk, and those with three or more long-term conditions are seven times more likely to develop depression, a known risk factor for suicide. Some treatments used to manage long-term conditions, such as insulin, provide easy access and lethal means for overdose. With some diseases, such as coronary heart disease and chronic obstructive airways disease, there is a higher suicide risk on, or immediately following, confirmation of the diagnosis (ibid.).

Protective Factors against Suicide

Protective factors promote resilience and mitigate the risk of suicidal behaviour. Clearly, timely access to effective mental health and voluntary services which can support the suicidal individual have significant impact on reducing risk. Psychological factors such as hopefulness, optimism, clear reasons for living, positive future thinking and optimism are all protective against suicide attempt among those with depression (McLean et al., 2008). Problem-solving and coping skills may be protective against suicidal behaviour among those who have attempted suicide. Social support, such as positive family relationships, connectedness and marriage have also been linked with lower rates of suicide. Employment has a protective effect against suicide, possibly due to collegiate social working relationships and a more favourable financial position.

Participation in religion and religious observances has often been cited as a protective factor against suicidal behaviour (Perlman et al., 2011). However, it is not clear if this is due to the support that may be offered by the religious community or possible moral sanctions against suicide.

Assessment of Current Suicide Risk

In assessing a current suicide risk, the service user should be asked directly about suicide but it is vital that this is done sensitively and compassionately. There is no evidence that doing so increases the risk. When assessing the risk of suicide, it is important to consider the history of the service user (see Chapter 7), alongside the static and dynamic risk and protective factors (outlined above) contributing to the current presentation. In assessing the current level of risk, it is vital that the assessor considers three key areas: ideation, intentions and plans.

1. Assess Ideation

Has the service user had any current thoughts of ending their life or of suicide?

Questions can be direct, indirect or normalising.

Direct questions ask about suicide in a frank and open way, for example:

- 'Have you been thinking of killing yourself?'

This questioning style can be appropriate in many situations because it is clear and unambiguous. However, such direct questioning may seem rather insensitive and threatening, which may discourage the person from discussing their current feelings and, at such times, ask the question in a modified form. These *indirect* questions imply or lead to the subject of suicide, for example:

- 'Have you been thinking of ending it all?'
- 'Have you felt like harming yourself recently?'

This questioning style may seem more gentle and can be useful in broaching a sensitive subject but it can lack clarity. It is important therefore to follow up such questioning to clarify ideas of suicide, for example:

- 'Do you mean that you have thoughts of suicide?'

Normalising questions bring up the subject of suicide in the context of the situation, for example:

- 'You must be very stressed at the moment, sometimes people in this situation think about killing themselves. Is this something you've considered?'

It is also important to assess the frequency and intensity of the suicidal thoughts. The thoughts may be occasional and fleeting in nature, or may be frequent, strong, overwhelming thoughts that would indicate an increased risk. It should be clarified if the thoughts come from an internal source (i.e. the individual's own thoughts) or if there is any evidence of command hallucinatory experiences indicative of a psychotic disorder.

2. Assess Intentions

If thoughts of suicide are present, does the person intend to act on them?

If a person has suicidal ideation, then it is important to assess their intention to commit suicide. Direct questions that may be helpful as a starting point for a conversation about the intent include:

- Do you think you will act on these thoughts?
- Do you think you will kill yourself?

The Pierce Suicide Intent Scale (Pierce, 1977) can be useful as a structured assessment of a recent apparent suicide attempt. The aim is to understand the circumstances surrounding the attempt, as shown in Table 9.3.

Table 9.3 Pierce Suicide Intent Scale

Circumstances		Score
Isolation	Someone was present at the time the attempt was made	0
	Someone was nearby or on the telephone	1
	No one was nearby	2
Timing	The attempt was timed so that intervention was possible	0
	Intervention was unlikely	1
	Intervention was highly unlikely	2
Precautions against rescue	There were no precautions taken against discovery	0
	Precautions were passive (e.g. alone in room, door unlocked)	1
	Active precautions	2
Acting to gain help	Someone was notified	0
	Contacted someone, but did not explicitly tell them	1
	No contact with anyone	2
Final acts in anticipation of death	No final acts	0
	Partial preparation	1
	Definite plans (e.g. writing a will, insurance, gifts)	2
Suicide note	No suicide note written	0
	Note written but torn up	1
	Presence of note	2

Self-report		Score
Lethality	The person thought what they did would not kill them	0
	Person is unsure that the chosen method was lethal	1
	Believed it would kill them	2
Premeditation	The attempt was impulsive	0
	The attempt was considered for <1 hour	1
	Considered for <1 day	2
	Considered for >1 day	3
Stated intent	The person reports that they did not want to die	0
	Unsure	1
	Wanted to die	2
Reaction to act	The person reports that they are glad they have recovered	0
	Uncertain	1
	Sorry they were unsuccessful	2

Medical risk score		Score
Predictable outcome	Survival certain	0
	Death unlikely	1
	Death likely	2
Death without medical treatment	No	0
	Uncertain	1
	Yes	2

Source: Adapted from Pierce (1977)

The maximum score for the Pierce Suicide Intent Scale is therefore 25, with the level of intent/risk graded as follows:

- Less than 4 = low intent/risk
- 4–10 = medium intent/risk
- More than 10 = high intent/risk

3. Assess Plans

If thoughts of suicide and intentions are present, it is important then to consider:

- Has the person had thoughts of, or made a plan of, how they will actually kill themselves?
- If so, how detailed is the plan?
- What is the potential lethality of the means?
- Do they have access to the chosen means?
- Are they readily available?
- Have they recently written or planned a suicide note?
- Have they made any moves to distance themselves from friends and/or relatives?
- Or have they made any preparations in anticipation of dying, for example giving away property or rewriting their will?

In general, a detailed and well-prepared plan indicates a degree of thought and possible rumination on the act, suggestive of a greater risk as is the availability and lethality of means.

Any assessment of ideation, intention and plans must be understood in the context of the person's current situation, along with an assessment of the static and dynamic factors, including active mental health symptoms. It is also important to note that if a person is not disclosing thoughts, plans and intentions, it does not mean that a risk is not present.

Self-Neglect

People who neglect their own personal and household hygiene and health are familiar to mental health staff (Lauder, 2005), and it is therefore a significant issue for mental health services and an important and challenging aspect of risk assessment.

Definitions of Self-Neglect

Self-neglect is 'a form of self-care deficit in which those self-care activities that are thought to be necessary to maintain a socially accepted standard of personal and household hygiene are not undertaken' (ibid.: 46). However, self-neglect may also include a failure to adequately manage personal finances; social and interpersonal neglect; poor adherence with treatment plans; and failures of people to protect themselves from sexual, financial and property abuse (ibid., 2001; Gunstone, 2003; Gibbons et al., 2006).

Self-neglect, of course, does not represent an all-or-nothing phenomenon but appears to exist on a continuum. The lower end of the self-neglect continuum may include issues such as a failure to look after one's diet; poor dental hygiene; not proactively seeking medical attention when an illness or condition is suspected; and so on. At the other end of the continuum, *severe self-neglect* may lead to a significant deterioration in physical and mental health such as: the hoarding of potentially hazardous or toxic rubbish and animals, both alive and dead; the continual neglect of rotting food; poor personal hygiene resulting in parasitic infestations, and other infections; recklessness arising from ignoring possible dangers from poorly maintained electrical appliances; and so on (Arluke et al., 2002; Gunstone, 2003; Lauder, 2001; Gibbons et al., 2006).

Risk Factors for Self-Neglect

Mental Illness

Self-neglect has been associated with various mental conditions such as obsessive-compulsive disorders (Maier, 2004); psychosis; depression; dementia (Halliday et al., 2000; Abrams et al., 2002); stress in later life (Clarke et al., 1975); and personality disorder (Damecour and Charron, 1998; Abrams et al., 2002). Self-neglect can also be found in those with frontal lobe atrophy, which can also be associated with aggression, hostility and paranoia (Orell et al., 1989). People who live in squalor also tend to have higher rates of mental conditions, often exacerbated by a co-morbid alcohol abuse (Halliday et al., 2000).

Mental illness, then, may be a clinical precursor to self-neglect. However, the links between psychiatric conditions and self-neglect are not always clear (Lauder, 1999a) as, for example, approximately 50 per cent of people who neglect themselves in the over-60s have no clinically diagnosed mental disorder (Macmillan and Shaw, 1966; Clarke et al., 1975). Whilst psychiatric experiences and the use of sedating psychiatric medication may contribute to some people's difficulties in coping with personal and household hygiene, finance, social interaction and concordance with treatment and so on, there is as yet no definitive evidence of a causal association between mental ill health and self-neglect (Vostanis and Dean, 1992).

Age and Gender

Significant associations may also exist between self-neglect and cognitive decline in older age (Macmillan and Shaw, 1966; Abrams et al., 2002), and this group, in particular, may experience social withdrawal (Hettiaratchy and Manthorpe, 1989), malnutrition, the hoarding of rubbish and severe neglect of personal hygiene (Clark et al., 1975).

However, self-neglect in younger adults (specifically those under 60 years of age) is poorly understood and poorly researched (Cooney and Hamid, 1995), so the self-neglect risk profile for these age groups is unclear. That is, it is not clear if there are specific risk factors for younger people with mental health problems who self-neglect that distinguish them from the general population (Lauder, 2005).

Psychosocial Factors

Psychosocial perspectives of self-neglect seek to understand and explain the phenomena rather than classify it as a symptom of some underlying mental disorder (Lauder 2001). For example, Bristow et al. (2001) found significant differences in the higher rates of self-neglect amongst admissions to inpatient mental health facilities in inner London areas compared with outer London. However, it is not clear if living in inner city/urban areas contributes to self-neglect or if people who are prone to self-neglect are drawn to those areas. Self-neglect may also occur where an individual becomes focused on, and perhaps over-involved with, the needs and welfare of others to the exclusion of their own personal needs (Fritz and Helgeson, 1998). Vostanis and Dean (1992) explored two cases of self-neglect in women aged 35 and 38. Both were unemployed and were described as having an emotionally detached upbringing from their family and relatives and no evidence of a treatable psychiatric illness was diagnosed. There were further similarities, in that both women had few contacts with friends, rejected help from outside agencies and were described as being often suspicious and quarrelsome. This supported previous findings on the social and interpersonal characteristics of those that self-neglect (Macmillan and Shaw, 1966).

However, consideration needs to be given to how assessors may interpret or perceive self-neglect (Lauder, 1999a). Social definitions and explanations of self-neglect are likely to involve individual values, culturally acceptable norms and perceptions of citizenship (Gunstone, 2003; Lauder 2001, 2005). As such, self-neglect may be perceived by assessors as a failure to engage in socially acceptable and culturally defined standards of personal and household hygiene (Lauder 2001):

> people who are 'dirty', 'unclean' and 'unhygienic' in Western Cultures are regarded as disordered, unhealthy and to be vanquished. (Lauder, 1999b: 60)

Self-neglect, then, may be seen as a violation of prevailing social norms (ibid., 2005) and, therefore, perceptions of acceptable levels of cleanliness and hygiene are likely to vary between individuals who are undertaking risk assessments of self-neglect (ibid., 2001). That is, mental health care practitioners are likely to make different judgements as to what constitutes self-neglect based, at least in part, on their own cultural values (Lauder, 2001). The implications are clear: health professionals who are making risk assessments of self-neglect need to be aware of what they consider 'normal and abnormal levels of cleanliness and hygiene' (Lauder, 1999b: 61). Furthermore, if risk assessments of self-neglect are culturally determined (Crowe and Carlyle, 2003), then perceptions may also vary, depending on the extent to which we assume those who self-neglect *choose* to do (Lauder, 2001). That is, whether we believe that a person's perceived self-neglect is an intentional decision on the part of the self-neglecting individual (Gibbons et al., 2006) or whether we assume that self-neglect results from the unintentional consequences of circumstances that are beyond the person's control (ibid.), such as experiencing mental health problems or cognitive decline.

Risk Assessment of Self-Neglect

There is a clear need for the early identification of self-neglect, not only so that early preventative action may be taken, but also because self-neglect may be part of a 'relapse signature' which might be suggestive of a service user's deteriorating mental state (Lauder, 1999a; Gunstone, 2003). Therefore, the regular monitoring of those at risk for nutrition and dietary intake, physical health status, self-care and hygiene, along with treatment concordance, is essential (Tierney et al., 2004).

Unfortunately, self-neglect may go 'undetected until either a pattern of behaviour is observed by health care personnel or the individual is acutely hospitalised in a state of severe neglect' (Gibbons et al., 2006: 11). However, Gunstone (2003) highlighted the significant problem that exists in the application of actuarial risk assessment tools, in that most have been developed for research, and do little to meet the everyday needs that emerge in individual cases. Some global or symptom-specific assessments, such as the Camberwell Assessment of Need (Phelan et al., 1995) or the Expanded Brief Psychiatric Rating Scale (Lukoff et al., 1986), may be helpful to indicate or describe a health care need.

Any risk assessment of self-neglect will need to develop an idiosyncratic profile of an individual, including details of the specific areas of neglect (such as poor hygiene; animal hoarding; lack of proper disposal of potentially hazardous or toxic rubbish; the continual neglect of rotting food; social and interpersonal neglect; poor adherence with treatment plans; recklessness; and failures of people to protect themselves from sexual, financial and property abuse). However, the assessment must also include details of the person's: culturally imbued beliefs surrounding the importance of hygiene and other factors; their ability to respond to their own perceived need; a clear baseline for their 'usual' standards of hygiene and variations from this baseline; and factors which might underpin a movement away from this baseline (Lauder, 1999a).

Violence

Risk Factors for Violence

The Health and Safety Executive (HSE, 2006) suggest that individual risk assessments of violence should be completed and regularly reviewed as part of the care planning process. The assessment should consider:

- The mental, emotional and physical condition of the person.
- The effect of medical conditions or ingestion of drugs, alcohol or medicines.
- Their stress levels.
- Whether they have a history of challenging, violent or aggressive behaviour.
- Whether they consider others a threat.

The factors should not be seen in isolation, but as complex, multiple interacting variables that contribute to increasing the likelihood of violent behaviour, such as family history, personal stressors (such as loss, marital break-up or bereavement), and socioeconomic factors (such as financial problems, debt and accommodation difficulties). We must not assume that the following variables are unique to this group and we must be aware that variables that increase the likelihood of violence in the general population will also affect those experiencing mental health problems. Risk factors thought to be associated with violence, some of which are discussed below, can be found in Table 9.4.

Table 9.4 Risk factors for violence

Demographic factors	Male
	Young age
	Socially disadvantaged neighbourhoods
	Lack of social support
	Employment problems
	Criminal peer group
Background history	Childhood maltreatment
	History of violence
	First violent at young age
	History of childhood conduct disorder
	History of non-violent criminality
Clinical history	Psychopathy
	Substance abuse
	Personality disorder
	Schizophrenia
	Executive dysfunction
	Non-compliance with treatment
Psychological and psychosocial factors	Anger
	Impulsivity
	Suspiciousness
	Morbid jealousy
	Criminal/violent attitudes
	Command hallucinations
	Lack of insight
	Current 'context'
	Threats of violence
	Interpersonal discord/instability
	Availability of weapons

Source: DH, 2007

History of Violence

People who have acted violently in the past are more likely than others to act violently in the future. Past violence is the single best predictor of future violence (Monahan et al., 2001). An exploration of the previous violence needs to be undertaken, with particular attention being paid to establishing any patterns and the circumstances surrounding past violent events – including triggers, stressors, health issues, contexts, motivations and so on. The risk of violence also increases with exposure to familial violence during childhood, parental physical abuse or criminal activity by a parent.

Age and Gender

Younger people tend to act more violently than older adults. Men tend to act more violently than women, with the latter, tending to direct violence towards family members at home (ibid.).

Socioeconomic Stress

Poverty and homelessness are widely thought to increase the risk of violence. However, recent research found no associations between childhood family income and subsequent violent criminality (Sariaslan et al., 2014).

Personal Stress

Being assaulted in the past year increases the risk of violence by the victim. People who have lost their job and/or experienced marital break-up or separation are more likely to become violent.

Mental Disorder

People experiencing hallucinations that command a violent act and those who are generally suspicious and angry may be more likely to become violent than people who do not experience these symptoms. Some forms of personality disorders (such as borderline personality disorder, antisocial personality disorder, conduct disorder), particularly where the person experiences emotional detachment, are strongly associated with violence. The MacArthur Violence Risk Assessment Study (Monahan et al., 2001), however, found that a diagnosis of a major mental disorder (especially schizophrenia) was associated with *lower* rates of violence overall.

Substance Use

The use of substances can be emotionally destabilising and can trigger violent behaviour by impairing judgement, exacerbating paranoid and hostile symptoms and reducing inhibitions. It is not surprising, therefore, that people who have a **dual diagnosis** are many times more likely than patients with a mental disorder alone to become violent (Monahan et al., 2001).

Risk Assessments of Violence

An appraisal of the various risk assessment tools for violence is outside the scope of this book but it is important to acknowledge that the predictive accuracy of any risk assessment tool varies, depending on the skills of the assessor and how they are used. In general, they tend to identify low-risk individuals with high levels of accuracy, but they should not be relied on for use as sole determinants of future violence (Fazel et al., 2012).

The use of some of these tools are restricted to specific occupational groups (e.g. psychologists) and may require formal training before they can be used, which may incur a charge, as might the purchasing of a licence for their use. For example, the HCR-20 (Version 3) (hcr-20.com) consists of 20 items, dividing risk assessment into historical factors, clinical factors and risk management factors. These indicate relevant issues in a service user's past history, evaluating the presence of contemporary dynamic issues in risk, and possible future risk management requirements. Each item is coded on a three-point scale ('absent', 'possibly present' or 'definitely present').

Violent People or Violent Situations?

The risk literature often portrays violence as a phenomena stemming from *within* the individual suggestive of a personality trait or a pathological symptom of an underlying 'disease'. As we have seen from the above discussion, risk assessments tend to focus on the dispositional, historical and clinical features of a violent individual reacting to a particular context. Risk assessments of violence, however, may involve a wider appreciation of the environmental, contextual, interpersonal and situational factors than the study of a decontextualised individual. That is, violence does not occur in isolation and we must recognise that stressful situations and contexts can provoke angry or possibly violent behaviour and that such reactions may not be reflective of a person's 'disposition' (McGrory and Trenoweth, 2008). Duxbury (2002) and Duxbury and Whittington (2005) also argue that the environment, both built and social, and organisational activities within inpatient services can impact on violent behaviour.

For Megargee, 'the degree of danger that an individual represents to himself or others varies markedly as a function of a number of variables' (1976: 5). Megargee proposed a formula to account for the complex interplay of intra-, inter-, situational risk factors and those protective variables that mitigate risk. These include:

- Risk factors that facilitate violent acts:
  - An individual's motivation to become violent (Mx).
  - The individual's past history of being reinforced for violent behaviour (H).
  - Factors within the situation which may facilitate violence (Sf).

- Risk factors that inhibit violent acts:
  - Factors which inhibit (I) violent act (a) against a victim (x) (Ia.x).
  - Factors within the situation which may inhibit violence (Si).

Megargee (ibid.) suggested that, when the inhibitions were stronger, there would be less likelihood of violence:

$$Mx + H + Sf < Ia.x + Si$$

and, where factors leading to violence were stronger than inhibitions, then violence would be more likely:

$$MX + H + Sf > Ia.x + Si$$

This model gives consideration to the patient's previous violent behaviour; incentives and disincentives to become violent; possible targets of the violent behaviour; and protective factors.

Megargree (ibid.) suggests that it is important to consider staff factors (Sf) that may also facilitate or inhibit violent behaviour. Negative staff–patient relationships, limit setting and controlling practices because of policy and organisational demands may also trigger episodes of violence (NICE, 2015). It has also been suggested that assessments of risk need to take into consideration the emotional and psychological state of the assessor. Tardiff, for example, suggests:

> a patient may be viewed as more dangerous than he actually is because of staff anxiety that is projected onto the patient. (1988: 543)

Similarly, there tends to be less violent behaviour in services that have well-trained and experienced staff working well together with good leadership and high morale (Royal College of Psychiatrists, 1998); and there tends to be more violence associated with services where there are staff who are inexperienced, poorly trained and authoritarian (Morrison, 1990; Lipscomb and Love, 1992). Furthermore, the assessment of violent, or potentially violent, behaviour needs to consider the environment in which the assessment takes place (which may be stressful and noisy). The presence of the individual who is making the assessment, and their actions, may increase or decrease the display of violent behaviour and, in turn, they may be personally affected by the risk, either emotionally or physically.

The National Institute for Health and Care Excellence (NICE) guidelines for *Violence and Aggression: Short-Term Management in Mental Health, Health and Community Settings* confirm that violence and aggression:

> depends on a combination of intrinsic factors, such as personality characteristics and intense mental distress, and extrinsic factors, such as the attitudes and behaviours of surrounding staff and service users, the physical setting and any restrictions that limit the service user's freedom. (2015: 4)

Therefore, it is evident that skilled risk assessment and management of violence and aggression must consider the intrinsic factors mentioned above but also the extrinsic factors such as clinical leadership and staff training, attitudes and behaviours, including: an ability to engage with service users and a person-centred approach to care; the involvement of people in their care; the recognition of escalating aggression and de-escalation to reduce the likelihood of violence; and ensuring that service users are offered appropriate therapies, physical activities and leisure pursuits (ibid.).

Safeguarding

While a full discussion of *safeguarding* is outside the scope of this book, it is important to highlight those issues that are particularly relevant to the psychosocial assessment process. Safeguarding is defined by the Care Quality Commission (CQC) as protecting people's health, well-being and human rights, and enabling them to live free from harm, abuse and neglect. This means that you may need to act upon some of the information that you are given in a psychosocial assessment, particularly where issues of risk are being discussed or where there are concerns of abuse, harm or neglect of vulnerable adults or children. If you are concerned about any information that you have received, then you should discuss this with the appropriate safeguarding lead or designate within your service. If there is no safeguarding lead, and you are concerned about a vulnerable child or adult, then you should contact the social care department at the appropriate local authority. If this is not possible, then you can contact the CQC on 03000 616161 or enquiries@cqc.org.uk. For further information, see the CQC website at: www.cqc.org.uk/content/safeguarding-people.

Chapter Summary

In this chapter, we have described and defined risk assessment and discussed the importance of risk assessment as a tool for enabling the management of risk through collaborative assessment and safety planning. In the risk assessment process, we should try wherever possible to involve and engage the service user. We have illustrated the principles of risk assessment by giving examples of three common areas in mental health care – suicide/self-harm, self-neglect, and violence. Risk assessments tend to explore factors *within* the individual but we argue that the situational factors that may facilitate and inhibit risk behaviours must also be considered. That is, in undertaking a comprehensive risk assessment, there is a need to consider risk in its broadest context and to consider risks posed to the individual as a result of having a mental health problem, including physical health, stigma, social situation, employment and finance that need to be tackled to minimise long-term risk.

EXERCISE

Risk assessments can sometimes fall into the trap of only considering the risk that the person poses to themselves or other people. However, it is important to recognise that service users themselves may be at risk from others. Jot down some risk that you feel mental health service users may be exposed to:

1. How might we assess these risks?

> ## CONSIDERATIONS FOR PRACTICE
>
> 1. What skills and values do you believe practitioners need to assess risk?
> 2. How might you involve the service user in the risk assessment process?
> 3. Risk assessments for self-neglect may not be routinely undertaken in clinical practice. Why might this be the case?

Further Reading

Department of Health (2007) *Best Practice in Managing Risk: Principles and Evidence for Best Practice in the Assessment and Management of Risk to Self and Others in Mental Health Services*. Available at: http://webarchive.nationalarchives.gov.uk/+/www.dh.gov.uk/prod_consum_dh/groups/dh_digitalassets/@dh/@en/documents/digitalasset/dh_076512.pdf (accessed 10 June 2016).

An essential document for identifying evidence-based best practice principles for risk assessment and management in health care. It identifies how best to work alongside service users in assessing and managing risk, and provides a framework for multi-professional working.

References

Abrams, R.C., Lachs, M., McAvay, G., Keohane, D.J. and Bruce, M.L. (2002) 'Predictors of self-neglect in community-dwelling elders', *American Journal of Psychiatry*, 159 (10): 1724–30.

Arluke, A., Frost, R., Luke, C., Messner, E., Nathanson, J., Patronek, G., Papazian, M. and Steketee, G. (2002) 'Health implications of animal hoarding', *Health and Social Work*, 27 (2): 125–32.

Barr, B., Taylor-Robinson, D., Scott-Samuel, A., McKee, M. and Stuckler, D. (2012) 'Suicides associated with the 2008–10 economic recession in England: time trend analysis', *British Medical Journal*, 345: e5142.

Boardman, J. and Roberts, G. (2014) *9. Risk, Safety and Recovery*. London: Centre for Mental Health and Mental Health Network, NHS Confederation.

Bristow, M., Kohen, D. and O'Mahony, G. (2001) 'Effects of social and behavioural factors in acute psychiatric admissions: a comparison between Inner and Outer London', *Journal of Mental Health*, 10 (1): 109–13.

Brown, S. and Langrish, M. (2011) 'Evaluation of a risk assessment tool to predict violent behaviour by patients detained in a psychiatric intensive care unit', *Journal of Psychiatric Intensive Care*, 8 (1): 35–41.

Clarke, A.N.G., Manikar, G.O. and Gray, I. (1975) 'Diogenes syndrome: a clinical study of gross neglect in old age', *The Lancet*, 1 (7903): 366–8.

Cooney, C. and Hamid, W. (1995) 'Review: diogenes syndrome', *Age and Aging*, 24 (5): 451–3.

Crowe, M. and Carlyle, D. (2003) 'Deconstructing risk assessment and management in mental health nursing', *Journal Of Advanced Nursing*, 43 (1): 19–27.

Daffern, M. (2006) 'The predictive validity and practical utility of structured schemes used to assess risk for aggression in psychiatric inpatient settings', *Aggression & Violent Behavior*, 12: 116–30.

Damecour, C. and Charron, M. (1998) 'Hoarding: a symptom, not a syndrome', *Journal of Clinical Psychiatry*, 59: 267–72.

Department of Health (2007) *Best Practice in Managing Risk: Principles and Evidence for Best Practice in the Assessment and Management of Risk to Self and Others in Mental Health Services*. London: DH.

Duxbury, J. (2002) 'An evaluation of staff and patients' views of and strategies employed to manage patient aggression and violence on one mental health unit', *Journal of Psychiatric and Mental Health Nursing*, 9: 325–37.

Duxbury, J. and Whittington, R. (2005) 'Causes and management of patient aggression and violence: staff and patient perspectives', *Journal of Advanced Nursing*, 50 (5): 469–78.

Fazel, S., Singh, J., Doll, H. and Grann, M. (2012) 'Use of risk assessment instruments to predict violence and antisocial behaviour in 73 samples involving 24 827 people: systematic review and meta-analysis', *British Medical Journal*, 345: e4692.

Fritz, H. and Helgeson, V. (1998) 'A theory of unmitigated communion', *Personality and Social Psychology Review*, 2 (3): 173–83.

Gibbons, S., Lauder, W. and Ludwick, R. (2006) 'Self-neglect: a proposed new NANDA diagnosis', *International Journal of Nursing Terminologies and Classifications*, 17 (1): 10–18.

Griffiths, C., Ladva, G., Brock, A. and Baker, A. (2008) 'Trends in suicide by marital status in England and Wales, 1982–2005', *Health Statistics Quarterly*, 37: 8–14.

Gunstone, S. (2003) 'Risk assessment and management of patients who self-neglect: a "Grey Area" for mental health workers', *Journal of Psychiatric and Mental Health Nursing*, 10: 287–96.

Halliday, G., Banerjee, S., Philpot, M. and Macdonald, A. (2000) 'Community study of people who live in squalor', *The Lancet*, 355: 882–6.

Hawton, K., Sutton, L., Haw, C., Sinclair, J. and Deeks, J.J. (2005a) 'Schizophrenia and suicide: systematic review of risk factors', *British Journal of Psychiatry*, 187 (1): 9–20.

Hawton, K., Sutton, L., Haw, C., Sinclair, J. and Harriss, L. (2005b) 'Suicide and attempted suicide in bipolar disorder: a systematic review of risk factors', *Journal of Clinical Psychiatry*, 66 (6): 693–704.

Health and Safety Executive (HSE) (2006) *Violence at Work*. Available at: www.hse.gov.uk/pubns/indg69.pdf (accessed 17 June 2016).

Hettiaratchy, P. and Manthorpe, J. (1989) 'The "hidden" nature of self-neglect', *Care of the Elderly*, 1 (1): 14–15.

HM Government and Department of Health (HMG/DH) (2012) *Preventing Suicide in England: A Cross-Government Outcomes Strategy to Save Lives*. Available at: www.gov.uk/government/uploads/system/uploads/attachment_data/file/430720/Preventing-Suicide-.pdf (accessed 20 June 2016).

Holmes, T. and Rahe, R. (1967) 'The Social Readjustment Rating Scale', *Journal of Psychosomatic Research*, 11 (2): 213–18.

Langan, J. (2010) 'Challenging assumptions about risk factors and role of screening for violence risk in the field of mental health', *Health, Risk & Society*, 12: 85–100.

Lauder, W. (1999a) 'Constructions of self-neglect: a multiple case study design', *Nursing Inquiry*, 6 (1): 48–57.

Lauder, W. (1999b) 'The medical model and other constructions of self-neglect', *International Journal of Nursing Practice*, 5: 58–63.

Lauder, W. (2001) 'The utility of self-care theory as a theoretical basis for self-neglect', *Journal of Advanced Nursing*, 34 (4): 545–51.

Lauder, W. (2005) 'Self-neglect: the role of judgement and applied ethics', *Nursing Standard*, 19 (18): 45–51.

Leitner, M. and Barr, W. (2006) *Systematic Review of Prevention and Intervention Strategies for Populations at High Risk of Engaging in Violent Behaviour: Final Project Report to the NHS National Forensic Mental R&D Programme*. London: DH.

Leitner, M. and Barr, W. (2011) 'Understanding and managing self-harm in mental health services', in R. Whittington and C. Logan (eds), *Self-Harm and Violence: Towards Best Practice in Managing Risk in Mental Health Services*. Chichester: Wiley.

Lipscomb, J.A. and Love, C.C. (1992) 'Violence towards health care workers: an emerging occupational hazard', *AAOHN Journal*, 40: 219–28.

Lukoff, D., Nuechterlein, K.H. and Ventura, J. (1986) 'Brief Psychiatric Rating Scale (expanded – 1986)', *Schizophrenia Bulletin*, 12: 594–602.

Macmillan, D. and Shaw, P. (1966) 'Senile breakdown in standards of personal and environmental cleanliness', *British Medical Journal*, 2: 1032–7.

Maier, T. (2004) 'On phenomenology and classification of hoarding: a review', *Acta Psychiatrica Scandinavica*, 110: 323–37.

McGrory, C. and Trenoweth, S. (2008) 'A systemic approach to violence risk assessment', in J. Lynch and S. Trenoweth (eds), *Contemporary Issues in Mental Health Nursing*. Chichester: John Wiley and Sons.

McLean, J., Maxwell, M., Platt, S., Harris, F. and Jepson, R. (2008) *Risk and Protective Factors for Suicide and Suicidal Behaviour: A Literature Review*. Available at: www.gov. scot/resource/doc/251539/0073687.pdf (accessed 10 November 2015).

Megargee, E. (1976) 'The prediction of dangerous behaviour', *Criminal Justice and Behaviour*, 3: 3–21.

Monahan, J., Steadman, H., Silver, E., Appelbaum, P., Robbins, P., Mulvey, E., Roth, L., Grisso, T. and Banks, S. (2001) *Rethinking Risk Assessment: The MacArthur Study of Mental Disorder and Violence*. New York: Oxford University Press.

Morrison, E. (1990) 'The tradition of toughness: a study of nonprofessional nursing care in psychiatric settings', *Image: Journal of Nursing Scholarship*, 22 (1): 32–8.

National Institute for Health and Care Excellence (NICE) (2015) *Violence and Aggression: Short-Term Management in Mental Health, Health and Community Settings*. Available at: www. nice.org.uk/guidance/ng10/resources/violence-and-aggression-shortterm-management-in-mental-health-health-and-community-settings-1837264712389 (accessed 10 February 2016).

Office for National Statistics (ONS) (2016) 'Suicides in the UK, 2014 registrations: registered deaths from suicide analysed by sex, age, area of usual residence of the deceased and suicide method', *Statistical Bulletin*. Available at: http://web.ons.gov.uk/ons/dcp171778_432185. pdf (accessed 24 July 2016).

Orrell, M., Sahakian, B. and Bergmann, K. (1989) 'Self-neglect and frontal lobe dysfunction', *British Journal of Psychiatry*, 155: 101–5.

Perlman, C.M., Neufeld, E., Martin, L., Goy, M. and Hirdes, J.P. (2011) *Suicide Risk Assessment Inventory: A Resource Guide for Canadian Health Care Organizations*. Toronto: Ontario Hospital Association and Canadian Patient Safety Institute.

Phelan, M., Slade, M., Thornicroft, G., Dunn, G., Holloway, F., Wykes, T., Strathdee, G., Loftus, L.P. McCrone, P. and Hayward P. (1995) 'The Camberwell Assessment of Need: the validity and reliability of an instrument to assess the needs of people with severe mental illness', *British Journal of Psychiatry*, 167 (5): 589–95, and doi 10.1192/bjp.167.5.589.

Pierce D.W. (1977) 'Suicidal intent in self-injury', *British Journal of Psychiatry*, 130: 377–85.

Royal College of Psychiatrists (RCP) (1998) *Management of Imminent Violence: Clinical Practice Guidelines to Support Mental Health Services*. London: RCP.

RCP (2008) *Rethinking Risk to Others in Mental Health Services*, College Report, CR150. London: RCP.

RCP (2010) *Self-Harm, Suicide and Risk: Helping People Who Self-Harm: Final Report of a Working Group*, CR158. London: RCP.

Sariaslan, A., Larsson, H., D'Onofrio, B., Långström, N. and Lichtenstein, P. (2014) 'Childhood family income, adolescent violent criminality and substance misuse: quasi-experimental total population study', *British Journal of Psychiatry*, 205 (4): 286–90.

Singh, J.P., Serper, M., Reinharth, J. and Fazel, S. (2011) 'Structured assessment of violence risk in schizophrenia and other psychiatric disorders: a systematic review of the validity, reliability and item content of 10 available instruments', *Schizophrenia Bulletin*, 37(5): 889–912.

Snowden, R.J., Gray, N.S., Taylor, J. and Fitzgerald, S. (2009) 'Assessing risk of future violence among forensic psychiatric inpatients with the classification of violence risk', *Psychiatric Services*, 60 (11): 1522–6.

Tardiff, K. (1988) 'Management of violent patient in an emergency situation', *Psychiatric Clinics Of North America*, 11: 539–49.

Tierney, M., Charles, J., Naglie, G., Jaglal, S., Kiss, A. and Fisher, R. (2004) 'Risk factors for harm in cognitively impaired seniors who live alone: a prospective study', *Journal of the American Geriatrics Society*, 52 (9): 1435–41.

University of Manchester (2014) *The National Confidential Inquiry into Suicide and Homicide by People with Mental Illness Annual Report*. Manchester: Centre for Mental Health and Safety, University of Manchester.

Vostanis, P. and Dean, C. (1992) 'Self-neglect in adult life', *British Journal of Psychiatry*, 161: 265–7.

Whittington, R. and Logan, C. (eds) (2011) *Self-Harm and Violence: Towards Best Practice in Managing Risk in Mental Health Services*. London: Wiley.

10

SUBSTANCE USE

MARY O'TOOLE

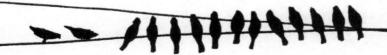

CHAPTER OVERVIEW

This chapter:

- Explores the concept of dual diagnosis and related terms.
- Gives an overview of the common drugs of misuse and their effects on mental health.
- Identifies the key components of a comprehensive assessment of a person with concurrent mental health and substance misuse problems.
- Highlights how brief interventions, including motivational interviewing, can form part of the assessment.

Introduction

Substance misuse is a broad term that refers to the harmful use of any psychotropic substance, including alcohol and either legal or illicit drugs. Substance misuse is generally (although not always) regarded as a problem if there is evidence of dependence (NICE, 2011). For a person to be considered dependent on a drug (including alcohol), they will have a strong desire or sense of compulsion to take the substance, with significant difficulties in controlling substance-taking behaviour in terms of its onset, termination or levels of use. They will experience a physiological withdrawal state when substance use has ceased or been reduced, and this will vary according to the characteristic withdrawal syndrome for the substance. There will be evidence of **tolerance** (the person will require increasing amounts of the substance in order to achieve the same effects). Generally speaking, there will be progressive neglect of other activities or interests because of **psychoactive substance** use, increased amount of time necessary to obtain or take the substance or to recover from its effects. The person is most likely to persist with substance use, despite clear evidence of overtly harmful consequences, such as harm to the liver through excessive drinking, depressive mood states consequent to periods of heavy substance use or drug-related impairment of cognitive functioning.

Dual Diagnosis

The term *dual diagnosis* has been used to describe varying combinations of physical, psychological or developmental conditions. However, for the purpose of this chapter, it is a term that has been used to describe people who experience coexisting mental health and substance use problems.

It is known that most misused substances increase **dopaminergic** activity in the brain (Koob and Volkow, 2010), and that mental health conditions such as schizophrenia and psychosis are characterised by an increase in dopaminergic transmission (Howes and Kapur, 2009). Most antipsychotic medications work by blocking dopamine receptors and therefore reducing dopamine activity, so, it can therefore be concluded that substance misuse is likely to increase symptoms of psychosis (such as hallucinations and delusions) and compromise the therapeutic effects of the antipsychotic medication.

Substance Misuse and Mental Health

Psychosis is a term used to describe a group of severe mental health disorders characterised by the presence of delusions and hallucinations that disrupt a person's perception, thoughts, emotions and behaviour. The main forms of psychosis are schizophrenia (including schizoaffective disorder, schizophreniform disorder and delusional disorder), bipolar disorder or other affective psychosis (NICE, 2011).

It is estimated that 40 to 50 per cent of people diagnosed with psychosis misuse substances at some point in their lifetime (NICE, 2011; Cleary et al., 2010), which is approximately double the rate seen in the general population. Levels of substance use that would be considered not particularly harmful in people without psychosis could have a significant impact on the mental health of an individual who has experienced, or is currently experiencing, psychotic symptoms. Indeed, substance misuse can be harmful without dependence among people with a coexisting psychosis.

People with coexisting substance misuse have a higher risk of relapse and hospitalisation, and have higher levels of unmet needs compared with other inpatients with psychosis who do not misuse substances (NICE, 2011; Hughes, 2006).

The reason that is most frequently cited for substance use in people with psychosis is as a way of coping with symptoms. However, for a third of people with psychosis, this amounts to harmful or dependent use (NICE, 2011). The outcome for people with psychosis and coexisting substance misuse is worse than for people without coexisting substance misuse, partly because the substances used may exacerbate the psychosis and partly because substances often interfere with pharmacological or psychological treatment.

Mental health problems and symptoms can frequently occur in individuals who use drugs. The symptoms vary according to the drug used and the route of administration. Most drugs will have detrimental effects on a person's mental state and may exacerbate already existing mental health problems. In addition, substance use is also associated with partial or non-adherence with medication, further increasing the likelihood of relapse (Mutsatsa, 2011).

Substance misuse among individuals with psychiatric disorders is associated with significantly poorer health and social outcomes than for individuals with a single disorder (NICE, 2011; Cleary et al., 2010). These are summarised in Table 10.1.

Table 10.1   Health and social outcomes for dual diagnosis

Health or social outcome	Example
Worsening psychiatric symptoms	Effects of stimulant drugs on psychotic symptoms; effects of alcohol on depressive symptoms
Poor physical health	Liver damage; HIV and other blood-borne viruses; poor nutrition; smoking-related conditions
Poor medication adherence	Non-adherence due to potentially chaotic lifestyle; drugs may interfere with pharmacological action of prescribed medication
Homelessness/rooflessness	Lack of income, stability and generally chaotic lifestyle
Lack of engagement/drop out from services	Lack of coordination between addictions and mental health services; chaotic lifestyle; stigma; reluctance to engage due to fear of recrimination
Family problems	Family estrangement; stigma
Increased contact with criminal justice system	Increase in acquisitive crime to pay for drugs/alcohol

A Complex Relationship

The relationship between psychosis and substance use is complex, as it is often unclear whether the individual is experiencing psychosis as a result of substance misuse or whether they are using substances as a consequence of their psychosis. Indeed, many individuals would argue that their substance use can serve to ease their symptoms, whilst others have proposed that substance use can exacerbate those symptoms. Evidence suggests that substance use, intoxication, withdrawal and dependence may all lead to, or exacerbate, mental health symptoms. Conversely, mental health problems may lead to substance use and dependence (DH, 2002; Crome et al., 2009).

Historically, there has been much discussion around the concept of 'true' dual diagnosis. However, as Crome et al. (2009) suggest, individuals may present during an episode of intoxication or withdrawal; may be dependent on one or more substances; and may suffer from more than one mental health symptom or condition. The question of whether a person is experiencing 'true' dual diagnosis is therefore largely meaningless for service users who may be excluded from help as a result. In addition, a preoccupation with 'what comes first' is unhelpful and the aim of any treatment plan should be to treat the person holistically.

Four distinct relationships within dual diagnosis have been recognised (DH, 2002; Crome et al., 2009), and these are summarised in Table 10.2.

Table 10.2   Relationships within dual diagnosis

1.	Mental conditions precipitating or leading to substance misuse (e.g. a person with severe anxiety is prescribed a benzodiazepine. The person begins taking four-times the prescribed dose to alleviate symptoms. The person becomes dependent)
2.	Substance misuse worsening or altering the course of a condition
3.	Intoxication and/or substance dependence leading to psychological symptoms
4.	Substance misuse and/or withdrawal leading to psychiatric symptoms or conditions

Common Substances of Misuse

Substances have often been categorised according to their effects on the body. So, for example, cocaine, crack cocaine and amphetamines are categorised as stimulants. Alcohol, benzodiazepines, cannabis and opiates such as heroin would be categorised as sedatives. Acid, LSD and ecstasy are categorised as hallucinogens. However, it is important to note that these are slightly nebulous categories because drugs can react in different ways for each individual, particularly if they are mixed with other drugs and/or alcohol.

Table 10.3 summarises some of the key mental health problems and symptoms associated with some of the common drugs of misuse.

Table 10.3   Drugs and their associated mental health problems

Drug	Associated mental health problems
Heroin (and other opiates)	Anxiety, depression, suicidal ideation, overdose, personality disorder
Cannabis	Anxiety, restlessness, thought disorder, paranoia
Cocaine, crack cocaine	Psychosis, persecutory delusions, paranoia, depression, sleep disturbance
GHB (gammahydroxybutrate) and GBL (gammabutyrolactone)	Sedative (very dangerous when mixed with alcohol) disinhibition, confusion, paranoia
Ecstasy (MDMA)	Anxiety, panic, paranoia, psychosis
Amphetamine	Thought disorder, hallucinations, paranoia, restlessness, sleep disturbance

New Psychoactive Substances (Legal Highs)

A more recent and worrying development is the advent of new psychoactive sub-stances (NPS, formerly known as 'legal highs'). NPS are compound substances which produce similar effects to other illegal drugs such as cocaine, cannabis and ecstasy. These substances were banned on 6 April 2016 under the Psychoactive Substances Act 2016. Prior to the ban, they were very easily available and affordable online or in legal high shops. Today, possession of an NPS is not an offence, but possession with an intent to supply can lead to seven years imprisonment and/or a fine. NPS are constantly being developed and manufactured and, as such, very little is known about their potency, adverse effects and long-term effects as research is still in its infancy. NPS have already been linked to numerous emergency hospital admissions and some deaths.

As with other drugs, NPS can be described according to their effects. The three main categories of NPS are stimulants, sedatives and hallucinogens, and they generally come in the form of pills, powders, liquids or smoking material. There is wide variation in the appearance of these substances and their names. They are often presented in brightly coloured packaging with interesting names (clockwork orange, white pearls). However, this does not reflect the fact that they are a highly potent and potentially dangerous psychoactive substance, fur-ther increasing the risk of harm as potential users will not necessarily realise the risk they are taking.

NPS are normally taken as a pill, snorted, smoked or injected. The same risks are associated with injecting NPS as with injecting any illegal drugs. For example, any drug that is injected direct into a vein will hit the blood stream rapidly and the effect will be immediate. If little is known about the NPS and its potency, then this is a very risky practice as the drug may reach harmful, or even fatal, levels in a matter of seconds. There are also the additional risks associated with the injecting process, such as blood clots and abscesses and transmission of blood-borne viruses such as HIV and hepatitis C.

Many of the effects of NPS have been described as similar to those of other illegal substances. Table 10.4 summarises some of the key mental health problems and symptoms associated with NPS.

Table 10.4 New psychoactive substances (NPS, formerly known as 'legal highs') and their associated mental health problems

Type of NPS	Effects	Associated mental health problems/adverse effects
Stimulant (e.g. BZP, mephedrone (meow meow), MPDV, NRG-1, Benzo Fury, MDAI, ethylphenidate)	Act like amphetamines, cocaine, ecstasy. Makes user feel overconfident and disinhibited	Can induce feelings of anxiety, panic, confusion, paranoia; can cause or exacerbate psychosis. User may feel low for a time after use

Type of NPS	Effects	Associated mental health problems/adverse effects
Sedative (e.g. etizolam, pyrazolam and flubromazepam)	Act like cannabis, benzodiazepines, GHB/GBL. Reduces inhibitions and concentration, slows down reactions and makes user feel lethargic, forgetful or physically unsteady Can also cause unconsciousness, coma and death, if mixed with alcohol and/or with other sedatives	Can induce feelings of anxiety, particularly after stopping Withdrawal can be dangerous and may require medical attention
Hallucinogenic (e.g. 25i-NBOMe, Bromo-Dragonfly)	Act like LSD, magic mushrooms, ketamine. Can cause strong hallucinatory reaction (trip) Some NPS create strong dissociative effects, which make user feel like their mind and body are separated	Can cause confusion, panics and hallucinations ('bad trips'); erratic behaviour; risk-taking; self-harm; impaired judgement

Cannabis and Psychosis

Cannabis is the most widely used illicit substance in the UK and frequent use of cannabis is about twice as likely amongst young people. Recent figures indicate that nearly 5.3 million 16–24-year-olds have used it in the UK in the last year (Royal College of Psychiatrists, 2014). There has been much debate with regard to the link between cannabis and psychosis, and research over the last 10 years it has been suggested that it can have serious consequences for some people, particularly those who are genetically vulnerable to developing a psychotic illness.

In recent years, a stronger form of cannabis known as 'skunk' has become popular. It has a much higher concentration of THC (tetrahydrocannabinol), the main active ingredient, than other more traditional herbal varieties. For many people, the effects of smoking cannabis are quite pleasant and can make the user feel relaxed and happy. However, when higher amounts are consumed, it can have the opposite effect by increasing anxiety. Other effects include confusion, hallucinations, anxiety and paranoia. In some people, these effects last a few hours but others suffer longer-term consequences.

Evidence suggests that people with mental health problems, including depression and psychosis, are more likely to use cannabis or have used it for long periods of time in the past. Regular use of the drug has appeared to double the risk of developing a psychotic episode or long-term schizophrenia (Patton et al., 2002; RCP, 2014). A key question within this field of research is whether cannabis causes depression and schizophrenia or whether people with these disorders use it as a medication? Indeed, there does seem to be a clear link between early cannabis use and later mental health problems in those with a genetic vulnerability, particularly when cannabis is used by adolescents. It has been suggested that the reason that adolescents are particularly vulnerable is that the brain is still developing in the teenage years and up to the age of about 20. Heavy use of cannabis may interfere with neural development resulting in long-term psychological effects.

Alcohol and Depression

Alcohol consumption has long been linked to depression or low mood. Indeed, it is known that regular drinking lowers the levels of serotonin in the brain – a chemical that helps to regulate mood (RCP, 2013; DH, 2012). Excessive alcohol consumption may be either a cause or a consequence of depression. A person may use alcohol to alleviate feelings of anxiety and depression; as tolerance to alcohol increases, so will consumption. Furthermore, alcohol is likely to interrupt the pharmacological action of anti-depressants, thus reducing their effectiveness. People who consume excessive alcohol are more at risk of suicide and self-harm (Raistrick et al., 2006).

Assessment of Substance Misuse

A comprehensive and thorough assessment is essential for individuals presenting with coexisting mental health and substance use problems. Before considering assessment in any detail, it is important to highlight that despite successful national campaigns pioneered by organisations such as Mind and Rethink, there is still considerable stigma and lack of understanding associated with mental health problems as well as substance misuse. Indeed, stigma and lack of understanding can even occur within health care settings and between health care professionals. Individuals who have both conditions may well encounter discrimination as a result of this (NICE, 2011). Social isolation, stigmatisation and social exclusion are likely to be common experiences, as well as generally poor provision in some areas and for some groups of people (Crome et al., 2009). Moreover, a person seeking help may experience feelings of shame and fear.

It is vital, therefore, that we convey a non-judgemental attitude and that the assessment is conducted collaboratively with the service user and families (if appropriate) in an atmosphere of warmth, empathy and respect. Effective written and verbal communication is vital for a person with coexisting mental health and substance misuse problems. This applies to communication between health care workers and service users and their family (if appropriate) and also between health care professionals. Service users and their family should have a clear plan in place with regard to whom they need to contact in a crisis or indeed a routine situation.

Information Gathering

An assessment of a person with coexisting mental health and substance misuse problems should be comprehensive and cover each area of a person's life in as much detail as possible.

There are a number of key areas that should always be included in any assessment and these are summarised in Table 10.5.

Table 10.5 Assessment of person with coexisting mental health and substance misuse problems

Current substance-misuse related physical health problems	Blood-borne viruses (HIV, hepatitis C)
	Circulatory and wound problems (relating to frequent injecting)
Substance misuse related offending behaviour	Criminal record
	Pending court cases
Accommodation	Including history of homelessness
	Stability of current living arrangements
Current substance misuse	Particular substance(s) used
	Quantity/pattern of use
	Route of administration
	Duration of current level of use
	Cigarette smoker?
	Supply issues
Past substance misuse	History of substance misuse
	General impact on their life and health
	Previous treatments
	Previous experience/responses to treatment
Current alcohol use	Drink of choice?
	How many units/drinks?
	What time do you start/stop?
	Withdrawal symptoms?
	Ever had seizures?
Current view of treatment	Treatment preferences/goals
	Personal strengths and weaknesses
	Readiness to change their substance use/motivation

The assessment may need to take place over several meetings to gain a full picture of the person and their needs. This will also help to develop trust and promote engagement. Indeed, a person may not be able to endure an assessment session that lasts longer that an hour. However, it is worth noting that this service user group will often lead quite chaotic and complicated lives and, as such, it is important to keep in mind that the initial assessment may be your only contact with that person. It is important, therefore, to maximise your time and take opportunities for brief interventions – this will be discussed in more detail in the following section. If the service user agrees, then discussion and collaboration with family members and supportive friends is also useful.

As well as obtaining detail with regard to substance use, it is important to explore with the service user situations or states when he or she is vulnerable to drug use and to explore alternative coping strategies. If possible, it is beneficial to encourage the service user to make links with symptoms of their mental health problem and effects of the drug. For example, the service user may wish to think about the effect of the drug on symptoms such as hallucinations or low mood.

Assessment Tools and Approaches

There are a number of assessment tools in existence for substance misuse as well as mental health, and their uptake and use vary nationally. Most substance misuse assessment tools will assess severity of dependence and levels of use (Opiate Treatment Index, Darke et al., 1991; AUDIT, Babor et al., 1992; CAGE, Ewing, 1984); whilst most mental health tools will focus on symptoms and side effects of medication (PHQ-9, Kroenke et al., 2001; LUNSERS, Day et al., 1995). There are no widely recognised tools designed specifically for dual diagnosis.

Standardised assessment tools should only ever be used in conjunction with a comprehensive face-to-face assessment and should be viewed as additional information to complement the main assessment. Assessment tools are useful for giving a baseline and also to monitor any changes in a person's symptoms, substance use or severity of dependence. A self-assessment tool may be useful for initial engagement with a person and may serve as a guide or a structure for further in-depth assessment.

Timeline

Using a timeline (see Chapter 4 for more details) can be really simple but very effective, particularly for individuals with coexisting mental health and substance misuse problems. The service user can mark key points in their life along a timeline (see Figure 10.1).

For example, when they first noticed that they were unwell; when they were prescribed medication and which type; when they first started using each substance; when their symptoms were worse or better. You and the service user can then look at whether there are any links in events. For example, the service user may notice that when they were using less alcohol, their mood seemed more stable. The service user who uses cannabis may make links between increased use and exacerbation of symptoms or even hospital admission.

started new job	not sleeping well	feeling anxious	went off sick	saw GP/CPN	signed off for one month	back to socialising	back to work
taking meds low-level drinking	stopped/ reduced meds	drinking more alcohol	meds occasionally and drinking ⁺⁺	advised re meds	no drinking and taking meds	sleeping well taking meds	
Feb 2016	March 2016		April 2016	May 2016		June 2016	July 2016

Figure 10.1   Example of a timeline

Diary

A diary is also a really useful way of tracking thoughts, feelings and behaviours, particularly in terms of drug taking and/or alcohol consumption. Your service user should be encouraged to keep a daily diary (written or electronic) and record as much information as possible on each day:

- What type(s) of substance is used (including alcohol).
- How much of each substance.
- What time of the day did you start using?
- What time of the day did you stop (or did you 'crash out')?
- Who were you with, or were you alone?
- Where were you? (At home? In the pub? At your mate's house?)
- How did you feel before you started using on that day?
- How did you feel while using? (Happy, sad, voices? Good or bad thoughts? Angry? Bored?)
- How did you feel the next day?

The service user can then bring their diary to your next meeting and use this to explore patterns in behaviour and potential consequences of substance or alcohol use on their mental and physical health. This can also be a really good way of providing insight into reasons and situations that may lead to using.

Decisional Balance Chart (Pros and Cons Chart)

A decisional balance chart (pros and cons chart, decision matrix) can be a useful way of exploring the good and not so good aspects of substance use. It can be as simple as writing a list on a piece of paper or a more complex arrangement. This can be done during an assessment/session and you can encourage your service user to think of the advantages (or pros) of continuing to use a substance versus the disadvantages (or cons) of usage. This can be an excellent starting point for a brief intervention or helping the person to think about addressing substance misuse issues. If, at assessment, the individual appeared determined and ready to make changes, then they may be referred to the appropriate service.

Brief Interventions

The assessment process provides an ideal opportunity for opportunistic brief interventions. For example, a person who is experiencing depression may be drinking well above the recommended limits of alcohol but be unaware of the potential harm on his physical and mental health. He may not have had the opportunity or inclination to discuss this with any health care professional previously. Similarly, a person with schizophrenia may smoke cannabis to help him relax but be unaware of the potential for cannabis to exacerbate psychotic symptoms. Even highlighting the issue in a non-judgemental and supportive manner may help that person to begin to think about their drinking behaviour and begin to take steps to change. Simply raising a person's awareness with regard to the link between alcohol and mood (or cannabis and psychosis) may be enough to start that person thinking about changing their behaviour.

Assessment of Withdrawal

Withdrawal from substances can be very distressing for the user, and potentially life-threatening in the case of alcohol. It is therefore important to recognise if a person is withdrawing (either deliberately or inadvertently) from a substance to which they are physiologically addicted.

Alcohol Withdrawal

Acute alcohol withdrawal occurs if a dependent drinker suddenly stops drinking. Symptoms can begin as soon as two hours after the last drink and can persist (in mild form) for weeks. Symptoms can range from mild anxiety and shakiness to severe symptoms such as seizures and **delirium tremens** (so-called **DTs**), both of which are potentially life-threatening. The symptoms of DTs include confusion, tachycardia and a high fever, and occurs in 1–5 per cent of cases.

Assessment of Alcohol Withdrawal

Alcohol withdrawal can be assessed using the Clinical Institute Withdrawal Assessment of Alcohol Scale, Revised (CIWA-Ar) (Sullivan et al., 1989). This is a 10-point questionnaire, using a combination of objective and subjective observations about the person's withdrawal symptoms. The scale can be repeated frequently (hourly in the first 24 hours and then 4-hourly) and the person's score can then be titrated against the dose of medication given to facilitate withdrawal (usually diazepam or chlordiazepoxide).

Opiate Withdrawal

Opiate withdrawal occurs if a dependent opiate user stops using. Untreated, it can last for up to a week, peaking after 3–4 days. Although highly unpleasant, opiate withdrawal is not considered a life-threatening condition. Opiate overdose, however, is. Generally, the signs of opiate withdrawal include sweating, running eyes and nose, sneezing, yawning, restlessness, insomnia, gooseflesh, dilated pupils, flushing, shivering, muscle twitching, pains in muscles and joints, nausea and vomiting, abdominal cramps, diarrhoea, tachycardia, raised blood pressure (BP) and low-grade fever.

Assessment of Opiate Withdrawal

Opiate withdrawal can be assessed using the Clinical Opiate Withdrawal Scale (COWS) (Wesson and Ling, 2003). This is an 11-item scale, designed to be administered by a clinician. Its purpose is to rate common signs and symptoms of opiate withdrawal and monitor these symptoms over time. Scores for the complete scale can be used to help clinicians determine the stage or severity of opiate withdrawal and assess the level of physical dependence on opioids. Symptoms of withdrawal can be treated with buprenorphine (Subutex) or methadone – doses can be titrated according to severity of withdrawal within the first 24 hours.

Reviewing Changes

Whilst a detailed and comprehensive assessment is important at the start of a person's treatment journey, it is vital that any changes are reviewed regularly with regard to both mental health and substance use. A regular review is also a further opportunity for brief intervention if a person is difficult to engage. This is summarised in Table 10.6.

Table 10.6 Reviewing changes

Personal circumstances	Changes in accommodation (homelessness)
	Benefits still being paid?
	Changes in family circumstances (estrangement)
Substance misuse	Is the person taking more of a particular drug to achieve the same effect (change in tolerance level)? Are they using a different route of administration (smoking, injecting)?
	Are they drinking more/less alcohol?
	Have they added or omitted a drug to their drug-taking routine?
Mental health	Have they developed symptoms (paranoia, low mood) or have things improved? Are they still taking prescribed medication?
	Any changes to risk of self-harm/harm to others?
Physical health	Development of physical health problems (blood-borne viruses, diabetes, altered liver function)
	Evidence of withdrawal syndrome?
	Interaction of drug with prescribed medication?

Chapter Summary

There are a number of commonly misused drugs that have a detrimental effect on mental health. Links have been made between psychosis, cannabis and novel psychoactive substances, as well as alcohol and depression. The rate of substance misuse amongst people with mental health problems is higher than that seen in the general population – for example, 40–50 per cent of people with psychosis misuse substances at some point in their lifetime, which is approximately double the rate seen in the general population (NICE, 2011).

People with coexisting mental health and substance use problems will often experience a significant number of negative health and social outcomes, as well as a high level of unmet needs, and will benefit from a comprehensive, collaborative and sensitive assessment of their needs.

The assessment process provides an ideal opportunity for opportunistic brief interventions. A number of practical tools can aid the assessment and information gathering. In this chapter, we have explored substance misuse and the concept of dual diagnosis. We have given an overview of the common drugs of misuse and given some detail with regard to specific effects on a person's mental health. We have identified the key components of a comprehensive assessment of a person with concurrent mental health and substance misuse problems, highlighting the importance of communication, information gathering, ongoing review and the use of standardised assessment tools. We have also demonstrated how brief interventions can form part of the assessment.

EXERCISE

CASE STUDIES

ANGELA

Angela has been diagnosed with severe anxiety and has been prescribed diazepam (5 mg, three times a day) for two weeks to help alleviate her symptoms so that she may engage in a course of **cognitive behavioural therapy (CBT)**. After two days on diazepam, Angela is feeling a lot less anxious and really likes the slightly detached feeling she is experiencing. She receives a call from the GP, telling her that, unfortunately, she cannot start her CBT for another two weeks due to high demand in her area. The GP is happy for Angela to continue on the diazepam and encourages her to engage in an online programme to help with her anxiety. Angela does not really feel she benefits from the online programme but she is becoming increasingly reliant on the diazepam and gradually increases her dose (without consulting the GP). Angela finds that she is able to obtain a further supply of diazepam online (grey market) and is now taking four times her original prescribed dose.

Reflect on this case study and consider the following questions:

1. According to the Department of Health categories, which type of dual diagnosis does this represent?
2. What are the challenges when working with Angela?
3. Why is the practitioner's attitude important in the assessment process?

CHARLES

Charles was diagnosed with schizophrenia in his early twenties. Now 33, he has had a number of admissions to hospital and, until recently, has been feeling relatively well and living independently for the last year. Charles hears voices, which are often relent-less and persecutory in nature. He is prescribed olanzapine (10 mg daily), which he sometimes believes to be effective, although would rather not have to take medication at all and will quite often miss a dose. Charles smokes cannabis regularly (around four or five joints a day, generally from 3 p.m. in the afternoon and throughout the evening). Smoking cannabis normally makes him feel relaxed and helps him sleep and, although he still hears the voices, they do not bother him so much if he has had cannabis. Charles has recently split up from his girlfriend of 10 years, which was a major blow for him. Since then, he has been smoking more cannabis (up to seven joints a night) and also drinking alcohol (strong lager and some vodka). In the last week, Charles has reported some quite worrying intrusive thoughts relating to his neighbours – he has started to believe that they want him to leave and are recording his every move. His voices have become relentless again and his sleep is disturbed. He is still willing to meet with his community nurse, with whom he has a good relationship.

Reflect on this case study and consider the following questions:

1. What do you know about the link between cannabis and psychosis – can you find any current research relating to this area?
2. How might alcohol affect Charles's mental health?
3. How might you be able to help Charles – what steps might you take to try and raise his awareness with regard to the link between cannabis and psychosis and possible solutions?

CONSIDERATIONS FOR PRACTICE

1. What are the signs that a person may have been using drugs and/or alcohol?
2. What are the challenges you might encounter when working with service users who use new psychoactive substances?

Further Reading

Drugwise: www.drugwise.org.uk/ (accessed 25 June 2016).

Drugwise is an excellent resource, frequently updated with topical, evidence-based and non-judgemental information relating to drugs, alcohol and tobacco.

National Institute for Health and Care Excellence (NICE) (2011) Clinical Guideline 120 [CG120]: *Psychosis with Coexisting Substance Misuse: Assessment and Management in Adults and Young People.* Available at: guidance.nice.org.uk/cg120 (accessed 10 October 2015).

This is a comprehensive overview of the key issues relating to substance misuse and psychosis – it is definitely worth familiarising yourself with this guideline.

National Treatment Agency: www.nta.nhs.uk/ (accessed 23 June 2016).

Now part of Public Health England, the National Treatment Agency has lots of information on its website about drugs and the various treatment options available.

Talk to Frank: www.talktofrank.com (accessed 1 July 2016).

An excellent guide to substance use, including an A–Z of all substances and the different slang terms in use. It also includes photos of what the drug looks like and details on the physical and psychological effects.

References

Babor, T.F., de la Fuente, J.R., Saunders, J. and Grant, M. (1992) *The Alcohol Use Disorders Identification Test (AUDIT): Guidelines for Use in Primary Health Care*. Geneva: World Health Organization.

Cleary, M., Hunt, G.E., Matheson, S.L., Siegfried, N. and Walter, G. (2010) *Psychosocial Interventions for People with Both Severe Mental Illness and Substance Misuse (Review)*. The Cochrane Collaboration. London: John Wiley & Sons.

Crome, I., Chambers, P., Frisher, M., Bloor, R. and Roberts, D. (2009) *The Relationship between Dual Diagnosis: Substance Misuse and Dealing with Mental Health Issues*. Research Briefing 30. London: Social Care Institute for Excellence. Available at: www.scie. org.uk (accessed 17 September 2015).

Darke, S., Ward, J., Hall, W., Heather, N. and Wodak, A. (1991) *The Opiate Treatment Index (OTI) Researcher's Manual*. National Drug and Alcohol Research Centre Technical Report No. 11. Sydney: National Drug and Alcohol Research Centre.

Day, J.C., Wood, G., Dewey, M. and Bentall, R.P. (1995) 'A self-rating scale for measuring neuroleptic side-effects: validation in a group of schizophrenic patients', *British Journal of Psychiatry*, 166 (5): 650–3.

Department of Health (2002) *Mental Health Policy Implementation Guide: Dual Diagnosis Good Practice Guide*. London: DH.

Department of Health (2012) *Alcohol Needs Research Assessment Project (ANARP): The 2004 National Alcohol Needs Assessment for England*. London: DH.

Ewing, J.A. (1984) 'Detecting alcoholism: the CAGE questionnaire', *Journal of the American Medical Association*, 252 (14): 1905–7.

Howes, O.D. and Kapur, S. (2009) 'The dopamine hypothesis of schizophrenia – version 111 – the final common pathway', *Schizophrenia Bulletin*, 35 (3): 549–62.

Hughes, L. (2006) *Closing the Gap: A Capability Framework for Working Effectively with People with Combined Mental Health and Substance Misuse Problems (Dual Diagnosis)*. Lincoln: Centre for Clinical and Academic Workforce Innovation, University of Lincoln.

Koob, G.F. and Volkow, N.D. (2010) 'Neurocircuitry of addiction', *Neuropsychopharmacology*, 35 (1): 217–38.

Kroenke, K., Spitzer, R.L. and Williams, J.B. (2001) 'The PHQ-9: validity of a brief depression severity measure', *Journal of Internal Medicine*, 16 (9): 606–13.

Mutsatsa, S. (2011) *Medicines Management in Mental Health Nursing*. London: Sage.

National Institute for Health and Care Excellence (NICE) (2011) *Psychosis with Coexisting Substance Misuse: Assessment and Management in Adults and Young People*, Clinical Guideline 120 [CG120]. Available at: guidance.nice.org.uk/cg120 (accessed 23 May 2016).

Patton, G.C., Coffey, C., Carlin, J.B., Degenhardt, L., Lynskey, M. and Hall, W. (2002) 'Cannabis use and mental health in young people: cohort study', *British Medical Journal*, 325: 1195–8.

Raistrick, D., Heather, N. and Godfrey, C. (2006) *Review of the Effectiveness of Treatment for Alcohol Problems*. London: National Treatment Agency.

Royal College of Psychiatrists (RCP) (2013) *Alcohol and Depression*. www.rcpsych.ac.uk/
    healthadvice/problemsdisorders/alcoholdepression.aspx (accessed 23 May 2016).
RCP (2014) *Cannabis and Mental Health*. Available at: www.rcpsych.ac.uk/mentalhealthinfo/
    problems/alcoholanddrugs/cannabis.aspx (accessed 23 May 2016).
Sullivan, J.T.; Sykora, K.; Schneiderman, J.; Naranjo, C.A.; and Sellers, E.M. Assessment of
    alcohol withdrawal: The revised Clinical Institute Withdrawal Assessment for Alcohol
    scale (CIWA-Ar). British Journal of Addiction 84:1353–1357, 1989.
Wesson, D.R. and Ling, W. (2003) 'The Clinical Opiate Withdrawal Scale (COWS)', *Journal
    of Psychoactive Drugs*, 35 (2): 253–9.

11

STRENGTHS AND MENTAL WELL-BEING

STEVE TRENOWETH

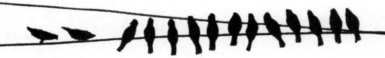

CHAPTER OVERVIEW

This chapter:

- Considers those factors that assist in protecting an individual from psychological harm and in promoting mental health following a crisis.
- Discusses factors that are related to an individual's mental well-being, satisfaction and happiness, and help the person to **flourish** and give a sense of meaning and purpose to their lives.
- Outlines the general approaches to the assessment of mental well-being and the classification of an individual's strengths, abilities and talents.
- Considers specific issues of hope, self-efficacy, resilience and positive relationships.

Introduction

Psychosocial assessments should consider not only the difficulties and challenges that a person may be facing in their life, but also those factors that help them to cope with and manage their current troubles. It is important, therefore, to take account of and understand both a person's positive and negative experiences (Westbrook, 1976). In this chapter, we discuss those factors that seem to *protect* individuals from psychological harm and promote their mental well-being and satisfaction with life.

In psychological terms, *strengths* are broadly those features of ourselves and/or our environment that are the capital which we can draw on to *protect* us in times of adversity. Like personal wealth, some people are richer in such capital than others.

As we saw in Chapter 4, the Stress Vulnerability model (Zubin and Spring, 1977) reminds us of the factors which impact on our ability to cope with challenging circumstances in our lives. In this model, exogenous stressors (such as bereavements, divorce, marriage, childbirth and so on) may precipitate a crisis, and may pose challenges for an individual's ability to cope and adapt to such stresses and subsequently readjust their lives. An individual's vulnerability to stress varies with the extent of the level of *inborn* (for example, the genetic and 'internal environment' of the individual) and *acquired factors* (for example, trauma, drug and alcohol use and so on). Such factors may *predispose* us to mental distress. Factors which are seen to be helpful and protective to the individual (such as our coping abilities, helpful beliefs, positive relationships and social networks, personal strengths and talents) can reduce our vulnerability to psychological and psychiatric distress at times of adversity and promote resilience. Likewise, factors that are unhelpful (such as maladaptive coping mechanisms, social isolation and so on) can increase our vulnerability at times of stress and may lead to a crisis for a person's mental health and well-being. Amongst vulnerable people, a failure to cope and adapt to such stresses may place their mental health under strain and increase the likelihood of exacerbation of their condition or a relapse.

In this chapter, a number of tools and tests are described and the reader is encouraged to research further to identify other tests which may also be suitable for use in particular cases.

Strengths

What are strengths? For Park et al., our character strengths are 'positive traits reflected in thoughts, feelings, and behaviours' that are associated with mental well-being (2004: 603). Strengths are the personal and **social capital** that support our *resilience* and our ability to *cope* at times of uncertainty, *protecting* us from psychological harm, and thereby allowing us to 'flourish'. An individual who is 'flourishing', in this sense, may be seen as someone who is *thriving* in their world. The person may feel that they are in charge of their lives, with a sense of *autonomy*, and that they believe that they have the personal and social resources and abilities to be *resilient* and *cope* with life's troubles. There might be a sense of *personal accomplishment*, *environmental mastery* (that is, an ability to feel in control of our lives and situation) and *personal growth*. A person may feel that their *talents*, *knowledge* and *skills* are strengths in that they provide *opportunities* for them to meet their *aspirations* or pursue their personal *interests* (Reeve, 2009).

Mental Well-Being

Mental well-being is a complex and multidimensional concept. It is generally considered, however, that our mental well-being is subjective and comprises happiness, hope and optimism and life satisfaction, positive psychological functioning, resilience to adversity, autonomy and a sense of control over one's life, self-awareness and acceptance, and supportive and interpersonal relationships. Mental well-being facilitates our personal growth and supports a personally satisfying life, which is purposeful and meaningful, and capable of reaching its full potential (Ryff and Keyes, 1995; Stewart-Brown and Janmohamed, 2008; Jenkins et al., 2008).

For the World Health Organization (WHO), health is 'not merely the absence of disease or infirmity' (1946). It further defines mental health as:

> a state of well-being in which the individual realises his or her own abilities, can cope with the normal stresses of life, can work productively and fruitfully, and is able to make a contribution to his or her community. (Ibid.)

However, there often exists confusion over what the term 'mental health' actually means (Stewart-Brown and Janmohamed, 2008). Many people now prefer the term 'mental well-being', defined by the mental health strategy for England *No Health without Mental Health* by the Department of Health as:

> A positive state of mind and body, feeling safe and able to cope, with a sense of connection with people, communities and the wider environment. (2011: 90)

These definitions recognise the personal and subjective nature of one's experience of mental health and well-being. A person with a positive sense of mental well-being may be satisfied with their life overall and also feel physically healthy. It also reflects feelings of security and our ability to function, cope within, and make a contribution to society, recognising the social nature of our functioning as human beings.

An individual's personal sense of mental well-being is therefore likely to be associated with their construing of positive satisfying, interpersonal relationships in their lives (Viney, 1981, 1983). Furthermore, a person who feels that they have a positive sense of mental well-being may also have a sense of self-reliance, with feelings of personal competence, self-efficacy and agency, and may perceive themselves as having self-determined intentions, plans and goals, which they feel are within their grasp (Viney, 1986). They may express a positive sense of striving or trying to achieve these goals, and an ability to overcome or influence others or the environment (Westbrook and Viney, 1980; Viney, 1981).

People who have a positive sense of mental well-being often describe a sense of purpose and meaning in their lives. There is an acceptance of their life, along with its highs and lows of life's events. People may describe a sense of resilience, in that they may have relevant skills, abilities and resources to cope with and bounce back after adversity.

Conversely, people may perceive themselves as lacking self-determination, in that they express feelings of helplessness, with a lack of personal agency and feelings of being a victim of circumstance. They may describe a sense of being controlled, forced, prevented by, or at the mercy of, things which are outside of their influence (Westbrook and Viney, 1980; Viney, 1981) or that they have little hope of being able to reach their goals.

For Carol Ryff (1989; Ryff and Keyes, 1995), psychological mental well-being is a multifaceted concept embracing:

- Self-acceptance (a positive attitude towards one's personal history and current self, acknowledging and accepting one's abilities and limitations).
- The establishment of positive, warm, close, supportive and trusting interpersonal relationships (including an ability to compromise; have empathy and compassion for others; and have an understanding of the ebb and flow of human relationships).
- A sense of self-determination and autonomy (including an ability to be assertive and judge one's self by personal standards).
- The ability to master complex environments (including a sense of personal competence in managing one's personal world).
- Having a purpose in life (including a sense of personal meaningful goals and reasons for living).
- Ongoing development as a person (including being open to new experiences and self-improvement).

The components of mental well-being are summarised in Figure 11.1 and discussed below.

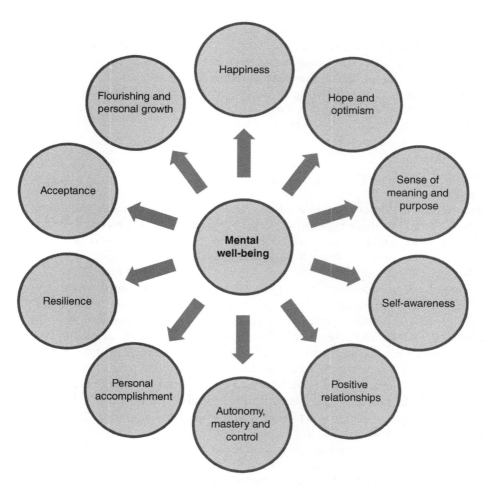

Figure 11.1 Components of mental well-being

Assessing Protective Factors

In this section, we will discus some of those factors that help to protect the individual.

Strength-Focused Conversations

While there are some approaches that can be used to structure discussions and assessments of an individual's perceived strengths and mental well-being, it is vital for a person to be offered the opportunity just to talk about the good things in their lives. Of course, at times of particular distress, a person may feel that their life was once more positive than it is now but such experiences are now elusive. This makes the need for such discussions and assessments to be undertaken sympathetically and sensitively.

A general conversation can help the person to express what they consider to be their personal and social capital whilst imposing a minimum amount of structure by an interviewer. This may also help the person to consider the balance between positive and negative aspects of their lives and to re-evaluate their experiences and to consider that there are a number of personal and social resources that may be available to them, but which they may have not considered.

Peter Watkins (2001) identifies a person-centred approach to 'assessment' and highlights a number of positively toned questions to help structure a general conversation about strengths and well-being (Table 11.1).

Assessing Strengths

Attempting to identify an individual's strengths and abilities is a challenge as people often find it is easier (and quicker) to describe their perceived weaknesses (Snyder et al., 2011). This is also a challenge perhaps for mental health practitioners who are most used to assessing psychological deficits (Peterson and Seligman, 2004).

There have been a number of approaches that have attempted to assist people to identify their strengths, abilities and talents, such as personal diaries and reflective journals in which the person is encouraged to give a positive and negative appraisal of their responses to situations and events for later discussion with an interviewer. There are also a number of rating scales that have been developed. For example, the Clifton Strengths Finder (Buckingham and Clifton, 2001; available at: www.strengthsfinder.com for purchase) is a self-report questionnaire that identifies 34 strength themes such as *communication* (the ability to put one's thoughts into action), *restorative* (being able to resolve challenges) and *analytical* (understanding reasons and causes).

Other self-report questionnaires include the only free, online and psychometrically valid measure of strengths in the world, referred to colloquially as the VIA Survey (VIA Inventory of Strengths, or for young people, the VIA Youth Survey).

Table 11.1   A strengths-orientated conversation

What in your life do you find inspiring?	What sort of help do you think you need?	Could you say a little about the good things in your life, the things that are OK?
• What are some of the things in your life that give it meaning? • What sorts of experiences have brought a sense of joy or peace to your life? • Where do you go/what do you do when you want to find a sense of peacefulness?	• When you've felt like this before, what has helped you most? • Is there anything you can do to help yourself to get through this? • Who do you turn to if you need help? • How do you think I/we can help? • What would help you the most at the moment? • What makes it easier for you to cope? • Is there one thing that would possibly be helpful now that we can work on?	• What are the things in your life that you get satisfaction from? • What are some of the things that you enjoy/are interested in? • What are you good at? What would the person who knows you best say that you are good at? What would they say are your good points? • What are some of the things that you've done that you are proud of? • Who are the people who are important in your life? • Have there been times when other people have had to rely on you/when you've helped others out? • Tell me about a time in your life when you felt happy. • What's the best job you've ever had? What sort of work would you like to do? • How do you look after yourself/stay well? • How do you relax? • What's kept you going through all the difficult times? What helps? What do other people do that helps? • What are some of your hopes for the future? • If I met you a few years back, what would I have noticed about you that would be different from now?

Source: Adapted from Watkins (2001)

The VIA Survey comprises 120 questions, takes approximately 15 minutes and generates a personalised rank order of character strengths from 1 to 24, along with definitions. It has been translated into 34 languages and has been taken by over 4 million people. It is found at the VIA Institute on Character's website at: www.viacharacter.org. These surveys seek to reveal an individual's personal strengths (see Table 11.2). This helps people to understand their characters better and, subsequently, to take advantage of their positive personal qualities in enhancing their everyday life (Snyder et al., 2011).

Of the strengths identified in Table 11.2, it seems that hope, zest for life, gratitude, love and curiosity are the ones which are most substantially related to satisfaction with one's life (Park et al., 2004).

Table 11.2   The VIA Classification of Character Strengths

Appreciation of beauty and excellence (awe, wonder, elevation)	Noticing and appreciating beauty, excellence, and/or skilled performance in all domains of life, from nature to art to mathematics to science to everyday experience
Bravery (valour)	*Not* shrinking from threat, challenge, difficulty, or pain; speaking up for what is right even if there is opposition; acting on convictions even if unpopular; includes physical bravery but is not limited to it
Citizenship (social responsibility, loyalty, teamwork)	Working well as a member of a group or team; being loyal to the group; doing one's share
Creativity (originality, ingenuity)	Thinking of novel and productive ways to do things; includes artistic achievement but is not limited to it
Curiosity (interest, novelty-seeking, openness to experience)	Taking an interest in all of ongoing experience; finding all subjects and topics fascinating; exploring and discovering
Fairness	Treating all people the same according to notions of fairness and justice; not letting personal feelings bias decisions about others; giving everyone a fair chance
Forgiveness and mercy	Forgiving those who have done wrong; giving people a second chance; not being vengeful
Gratitude	Being aware of and thankful for the good things that happen; taking time to express thanks
Hope (optimism, future-mindedness, future orientation)	Expecting the best in the future and working to achieve it; believing that a good future is something that can be brought about
Humour (playfulness)	Liking to laugh and tease; bringing smiles to other people; seeing the light side; making (not necessarily telling) jokes
Integrity (authenticity, honesty)	Speaking the truth but more broadly presenting oneself in a genuine way; being without pretense; taking responsibility for one's feelings and actions
Judgement (open-mindedness, critical thinking)	Thinking things through and examining them from all sides; not jumping to conclusions; being able to change one's mind in light of evidence; weighing all evidence fairly
Kindness (generosity, nurturance, care, compassion, altruistic love, 'niceness')	Doing favours and good deeds for others; helping them; taking care of them
Leadership	Encouraging a group of which one is a member to get things done and at the same time maintaining good relations within the group; organising group activities and seeing that they happen
Love	Valuing close relations with others, in particular those in which sharing and caring are reciprocated; being close to people

Love of learning	Mastering new skills, topics, and bodies of knowledge, whether on one's own or formally; obviously related to the strength of curiosity but goes beyond it to describe the tendency to add *systematically* to what one knows
Modesty and humility	Letting one's accomplishments speak for themselves; *not* seeking the spotlight; *not* regarding oneself as more special than one is
Persistence (perseverance, industriousness)	Finishing what one starts; persisting in a course of action in spite of obstacles; 'getting it out the door'; taking pleasure in completing tasks
Prudence	Being careful about one's choices; not taking undue risks; not saying or doing things that might later be regretted
Self-regulation (self-control)	Regulating what one feels and does; being disciplined; controlling one's appetites and emotions
Social intelligence (emotional intelligence, personal intelligence)	Being aware of the motives and feelings of other people and oneself; knowing what to do to fit into different social situations; knowing what makes other people tick
Spirituality (religiousness, faith, purpose)	Having coherent beliefs about the higher purpose and meaning of the universe; knowing where one fits within the larger scheme; having beliefs about the meaning of life that shape conduct and provide comfort
Zest (vitality, enthusiasm, vigour, energy)	Approaching life with excitement and energy; not doing things halfway or halfheartedly; living life as an adventure; feeling alive and activated

Reproduced with permission: © VIA Institute on Character 2004–2017

Acknowledgement: VIA Classification of Character Strengths is copyright VIA Institute on Character, 2004–2017. Used with permission. All rights reserved. www.viacharacter.org

Assessing Mental Well-Being

The Warwick-Edinburgh Mental Well-Being Scale (WEMWBS) (available after registration at: http://www2.warwick.ac.uk/fac/med/research/platform/wemwbs/) is a recently developed rating scale for use amongst adults over the age of 16 years, which aims to measure mental well-being. It is a 14-item self-report scale, capturing perceptions of subjective mental well-being and positive mental health during the previous fortnight. Responses are scored on a 1–5 Likert scale (where 1 is 'none of the time', to 5 'all of the time'). Scores are summed up and the range is 14 to a maximum of 70. Higher scores are associated with greater subjective feelings of mental well-being.

Assessing Happiness

Positive mental well-being is often associated with happy, enjoyable experiences (Viney and Henry 2002). However, *happiness* is an elusive, complex and metaphysical concept. What exactly is happiness? Are there qualities of happiness that do not vary between individuals and cultures? How do we, as human beings, 'become' happy? Can we ever be truly happy all the time? These questions have clear implications for any strength-focused assessment – if we are unable to be clear and to define our terms, it will not be possible to capture the phenomenon as a human experience. What is clear, however, is that happiness is a personal and subjective experience.

There is a debate between people who see happiness as a function of one's personality (that is, relatively stable personal 'set points' and predispositions for happiness), or that one's happiness is less stable, reflective of positive/negative experiences within which one finds oneself. It seems, therefore, that any assessment of happiness must consider both personality and situational variables (Snyder et al., 2011).

For Seligman (2002), true happiness is an enduring experience. This is to be compared with the pursuit of hedonistic experiences, characterised by transient, momentary and fleeting pleasures:

> Momentary happiness can easily be increased by any number of uplifts, such as chocolate, a comedy film, a back rub, flowers or a new blouse. (Seligman, 2002: 45)

The type of happiness that Seligman (ibid.: 45) has in mind is one that is 'authentic' and complex, as suggested by his formula:

$$H = S + C + V$$

Where:

- H is enduring happiness.
- S is our biological, genetic *set point*, although to determine our range of potential happiness.
- C are the circumstances in which we find ourselves that can influence our happiness.
- V are those voluntary factors that we can control.

That is, lasting happiness (H) is related to our life conditions (C) and our perceived ability to influence our environment and the choices we make (V) but, crucially, that there is a happiness point (S) to which we eventually return after good or bad news (our 'set point').

The four-item Subjective Happiness Scale (Lyubomirsky and Lepper, 1999) is scored on a 7-point Likert scale, and helps us to understand an individual's overall, global level of happiness or, to put this another way, whether a person is generally happy or not. The person is also invited to compare their level of perceived happiness with others and whether or not they feel that they enjoy life, regardless of what is going on around them. The average score is taken with a possible range of 1.0 to 7.0. Using this scale, it has been found that the average score for adult American partici-pants is 4.8 with a range of 3.8 to 5.8 (Seligman, 2002). In America, at least, people perceive themselves to be generally happy!

Seligman (ibid.) reviewed research over 35 years and identified external circumstances that can affect our level of subjective happiness. People who live in a relatively wealthy democracy (as opposed to an impoverished dictatorship) tend to be happier; as do people who are married; those have avoided negative experiences or negative emotions; and those who belong to a religion. Money, health, level of education and race do not appear to have any effect in our subjective happiness. It appears that our subjective attitude towards such circumstances (for example, if we feel personally impoverished or are dissatisfied with our level of health or ability or the things we feel we *should* have) rather than objective criteria (such as how much money we have in the bank, fitness level and so on) which matters most (ibid.).

Finally, Seligman (ibid.) considers the influence of those factors that are under our voluntary control (the V variable in his happiness equation) which can influence happiness. Here, Seligman identifies variables relating to our satisfaction with the past (see the section below on 'Assessing Satisfaction with Life'), present and future (see the section on 'Hope'). With regards to satisfaction with the present, Seligman distinguishes between *pleasures* ("delights that have clear sensory or strong emotional components ... ecstasy, thrills, orgasm, delight, mirth, exuberance, and comfort'", ibid.: 102) and *gratifications* (personally satisfying activities which engage and absorb us, when we are in touch with our strengths). For Csikszentmihalyi (1975), happiness 'flows' from a positive psychological state, where our personal skills are optimally and appropriately challenged and tested by tasks in our daily lives. We become so involved and immersed in a task, which tests us, that we lose all sense of time. This allows us to learn, develop and grow as individuals and to develop a personal sense of satisfaction in accomplishment.

Assessing Satisfaction with Life

The Satisfaction with Life Scale (SWLS) (Diener et al., 1985) is a five-item self-report scale, which respondents rate on a 7-point scale:

1 = Strongly Disagree

2 = Disagree

3 = Slightly Disagree

4 = Neither Agree nor Disagree

5 = Slightly Agree

6 = Agree

7 = Strongly Agree

The items are described in Table 11.3.

Table 11.3   The Satisfaction with Life Scale (SWLS)

Items	Scoring
1. In most ways my life is close to my ideal.	30–35 Very High Score; Highly Satisfied
2. The conditions of my life are excellent.	25–29 High Score
3. I am satisfied with life.	20–24 Average Score
4. So far, I have gotten the important things I want in life.	15–19 Slightly Below Average in Life Satisfaction
5. If I could live my life over, I would change almost nothing.	10–14 Dissatisfied
	5–9 Extremely Dissatisfied

Reproduced with permission: © Ed Diener et al. (1985)

Acknowledgement: © Ed Diener, Robert A. Emmons, Randy J. Larsen and Sharon Griffin as noted in the 1985 article in the *Journal of Personality Assessment*

The scores range is 5–35, with higher scores revealing greater levels of reported satisfaction with life. For those who score the highest range (in the 30–35 range), life is perceived as enjoyable and domains of life (such as work, family and personal development) are going well. Those with high scores may feel that their life is mostly good and may be motivated to improve less successful areas of their lives. For people whose scores are average (that is, average within economically developed countries), where most of the population live, life is generally good and there is an air of satisfaction, but there is also room for improvement. For those who feel less satisfied with their lives (in the 15–19 range), there are some small but, nonetheless, significant areas of life which are a source of dissatisfaction. This may be due to some recent, temporary changes in their lives that bring temporary dissatisfaction, which may improve. For people who express dissatisfaction or extreme dissatisfaction with their lives, life has become challenging. There may be significant problems at home or at work, or there may be significant life events such as bereavements, divorce or redundancy. Persistently low life satisfaction may indicate a chronic condition, where the person may need support to make positive changes to their lives. It might be, for example, that the individual finds it difficult to let go of an unhappy past or are unable to forgive perceived past wrongs (Seligman, 2002).

For Diener et al., a person's general satisfaction with life reflects an individual's personal evaluation of those aspects of their own life that are seen as important and 'not upon some criterion which is judged to be important by the researcher' (1985: 71). To this end, the SWLS should be seen as a general starting point for further discussions on sources of satisfaction and dissatisfaction in their life.

Assessing Hope

Hope is an important concept in modern approaches to mental health care (Kylmä et al., 2006; Cutcliffe and Koehn, 2007; Shepherd et al., 2008), and is considered the 'catalyst that facilitates behavioural change with the client'

(Hellman et al., 2013: 727). Furthermore, hope may also enhance our sense of self-compassion, skills in personal relationships and life satisfaction (Umphrey and Sherblom, 2014).

For Snyder et al., hope is: 'goal-directed thinking in which the person utilises pathways thinking (the perceived capacity to find routes to desired goals) and agency thinking (the requisite motivations to use those routes)' (2011: 185). So, a person who is hopeful has knowledge of their own personally valued goals, which they are motivated to strive for, and a sense of their own ability to positively and persistently work towards those goals. It also follows that hopeful people are likely to have a sense that, if one particular route to their goal is blocked or unfruitful, then they will be able to find others pathways. Furthermore, they are likely to have a zest and an optimism that their efforts to goal attainment will be worthwhile.

The Adult Hope Scale (Snyder et al., 1991) is a self-report 12-item test using an 8-point Likert scale, from 'Definitely False' to 'Definitely True', which seeks to capture an individual's sense of hope. There are two subscales: *agency* (such as the perceived ability to pursue and achieve our personal goals); and *pathways* (such as the ability to problem-solve and pursue the things that we feel are important in our lives).

The scale has been extensively studied and used widely in research and clinical practice (Snyder et al., 1991), and is generally considered to have 'value as a measurement tool toward our understanding of optimum human functioning' (Hellman et al., 2013: 728).

Assessing Self-Efficacy

Self-efficacy may be seen as:

> beliefs in one's capabilities to mobilise the motivation, cognitive resources, and courses of action needed to meet given situational demands. (Wood and Bandura, 1989: 408)

In essence, then, self-efficacy may be seen as the person's perception of their own capacity and capability to succeed in particular tasks, or 'specific self-efficacy' (SSE).

There have been concerns, however, that SSE may be ephemeral and unstable, being influenced by an individual's motivation. More recently, self-efficacy has been seen as a broader concept, encompassing the person's belief in their abilities across a wide range of situations and contexts (Chen et al., 2001). This 'general self-efficacy' (GSE) may develop from past successes and failures across our lifespan, and it is suggested that this, in turn, influences the perceptions of our abilities in specific situations.

The New General Self-Efficacy Scale (NGSE) (ibid.) is an 8-item, self-report measure that seeks to capture GSE, that is, how people view their capabilities of meeting the demands from tasks across a range of situations (see Table 11.4).

Table 11.4   Items on the New General Self-Efficacy Scale (NGSE)

1.	I will be able to achieve most of the goals that I have set for myself.
2.	When facing difficult tasks, I am certain that I will accomplish them.
3.	In general, I think that I can obtain outcomes that are important to me.
4.	I believe I can succeed at almost any endeavour to which I set my mind.
5.	I will be able to successfully overcome many challenges.
6.	I am confident that I can perform effectively on many different tasks.
7.	Compared to other people, I can do most tasks very well.
8.	Even when things are tough, I can perform quite well.

Source: Chen et al. (2001: 79)

The NGSE is rated on a 5-point scale from 'Strongly Disagree' (which scores 1) to 'Strongly Agree (which scores 5).

Assessing Resilience

Resilience is the 'ability to bounce back or positively adapt in the face of significant adversity or risk' (Snyder et al., 2011: 114). Of course, the issue here is to consider to what people are actually 'bouncing back'? There is a danger of specifying what may be considered within the normal range of human functioning and we should take into account that any measure of resilience considers the individual and cultural context of individuals (ibid.).

For Friedli (2009), there are three broad dimensions that support resilience and confer protection at times of adversity:

- *Environmental resources*: Features of the natural and built environment that support communal capacity for resilience (not discussed in this book).
- *Social resources*: Social networks and family life that enhance resilience amongst people and communities (see below).
- *Personal emotional and cognitive resources*: That support and contribute to developing resilience amongst individuals, such as good mental health – factors which undermine personal resilience include mental distress, low levels of mental well-being and neglect of self and others and a range of unhelpful coping mechanisms and self-harming behaviours, including self-sedation and, e.g., self-medication through alcohol and drugs, high fat and sugar consumption.

Tools which seek to understand an individual's perception of their own resilience include the Brief Resilience Scale (Smith et al., 2008) and the Connor-Davidson Resilience Scale (CD-RISC) (Connor and Davidson, 2003). These scales ask the individual to consider their ability to bounce back and recover after hard times and stressful events. The CD-RISC scale contains 25 items. There is a 5-point range of responses, based on how the respondent felt over the past month (where: 0 = Not True at All; 1 = Rarely True; 2 = Sometimes True; 3 = Often True; and 4 = True Nearly

All of the Time). The range of total scores is 0–100, and higher scores reflect greater reported resilience (the scale is available at: www.connordavidson-resiliencescale. com/index.php).

Assessing Positive Relationships

For many people, positive interpersonal relationships are assets that *protect* them from psychological harm and distress, *promote* their mental well-being and satisfaction with life and *support* resilience at times of adversity (Friedli, 2009). Furthermore, interpersonal support may protect people from significant consequences of major physical illness (Sherbourne and Stewart, 1991; Moser et al., 2012).

Our social well-being often stems from positive interpersonal relationships and social support. Danzinger (1976) identified a classification of positive relationships based on:

- *Solidarity*: A sense of belonging and interpersonal integration, social acceptance within a community and a common commitment between people and sharing resources.
- *Intimacy*: People relating to one another as sources of personal satisfaction, including kindness, altruism, love, empathy and attachment.
- *Influence*: Recognising the relevance of social status and standing within a community or group.

The Medical Outcomes Social Support Survey (MOS-SS) (Sherbourne and Stewart, 1991) is a brief 19-item test that seeks to capture the quantity and quality of companionship and affection, assistance and other types of social support. An online version can be found at: www.rand.org/health/surveys_tools/mos/social-support/ survey-instrument.html and guidance on scoring the test can be found at: www. rand.org/health/surveys_tools/mos/social-support/scoring.html.

Problems with Assessing Strengths and Mental Well-being

There are, of course, many issues to consider when assessing strengths and well-being. Sometimes, it can be easier for us all to recall the qualities, skills, abilities and talents that we don't have than those that we do! This, of course, can be even more trying for people who are currently experiencing mental distress (of course, an individual who is experiencing an elated mood may also lack accuracy). Additionally, there may be gender and cultural influences that discourage discussions of such matters. At such times, discussion with friends and families may be fruitful, and indirect questioning may be helpful.

Such discussions can lead to important self-discovery that may lead to reflection and a positive appraisal of our skills and talents. The **Johari window** suggests that there are some elements of our self: to which we are blind (i.e. not known to us, but known to others); that are hidden (i.e. known to us, but not known to others); and that are unknown (i.e. not known to us or others). The process of mental health assessment can, therefore, be potentially revelatory as the individual may become aware of those aspects of self which have been previously blind or unknown to them. Another important element of an assessment of strengths is the potential problem of capturing variables that are subjective. Self-report can be biased and is subject to errors, such as imperfect recall of previous and state-dependent memory, the tendency to recall events and experiences better when the person is in the same state as when the memories were formed. That is, happy events are best recalled when we are happy, and sad events are easier to bring to mind when we are sad.

It is generally considered that aspects of our personality are relatively stable and enduring over our adult lives, in that we return to a 'set point' following positive and negative experiences. Of course, this does not mean that we cannot develop new strengths and talents or hone existing ones by acquiring new skills and knowledge. However, our strengths may be compromised at different points in our lives by our life experiences and the situations, conditions and contexts in which we find ourselves, and, at such times, our personal resilience and our ability to cope with life's problems may be compromised. There may also be a motivational component to our strengths that may be influenced by our goals in any given situation (Snyder et al., 2011).

Chapter Summary

In this chapter, we have explored factors that assist in protecting an individual from psychological harm and in promoting mental health following a crisis. We also discussed factors that relate to an individual's mental well-being, satisfaction and happiness and help the person to flourish and give a sense of meaning and purpose to their lives. We discussed the general approaches to the assessment of mental well-being and the classification of an individual's strengths, abilities and talents before considering specific issues of hope, self-efficacy, resilience and positive relationships.

EXERCISE

1. Do you consider yourself to be mentally healthy at the moment? What criteria are you using to judge this? What might need to happen to change how you are currently feeling about your mental health?
2. What gives your life meaning?
3. Reflect on and list those factors in your life that promote your resilience. How do you cope with difficult issues in your life? What protects you from psychological harm?

CONSIDERATIONS FOR PRACTICE

1. How could you help a person who is low in mood and/or has lost all confidence in themselves to consider their skills talents and abilities?
2. How could you encourage and support an individual to develop a latent talent, should they, of course, wish to?
3. How do we help people to develop a sense of citizenship to support their connection with community life?

Further Reading

Lopez, S., Pedrotti, J. and Snyder, C. (2014) *Positive Psychology: The Scientific and Practical Explorations of Human Strengths*, 3rd edn. Los Angeles, CA: Sage.

An excellent, comprehensive and crucially applied text that is clear and easy to read. It focuses on positive psychology but is suitable for all practitioners working in mental health, and who want to develop their skills and knowledge about working positively with service users. There are clear synergies here with the recovery approach.

References

Buckingham, M. and Clifton, D.O. (2001) *Now, Discover Your Strengths: How to Develop Your Talents and Those of the People You Manage*. London: Simon & Schuster.

Chen, G., Gully, S.M. and Eden, D. (2001) 'Validation of a New General Self-Efficacy Scale', *Organizational Research Methods*, 4 (1): 62–83.

Connor, K. and Davidson, J. (2003) 'Development of a new resilience scale: the Connor-Davidson Resilience Scale (CD-RISC) Depress Anxiety', 18 (2):76–82.

Csikszentmihalyi, M. (1975) *Beyond Boredom and Anxiety: Experiencing Flow in Work and Play*. San Francisco, CA: Jossey-Bass.

Cutcliffe J.R. and Koehn C.V. (2007) 'Hope and interpersonal psychiatric/mental health nursing: a systematic review of the literature – Part II', *Journal of Psychiatric and Mental Health Nursing*, 14: 141–7.

Danzinger, K. (1976) *Interpersonal Communication*. Oxford: Pergamon Press.

Department of Health (2011) *No Health without Mental Health*. Available at: www.gov.uk/government/uploads/system/uploads/attachment_data/file/213761/dh_124058.pdf (accessed 18 June 2016).

Diener, E., Emmons, R.A., Larsen, R.J. and Griffin, S. (1985) 'The Satisfaction with Life Scale', *Journal of Personality Assessment*, 49 (1): 71–5.

Friedli, L. (2009) *Mental Health, Resilience and Inequalities*. Copenhagen: World Health Organization Europe.

Hellman, C.M., Pittman, M.K. and Munoz, R.T. (2013) 'The first twenty-years of the will and the way: an examination of score reliability distribution on Snyder's Dispositional Hope Scale', *Journal of Happiness Studies*, 14: 723–9.

Jenkins, R., Meltzer, H., Jones, P.B., Brugha,T., Bebbington, P., Farrell, M., Crepaz-Keay, D. and Knapp, M. (2008) *Foresight Mental Capital and Wellbeing Project (2008). Mental Health: Future Challenges.* London: Government Office for Science.

Kylmä, J., Juvakka, T., Nikkonen, M., Korhonen, T. and Isohanni, M. (2006) 'Hope and schizophrenia: an integrative review', *Journal of Psychiatric and Mental Health Nursing*, 13: 651–64.

Lyubomirsky, S. and Lepper, H. (1999) 'A measure of subjective happiness: preliminary reliability and construct validation', *Social Indicators Research*, 46: 137–55.

Moser, M., Stuck, A., Silliman, R., Ganz, P. and Clough-Gorr, K. (2012) 'The eight-item modified Medical Outcomes Study Social Support Survey: psychometric evaluation showed excellent performance, *Journal of Clinical Epidemiology*, 65: 1107–16.

Park, N., Peterson, C. and Seligman, M. (2004) 'Strengths of character and well-being', *Journal of Social and Clinical Psychology*, 23 (5): 603–19.

Peterson, C. and Seligman, M.E.P. (2004) *Character Strengths and Virtues: A Classification and Handbook.* New York: Oxford University Press and Washington, DC: American Psychological Association.

Reeve, J. (2009) *Understanding Motivation and Emotion*, 5th edn. Hoboken, NJ: John Wiley & Sons.

Ryff, C. (1989) 'Happiness is everything, or is it? Explorations on the meaning of psychological well-being', *Journal of Personality and Social Psychology*, 57: 1069–81.

Ryff, C. and Keyes, C. (1995) 'The structure of psychological well-being revisited', *Journal of Personality and Social Psychology*, 69: 719–27.

Seligman, M. (2002) *Authentic Happiness.* London: Nicholas Brearley.

Shepherd, S., Boardman, J. and Slade, M. (2008) *Making Recovery a Reality.* London: Sainsbury Centre for Mental Health.

Sherbourne, C. and Stewart, A. (1991) The MOS social support survey', *Social Science & Medicine*, 32 (6): 705–14.

Smith, B., Dalen, J., Wiggins, K., Tooley, E., Christopher, P. and Bernard, J. (2008) 'The brief resilience scale: assessing the ability to bounce back', *International Journal of Behavioral Medicine*, 15 (3): 194–200, and doi 10.1080/10705500802222972.

Snyder, C.R., Harris, C., Anderson, J.R., Holleran, S.A., Irving, L.M., Sigmon, S.T., et al. (1991) 'The will and the ways: development and validation of an individual-differences measure of hope', *Journal of Personality and Social Psychology*, 60: 570–585.

Snyder, R., Lopez, S. and Pedrotti, J. (2011) *Positive Psychology: The Scientific and Practical Explorations of Human Strengths.* 2nd edn. Thousand Oaks, CA: Sage.

Stewart-Brown, S. and Janmohamed, K. (2008) *Warwick-Edinburgh Mental Well-being Scale (WEMWBS): User Guide Version 1.* Available at: www.mentalhealthpromotion.net/resources/user-guide.pdf (accessed 24 June 2016).

Umphrey, L.R. and Sherblom, J.C. (2014) 'The relationship of hope to self-compassion, relational social skill, communication apprehension, and life satisfaction', *International Journal of Wellbeing*, 4 (2): 1–18.

Viney, L.L. (1981) 'Experimenting with experience: a psychotherapeutic case study', *Psychotherapy: Theory, Research and Practice*, 18 (2): 271–8.

Viney, L.L. (1983) 'The assessment of psychological states through content analysis of verbal communications', *Psychological Bulletin*, 94 (3): 542–63

Viney, L.L. (1986) 'Expression of positive emotion by people who are physically ill: is it evidence of defending or coping?', in L.A. Gottschalk, F. Lolas and L.L. Viney (eds), *Content Analysis of Verbal Behaviour: Significance in Clinical Medicine and Psychiatry.* Berlin: Springer-Verlag.

Viney, L.L. and Henry, R.M. (2002) 'Evaluating personal construct and psychodynamic group work with adolescent offenders and nonoffenders', in R.A. Neimeyer and G.J. Neimeyer (eds), *Advances in Personal Construct Psychology: New Directions and Perspectives.* Westport, CT: Praeger.

Watkins, P. (2001) *Mental Health Nursing: The Art of Compassionate Care*. Edinburgh: Butterworth Heinemann.

Westbrook, M.T. (1976) 'Positive affect: a method of content analysis for verbal samples', *Journal of Consulting and Clinical Psychology*, 44 (5): 715–19.

Westbrook, M.T. and Viney, L.L. (1980) 'Scales for measuring people's perception of themselves as origins and pawns', *Journal of Personality Assessment*, 44 (2): 167–74.

Wood, R. and Bandura, A. (1989) 'Impact of conceptions of ability on self-regulatory mechanisms and complex decision making', *Journal of Personality and Social Psychology*, 56: 407–15.

World Health Organization (WHO) (1946) International Health Conference, New York, 19 June–22 July. Official Records of the World Health Organization, No. 2, p. 100. Geneva: WHO.

WHO (2014) *Mental Health: A State of Wellbeing*. Available at: www.who.int/features/factfiles/mental_health/en/ (accessed 24 May 2016).

Zubin, J. and Spring, B. (1977) 'Vulnerability: a new view of schizophrenia', *Journal of Abnormal Psychology*, 86: 103–26.

PART 3

ANALYSING AND INTEGRATING ASSESSMENT INFORMATION

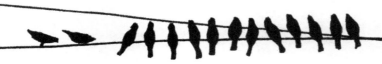

12

CASE CONCEPTUALISATION

NICKI MOONE, JACKIE GLENISTER AND BRIAN THOMSON

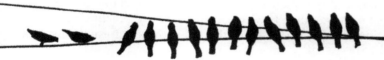

CHAPTER OVERVIEW

This chapter:

- Provides an overview of the value of developing a case conceptualisation.
- Highlights how the process of developing a case conceptualisation enables the use of a recovery approach and builds on the service user's narrative.
- Identifies the central features of a case conceptualisation and presents a model for developing a shared understanding with a service user using a template based on central themes explored in previous chapters.
- Highlights key considerations when developing the case conceptualisation with a service user.
- Demonstrates how the case conceptualisation is used to underpin the development of strengths and needs statements and to define goals with the service user.

Introduction

The terms of **case formulation** and 'case conceptualisation' are interlinked and are often used interchangeably. However, it is important to recognise a distinction between these concepts. Whereas case formulations tend to underpin specific interventions and therapies, case conceptualisations focus attention on the person's recovery journey in light of the their personal narrative alongside findings from the assessments undertaken. Using a case conceptualisation enables both the service user and the practitioner to begin to make sense of the wider picture and begin the process of identifying needs and building on the person's strengths.

Broadly speaking, therefore, the case conceptualisation should:

- Help to normalise a service user's experiences.
- Offer a clear picture of the factors that may have impacted on overall health and functioning.
- Help to arrange large amounts of complex information gathered during the assessment phase.
- Use the stress vulnerability explanation to understand presenting problem/s.
- Develop a shared understanding between service user and practitioner.
- Lay the foundations for identifying strengths and needs and formulating goals.

Case conceptualisation, identifying strengths and formulating needs (Chapter 13) and goal statements (Chapter 14) are all interlinked, as represented in Figure 12.1.

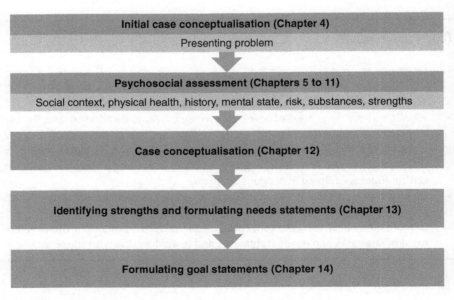

Figure 12.1   Key stages of the psychosocial approach

Key Skills in Case Conceptualisation

Developing a meaningful case conceptualisation is a skilled process, requiring consider-able technical knowledge and skill in assisting the service user to begin to make sense of their experiences and work towards ongoing recovery. As discussed in previous chapters, there are therapeutic skills that are needed to ensure a person-centred approach in order to facilitate and guide the discussion. Therefore, core skills of agenda setting, communication, active listening, using reflective statements, questioning and affirmation are key to the process. The mental health practitioner needs to be mindful of attention to detail, and be able to analyse and synthesise information that has been gathered throughout the assessment process. Skills of negotiation and collaboration with the service user will ensure that the case conceptualisation develops to underpin the development of strengths and needs statements and the formulation of goals.

Preparing for the Case Conceptualisation

As with any session with a service user, consideration needs to be given to the venue within which it will take place, that is, as discussed in Chapter 2. In line with a sys-tematic approach to the assessment process, time and consideration needs to be given to ensure adequate preparation on the part of the mental health practitioner. Using a 'funnelling approach' (see Chapter 2), the practitioner will have begun to draw together information that has significance to the presenting problem/s and factors that influence/impact on health and functioning. To give value to the wealth of infor-mation that has been shared during the assessment process as a whole, it is useful to sketch initial thoughts before the meeting with the service user. This ensures that all areas covered during the assessment process are given adequate consideration and ensures that there are no oversights during the initial case conceptualisation.

Introducing the Case Conceptualisation

When thinking about developing the case conceptualisation with the service user, attention needs to be given to helping the service user understand and begin to link together component parts of their experiences. It is important to revisit previous sessions and collate information gathered in a comprehensive manner.

We advise starting with a normalising rationale. Here, the practitioner uses thera-peutic skills to show empathy and understanding and demonstrate sensitivity. They will help the service user to reflect on experiences and recognise that their reactions are completely understandable, and they will be mindful not to minimise the ser-vice user's experiences and the distress that they have experienced. Throughout the case conceptualisation, the practitioner will use the information gathered during the assessment process to highlight to the service user that everyone has different apti-tudes to remain well in the face of personal and environmental stressors, as suggested by the Stress Vulnerability model (Zubin and Spring, 1977). The practitioner should acknowledge the value of the service user's cooperation with the assessment process.

It is critical to use language that conveys sensitivity towards past and present experiences and to ensure that the statements made are clear and in a language that makes sense to both the service user and yourself. For example:

> Over the last few weeks, we have begun to share information and to get a clearer picture of what has been happening for you ... It has been really useful to have taken the time to understand your ideas and how you feel about what has been going on for you lately ... I know that it has not always been easy to think about things that have been distressing for you, but the thing that has struck me is that you have much strength and this has enabled you to cope with situations that most people would find difficult ... I have begun to try to draw together what I believe to be key factors that are important to you ... By using this template, we can begin to make more sense of what has been happening ... The idea behind this is that, by looking at a visual representation of all we have discussed and explored recently, it becomes easier to understand the connections between the component parts... and, importantly, how best to proceed ... I am hoping today that we can begin to get a sense of how best to proceed, alongside how best to build on your strengths ...

Case Conceptualisation Format

As can be seen in Figure 12.2, the use of a structured approach to a case conceptualisation can help draw together key information and help the service user begin a process of making sense of their experiences. Using the session to begin to bullet-point key information can prove a valuable exercise in making connections between

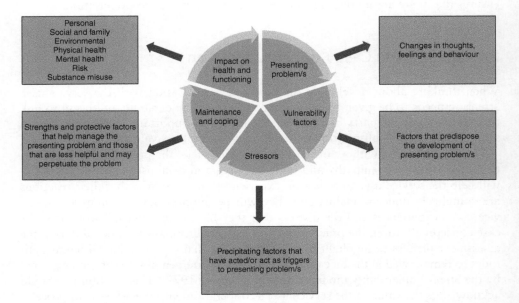

Figure 12.2   The format of a case conceptualisation

factors that have contributed to the presenting problem/s and potential areas of needs alongside strengths and protective factors. A template (adapted from the work of Birchwood et al., 1992; and Kingdon and Turkington, 2005) for your use in practice is at the end of this chapter (see Appendix 12.1).

Throughout this chapter (and the following Chapters 13 and 14), we will be looking at a case scenario involving Emily. This is a fictional person, who is a composite of many service users we have worked with which will help to illustrate and apply the key skills and techniques. An overview of Emily's case is presented in Case Scenario 12.1.

CASE SCENARIO 12.1   EMILY

Emily was a premature baby and required specialist treatment for the first month of her life. She developed a speech problem as she matured, and mentioned when completing the timeline that she did not speak until much later than her peers. She received speech and language therapy, which helped, but she can remember feeling different from her friends as she had to be taken out of class at school to receive this treatment. She remembers being bullied from pre-school age. Her father's friend sexually abused Emily as a child. Emily also attended a special school at primary school age due to her speech problems and she remembers feeling depressed from a very young age. Emily moved out of the family home after school at the age of 16 to gain more independence, however she ended up living in a hostel. This environment led her to experiment with drugs, mainly cannabis. Emily talks about the fact that she had numerous relationships with different men within the hostel environment and that these relationships were never stable or supportive. She mentioned that she never talked about her past issues or her low mood to others. She moved accommodation regularly from hostels to temporary flats. She eventually started a college course and was studying maths, English and childcare and was working part-time at a nursery, but she struggled to maintain this due to the multiple demands and eventually stopped the course and lost her job. This was around the time that she had her first episode of psychosis and ended up in hospital under section. She does not remember a lot about the circumstances leading to her admission, but she does remember not being in touch with reality and believing that her family and friends were aliens whom she couldn't trust. Emily currently lives within a supported housing project with other people who have mental health problems. She receives a monthly antipsychotic medication in the form of a **depot**, which she receives through her GP practice. Her **long-term goal** is to work with children within a nursery setting, which she did before her first episode of psychosis. Emily likes shopping, especially for handbags, and has one close friend (Sue) whom she used to go into town with but recently she has not felt able to meet up with her.

Developing the Case Conceptualisation

Presenting Problem(s)

As discussed in Chapter 4, there are various factors that can impact on a person's overall functioning and health. The presenting problem/s can include psychiatric symptoms (changes in thinking, feeling and behaving), emotions, bodily sensations, problem behaviours. During the initial assessments, you will have begun to draw together a clear picture of the presenting problem/s and will have begun the process of helping the service user have a clear understanding of why and how the current presentation is as it is. A comprehensive picture begins to develop as consideration is given to: vulnerability factors, stressors, helpful and unhelpful coping, strengths, maintenance factors and overall functioning.

It is important that you have the correct understanding of the presenting problem. When you share the case conceptualisation, you will revisit and clarify discussions had with the service user. It is important to sketch out your initial ideas beforehand, but remember that this is collaborative in nature and it is vital that you obtain feedback from the service user. This helps to ensure your shared understandings and that any inaccuracies or misunderstandings can be corrected. For example:

- It can be difficult to think about how distressing things are/have been. Although, by trying to understand this, we can begin to think about developing a plan to build on your strengths.
- How do you feel about what I have said, Emily?
- Do you think what I have said accurately captures the situation for you?
- Is there anything that we have not included?
- As we move on to the other areas, we will begin to make connections between factors that play a role in how you have been.
- When I read this, I am struck by how distressing things have been for you and that, despite this, you have …

Following the assessment process and the service user narrative, there will usually be a clear sense of the presenting problem. In summarising the presenting problem, it is important to use language that is simple and clear and uses the service user's own words. Therefore, rather than a list of symptoms, statements like 'feeling very low in mood' are preferential to 'depressed'. Using Emily's case as an example, the completed template box for her presenting problem(s) may look like Table 12.1.

Table 12.1   Emily's presenting problem

Presenting problem/s (changes in thoughts, feelings and behaviour)
Feeling unable to do things, having no energy and struggling to get things done
Feeling very low in mood
Spending long periods on my own and feeling very lonely, not going out much
I have ideas that I am being watched, I feel suspicious
Struggling to look after myself

Vulnerability (Predisposing Factors)

As previously discussed, a service user's mental health can be determined by a number of interactions between biological, environmental and social factors, known as 'predisposing factors', which increases a person's vulnerability to illness. Using a normalising rationale, discussion can help the service user understand how in certain conditions we can all develop difficulties and that some factors in life have increased their vulnerability to do so. Simply put, individuals with high vulnerability can develop symptoms with relatively low levels of stress, people with low vulnerability can develop symptoms with higher levels of stress, and the presence of protective factors and coping skills can influence the recovery journey. Potential vulnerability factors will have been explored as part of the psychosocial assessment process and this can include; genetic predisposition, developmental problems, anomalies in cognitive processing, substance use, head injury and childhood trauma.

It is important that you have the correct understanding of the vulnerability factors pertinent to the service user. When you share this part of the case conceptualisation, you will discuss important experiences and issues that have increased the service user's vulnerability. Therefore, sensitivity and empathy are essential to highlight the role that these factors will have played. It is important to sketch out your initial thoughts beforehand, but remember that the wording may be critical for the service user. Major events cannot be ignored but be mindful of how you deal with them during your discussions. This helps to ensure a shared understanding and convey a sense of hope and the role that resilience has played for the service user.

For example:

- In our discussions, we have talked about how past experiences have increased your predisposition/vulnerability and I have started to think about how we can summarise them to begin understanding the role that they have played. It can be hard to think about how difficult past events have been for you. By trying to understand this, though, we can begin to think about how you have coped and, importantly, how we can build on the strengths that you have.
- I am struck when I read this of how well you have coped, and that most people would have found this hard to deal with.
- How do you feel about what I have said Emily?
- Do you think what I have said accurately captures the situation for you?
- Is there anything that we have not included?

When drawing together vulnerability factors, it is important to convey sensitivity. Use skills that show understanding and do not minimise the service user's experiences. It is important to think about wording and the use of language to convey a sense of hope. Looking at a list of distressing life events can be difficult for some service users and they may prefer statements such as 'very difficult experiences to deal with in childhood' to 'sexually abused as a young child'. Using Emily's case as an example, the completed template box may look like Table 12.2.

Table 12.2   Emily's vulnerability/predisposing factors

Reaching development milestones later than peers, attended special school

Difficult experiences at school being bullied

Traumatic experiences in childhood

Early use of cannabis

Stressors (Precipitating Factors)

When discussing stressors, the service user and the practitioner explore longer-term stressors and precipitating factors and events that have led to presenting problem/s. The aim here is to use the service user's narrative to begin to increase understanding of how events/stressors have played a role in current presentation (Persons, 2012). At times of distress, it can be difficult to ascertain what events or situations are connected and how this can manifest as changes in thinking, feeling and behaviour. The discussion centres on drawing together previous discussions to highlight factors that have precipitated presenting problem/s. By doing this, you begin the process of helping the service user give meaning to experiences and highlight how this understanding can build on strengths and identify needs. As with all stages of developing the case conceptualisation, time is taken to clarify and identify important factors. As with previous examples in this section, it is critical to remember that the overall purpose is to help the service user to begin to make sense of their experiences. Attention therefore needs to be given to using a normalising rationale in discussion and how best to build on strengths to manage stressors and to build on areas of need.

For example:

- You have had a difficult time recently and I'm sure many people who have had your experiences in recent weeks would feel as you do.
- I have begun to list the recent factors that I believe have been significant for you and may have contributed to how you are feeling now.
- Recently, these are some of the things which have happened which may be related to your presenting problem ... Would you agree?

Use skills to help the service user understand events that led up to the current situation. An important part of this is to help make connections between the sequence of events and the presenting problem. By doing this, you begin the process of helping the service user give meaning to experiences, and how this understanding can build on strengths and identify needs. Using Emily's case as an example, the completed template box may look like Table 12.3.

Table 12.3   Emily's stressors/precipitating factors

Starting a college course
Working in a stressful and demanding job in a nursery
Leaving your job
Stopping the college course
Arguments with family – couldn't trust them
Accommodation issues

Maintenance and Coping (Protective and Perpetuating Factors)

It is important to acknowledge both helpful and less helpful strategies that the service user has to manage and cope with their experiences. Helpful strategies and adaptive coping skills are likely to be protective. However, maladaptive coping skills may initially seem to be helpful but are likely to perpetuate a problem, preventing its resolution, and are ultimately likely to be unhelpful.

In line with previous discussions and assessments of the person's strengths and well-being, the practitioner helps the service user make sense of how these factors have direct links to overall functioning. It is important that the practitioner is aware that several areas need to be considered to ensure that discussions and subsequent case conceptualisation reflect the service user's narrative and the information that has been gathered during the assessment process, namely:

- Appraisal:

  - What is the service user's judgement of their protective factors?
  - How does the service user feel about the perpetuating factors?
  - How does the service user consider these factors in relation to current and ongoing health and functioning?

- Availability of coping resources:

  - What resources does the service user have access to?
  - Are they sufficient?
  - Do they have a social support network?
  - Are there any groups they can attend?

- Coping strategies:

  - What coping skills does the service user have that are helpful to ongoing health and well-being?
  - What helpful strategies is the service user using to cope and how do they feel about them?
  - What unhelpful strategies is the service user using to cope and how do they feel about them?

- Environment:

  - What is the service user's situation and their surrounding?
  - How does this impact on their protective and perpetuating factors?

- Social situation:

  - What is the service user's social situation?
  - Do they have family?
  - Do they have friends?
  - How does their social situation impact on protective and perpetuating factors?

For example:

- In our discussions, we have talked about how you have coped with your experiences and how you use a range of coping strategies to manage your ongoing health. I think we agree that there are some things you do that are really helpful and warrant further attention and others that may be deemed less helpful in the longer term. By trying to understand this, though, we can begin to think about how you have coped and, importantly, how we can build on the strengths that you have. It is also important that we think about what is available to you to support you, the important people in your life, your current situation and support network.
- How you have coped with the stressors in your life recently has been very difficult for you. We have talked through some of the ongoing stress that you have and also some of the recent events that may have contributed to your recent ... presenting problem/s.
- When I read this, I am struck by how well you have coped and that most people would have found this hard to deal with.
- How do you feel about what I have said, Emily?
- Do you think that this is a clear reflection of helpful and unhelpful factors?
- Is there anything that we have not included?

The use of language is critical to ensure that you convey sensitivity and are not critical of less helpful strategies. It is useful to gently help the service user make links between less helpful strategies and the presenting problem/s and impact on overall functioning. Helpful strategies or coping skills are those that may be useful for the service user to do more of. It is an opportunity to explore strengths and resilience, and to help the person to think about how they might capitalise on their coping skills and abilities. Using Emily's case as an example, the completed template box may look like Table 12.4.

Table 12.4   Maintenance and coping: Emily's protective and precipitating factors

Things that are helpful	Things that may be less helpful
I have friends, Sue is my best friend	I sometimes use substances if I am distressed
I am able to make friends	I can isolate myself from others and don't leave the house
I am motivated and keen to make changes and work towards recovery	Sometimes, I don't look after myself properly
I know myself and have insight into myself	Arguing with family
I have skills that I use to manage my distress and anxiety	Moving house frequently

Impact on Health and Functioning

In this part of the case conceptualisation, the service user and the practitioner consider the impact on overall health and functioning but also begin to articulate areas of need. The discussion includes exploring issues that impact on health and functioning and reiteration of areas of concern for the service user. This begins the process of identify-ing initial thoughts about possible **psychosocial interventions (PSI)**. Skills used ensure that both strengths and needs are highlighted in discussions.

Potential areas to be covered include those explored throughout previous chap-ters. Knowledge and skills are used by the practitioner to ensure that pertinent issues are included in the case conceptualisation, and that only issues pertinent to the client are included. This provides an opportunity for discussion to add detail to discussions on strengths and needs and the journey towards recovery.

It can be useful to use the following headings to think about how to structure discus-sions on the impact on health and functioning. In keeping with a recovery approach, attention needs to be given to instilling hope and capturing strengths alongside needs:

- Personal:

    o   What personal resources does the service user have?
    o   What coping strategies do they have?
    o   What motivates the service user?
    o   Does the service user have insight?
    o   Is there motivation to make changes?

- Social:

    o   What social networks does the service user have?
    o   Are they socially isolated?
    o   What is their social functioning?
    o   Does the service user want to build more social contacts?

- Family/relationships:

    o   Does the service user have close relationships?
    o   How do they feel about these relationships?
    o   Are there any issues with close or intimate relationships?

- Environmental:

    o   How does the service user feel about their situation, accommodation and their surroundings?
    o   What would the service user like to change?

- Physical health:

    o   Does the service user have any concerns about their physical health?
    o   Are there any concerns that warrant attention to improve overall physical health?

- Mental health:

    o   How does the service user feel about their treatment?
    o   Are they experiencing side effects from their medication?
    o   What coping skills does the service user have to manage their symptoms?

- Risk:

    o   Are there any risk factors that need consideration?
    o   How does service user feel about their risk?

- Substance Use:
  - o Are there are substances that the person is using?
  - o How frequent? How much? With whom? When?
  - o What are the reasons given for the substance use?
  - o Is the person aware of the impact of the substance on their health and functioning?

For example:

- In our discussions, we have talked through a lot of issues that have begun to help us make more sense of what has been happening for you. By thinking about getting an overall picture, I have started to think about how all that we have discussed has impacted on your health and how you function. I think that this can give us a sense of areas that are going well for you and also those that perhaps we need to think a bit more about. By trying to do this, we can begin to think about what the next steps are and how to work towards recovery.
- When I read this, I am struck by how well you have coped and that most people would have found this hard to deal with.
- How do you feel about what I have said, Emily?
- Do you think that what I have said accurately captures the situation for you?
- Is there anything that we have not included?

Using the person's own language, highlight those factors that appear to impact on health and functioning. This requires consideration of key areas previously discussed, areas of concern for the service user and initial thoughts about areas that may warrant attention. This begins the process of identifying initial thoughts about the person's needs and goals as a prelude to possible treatment and interventions. Using Emily's case as an example, the completed template box may look like Table 12.5.

Table 12.5   Impact on health and functioning

Personal	I really want to get well again and this keeps me motivated. I have got a lot of insight and this is good
Social	Sometimes, I feel quite lonely and scared about making new friends. I know I have the skills, though. Sue is my best friend and a real support to me
Family/ relationships	I sometimes struggle in my relationships with my family and close relationships and this makes me feel down, and makes me feel as though it is my fault
Environmental	I like living with other people, I like to know that there are others around me
Physical health	I am worried sometimes as I don't always look after myself and know that I don't always eat properly. I don't always go to the GP and I worry about my health
Mental health	I am beginning to develop some coping skills for my anxiety and am trying to think about ways of dealing with my suspicious thoughts. I don't like taking medication but can see that it helps
Risk	When I am unwell, I can be a risk to myself as I stop looking after myself. I also feel that I am easily led when I am unwell and have ended up in situations and relationships that make me feel bad
Substance use	I have used cannabis in the past and I am worried that I may experiment with drugs again, especially if I'm feeling vulnerable

Emily's full case conceptualisation can be found in Table 12.6.

Table 12.6 Emily's case conceptualisation

Presenting problem(s)	Vulnerability factors	Stressors	Helpful coping and protective factors	Unhelpful coping and perpetuating factors
Feeling unable to do things, having no energy and struggling to get things done Feeling very low in mood Spending long periods on my own and feeling very lonely, not going out much I have ideas that I am being watched, I feel suspicious Struggling to look after myself	Reaching development milestones later than peers Attended special school Difficult experiences at school being bullied Traumatic experiences in childhood Early use of cannabis	Starting a college course Working in a stressful and demanding job in a nursery Leaving the job Stopping the college course Arguments with family, problems with trust Accommodation issues	I have friends, Sue is my best friend I am able to make friends I am motivated and keen to make changes and work towards recovery I know myself and have insight into myself I have skills that I use to manage my distress and anxiety	I sometimes use substances if I am distressed I can isolate myself from others and don't leave the house Sometimes, I don't look after myself properly Arguing with family Moving house frequently

Impact on health and functioning

Personal: I really want to get well again and this keeps me motivated. I have got a lot of insight and this is good

Social: Sometimes, I feel quite lonely and scared about making new friends. I know I have the skills, though. Sue is my best friend and a real support to me

Family/relationships: I sometimes struggle in my relationships with my family and close relationships and this makes me feel down, and makes me feel as though it is my fault

Environmental: I like living with other people, I like to know that there are others around me

Physical health: I am worried sometimes as I don't always look after myself and know that I don't always eat properly. I don't always go to the GP and I worry about my health

Mental health: I feel anxious but I am trying to think about ways of dealing with my suspicious thoughts. I don't like taking medication but can see that it helps

Risk: When I am unwell, I can be a risk to myself as I stop looking after myself. I also feel that I am easily led when I am unwell and have ended up in situations and relationships that make me feel bad

Substance use: I have used cannabis in the past and I am worried that I may experiment with drugs again, especially if I'm feeling vulnerable

Closing the Case Conceptualisation Interview

Throughout the sharing of the case conceptualisation, the practitioner will use a range of supportive and therapeutic skills and knowledge to ensure that the case conceptualisation is developed in line with the service user narrative and the assessment process as a whole. The end product should provide a clear overview of the service user's experiences to date. The interview will have afforded an opportunity to identify both strengths and needs, and offer valuable insights into how best to proceed. As the session draws to a close, the practitioner needs to ensure that the service user has understood the purpose of the case conceptualisation and the value of the session is apparent to both parties. The summary should include discussion of how component parts link together and seek clarification from the service user. The practitioner should mention how forthcoming sessions will include building on strengths and needs alongside formulating goals and a plan of interventions.

Problems with Case Conceptualisations

There is a temptation when developing a case conceptualisation to overly prepare for the session and not give adequate attention to service user views. The case conceptualisation is as a result of collaboration between practitioner and service user during the assessment phase. It should not represent the practitioner's overview or understanding of the service user's experiences but instead seek to develop a shared understanding. The language used should reflect the service user's choice of words and should reflect sensitivity afforded to distressing experiences.

A template or instruction manual to guide and inform practice can be very useful. However, the practitioner needs to ensure that they feel adequately prepared for the session and that they do not overly rely on either the template or the practice suggestions made in this chapter. As practitioners, we all have different ways of conveying sensitivity towards service users and, likewise, different words that we use when talking with service users. It is always best to use a style that suits our style, rather than replicate words that we are not comfortable with. Finally, remember that the intention is to help the client begin to make sense and therefore use your judgement and be flexible in your approach.

Key Points in the Case Conceptualisation

- Acknowledge all the information that has been shared by the service user over previous sessions and how this can give a sense of how best to go forward.
- Use language that conveys sensitivity to the service user experiences.
- Use simple statements so that the case conceptualisation is clear and concise and therefore easier to make sense of experiences.
- Help the service user make connections between the different parts of the conceptualisation using stress vulnerability to normalise experiences and begin to understand both strengths and needs.

Chapter Summary

This chapter has sought to guide the practitioner through the process of developing a case conceptualisation. Using the service user's narrative and a recovery-focused approach, the case formulation is used to make sense of the service user's experiences. The chapter outlines how the wealth of information gathered during the assessment process can inform the process and make best use of the information. The chapter draws on the use of a normalising rationale to underpin the development of the case conceptualisation and highlights suggestions in the 'Considerations for Practice' section by providing example questions. Building on previous chapters, this chapter demonstrates how the case conceptualisation is used to underpin the development of strengths and needs statements and to define goals with the service user. Finally, a template and practice examples are used throughout the chapter, with reference to a case scenario to show the value of a collaborative case conceptualisation.

EXERCISE

Throughout this chapter, we have used a case scenario to illustrate how assessment information can be used to develop a case conceptualisation with Emily. Using this information and the template included in Appendix 12.1, begin to sketch out information to be included in the case conceptualisation:

1. What do you need to consider before meeting with a service user?
2. How will you explain the purpose of case conceptualisation with a service user?
3. Explain it to a colleague. Does it make sense to them?
4. How will you explain the links between the component parts to Emily?
5. How will the case conceptualisation help Emily set goals?

CONSIDERATIONS FOR PRACTICE

1. What purpose does case conceptualisation serve?
2. How does case conceptualisation help the service user and the practitioner make sense of experiences?
3. How does case formulation inform interventions?

References

Birchwood, M., MacMillan, F. and Smith, J. (1992) 'Early signs of relapse in schizophrenia: monitoring methodology', in D. Kavanagh (ed.), *Schizophrenia: an Interdisciplinary Handbook*. London: Chapman & Hall.

Kingdon, D.G. and Turkington, D. (2005) *Cognitive Therapy of Schizophrenia*. New York: Guilford Press.

Persons, J. (2012) *The Case Formulation Approach to Cognitive-Behaviour Therapy*. New York: Guilford Press.

Zubin, J. and Spring, B. (1977) 'Vulnerability: a new view of schizophrenia', *Journal of Abnormal Psychology*, 86: 103–26.

Appendix 12.1 Case Conceptualisation Template

Note: When using this template, it is important to make links between component parts. There is no order for completion and the intention is to develop understanding.

Presenting problem(s)	Vulnerability factors	Stressors	Helpful coping and protective factors	Unhelpful coping and perpetuating factors

Impact on health and functioning

Personal:

Social and family:

Environmental:

Physical health:

Mental health:

Risk:

Substance misuse:

13

IDENTIFYING STRENGTHS AND FORMULATING NEEDS STATEMENTS

VICKY NAIDOO

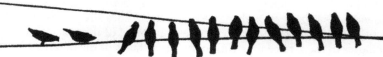

CHAPTER OVERVIEW

This chapter:

- Stresses the importance of gathering assessment information prior to formulating strength and needs statements.
- Highlights the recovery approach and achieving a collaborative relationship, and how this relates to shared understanding.
- Discusses the skilled techniques needed to identify strengths and formulate needs statements such as semi-structured interviews.
- Explains the process of identifying strengths and formulating needs statements in a structured and systematic way.

Introduction

This chapter demonstrates how to identify strengths and formulate needs statements, which leads directly on from the case conceptualisation stage (Chapter 12). This, in turn, will also support the formulation of goal statements (see Chapter 14) and subsequent care plans and psychosocial interventions and treatments.

Identifying strengths and formulating needs statements is a crucial phase in the service user's ongoing recovery (Beckwith and Crichton, 2010). It helps the service user and the practitioner to make sense of the current situation by revisiting information gathered during the various aspects of the assessment and case conceptualisation stages in order to identify a list of needs or 'problems' that are meaningful for the service user and their families.

Key Skills in Identifying Strengths and Formulating Needs Statements

Collaboration

In order to support this process, it is vital that a collaborative, therapeutic relationship is established between the practitioner and service user based on trust. Time needs to be spent to engage with the service user, and this includes: non-sessional-based conversation, humour and a relaxed atmosphere (Kingdon and Turkington, 2008). The term *befriending* is often used to describe the therapeutic relationship between practitioner and service user. Befriending is a professional friendship that includes shared boundaries between the practitioner and service user. It is the responsibility of the practitioner to explain these boundaries to the service user within the early stages of the therapeutic relationship. It is also important for the practitioner not to be overly boundaried within the relationship. The expectation is that the service user will have limited boundaries and will divulge their extremely personal experiences. If this is confronted with a cold practitioner, the therapeutic relationship will not sufficiently develop.

Collaboration is a key skill here. It is important that the service user's own language is used when completing formulations and when listing strengths and needs. This is to allow the service user to have a sense of ownership of their strengths and needs and also to help them with understanding the goal statements, which lead on to the interventions. The practitioner is required to be thoroughly prepared before this session, with the aim in mind to establish what problems currently cause the most difficulty within their day-to-day life.

It is also important to draw on good communication skills to demonstrate this shared understanding, for example, reflecting back or summarising what the service user has said to ensure the understanding is accurate (see Chapter 2). It is also important that the practitioner resists the temptation to list the needs statements that they think the service user should work on. Although the practitioner may believe that they know what the problems are, it needs to be the service user's list.

EXPERT VOICE

❝ An example of this was when I was working with a lady who heard the voice of God. I wanted to work on reducing the amount of times she heard this voice and the volume, and so recommended that we list this as a needs statement. However, this lady was not distressed by this voice and actually found it comforting as she believed this meant she was closer to God. ❞

To ensure the best recovery outcomes and successful collaboration, the service user's family and friends need to be included in the assessment and intervention process wherever possible (Patel et al., 2014). It could be a good opportunity to include them in identifying strengths and formulating needs as they will help to give collateral information as well as support the eventual goal setting stage. It is imperative that the service user is asked if they are happy to include family and/or friends and also the environment and logistics of including them, for example which session, location and boundaries.

Semi-Structured Interviewing

Identifying strengths and formulating needs statements consolidates the information gathered from assessment leading to tangible goals, which, in turn, guide subsequent interventions. One of the best ways to do this is to use a semi-structured interview as the method to analyse and synthesise assessment information. The advantage of a semi-structured interview is that the practitioner can have a set of structured questions already prepared; however, the interview itself can be flexible so as to allow the service user to expand on answers and to discuss in detail the results of the assessment.

EXPERT VOICE

What I tend to do is use a case conceptualisation template (see Chapter 12 and Appendix 12.1) and half fill it in, based on the results of the assessments. I then take this into the strengths and needs session and use it as a prompt for the semi-structured interview, and a way to ensure collaboration is achieved.

All the information gathered at assessment and case conceptualisation stages should be clearly presented at the start of the interview. The suggested format of the interview uses the 'funnelling technique' (see Chapter 12), which is often used in semi-structured interviews in the following format:

1.   Open Questions

In formulating needs statements, it is also important to start off reviewing the case conceptualisation (which you could also refer to as a *summary* if the term is confusing for the service user). Asking open questions starts the process of making sense of the assessment information and case conceptualisation, and allows discussion and reflection on what the service user feels are their current strengths and needs. It is important that the service user is invited to comment on the case conceptualisation to check that it is accurate from their point of view. It is also important that the practitioner shares their perspective and tentatively offers some suggestions about the way forward. Open questions may include:

- What do you make of this conceptualisation/summary?
- Having heard this summary, what do you feel are your current needs?

- Listening to your story, could I suggest that … also might be an issue for you at the moment? Would you agree?
- Are there any you feel are more of a priority for you at the moment?
- What are the good things for you at the moment?

2. Clarifying Questions

These questions allow the service user and practitioner to clarify and elaborate on perceived problems or issues to elicit more detail from the open questions. For example:

- Could I suggest that … seems important for you at the moment? Would you agree?
- Could you describe this problem in a bit more detail:

    o   When does this seem to be a problem for you?
    o   In what ways is it a problem for you, in particular?
    o   Who makes it better/worse?
    o   Anything else?

- What are the good things for you at the moment?

    o   What do you feel your strengths are?
    o   What and who might help us?
    o   When might they help us?

The FIND (Frequency, Intensity, Number, Duration) technique can also be used to obtain more specific details about a person's experience (see Figure 13.1).

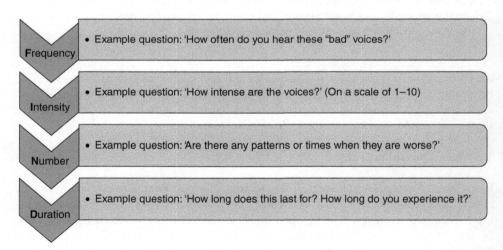

Figure 13.1   FIND technique of questioning

3. Summary

It is helpful to summarise and confirm the responses that were given by the service user to ensure that the practitioner's understanding is a true reflection of the answers. This also gives the service user an opportunity to give further details to their responses (Briddon et al., 2003).

Case Scenario – Emily

Look again at the case conceptualisation of Emily in Chapter 12 (see Table 12.5). From this, a list of needs for Emily may be negotiated and drawn up (see Table 13.1).

Table 13.1 Emily's list of needs

Number	Current Needs
1	Feeling low in mood
2	Struggling to motivate myself
3	Lost focus in my life
4	Frightened to go out
5	Having side effects of medication
6	Don't understand diagnosis or the way that I am
7	Feeling anxious around groups of new people
8	Feeling apathetic

EXPERT VOICE

❛You may be confronted with a lengthy list of needs following the assessment and case conceptualisation process. If it is not possible to address all of these needs, it is best to be guided by the service user and ask them which needs are the most distressing or the ones which they would like to work on the most, and start with these areas first.❜

Exploring a Need

The funnelling and FIND techniques described above can be used to explore and clarify needs and begin the process of prioritisation, as illustrated below, using Emily's case conceptualisation:

Practitioner: So, let's look a little more at your social life at the moment. It seems that recently you have lost contact with your friends and rarely leave the house. One of the themes when we look at the various assessments we have done together is that you say that you feel uncomfortable when you go out. Could you tell me a little bit more about that? (Open question)

Emily: I feel people are watching me when I go out.

Practitioner: Is there anything else that worries you when you go out? (Clarifying question)

Emily:	I can hear people talking about me.
Practitioner:	Can you tell me what they say to you? (Clarifying question)
Emily:	They say I'm evil and they are going to follow me.
Practitioner:	Is this every time you go out? (Frequency)
Emily:	Yes, every time.
Practitioner:	How bad is this for you on a scale of 1–10, where 1 is 'Not bad at all' and 10 is 'Unbearable'? (Intensity)
Emily:	I would say about 8. It's horrible.
Practitioner:	I'm sorry to hear that. Could you tell me if you noted any patterns or times of day when this happens? (Number)
Emily:	No – it's every time.
Practitioner:	When you go out, do you feel that people are watching you and talking about you all the time or some of the time? (Duration)
Emily:	All the time.
Practitioner:	Does anything or anyone help you to cope with this? (Identifying strengths)
Emily:	When I go out with my friend Sue, I feel a bit more confident. She is always there for me. I want to do something about this – I don't want to stay at home forever.
Practitioner:	Okay. So can I check if I understand what you have said? So far, you have said that you stay at home as you are afraid that people are watching you and that every time you have gone out you feel you have heard people telling you that you are evil and you will be followed. You feel you are motivated to cope with this and you feel that Sue may be able to help. Have I got this correct? (Summary)

So, in the first part of formulating needs statements, we have clarified and confirmed that Emily seems to have lost confidence in social situations, and feels frightened about going out and meeting new people. She says she hears voices of people telling her that she is evil, and that they will harm her constantly and consistently every time she goes out. She finds this very distressing. She feels that her friend Sue may be able to help, as she feels safe with her. This seems to be an area that Emily feels is a priority for her, so it would be appropriate to consider formulating a needs statement.

Formulation of Needs Statements

The next step is to formulate a need(s) into a statement that creates the foundation to set the goal for treatment (Beckwith and Crichton, 2010). As mentioned earlier, it is important to use the service user's own words when formulating the needs statement, as they will then own the needs and are more likely to engage in the intervention process. The needs statements should explore the impact and consequences of the problem, and how it affects the service user on a day-to-day basis.

The needs statement underpins goal statements, which will be explained in more detail in the next chapter (see Chapter 14). When formulating the goals for the service user from the needs statement, it is important not only to focus on the problems but also the strengths. These strengths may make up the service user's protective factors, which have helped them cope in the past, so it is equally important to identify these. Purely focusing on the problems could cause the service user to feel overwhelmed and unable to cope. By encouraging the service user to identify their strengths, they are more likely to feel empowered to tackle their areas of need, be left with feelings of hope and optimism and to become more self-reliant (Saleebey, 2001).

There are two key ways in which a needs statements can be structured:

1. The Antecedent-Behaviour-Consequence (ABC) Approach

In this ABC approach, the needs statement is formulated by identifying:

- *Needs Statement*: A clear summary of the need/problem.
- *Feared Consequence*: What does the service user fear may happen as a result of the need/problem?
- *Antecedent*: What happens before? Or, when is this a problem?
- *Behaviour*: What is done as a consequence of the need/problem?
- *Consequence*: What impact does this need/problem have?

An example of a needs statement using this method for Emily's scenario can be found in Table 13.2.

Table 13.2 Emily's needs statement using the ABC method

Needs statement	I have lost confidence and feel frightened about going out and meeting new people
Feared consequence	I will never be able to leave home
Antecedent	I hear voices of people telling me that I am evil and they will hurt me
Behaviour	I feel frightened all the time, avoid people and can't make friends
Consequence	I don't go out which makes me feel low in mood

2. The Kingdon and Turkington Model

Kingdon and Turkington (2008) provide another example of the way in which needs statements can be structured. This focuses on:

- *Need Definition*: A statement (or statements) in the person's own words which succinctly captures a current need.

- *Impact*: The effect that the need has on the person's day-to-day life and experience.
- *Consequence*: The influence that the need subsequently has on the person's behaviour, thoughts and feelings.

An example can be found in Figure 13.2.

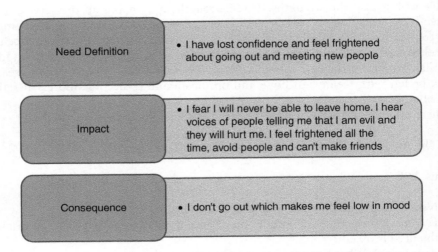

Need Definition
- I have lost confidence and feel frightened about going out and meeting new people

Impact
- I fear I will never be able to leave home. I hear voices of people telling me that I am evil and they will hurt me. I feel frightened all the time, avoid people and can't make friends

Consequence
- I don't go out which makes me feel low in mood

Figure 13.2   Emily's Needs Statements, using the Kingdon and Turkington (2008) Model

Errors in Need Formulation

Collaboration

The most important element to remember when identifying strengths and formulating needs statements is that it is a collaborative process. Try not to second-guess the needs or strengths of the service user and ensure that the service user's own language is used throughout the process.

Importance of Engagement

It is important to consider the literacy and understanding of the service user. Complicated language and words such as 'antecedent', 'conceptualisation' and so on could appear intimidating. Equally, presenting information in an overly simplistic way could also appear patronising to another service user. Ensure that time is taken during the engagement and assessment period to understand the context which the service user is coming from.

Chapter Summary

This chapter has aimed to give the reader an overview of identifying strengths and formulating needs statements as well as practical hints and tips on how to formulate them when working with service users. The chapter began with an overview of the approach within mental health care as this underpins all the assessment and intervention work that is carried out with our service users. It demonstrated some common techniques and the semi-structured interview style as the preferred model to collect the more detailed information required when formulating needs statements. The chapter then went on to discuss the importance of not just focusing on the service user's needs but also their strengths as this will ensure better recovery outcomes.

EXERCISE

1. With a colleague (and perhaps role playing, using the information supplied in Emily's case scenario), practice using the format techniques described in this chapter to identify strengths and formulate needs statements. Concentrate on developing the skills described in the funnelling and FIND techniques.

CONSIDERATIONS FOR PRACTICE

1. How might you involve family and friends in identifying strengths and formulating needs statements?
2. A good rapport and a supportive trusting relationship needs to be established before identifying strengths and formulating needs statements. Sensitivity is needed when discussing a person's needs. Given that mental health services can be very busy environments, how might you ensure that you spend sufficient time in developing a therapeutic alliance with a mental health service user?

Further Reading

Anthony, W. (1993) 'Recovery from mental illness', *Innovations and Research*, 2: 17–24.

Carers Trust (2013) *The Triangle of Care – Carers Included: A Guide to Best Practice in Mental Health Care in England*, 2nd edn. London: Carers Trust.

Corbin, J. and Morse, J.M. (2003) 'The unstructured interactive interview: issues of reciprocity and risks when dealing with sensitive topics', *Qualitative Inquiry*, 9: 335–54.

Kuipers, E. and Raune, D. (2000) 'The early development of expressed emotion and burden in the families of first onset psychosis', in M. Birchwood, D. Fowler and C. Jackson (eds), *Intervention in Psychosis: A Guide to Concepts, Evidence and Interventions*. Chichester: Wiley.

Lambert, M. (2014) *Bergin and Garfield's Handbook of Psychotherapy and Behaviour Change*, 6th edn. Chichester: Wiley.

Marshall, S., Deane, F., Crowe, T., White, A. and Kavanagh, D. (2013) 'Carers' hope, wellbeing and attitudes regarding recovery', *Community Mental Health Journal*, 49: 344–53.

National Institute for Health and Care Excellence (NICE) (2014) *Psychosis and Schizophrenia in Adults: Treatment and Management*. London: NICE.

Zubin, J. and Spring, B. (1977) 'Vulnerability: a new view of schizophrenia', *Journal of Abnormal Psychology*, 86: 103–26.

References

Beckwith, A. and Crichton, J. (2010) 'The negotiation of the problem statement in cognitive behavioural therapy', *Communication and Medicine*, 7 (1): 23–32.

Briddon, J., Richards D. and Lovell, K. (2003) 'Common mental health problems', *Journal of Community Nursing*, 17: 4–8.

Kingdon, D. and Turkington, D. (2008) *Cognitive Therapy of Schizophrenia*. London: Guilford Press.

Patel, M., Chawla, R., Krynicki, C., Rankin, P. and Upthegrove, R. (2014) 'Health beliefs and carer burden in first episode psychosis', *British Medical Centre Psychiatry*, 14: 171.

Saleebey, D. (2001) *The Strengths Perspective in Social Work Practice*, 3rd edn. Boston, MA: Allyn & Bacon.

14

FORMULATING GOAL STATEMENTS

ALISON ELLIOTT, JOHN BUTLER AND TRACEY KEARNS

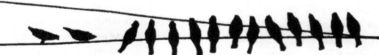

CHAPTER OVERVIEW

This chapter:

- Provides an understanding of goal formulation.
- Considers practical methods for engaging the individual/family member(s) in identifying and prioritising meaningful personal goals as a key component of the psychosocial approach.
- Considers helpful ways of reviewing and monitoring the achievement of goals.
- Promotes an awareness of strategies and resources that are helpful in overcoming difficulties/obstacles to goal formulation, thus supporting goal attainment.
- Offers some resources to support the practice of goal formulation and review.

Introduction

This chapter introduces the concept of goals and collaborative goal formulation as a key feature of psychosocial assessment and intervention, which follows directly on from identifying strengths and formulating needs statements (Chapter 13). It offers practitioners a practical approach to working alongside individuals to formulate meaningful **short-** and **long-term goals**, exploring how this can be achieved, and highlighting useful tips in the event of difficulties and obstacles.

The Importance of Goal Setting

Clear goal setting is an essential component of a psychosocial approach. This process not only allows the negotiation and agreement of subsequent therapies, care or treatments to address identified needs, but also allows the review of whether such interventions have had any impact on the distress/problems experienced by the individual (Laidlaw, 2015).

A 'goal' may be regarded as a desired outcome, as something that a person wishes to achieve, such as living independently, getting a job or getting married (Wright et al., 2014). Setting and working towards personal and meaningful goals is an effective way of focusing on issues that affect an individual, achieving a sense of value and managing stress, which enhances morale, motivation, sense of achievement and self-confidence, reduces distress and the sense of demoralisation and hopelessness, and thus promotes hope and recovery (Meyer et al., 2010; Powell, 2009; Westbrook et al., 2007; Wright et al., 2014).

Importantly, practitioners and teams who are trained in goal setting are more likely to set goals that service users/family members will be able and wish to meet, which is likely to have a positive impact upon recovery. As a notable example, Clarke et al. (2009) demonstrated improvements in the practice of goal setting following training, in areas such as: recovery focus; levels of goal attainment; and problem-solving the barriers to goal attainment.

Working Towards a Shared Understanding

Setting goals can be difficult, as many people lack a goal orientation in their lives. People may also be unsure about how best to set goals or they may fear, or have experienced, failure or disappointment. They may also have felt pressured to pursue the goals of others (Meyer et al., 2010; Powell, 2009). Furthermore, negotiating and agreeing goals with a couple or a family can prove challenging, as different and perhaps conflicting priorities may arise prior to reaching agreement. Establishing a good rapport and working relationship with the individual/family is a prerequisite to collaborative and meaningful goal setting, strengthening and facilitating decision-making.

As with case conceptualisation and the identification of strengths and the formulation of needs statements (see Chapters 12 and 13), the role of the practitioner takes the lead in facilitating and guiding this process. For goal setting to be meaningful, the practitioner clearly needs to adopt a style and approach consistent with some important principles for practice, including:

- *Collaborating* or working together with the person, assisting them to agree goals which are *personal* and *highly relevant* to their priority issues.
- *Helping* to focus the individual on a desired outcome that is achievable.
- *Enabling* the person to establish goals that are *clear* and *specific*.

This can be a difficult process. Consider, for example, the person who simply states: 'I want to feel better.' While this is, of course, a reasonable position for anyone to take, it is not clear what this actually means. If goals take the form of such vague, general and unfocused statements, they may never be achieved and may contribute to feelings of failure and hopelessness. It is therefore more helpful to set *specific* and *clear* goals. It is also essential that the person is encouraged and assisted to develop their own, personal and individualised goals. This expresses a commitment to act/do something, and promotes ownership and personal responsibility (Powell 2009).

Adequate time needs to be allocated for setting goals, being mindful of the potential difficulties that may arise. Negotiation is key during this process, ensuring the agreement of specific attainable goals, and providing the individual and practitioner with the opportunity to explore potential barriers and challenges to achieving the goals. Furthermore, when facilitating goal setting, it can be really helpful to use strategies such as open questions, positive reframing/rephrasing, reflecting upon previous positive experiences, considering the person's strengths, abilities and availability of support, and maintaining a focus on small steps. These strategies will enhance the chances of achievement/success and reduce the risk of failure, demoralisation and blame. For example, consider the individual who struggles to believe in their ability to achieve their goal, perhaps saying, 'I want to go to the shop, but I can't.' S/he could be encouraged to consider:

- What has helped in the past?
- Who has helped in the past?
- What/who would help me in achieving this goal of going to the shops?

Identifying and Prioritising Personal Goals

Goal setting is a meaningful intervention that may be structured as a series of steps (Meyer et al., 2010; Powell, 2009; Wright et al., 2014), as shown in Table 14.1.

It is therefore important to help the individual to consider both long- and short-term goals, which may be described as follows:

- *Short-term goals*: Tend to relate to the stages or steps that are necessary in achieving long-term goals, often being the first steps towards recovery, which are possible to achieve in the short term (e.g. a few weeks) – they may thus be viewed as process orientated.
- *Long-term goals*: Focus on what the individual would like to achieve in the longer term (e.g. 3–6 months), providing overall direction and hope, and usually focus on developing meaningful activities, e.g. a job, independent living, confiding/intimate relationships (Wright et al., 2009) – they may thus be viewed as desired outcomes (being outcome orientated), and are ideally recovery focused.

Although it is helpful to develop both short and long-term goals, it is important to realise that short-term goals are likely to be more helpful in the first instance, as these will have a greater chance of early success, and will therefore assist in further enhancing the individual's hope, morale and commitment to change (Morrison et al., 2004). A long-term goal, however, is aspirational and provides drive and motivation.

Table 14.1   The steps of goal setting

Step 1	Explore your interests and goals before you became unwell, thinking creatively about different areas of your life (e.g. family, home, work, study, leisure) in beginning to identify valued goals, or what you'd like to achieve/improve over the next few years
	As a critical first step in enhancing motivation to change, clarify what is important
Step 2	Review your emerging list, modifying or dropping those potential goals that are incompatible or unattainable (Powell, 2009)
Step 3	Identify a long-term recovery-focused personal goal, focusing on the desired outcome, and consider the benefits of change, e.g.: *How would things be better if you achieved this goal?* (Meyer et al., 2010; Treasure, 2004; Wright et al., 2014)
Step 4	Identify two or three related short-term or smaller manageable goals, and select one as your initial focus (Meyer et al., 2010; Wright et al., 2014)
Step 5	Create specific steps or committed actions for making changes and achieving each short-term goal (Meyer et al., 2010; Wright et al., 2014)
Step 6	Identify and plan for the obstacles or challenges that may need to be overcome (Powell, 2009)
Step 7	Steadily take steps towards the goal, gaining support and assistance as needed (Meyer et al., 2010)
Step 8	Recognise and celebrate effort and success, and overcoming obstacles (Meyer et al., 2010; Powell, 2009)

When negotiating goals, it is essential to clearly define and prioritise goals with the person. Negotiation and collaboration are key to reducing any potential conflict, clarifying the rationale and meaning of the goals that are agreed, and in agreeing priorities.

When prioritising, it is important to consider risk/urgency, the importance of the various goals, the individual's level of distress, or whether one goal needs to take precedence (Westbrook et al., 2007). To enhance a sense of ownership, hope and recovery, it is pivotal that the identified goals are generated by the individual and, wherever possible, written in their own words and a language that they can understand.

Forming Meaningful Goal Statements

Meaningful goals must be personalised, clear and specific. There are a number of methods that may be used to start to have meaningful conversations with people about their goals. Westbrook et al. (2007) and Wright et al. (2014), for example, recommend facilitating this process of identifying a meaningful goal by asking a few open questions, for example:

- What would be a meaningful change for you?
- What would you like things to be like?
- What would give you a sense of purpose?
- What would you like to be different?

In considering the formulation of meaningful goal statements focusing on addressing risk issues, Hart (2014) describes a helpful structure which involves considering:

- The concerned person – or, who will take responsibility for the action/solution.
- The objective – what will be achieved.
- The context/setting – the circumstances.
- The time frame.

Fox and Gamble (2006) suggest that forming a meaningful goal statement could be best facilitated by asking the individual to describe what they would like to achieve, encouraging them to describe something they would be doing (a positive change or alternative behaviour) that would indicate that the problem/issue is less severe or has been resolved. They also propose the use of a very helpful structure in formulating a clear and meaningful goal statement:

- Behaviour: What would the person like to do?
- Conditions: With whom? under what circumstances?
- Frequency: How often?
- Duration: For how long?

Expressing Goal Statements

The next stage would involve enabling the individual to phrase a goal statement, using the person's own words. Facilitating this process would involve reflecting back what s/he wishes to achieve, in clarifying, refining and fine-tuning the goal statement.

In developing meaningful goals, it is highly recommended that each goal is clearly expressed, to facilitate a meaningful review at key points. It is therefore important to ensure that each goal is consistent with a series of key criteria or principles, which have been summarised by several authors in the form of 'aide memoire' style acronyms, as shown in Figure 14.1 and described below.

			P			
S	M	A	R	T	E	N
P			O			
O			D			M
R		R	U	M	B	A
T			C			C
			T			R
						O
						S

Figure 14.1   Aide-memoires for expressing goals

These acronyms refer to:

- SMART = Specific, Measurable, Achievable, Relevant/Realistic and Time-limited (Wright et al., 2014)
- SMARTEN = Specific, Measurable, Achievable, Realistic, Time-orientated, Explicit and Negotiated (Padmore and Roberts, 2013)
- RUMBA = Relevant, Understandable, Measurable, Behavioural and Achievable
- SPORT = Specific, Person-centred, Observable, Realistic and Time-bound
- MACROS = Measurable, Achievable, Client-centred, Realistic, Outcome-written and Short (Barrett et al., 2012)
- PRODUCT = Person-centred, Recordable, Observable and measurable, Directive, Understandable and clear, Credible, Time-related (ibid.)

These variations of well-known acronyms clearly share and reinforce the importance of some common principles:

- *Realistic*: It is important to ensure that each goal is realistic, not too limited or over-ambitious, which may require some delicate negotiation with the individual (Westbrook et al., 2007), thus increasing the likelihood of completion – so, can you make it happen?
- *Understandable*: Each goal needs to be written in a simple way, such that the meaning is clear – so, does this make sense to you?
- *Measurable*: Clarifying how the goal will be measured allows for frequent and specific reviews of progress – so, how would you know that you've completed your goal?
- *Behavioural*: Describing something that the person would be doing – so, does it clarify the action that will be taken?
- *Achievable*: Negotiating what will be achievable, given the individual's own resources and abilities (e.g. skills, time, support from others, money, transport), focusing on what is within the person's control, rather than relying on the actions of others – so, is it possible for you to do?
- *Specific*: Ensuring that the goal is very clear to the individual and is tailored to need, clearly identifying what will be done – so, is your goal specific enough?
- *Time-bound*: Agreeing the time frame for completion allows for a focus on progression, although some flexibility is helpful – so, when will you have achieved your goal?

It is helpful to select and apply one of these aide memoires in ensuring that you have negotiated a meaningful goal, thus promoting the individual's success in actually achieving the goal. This may lead to modifying and strengthening the goal statement and/or further breaking down a goal into a series of sub-goals. In practice, as you collaboratively formulate a goal statement, explain the preferred aide memoire to the individual as a guide to testing and agreeing a meaningful goal.

So, looking back at Emily's story (which can be found in Case Scenario 12.1), and her needs statement (see Table 13.1 and Figure 13.2), a meaningful short-term and related long-term goal statement for Emily may look like the one in Table 14.2.

Table 14.2   Goal statement example (Emily) (using the 'behaviour, conditions, frequency and duration' method)

Short-term goal (6 weeks)

Behaviour	Conditions	Frequency	Duration
I would like to be able to go into town to do some shopping	with my friend Sue	twice a week	for at least 90 minutes each time

Long-term goal (6 months)

Behaviour	Conditions	Frequency	Duration
I would like to be able to go to college to attend childcare classes	on my own	three times each week	for each timetabled class (2 hours)

Reviewing and Monitoring Achievement

The risk of failure to achieve the agreed goals will increase if you are not clear, specific, realistic and time-orientated (Meyer et al., 2010). It is also very important to ensure opportunities for the frequent review and monitoring of progress in achieving agreed goals, for which several options may be considered.

Meyer et al. (ibid.), Powell (2009) and Wright et al. (2014) offer goal-monitoring record forms, which may be useful in explicitly recording and reviewing the setting and completion of goals. In addition to writing out a **SMART goal**, these goal-monitoring proformas also involve specifying a series of related action steps. A blank copy of a proforma is provided for your own use in Appendix 14.1, and see Table 14.3 as an example of how this might be used for Emily's case study. As shown in the example, the individual is involved in monitoring and rating how close they are to achieving their goal, using a simple **goal-attainment scaling** method.

Table 14.3   Example goal-monitoring record

Long-term goal

Instructions: Write down the goal you'd like to achieve over the next 3–6 months, considering how you'd like things to be different in terms of your feelings and behaviour

I would like to be able to go to college to attend childcare classes on my own, three times a week for each timetabled class (which last 2 hours)

Short-term goals

Instructions: Now break down your long-term goal into two or three smaller, manageable, short-term goals that you'd like to achieve over the next few weeks; then highlight the short-term goal that you'd first like to work on, by circling it

Goal 1   *I want to better structure my day, getting up by 9 a.m. each morning – within 2 weeks*

Goal 2   *I would like to apply for a childcare course at my local college – within 4 weeks*

(Continued)

Table 14.3 (Continued)

Goal 3	*I would like to be able to go into town to do some shopping with my friend Sue twice a week, for at least 90 minutes each time – within 6 weeks*

Steps: You may also find it helpful to write down a series of steps/actions that you need to take in achieving your chosen short-term goal

Step 1	*To review my medication with my psychiatrist*
Step 2	*To make a list of potentially helpful ways of coping and managing my anxiety about being around people*
Step 3	*To select two ways of coping with my anxiety and to try these out*
Step 4	*To monitor how well these coping strategies work through my diary*

Monitoring your progress

Write in the dates for review	*Instructions:* Using a 0–10 scale, rate how close you are to achieving your goal, by placing a mark on the scale below (0 = no progress; 5 = partially achieved; 10 = fully achieved)										
2 July	0	**1**	2	3	4	5	6	7	8	9	10
12 July	0	1	2	3	4	**5**	6	7	8	9	10
22 July	0	1	2	3	4	5	6	**7**	8	9	10

Monitoring performance and providing feedback has the potential to further enhance motivation and progress, allowing the person to consider what they hoped to achieve versus what they actually achieved (Clarke et al., 2006).

Supporting Goal Attainment: Identifying Strengths and Resources

Psychological well-being and goal attainment are closely associated and, according to Schindler and Sauerwald (2013), the support of friends and family is an influential factor in relation to goal attainment. It is important, therefore, to consider how goal attainment may be effectively supported by family/friends.

Here, it is necessary to explore the helpful and unhelpful relationships in relation to the desired goal, and potential difficulties with regard to achieving it. Ask the service user to consider those people who may be supportive of their goal attainment and those who may not be supportive or may sabotage goal attainment, with the aim of increasing contacts with more supportive people, thus making attainment more likely.

For Emily, it would appear that Sue is very helpful to her, therefore in terms of supporting goal attainment, it would be important to enlist Sue's help (with Emily's consent and assuming that Sue would be comfortable with this).

In addition to enlisting the support of family and friends, it is also helpful to record success and challenges (aided by the use of keeping a diary or journal, for example) and to ensure that progress towards the desired goal is monitored regularly. However, building in an awareness of times and situations when attainment may be more difficult or less likely (such as how stress can adversely affect motivation and impact upon symptoms) can be helpful to develop realistic contingency plans in supporting goal attainment. Other strategies can include the provision of information about local and online resources where service users and families may be able to access support (for examples, see the end of this chapter).

Identifying and Overcoming Difficulties and Obstacles

There may be occasions when the practitioner and individual do not agree on goals (for example, when an individual has been detained under the Mental Health Act who may want to be immediately discharged), which reinforces the need for sound therapeutic engagement and negotiation skills for practitioners, but also that goals should be achievable and relate to things over which the person has some control. It is also important to consider whether the service user has the resources they need in order to achieve their goals.

There are a number of methods to support the person to identify and overcome difficulties in achieving their goals.

Supporting Motivation

Motivation arises when there is a discrepancy between how people currently see themselves/their situation, and how they want things to be, e.g. wanting/achieving personal goals (Boudreaux and Ozer 2013; Westbrook et al., 2007; Wright et al., 2009). Motivation, however, diminishes if:

- A person finds it too difficult to identify specific goals due to feeling distressed.
- Agreed goals are set too low or too high, e.g. short-term goals seeming too simple or being inconsequential for the person, or being unable to progress long-term goals.
- There is too much pressure on the person to achieve the set goals.
- The person works on multiple or conflicting goals at the same time.
- Goals are poorly defined.

McKeown et al. (2002) suggest that practitioners should ensure that when working collaboratively with service users, goal statements are kept as simple as possible, using behavioural (measurable), clear and unambiguous wording. However, sometimes, activities and goals can be overwhelming, and so it can be useful to break down goals into specific and smaller steps, working at the person's own individual pace. Being specific, clear and concrete when setting goals also assists in identifying barriers or difficulties the individual may have in achieving them. However, it is also important to avoid framing goals in terms of how the service user would prefer *not* to be, e.g. *not* drinking, *not* feeling afraid or staying in all the time. Instead, service users should be asked to consider how they would like things to be or what they do want to do.

The Miracle Question

Using the **Miracle Question** (see Westbrook et al., 2007) can help this process, as described below:

> I'm going to ask you a question that sounds really strange, but it'd be really helpful if you could try and answer it as honestly as possible, is that OK?
>
> Imagine that you go to bed tonight and, while you are asleep, a miracle happens, which means that the problem you've come here with completely disappears. When you get up in the morning, how would you know that the problem had been solved? What sorts of things would be happening? What would you see? What would you be doing?

When following this up, it's important to ask for positive behavioural (measurable) descriptions – e.g. 'If you felt happier, what would you be doing?' – and to reinforce this by asking further questions such as 'What else?' questions and 'relationship questions' such as:

- What else would be happening?
- What would other people say or do?
- What would they think?
- How would other people notice that this miracle had happened and that you were different?
- What would they say?

It is important to appreciate that this process may be difficult for service users, and envisaging a future without problems might be challenging. However, the process can allow practitioners to raise service users' awareness of exceptions in their lives, as follows:

- I know that this miracle hasn't happened, but are there any, even really small, things that have already happened/are happening already?
- Tell me about a time when this problem wasn't so bad, what things were happening then?
- What was happening when you dealt with this more/most successfully?
- Are there times when this problem is not as apparent? What did you do to influence this?

Chaining

Another potentially useful strategy is that of **chaining**, which, according to Grist, 'allows for the motivation muscle to be stretched' by linking smaller activities to an ultimate goal (2015: 119). This allows the person to see the impact of their behaviours, thoughts and feelings on their goals. Consider the example of Emily in relation to going to the supermarket (see Figure 14.2).

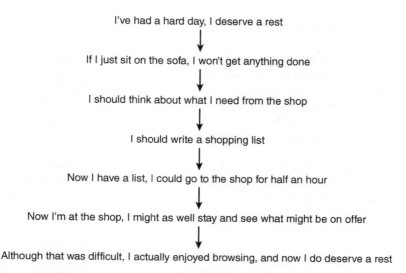

I've had a hard day, I deserve a rest

↓

If I just sit on the sofa, I won't get anything done

↓

I should think about what I need from the shop

↓

I should write a shopping list

↓

Now I have a list, I could go to the shop for half an hour

↓

Now I'm at the shop, I might as well stay and see what might be on offer

↓

Although that was difficult, I actually enjoyed browsing, and now I do deserve a rest

Figure 14.2   An example of chaining

Remember: one of the key barriers to service users achieving their goals, and therefore making disengagement more likely, is that goals have been poorly articulated and written.

Formulating Goals: 10 Key Points

- A goal may be regarded as a desired outcome, as something that you wish to achieve.
- Goal setting involves a series of structured steps.
- Establishing a good rapport and working relationship with the individual/ family is a prerequisite to collaborative and meaningful goal setting.
- Short- and long-term goals should be specific, highly relevant and personalised.
- Working towards short-term goals is likely to be more helpful, offering a greater chance of early success, and further enhancing motivation and commitment to change.
- When formulating goal statements, succinctly define the behaviour in positive terms (i.e. what the person will aim to do, rather than what they will aim *not* to do) and, as relevant, capture any required conditions, the frequency and the duration.
- Test and fine-tune goal statements by using an aide memoire, such as SMART.
- Ensure opportunities for the frequent review of progress in achieving agreed goals.
- Consider accessing the support of friends, family and other resources in progressing agreed goals.
- Consider the use of helpful practical strategies in overcoming difficulties, challenges and obstacles – e.g. breaking goals down into smaller manageable goals, use of the Miracle Question and chaining techniques.

Chapter Summary

We have considered the place of goal setting within the contemporary practice of psychosocial and mental health assessment. We have presented a series of practical methods for the negotiation of personalised, recovery-focused meaningful goals, and considered the importance of frequent monitoring and review. In discussing a series of potential difficulties and challenges, we have highlighted a number of helpful practical strategies and signposted some potentially helpful resources.

In ensuring a positive experience for the individual, we recommend that practitioners adopt a highly collaborative, flexible and creative approach in actively engaging the individual and their family members in identifying and achieving their personal goals.

EXERCISES

1. Review Emily's case conceptualisation (see Table 12.6) and try to identify more examples of short- and long-term goals.
2. Try proposing some steps that Emily could take to achieve short-term goals, as described in Table 14.1 How would you ensure that you collaborate with Emily on this and also ensure that short-term goals are clearly negotiated?
3. Taking time to review this chapter, critically review the following goal statements, considering the extent to which each goal is SMART and, if appropriate, propose an example of a better phrased and SMARTer goal statement:

   - For Gillian to sleep better at night.
   - For Julie to remain stable in mood.
   - Julie will be symptom free.
   - Jim would like to have quality time with his wife.
   - For Melanie to comply with her medication.

You may find it helpful to relate these goal statements to particular individuals drawn from own your clinical experience. Once you have proposed your own alternative goals, consider the examples provided in Appendix 14.2.

4. Case Study: Luke

Reviewing the practice recommendations that have been made in this chapter, consider the following short case study and identify some precipitating factors and presenting problems (see Chapter 4) for Luke and his wife. Then, propose one or two meaningful goals both for Luke and for his wife:

   Luke is a 29-year-old man who is married with a young daughter. He is unemployed after being made redundant, is experiencing financial difficulties and smokes cannabis on a regular basis. Prior to Luke's relapse, his father died suddenly. Luke spends the majority of his time in his house. He finds it difficult to trust others because he believes that someone is going to harm him or his family. As a result of this, Luke has stopped socialising with his friends, although he does communicate with them via social media as he believes no harm can come to him this way. Luke occasionally goes out with his wife and daughter shopping, but he finds this very difficult and has had to leave due to severe anxiety and paranoia. As a consequence of Luke's withdrawal, his wife's social activity has also reduced. They often used to have meals with friends in the house and have regular gatherings with the family.

Appendix 14.1 Goal-Monitoring Record

Long-term goal

Instructions: Write down the goal you'd like to achieve over the next 3–6 months, considering how you'd like things to be different in terms of your feelings and behaviour

Short-term goals

Instructions: Now break down your long-term goal into two or three smaller, manageable, short-term goals that you'd like to achieve over the next few weeks; then highlight the short-term goal that you'd first like to work on, by circling it

Goal 1

Goal 2

Goal 3

Steps: You may also find it helpful to write down a series of steps/actions that you need to take in achieving your chosen short-term goals

Step 1

Step 2

Step 3

Step 4

Monitoring your progress

Write in dates for review

Instructions: Using a 0–10 scale, rate how close you are to achieving your goal, by placing a mark on the scale below (0 = No Progress; 5 = Partially Achieved; 10 = Fully Achieved)

0	1	2	3	4	5	6	7	8	9	10
0	1	2	3	4	5	6	7	8	9	10
0	1	2	3	4	5	6	7	8	9	10
0	1	2	3	4	5	6	7	8	9	10

Appendix 14.2 Some Alternative Goal Statements

As more meaningful alternatives to the stated goals in Exercise 3 (see Exercises section above), consider the following examples:

1. Gillian would like to have seven hours of sleep each night, during the majority of nights – over the next two weeks.
2. Julie would like to be able to recognise and manage the changes in her mood – within three weeks.
3. Julie would like to learn ways of coping with the voices – within four weeks. Julie would like the voices to be less frequent, less intense and less distressing – within four weeks.
4. Jim would like to go out with Gillian for a meal in a restaurant – within the next two weeks. Jim would like to go to the cinema with Gillian – within the next seven days.
5. Melanie would like to understand more about her prescribed medication – within two weeks. Melanie would like any side effects of her medication to be resolved or managed – within six weeks.

How do these examples compare with your own suggestions?

Further Reading

Gamble, C. and Brennan, G. (2006) *Working with Serious Mental Illness: A Manual for Clinical Practice*, 2nd edn. Edinburgh: Elsevier.

A popular text among mental health practitioners who are working with those who experience a serious mental illness. Jayne Fox and Catherine Gamble explain their method of formulating problem and goal statements in chapter 9.

Powell, T. (2009) *The Mental Health Handbook: A Cognitive-Behavioural Approach*, 3rd edn. Milton Keynes: Speechmark.

A really helpful text, this provides a set of practical resources and handouts to support therapeutic assessment and intervention, primarily based on the cognitive behavioural approach. A CD-ROM resource is provided with the handbook, which includes materials on goal planning.

Westbrook, D., Kennerley, H. and Kirk, J. (2007) *An Introduction to Cognitive Behaviour Therapy: Skills and Applications*. London: Sage.

A popular text among mental health practitioners interested in the application of cognitive behavioural intervention. A helpful section is included on the use of the Miracle Question as a strategy to facilitating goal setting in chapter 11.

Wright, N.P., Turkington, D., Kelly, O.P., Davies, D., Jacobs, A.M. and Hopton, J. (2014) *Treating Psychosis: A Clinician's Guide to Integrating Acceptance and Commitment Therapy, Compassion Focused Therapy and Mindfulness Approaches within the Cognitive Behaviour Therapy Tradition*. Oaklands, CA: New Harbinger.

Focusing on the use of an integrative approach for working with service users with psychosis, this clinical guide sets out practical interventions and exercises, supported by sample resources and downloadable tools, which include goal setting.

For Service Users and Families

healthtalk: www.healthtalk.org/peoples-experiences/mental-health/experiences-psychosis/
   topics

This has useful information about psychosis, causes, treatments and coping strategies.

Mental Health Foundation: www.mentalhealth.org.uk

The Mental Health Foundation provides information about a range of mental health problems, as well as being involved in research and policy development.

Mind: www.mind.org.uk

The organisation Mind provides information about a range of mental health problems and rights and where support can be accessed.

MoodJuice: www.moodjuice.scot.nhs.uk

A Scotland-based website designed to help people think about emotional problems and work towards solving them. It provides information and links to local resources for a range of issues, e.g. benefit and debt advice, health-related information, organisations and services and self-help guides.

NHS choices Moodzone: www.nhs.uk/Conditions/stress-anxiety-depression/Pages/low-
   mood-stress-anxiety.aspx

The 'Moodzone' has information about common mental health problems and tips on improving mental well-being, as well as links to other potentially useful information.

Psychology Tools: http://self-help.tools

Provides free downloadable self-help tools, information about CBT and advice about how to find an appropriate therapist.

Rethink Mental Illness: www.rethink.org

Rethink provides information and advice in relation to living with mental illness, has a range of services and support groups nationally, and campaigns to improve policy in relation to mental health.

Self Help UK: www.self-help.org.uk

A free searchable database of over 1000 self-help organisations, support groups and charities across the UK that provide support, guidance and advice to service users, families/carers and their relatives. The groups and organisations cover a range of medical conditions, diseases and treatments.

SelfHelp: www.selfhelpservices.org.uk

A North England-based user-led mental health charity, which provides a range of support, services and opportunities for people living with common mental health problems such as anxiety, depression, phobias and panic attacks. At least 60 per cent of the staff have had personal or lived experience of a common mental health problem.

Turning Point: www.turning-point.co.uk

This is a social enterprise, providing services which focus on improving lives for people, especially those with complex needs, across mental health, learning disability, substance misuse, primary care, the criminal justice system and employment.

For Practitioners

Centre for Clinical Interventions: www.cci.health.wa.gov.au/resources/index.cfm

Free downloadable resources to assist in providing interventions for mental health problems. The resources aim to provide general information about various mental health problems, as well as techniques that focus on a cognitive behavioural approach to managing difficulties.

getselfhelp: www.getselfhelp.co.uk

Has free downloadable information leaflets, handouts and tools.

healthypsych: http://healthypsych.com/psychology-tools-series

This has 20 free downloadable practical psychology tools based on cognitive behavioural science and mindfulness-based theory.

Psychology Tools: http://psychology.tools/

Has free downloadable information about a range of therapeutic approaches and techniques to a range of problems, in a range of different languages.

Therapist Aid: www.therapistaid.com

Has free downloadable resources such as worksheets, videos and guides.

References

Barrett, D., Wilson, B. and Woollands, A. (2012) *Care Planning: A Guide for Nurses*. Harlow: Pearson Education, see chapter 2, 'ASPIRE: the problem-solving approach to care delivery' pp. 19–40.

Boudreaux, M.J. and Ozer, D.J. (2013) 'Goal conflict, goal striving, and psychological well-being', *Motivation and Emotion*, 37: 433–43.

Clarke, S.P., Crowe, T.P., Oades, L.G. and Deane, F.P. (2009) 'Do goal-setting interventions improve the quality of goals in mental health services?', *Psychiatric Rehabilitation Journal*, 32 (4): 292–9.

Clarke, S.P., Oades, L.G., Crowe, T.P. and Deane, F.P. (2006) 'Collaborative goal technology: theory and practice', *Psychiatric Rehabilitation Journal*, 30 (2): 129–36.

Fox, J. and Gamble, C. (2006) 'Consolidating the assessment process: the semi-structured interview', in C. Gamble and G. Brennan (eds), *Working with Serious Mental Illness: A Manual for Clinical Practice*, 2nd edn. London: Elsevier.

Grist, S. (2015) 'Why should I get fit? Physical activity as an intervention', in S. Walker (ed.), *Psychosocial Interventions in Mental Health Nursing*. London: Sage.

Hart, C. (2014) *A Pocket Guide to Risk Assessment & Management in Mental Health*. London: Routledge.

Laidlaw, K. (2015) *CBT for Older People: An Introduction*. London: Sage.

McKeown, M., McCann, G. and Forster, J. (2002) 'Psychosocial interventions in institutional settings', in N. Harris, S. Williams and T. Bradshaw (eds), *Psychosocial Interventions for People with Schizophrenia: A Practical Guide for Mental Health Workers*. Basingstoke: Palgrave Macmillan.

Meyer, P.S., Gingerich, S. and Mueser, K.T. (2010) 'A guide to implementation and clinical practice of illness management and recovery for people with schizophrenia', in A. Rubin, D.W. Springer and K. Trawver (eds), *Psychosocial Treatment of Schizophrenia: A Clinician's Guide to Evidence-Based Practice*. Hoboken, NJ: John Wiley.

Morrison, A.P., Renton, J.C., Dunn, H., Williams, S. and Bentall, R.P. (2004) *Cognitive Therapy for Psychosis: A Formulation-Based Approach*. Hove and New York: Brunner-Routledge.

Padmore, J. and Roberts, C. (2013) 'Care planning', in I. Norman and I. Ryrie (eds), *The Art & Science of Mental Health Nursing: Principles and Practice*, 3rd edn. Maidenhead: Open University Press.

Powell, T. (2009) *The Mental Health Handbook: A Cognitive-Behavioural Approach*, 3rd edn. Milton Keynes: Speechmark.

Schindler, V.P. and Sauerwald, C. (2013) 'Outcomes of a 4-year program with higher education and employment goals for individuals diagnosed with mental illness', *Work*, 46: 325–36.

Treasure, J. (2004) 'Motivational interviewing', *Advances in Psychiatric Treatment*, 10 (5): 331–7, and doi 10.1192/apt.10.5.331.

Westbrook, D., Kennerley, H. and Kirk, J. (2007) *An Introduction to Cognitive Behaviour Therapy: Skills and Applications*. London: Sage.

Wright, J.H., Turkington, D., Kingdon, D. and Ramirez Basco, M. (2009) *Cognitive-Behaviour Therapy for Severe Mental Illness*. London: American Psychiatric.

Wright, N.P., Turkington, D., Kelly, O.P., Davies, D., Jacobs, A.M. and Hopton, J. (2014) *Treating Psychosis: A Clinician's Guide to Integrating Acceptance and Commitment Therapy, Compassion Focused Therapy and Mindfulness Approaches within the Cognitive Behaviour Therapy Tradition*. Oaklands, CA: New Harbinger.

GLOSSARY

active listening   conscious responsive listening which acknowledges and demonstrates to a speaker – via verbal and non-verbal behaviour – that their communication has been heard

ascites   free fluid, often yellowish in colour, that is in the peritoneal cavity

atopic eczema   eczema with an unidentified cause

Beliefs About Voices Questionnaire (BAVQ)   self-report measure of a service user's beliefs, emotions and behaviour towards their auditory hallucinations

Body Mass Index (BMI)   the weight of the person (kg) is divided by the square of their height (m)

Brief Psychiatric Rating Scale (BPRS)   an assessment scale which practitioners can use to measure psychiatric symptoms

case conceptualisation   a framework which encompasses all the information gathered through the engagement and assessment stages. It forms the basis for the service user to understand the reasons for: their illness; a hypothesis or theory about a client's current problems; a way of integrating information gathered through the assessment phase, in reaching a shared understanding of the themes and issues concerning the individual's and/or family's presenting issues, needs and strengths, which become the focus and guide for intervention

case formulation   a framework which encompasses all the information gathered through the engagement and assessment stages that form the basis of therapy and treatment

CAT (computerised axial tomography)   a computerised technique that can examine a cross-section of the body. Also known as a CT scan

chaining   a method of linking smaller activities to an ultimate goal

chest X-ray   electromagnetic waves are utilised to view the image of the internal chest cavity

clarifying assessment   assessments that seek a deeper understanding of a person's experience through more detailed questioning or the use of specific rating scales

clinician-administered   psychometric tools and rating scales which are administered by practitioners

cognitive behavioural therapy (CBT)   a type of therapy that aims to solve unhelpful thinking patterns, by using a combination of behavioural and cognitive interventions

concurrent validity   a type of validity where a measurement instrument produces the same findings as the 'gold standard' instrument

congruence   genuineness and authenticity

construct validity   relates to the ability of the measurement instrument to measure the theoretical underpinning constructs from which the instrument was designed

content validity   a type of validity that is more rigorous than face validity and relates to the extent and breadth to which the content of a measurement instrument measures the aspects of the construct it alleges to measure

criterion validity   relates to the extent to which a measurement instrument produces the same findings as an established and already validated instrument

Cushing's syndrome   a condition where there is over-secretion by the adrenal cortex

cyanosis   individuals present with a bluish tinge to their skin and mucous membranes which is due to inadequate oxygenation of the blood

deep vein thrombosis (DVT)   a blood clot that has formed in the deep veins of the lower leg

delirium tremens (so-called **DTs**)   severe symptoms experienced during withdrawal from chronic alcohol use, involving tremors, hallucinations, anxiety and disorientation

dependence   occurs when the body adapts to prolonged use of a drug and where the person experiences withdrawal in its absence

depot   an injection which is given deep within the muscle to allow for longer absorption and is therefore longer-acting

diabetes mellitus   a metabolic disease where the body is not able to regulate blood sugar levels due to an inability to produce insulin

dopaminergic   related to the action of dopamine, a neurotransmitter

Doppler   a device that measures the frequency of blood flow, e.g. in the leg

dual diagnosis   co-morbidity of two illnesses or conditions, commonly a mental condition with substance misuse

dyspnoea   laboured breathing

effusion   water on the knee (or other joints)

empathy   the ability to share another person's point of view

epilepsy   convulsive attacks caused by a number of conditions which are due to disordered electrical activity in the brain

exogenous stressors   stress which derives from outside the body such as life-event stress

external reliability   consistency over time and between different raters using the same measurement instrument

face validity   a basic form of validity and an intuitive and subjective evaluation

femoral   the artery that runs from the groin to the knee

flexures   a bend or curve such as the back of the knee

flourishing   thriving

funnelling approach   an interviewing approach which starts off with broad questions before seeking clarification through asking more specific and detailed questions

global assessments   broad assessments of a person's overall holistic needs

glomerular disease   refers to the kidney's inability to maintain a balance of specific substances in the blood stream

glycosuria   glucose is present in the urine, one indicator of diabetes

goal   a desired outcome, or something that you wish to achieve

goal attainment scaling   a method for evaluating progress towards goals, which involves the use of a personal rating tool/scaling technique

goal statement   a personally meaningful, structured statement outlining the short- and long-term goals of a person based on identified needs or problems

head-to-toe systems approach   a structured, systems-based approach to physical health assessment

hyperlipidaemia   high blood lipid levels

hyperparathyroidism   excessive activity of the parathyroids

hypertension   elevated blood pressure

hyperthyroidism excessive activity of the thyroid gland

hypothetical questions questions regarding situations, statements or about something imaginary, rather than something real

hypothyroidism insufficiency of thyroid secretion

initial conceptualisation an initial outline of a case conceptualisation usually made on first contact with a person presenting for assessment

internal reliability the consistency within the measurement instrument itself

jaundice bile pigment in the blood that causes a yellow discolouration of the skin and conjunctivae

Johari window a tool for improving self-awareness and understanding between individuals

life-course approach an approach which looks back over an individual's life and experiences (including social, economic and cultural contexts) for an understanding of current patterns of health and illness

long-term goal a recovery-focused desired outcome that can be achieved in the longer term, within 3–6 months or sometimes longer, such as gaining employment or independent living

Magnetic Resonance Imaging (MRI) an imaging technique used to obtain cross-section images of the body in any plane

Miracle Question a specific goal-orientated strategy from Brief Solution Focused Therapy, which involves considering indicators of positive change following the imagined experience of a 'miracle' that resulted in the presenting problem disappearing

motivational interviewing a person-centred counselling technique supporting health behaviour change

multiple sclerosis a chronic and progressive disease which is characterised by patches of demyelination throughout the spinal cord and brain

myocardial infarction (MI) cardiac arrest which requires urgent intervention, including ABC (Airway, Breathing, Circulation) assessment and urgent assistance

needs statement a structured statement which clearly articulates a person's need or problem

nerve conduction studies utilised to assess a number of facets, including nerve impulses

nocturia the production of large quantities of urine at night

nocturnal dyspnoea   laboured breathing at night

normalising rationale   an affirming statement which aims to identify the commonality of a person's experiences

oedema   an excessive amount of fluid in the body tissues

ordinal   rank ordering

orthopnoea   breathing is laboured unless in an upright position such as sitting

oxygen saturation   the level of oxygen in the blood

paroxysmal nocturnal dyspnoea   reoccurring laboured breathing at night

perpetuating factors   factors which maintain a problem

personal recovery outcomes   health care outcomes which are defined by the individual as opposed to mental health practitioners or services

polycystic ovary syndrome (PCOS)   numerous cysts in the ovaries

polyuria   abnormally large outputs of urine

popliteal dorsis pedi   a blood vessel of the lower limb that carries oxygenated blood to the dorsal surface of the foot

posterior tibial artery   carries blood to the posterior compartment of the leg

precipitating factors   factors which have preceded a person's current problem

predictive validity   measurement instrument that accurately predicts an event or phenomena such as changes in, for example, psychotic symptoms, relapse, recovery, self-harm or the development of a specific condition

predisposing factors   factors in a person's previous history and experience which have increased their vulnerability to mental health or other health care problems

presenting problem   the person's current problem

prosocial activities   voluntary activities to promote social activities to benefit an individual or group

protective factors   mitigating factors which support the person

proteinuria   an excess of serum proteins in the urine

psoriasis   a chronic skin condition characterised by large plaques

psychoactive substance   any substance which alters brain functioning

psychoeducation   learning which is offered to service users and their families who suffer from mental illness. This education can come in many forms, including written and oral information, techniques and behavioural interventions

psychometric tools   tests which measure properties of mental capacities

psychosocial interventions (PSI)   evidence-based interventions which are underpinned by psychological tools to support individuals in their recovery

recovery approach   an approach to mental health care that stresses the holistic and biopsychosocial approaches whilst emphasising individual and personal pathways of recovery

Recovery Star™   an assessment and outcome measure which highlights 10 areas of need and asks the service user to rate themselves in each area. It can be repeated to show progress

reflexive   a bidirectional influence in which the cause and effect influence each other

reliability   in statistics, an overall consistency of a measure

remote patient monitoring (RPM)   the monitoring of a patient's symptoms at a distance, using medical sensing devices, often in the patient's own home

rheumatoid arthritis   a chronic, progressive inflammation of one or more joints

schizophrenia   a severe mental disorder which is characterised by a loss of reality. This includes symptoms of hallucinations and delusions as well as a deterioration in function and activities of daily living

self-efficacy   the perception of the person's own abilities to achieve

self-report   assessment information of an individual which is collected by the individual themselves

sensitivity   the ability of a tool to reveal a true positive rate

short-term goal   a process-orientated stage or step towards a longer-term goal that can typically be achieved within a few weeks and is often the first step towards recovery

SMART goal   referring to the use of the well known SMART (Specific, Measurable, Achievable/Attainable, Relevant/Realistic and Time-bound) acronym for testing the quality and value of a personal goal statement. Alternative acronyms include RUMBA and SPORT

social capital   the totality of an individual's social, community and interpersonal resources

Social Functioning Scale (SFS)   assesses the daily functioning of an individual with a mental illness. This includes social relationships, interpersonal skills and activities of daily living

sociogram   a diagram of a person's social contacts and networks

specificity   the ability of a tool to reveal a true negative rate

subarachnoid/intracranial haemorrhage   bleeding into the subarachnoid space

synovitis   inflammation of the membrane which lines joints

tachycardia   abnormally rapid action of the heart which results in an increased pulse rate

telemental health (TMH)   the provision of mental health care from a distance, including mental health assessment, treatment, education, monitoring and collaboration

telephone triage   assessment undertaken over a telephone, often in a crisis and accompanied by health care advice, guidance, treatment and/or support

thyrotoxicosis   *see* hyperthyroidism

timeline   representation of chronological events in a person's life

tolerance   the body's diminished responsiveness to a drug

torticollis   also known as 'wry neck', when the cervical muscles contract causing torsion

ultrasonography   the deep structures of the body are visualised by a radiological technique

ultrasound   interior organs of the body are examined by ultrasonic waves

unconditional positive regard   a non-judgemental, positive attitude to another

validity   the extent to which a study measures what it is supposed to measure

white cell count   can be raised due to certain infections (leukocytosis)

INDEX